EMBRYONIC ORIGINS OF DEFECTIVE HEART DEVELOPMENT

ANNALS OF THE NEW YORK ACADEMY OF SCIENCES
Volume 588

EMBRYONIC ORIGINS OF DEFECTIVE HEART DEVELOPMENT

Edited by Dale E. Bockman and Margaret L. Kirby

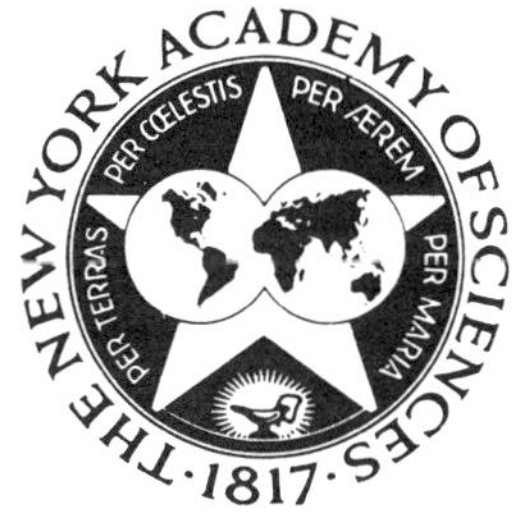

The New York Academy of Sciences
New York, New York
1990

Library of Congress Cataloging-in-Publication Data

Embryonic origins of defective heart development / edited
  by Dale E. Bockman and Margaret L. Kirby.
      p.   cm. — (Annals of the New York Academy of
Sciences. ISSN 0077-8923 ; v. 588)
    The result of a conference held in Arlington, Va., May 4-
6, 1989, by the New York Academy of Sciences.
    Includes bibliographical references.
    ISBN 0-89766-571-6 (alk. paper). — ISBN 0-89766-572-4
(pbk. : alk. paper)
    1. Heart—Abnormalities—Etiology—Congresses. 2.
Heart—Growth—Molecular aspects—Congresses. I.
Bockman, Dale E. II. Kirby, Margaret L. III. New York
Academy of Sciences. IV. Series.
    [DNLM: 1. Heart—embryology—congresses. 2. Heart
Defects, Congenital—etiology—congresses. W1 AN626YL v.
588 / WG 220 E53 1989]
    Q11.N5   vol. 588
    [RC687]
    500 s—dc20
    [616.1'2043]
    DNLM/DLC
    for Library of Congress   90-5807
                                                   CIP

PCP
Printed in the United States of America
ISBN 0-89766-571-6 (cloth)
ISBN 0-89766-572-4 (paper)
ISSN 0077-8923

ANNALS OF THE NEW YORK ACADEMY OF SCIENCES

Volume 588
April 9, 1990

EMBRYONIC ORIGINS OF DEFECTIVE HEART DEVELOPMENT [a]

Editors and Conference Organizers
DALE E. BOCKMAN AND MARGARET L. KIRBY

Ad Hoc Advisors
CONSTANCE WEINSTEIN AND TONY L. CREAZZO

Advisory Board
HENRY GREENBERG, JENE M. JONAKAIT, CHARLES NICHOLSON,
AND FLEUR STRAND

CONTENTS

[a] This volume is the result of a conference entitled **Embryonic Origins of Defective Heart Development,** held in Arlington, Virginia on May 4-6, 1989, by the New York Academy of Sciences.

Financial assistance was received from:

- AMERICAN HEART ASSOCIATION
- ICI PHARMACEUTICALS
- NATIONAL HEART, LUNG, AND BLOOD INSTITUTE, NIH
- PARKE-DAVIS, PHARMACEUTICAL RESEARCH DIVISION, WARNER-LAMBERT COMPANY
- PFIZER PHARMACEUTICALS

Introductory Remarks

DALE E. BOCKMAN

Department of Anatomy
Medical College of Georgia
Augusta, Georgia 30912-2000

The critical stages that mark the establishment of the basic constituents of the heart and major vessels are the result of a dynamic interaction of genetic capabilities and continually changing local microenvironments. These events start at a very early stage, and there is a continuing interplay among emerging structural elements, their functional manifestations, and control mechanisms that regulate and direct development. Insufficient quantities of germinal elements and improper timing of cellular interactions and other controls lead to defective development. Environmental agents may trigger defective development by acting through these mechanisms.

Defective cardiovascular development traditionally has become evident at birth. More modern techniques allow detection *in utero* and provide the advantage of forewarning of therapeutic measures that must be taken. The proportion of cardiac defects at birth, however, remains about the same, and our knowledge of the root cause of these defects remains inadequate. Fortunately, new approaches have become possible recently because of newly developed animal models and the development of technologies and techniques necessary to probe the nature of basic mechanisms, as well as the interaction of control mechanisms that guide development. Some of these characteristics are shared in common with other developing systems, and some are unique to cardiovascular development.

The investigators in the multiple disciplines through which increased knowledge of cardiovascular development may be gained do not necessarily interact personally in their customary meetings. Thus critical conceptual connections that might be made when investigators from different disciplines share information could be missed or at least delayed. This conference on embryonic origins of defective heart development was planned to help forge these connections. Furthermore, the focus of the conference remained on biological questions and functions of the developing cardiovascular system, a perspective that may be missing in annual meetings of some of the pertinent disciplines.

Four main goals were realized in this conference. First, experienced and new investigators were brought together to establish the state of combined knowledge, as of 1989, concerning normal and abnormal embryonic development of the heart and related structures. Second, the conference provided a forum in which both realized and potential contributions from a number of different technologies and techniques could be presented, discussed, and integrated. Third, this gathering identified problems central to the understanding of normal and defective development of the heart, to allow formulation of approaches likely to yield solutions to these problems. Fourth, this meeting provided a milieu for the stimulation of future collaborations among investigators from the diverse fields represented.

The investigations reported at this conference were conducted by scientists who approach the cardiovascular system from different perspectives. The latest insights into development of specific regions of the heart, outflow tract, and vessels were presented along with hemodynamics and neural control. The importance of the extracellular matrix and cell-cell interactions was presented. Membrane and control phenomena, including the role of membrane channels, were integrated with the molecular biology of cardiovascular components and with angiogenesis. Normal development was contrasted with cardiovascular dysmorphogenesis, highlighting recent advances using new models of cardiac malformation.

Collectively, the reports of the conference document the inclusion of the latest investigative techniques with more traditional ways of trying to understand the fundamental changes that cause abnormal cardiovascular development. Surely new insights will derive from this combination.

Overview of Problems and Approaches in Heart Development

MARGARET L. KIRBY

Department of Anatomy
Medical College of Georgia
Augusta, Georgia 30912-2000

HISTORICAL PERSPECTIVE

Development of the heart has fascinated scientists and philosophers for centuries and has left the legacy of an impressive body of literature that describes in detail the morphological development of hearts in various species of animals. Morphologists have had the edge over other scientists studying normal heart development because they have had the technical advantage in their ability to assess small tissues.

Until the last few years, pathologists and pediatric cardiologists have described congenital heart defects in fully developed hearts obtained from autopsies and inferred the embryogenesis of those defects that occurred several months or years earlier. Very few studies using experimental and prospective methods were available to describe the origins of defective heart development. Shaner's studies in the 1940s and 1950s stand out because he searched thousands of embryos to find those in the process of developing abnormal hearts.[1] Unfortunately, the search involved fixing the heart in time for a morphological analysis, and there was no chance of studying structure/ function relationships during cardiac dysmorphogenesis.

The first models of congenital heart disease began to appear in the 1940s and 1950s when teratologists identified specific teratogens that produced embryos with congenital heart defects.[2,3] Many of these teratogens produced constellations of defects in which the heart defect was part of a spectrum of defects. Frequently the heart defect was a minor part of the spectrum and was found in a relatively small percentage of affected embryos. In the mammal, dextroamphetamine, several azo dyes, and X-rays produced cardiac and aortic arch anomalies. Vitamin A deficiency as well as excess, caused complex malformations of the face and heart, with a high incidence of ocular and genitourinary anomalies.[4-6] Trypan blue exposure in gestating rats and mice resulted in anophthalmia or microphthalmia and shortening of the vertebral column, transposition of the great vessels, and other malformations of the heart and great vessels.[7] The teratogen of scientists' dreams was one that produced 100% incidence of predictable heart defects with few or no other congenital anomalies.

Producing heart defects with teratogens reached its pinnacle in the mid 1970s with the discovery of bis-diamine.[8] Bis-diamine, or fertilysin, produces 100% incidence of persistent truncus arteriosus in rat fetuses exposed to the drug during early gestation.[9] It also produces hypoplastic or aplastic thymus and hence a fetus with all the major characteristics of DiGeorge syndrome described in children.[10]

The last ten years have seen the advent of many new and exciting models of congenital heart disease. A number of teratogens are currently in use. Dr. Miyagawa and other Japanese investigators have shown that nimustine hydrochloride causes a high incidence of dextroposed aorta and persistent truncus arteriosus in rats and chicks.[11,12] Dr. Bruyere and Dr. Gilbert have used caffeine to produce heart defects that they have studied using cinephotography.[13]

Dr. Patterson, using his breed of keeshond dogs, has been instrumental in studying the embryogenesis of persistent truncus arteriosus.[14] Dr. Layton developed a genetic mouse model of situs inversus in which he and Dr. Manasek are studying looping, a phenomenon that remains unexplained.[15] The latest of the genetic models belongs to Dr. Morrison-Graham and Dr. Weston who have developed a number of mouse models with an abnormal extracellular matrix.[16] One of these, the Patch mouse, has serious heart defects that may be the result of the inability of the mesenchyme and ectomesenchyme to migrate in the heart.

Finally, our own model of heart defects using neural crest ablation has proved to be very reliable in the production of predictable heart defects and is lending itself to study during the process of heart dysmorphogenesis.[17]

With the abundance of models for heart dysmorphogenesis, it should no longer be necessary to infer pathogenesis from a fully developed, abnormal heart. We are now able to follow the dysmorphogenesis of a number of cardiac anomalies as a dynamic process. This should leave us much wiser about normal processes necessary for heart development as well as detailed structural/functional sequences occurring in cardiac dysmorphogenesis.

Although a number of investigators have incorporated models of cardiac dysmorphogenesis into their investigations on heart development, most of the work on heart development is still in normal developing hearts. The reason for this is that although gross morphological development has been explored and described very thoroughly, little is known about the underlying causes and processes. We just do not know enough about normal development to understand which processes are altered during abnormal development and their significance. Many complicated tissue interactions and cell migrations occur, and it is very difficult to study them in these tiny developing organs that must maintain an embryo at the same time they are themselves developing.

In order to show some of the more prominent areas that researchers in heart development have on their minds, I would like to review briefly the last two conferences on heart development.

SOME DETAILS OF THE PREVIOUS MEETINGS

The last meeting devoted to heart development in the United States was a workshop held in December 1984, sponsored by the National Heart, Lung, and Blood Institute, and the National Institutes of Health as a means of identifying important areas of normal cardiac development to be targeted for a Request for Applications. That meeting was divided into eight main topics as seen in TABLE 1. At the meeting, the new technologies of molecular biology were being applied to muscle development by Dr. Nadal-Ginard and Dr. Zak and their colleagues, and a tremendous amount of new information was available about contractile protein isoforms in normal and abnormal hearts.[18,19] Cell adhesion molecules were described by Dr. Hoffman in the developing heart and their importance in controlling morphogenesis was being explored.[20] Dr. Clark had reported on the relationship between cardiac function and heart growth in the chick embryo, and using state of the art technology he and Dr. Wagman showed that the Starling relationship is an initial control mechanism for the embryonic circulation.[21,22]

More recently, in November 1988, The Third Symposium on Etiology and Morphogenesis of Congenital Heart Disease was held at The Heart Institute of Japan in Tokyo. This meeting was organized by Dr. Takao and his colleagues and sponsored by the Sankei Press, the International Society and Federation of Cardiology, and the Japan Research Promotion Society for Cardiovascular Diseases. The topical organization of that meeting was similar to the one in 1984 with a slight shift in emphasis (TABLE 2). The first part of the Japanese meeting was devoted to development of the molecular basis of the myocardium and myofibrillar assembly followed by discussions of development of the myocardial cytoskeleton. A session on the neural crest was followed by discussions of the extracellular matrix and septation of the atrioventricular (AV) region and outflow tract. The second day was devoted to physiological aspects of the development of the heart and circulation, pathogenesis of congenital heart

TABLE 1. Major Topics for the Conference Entitled Selected Topics in Cardiac Morphogenesis[a]

1. Protein synthesis and muscle development
2. Cell division, cell to cell interaction, and cell aggregation and migration
3. Differentiation; role of the extracellular matrix
4. Development, structure, and function of the contractile apparatus
5. Formation of the primary cardiac tube, initiation of contraction and hemodynamic effects
6. Partitioning of the heart and valvular development
7. Physiological development of the heart
8. Functional aspects of cardiac development

[a] Held in December 1984 in Alexandria, Virginia.

disease along with etiology and epidemiology of congenital heart disease. The final day of the meeting was devoted to the morphology of congenital defects in human hearts with a primary focus on AV septal defects and the heart in situs inversus.

It would be impossible to summarize all of the exciting results reported at the Tokyo meeting. I have singled out a few highlights that were most interesting to me, however. Dr. Fischman and colleagues reported on the appearance of sarcomeric myosin in stage 7-8 chick embryos using a monoclonal antibody specific for the rod region of sarcomeric myosin heavy chain. Using other markers he was able to determine myocardial cell polarity with regionally segregated domains of plasma membrane. Myosin distribution in these cells occurs in the region of the terminal web substantially before the onset of the heartbeat. Dr. Tokuyasu showed, using [³H]thymidine labeling, that as the myocardial wall thickens during the first day of blood flow generation, mitosis occurs much more frequently in the outermost cell layer of the myocardial wall than in the rest of the wall, suggesting a polarization of the myocardium such that the myocytes that are the oldest and therefore the most highly developed structurally will be found along the inner surface of the myocardial wall. In a poster presentation, Dr. Ikeda and colleagues reported on the reactivity of Leu-7 in human embryos in the regions of the presumptive sinoatrial and AV nodes as well as the His bundle. Because Leu-7 is a marker for the early neural crest, this suggests a neural crest origin for the conduction system in the heart. Dr. Markwald reported on the induction of AV, but not ventricular endothelium, to transform into mesenchyme under the influence of adheron-like particles containing fibronectin and glycoproteins. This transformation could be prevented by an antibody directed against these particles. Dr. Kamino and colleagues, using voltage-sensitive dyes, have optically demonstrated the occurrence of action potential, and development of pacemaker potential and cardiac rhythm generation in embryonic precontractile chick heart. Spontaneous electrical activity begins in the perfused cardiac primordia at the 6th and early 7th somite stages. By stage 9 the pacemaking area becomes confined to the left preatrial tissues. Dr. Nakazawa and colleagues have examined the effect of acetylcholine, isoproterenol, and caffeine on heart rate, blood pressure, and dorsal aortic flow in rat embryos. They found that there were different responses in the rat embryo as compared to the chick embryo. Interestingly, none of these agents affected blood pressure in the rat, whereas blood pressure in the chick was always affected. This is perhaps due to the reservoir capacity of the placenta in mammalian embryos.

MAJOR PROBLEMS

A number of major problems remain to be resolved. If you look at the major subdivisions of topics from the last three meetings featuring heart development, you can see that the topics have not changed (see TABLE 3 for the current meeting), even though the emphasis of each meeting is slightly different because of the particular interests of the organizers. The topics include, but are not limited to, origins and tissue specificity, cell lineage, determination and plasticity, epicardium and coronary circulation, mesenchyme (extracardiac and endocardially derived), connective tissue development, neural crest, extracardiac vessels (aortic arch arteries and veins), and hemodynamics (structure/function relationships). A number of issues concern myocardial development, including development of the contractile apparatus, electrical properties (ion channel regulation; K and Na currents), development of Ca^{2+} regulation (T tubules, sarcoplasmic reticulum (SR), control of release, electrical coupling), pharmacological sensitivity and innervation (autonomic control), metabolism (energy production), and development of the conduction system. At present we still barely know when things happen, much less how they are influenced by other developmental events and how they influence each other.

TABLE 2. Major Topics for the Third Symposium on Etiology and Morphogenesis of Congenital Heart Disease[a]

1. Cellular and molecular basis of cardiovascular morphogenesis
2. Extracellular matrix, cell migration, and interaction
3. Physiological aspects of developing heart
4. Pathogenesis of congenital heart disease
5. Etiology and epidemiology of congenital heart disease
6. Morphogenesis of congenital heart disease

[a] Held in November 1988 at Tokyo Women's Medical College in Tokyo, Japan.

TABLE 3. Major Topics for Embryonic Origins of Defective Heart Development[a]

1. Normal and defective development of the heart and related structures
2. Cell-cell interactions and extracellular matrix
3. Membrane and control phenomena
4. Membrane channels
5. Molecular biology, contractile proteins, and angiogenesis
6. Experimentally induced developmental defects

[a] Held in May 1989 in Arlington, Virginia.

SUGGESTED BROAD APPROACHES FOR SOLVING THE PROBLEMS

It is difficult for me to suggest approaches to solving these problems to a group of investigators who have much more experience in the field and understand many of the problems better than I do. Our own approach has been moderately successful, and I would like to outline it. We have chosen the neural crest ablation model in chick embryos and have organized our work in projects around this model. We are able to produce persistent truncus arteriosus (PTA), and dextroposed aorta (DPA), which seem to develop by way of different mechanisms. In PTA the outflow septation is absent, whereas in DPA, we think, hemodynamics are altered, causing malalignment of the cardiac septa. Our projects are organized along broad outlines containing each individual's expertise: morphological development, elastin production, ion channels, and innervation. The centerpiece of this program is our hemodynamics project, which interacts with all of the other units.

I am not suggesting that anyone interested in heart development should work in a multidisciplinary group and that individuals cannot make significant contributions. But as with everything else these days, neither individuals nor groups will get very far without a significant commitment to a holistic approach to heart development.

At the same time, even though the problems have not changed in the last five years, technology has progressed at a monumental rate. We must snap up new methods and apply them quickly to heart development. Molecular biology has been very successfully applied to studies of myocardial contractile proteins, and some molecular studies are being done on connective tissue development and the extracellular matrix. It is also important to continue combining our advancing knowledge of cellular and molecular events with the physiological status of the developing cardiovascular system.

THE FUTURE

Somehow, I do not think that the major subdivisions of the next meeting on heart development in four or five years will have changed very much. I hope that progress will be made in combining structural/molecular/functional relationships in normal development as well as in the process of cardiac dysmorphogenesis. The techniques of molecular biology are now available for general use and have already started a revolution in experimental embryology.

The future of the group that I work with lies in the application of molecular biological techniques to neural crest migration and differentiation in order to identify specific genes that are expressed for normal heart development. My dream is to be able to alter selectively, or turn off, single genes in the cardiac neural crest and to follow the ensuing anatomical and physiological events in heart development.

It is up to us to see that the best of the new technology is applied to our own areas of heart development. Molecular biology is perhaps the most spectacular of the new technologies, but it is certainly not the only one, nor is it necessarily the most important. We are now in possession of an impressive armamentarium with which to probe the mysteries of heart development, and the future is in our hands.

REFERENCES

1. SHANER, R. F. 1951. Complete and corrected transposition of the aorta, pulmonary artery and ventricles in pig embryos, and a case of corrected transposition in a child. Am. J. Anat. **88:** 35-62.
2. SHEPARD, T. H. 1973. Catalog of Teratogenic agents. Johns Hopkins Press, Baltimore, MD.
3. WARKANY, J. 1971. Congenital malformations. Year Book Med Publishers, Chicago, IL.
4. WILSON, J. G. & J. WARKANY. 1949. Aortic arch cardiac anomalies in the offspring of Vitamin A deficient rats. Am. J. Anat. **85:** 113-155.
5. KALTER, H. & J. WARKANY. 1961. Experimental production of congenital malformations in strains of inbred mice by maternal treatment with hypervitaminosis A. Am. J. Pathol. **38:** 1-21.
6. LANGMAN, J. & G. W. WELCH. 1966. Effect of vitamin A on development of the central nervous system. J. Comp. Neurol. **128:** 1-16.
7. WILSON, J. G. 1955. Teratogenic activity of several azo dyes chemically related to trypan blue. Anat. Rec. **123:** 313-333.
8. TALEPOROS, P., M. P. SALGO & G. OSTER. 1978. Teratogenic action of a bis(dichloroacetyl)diamine on rats: Patterns of malformations produced in high incidence at time-limited periods of development. Teratology **18:** 5-16.
9. OKAMOTO, N., Y. SATOW, J. Y. LEE, H. SUMIDA, K. HAYAKAWA, S. OHDO & T. OKISHIMA. 1984. Morphology and pathogenesis of the cardiovascular anomalies induced by bis-(dichloroacetyl)diamine in rats. *In* Congenital Heart Disease: Causes and Processes. J. J. Nora & A. Takao, Eds. Futura. Mount Kisco, NY.
10. IKEDA, T., T. MATSUO, K. KAWAMOTO, K. IWASAKI & T. JUBASHI. 1984. Bis-diamine-induced defects of the branchial apparatus in rats. *In* Congenital Heart Disease: Causes and Processes. J. J. Nora & A. Takao, Eds. Futura. Mount Kisco, NY.
11. MIYAGAWA, S. & M. L. KIRBY. 1989. Pathogenesis of persistent truncus arteriosus induced by nimustine hydrochloride in the chick embryo. Teratology **39:** 287-294.
12. MIYAGAWA, S., ANDO, M. & A. TAKAO. 1988. Cardiovascular anomalies produced by nimustine hydrochloride in the rat fetus. Teratology **38:** 553-558.
13. BRUYERE, H. J., B. J. MICHAUD, E. F. GILBERT & J. D. FOLTS. 1987. The effects of cardioteratogenic doses of caffeine on cardiac function in the 3-day chick embryo. J. Appl. Toxicol. **7:** 197-203.
14. VAN MIEROP, L. H. S., D. F. PATTERSON & W. R. SCHNARR. 1977. Hereditary conotruncal septal defects in Keeshond dogs: Embryologic studies. Am. J. Cardiol. **40:** 936-950.
15. LAYTON, W. M. 1984. The biology of asymmetry and the development of the cardiac loop. *In* Cardiac Morphogenesis. V. J. Ferrans, G. Rosenquist & C. Weinstein, Eds. Elsevier. New York.
16. MORRISON-GRAHAM, K. & J. A. WESTON. 1989. Mouse mutants provide new insights into the role of extracellular matrix in cell migration and differentiation. Trends Genet. **5:** 116-121.

17. KIRBY, M. L. 1988. Role of extracardiac factors in heart development. Experientia **44:** 944-950.
18. MAHDAVI, V., R. MATSUOKA & B. NADAL-GINARD. 1984. Molecular characterization and expression of the cardiac α- and β-myosin heavy chain genes. *In* Cardiac Morphogenesis. V. J. Ferrans, G. Rosenquist & C. Weinstein, Eds. Elsevier. New York.
19. NAG, A. C., M. CHENG & R. H. ZAK. 1984. Cell proliferation and expression of myosin isoforms in cardiac muscle cells in culture. *In* Cardiac Morphogenesis. V. J. Ferrans, G. Rosenquist & C. Weinstein, Eds. Elsevier. New York.
20. HOFFMAN, S., M. GRUMET & G. M. EDELMAN. 1984. Cell adhesion molecules in the histogenesis of nerve and muscle. *In* Cardiac Morphogenesis. V. J. Ferrans, G. Rosenquist & C. Weinstein, Eds. Elsevier. New York.
21. CLARK, E. B. 1984. Ventricular function and cardiac growth in the chick embryo. *In* Cardiac Morphogenesis. V. J. Ferrans, G. Rosenquist & C. Weinstein, Eds. Elsevier. New York.
22. WAGMAN, A. J. & E. B. CLARK. 1984. The Frank-Starling relationship in the embryo. *In* Cardiac Morphogenesis. V. J. Ferrans, G. Rosenquist & C. Weinstein, Eds. Elsevier. New York.

Introduction to Congenital Heart Disease

LODEWYK H. S. VAN MIEROP

Department of Pediatrics
University of Florida College of Medicine
Gainesville, Florida 32610

The story of congenital heart disease as a medical problem is of quite recent vintage. Prior to 1940 there was little interest on the part of clinicians in congenital cardiac anomalies because there was little or nothing that could be done for children afflicted with such anomalies. In his book *The Principles and Practice of Medicine,* published in 1892, William Osler[1] states that "these have only limited clinical interest, as in a large proportion of the cases the anomaly is not compatible with life, and in others nothing can be done to remedy the defect or even to relieve the symptoms." The entire discussion under the heading "Congenital Affections of the Heart" takes up four of the 71 pages devoted to "Diseases of the Heart."

Five years later a pediatrician, L. Emmett Holt,[2] in his book *The Diseases of Infancy and Childhood* could do little better: "No treatment is of the slightest avail in diminishing the amount of deformity or promoting the closure of any of the abnormal openings." For that matter, surgeons of that time were not any more encouraging or enterprising. In 1883 the famous Viennese surgeon Theodor Billroth stated: "Let no man who hopes to retain the respect of his medical brethren dare to operate on the human heart," and Sir Stephen Paget, another leading surgeon of the time, predicted dourly, in 1896, that "the heart alone of all viscera has reached the limits set by Nature to surgery. No new method and no new technique can overcome the natural obstacles surrounding a wound of the heart." That very same year Ludwig Rehn of Frankfurt, Germany, successfully sutured a stabwound of the heart and proved Paget's pronouncement one of the monumental miscalculations in medicine.

Occasional cases of cardiac anomalies were reported prior to the turn of the century, mainly as curiosities. Some authors marveled at the (perceived) anatomical similarities between such cases and the hearts of lower vertebrates and considered them atavisms (throwbacks). Systematic studies of the pathological anatomy of congenital cardiac defects, such as the monographs by Peacock,[3] Rokitanski,[4] Mönckeberg,[5] and Abbott,[6] were not published until the latter half of the 19th or early part of the 20th century. Some authors, including Rokitanski and Alexander Spitzer,[7] proposed theories as to their pathogenesis. In part these were based on what was then known about cardiovascular embryology and comparative anatomy, and in part on deductive reasoning.

The real impetus for the study of the clinical manifestations of congenital heart disease was provided primarily by two factors. One was the appointment of Helen B. Taussig, after graduation from medical school in 1927 and two additional years of training, as head of the Harriet Lane Home for children with rheumatic and congenital heart disease. Not content with simply providing custodial care, she worked out the criteria for the clinical diagnosis of many of the anomalies. The other was the birth of cardiac surgery; rapid advances in this field changed the problem from a theoretical to a very practical one. Cardiologists and, somewhat later, pediatricians had to scramble rather suddenly to catch up and keep up with their surgical colleagues.

In 1938 Robert Gross[8] successfully ligated a patent ductus arteriosus, the first operation for a congenital cardiovascular defect. In 1944 Alfred Blalock[9] performed the first shunt operation for tetralogy of Fallot, a procedure developed at the suggestion of Taussig, who had observed that children with tetralogy did much better clinically if they also had a patent ductus. This relatively simple operation, which has become known as the Blalock-Taussig procedure, transformed severely disabled, unhappy cyanotic children almost overnight into functioning, cheerful, and nearly acyanotic kids who could play with other children and go to school. It captured the imagination not only of physicians but also of the media and the public and probably did more to stimulate further developments in the diagnosis and treatment of congenital heart disease than any other procedure. The third anomaly to yield to surgical ingenuity was coarctation of the aorta, corrected almost simultaneously in 1945 by Gross[10] in the United States and Clarence Crafoord[11] in Sweden.

All three procedures involved vascular, extracardiac structures. Although subsequently a few intracardiac anomalies such as atrial septal defect, pulmonary valvar and subvalvar stenosis, and aortic stenosis were corrected using "closed" methods, hypothermia, or cross circulation, it was the development of the heart-lung machine that led to the spectacular and explosive advances in the correction or at least palliation of nearly all, even very complex, cardiac defects. These in turn, however, would not have been possible without new conceptual and technological developments, such as the work by Alexis Carrel and his able assistant, Charles Lindbergh (of later aviation fame); the discovery of blood types by Landsteiner and Wiener;[12,13] the discovery of heparin by a medical student, J. McLean, and subsequently characterized and named by Howell and Holt;[14] the invention of endotracheal intubation and anesthesia by Magill;[15] and the discovery of penicillin by Fleming.[16] Other important factors were the invention of plastics and the Second World War, which, as has been the case in earlier wars, stimulated many technological advances.

John Gibbon[17] was the first to correct an intracardiac anomaly, an atrial septal defect, using a heart-lung machine developed by him and his wife, Mary. Unfortunately the next two patients died and Gibbon made no further efforts. DeWall and associates developed the bubble oxygenator, descendants of which are now generally used. The original model can be considered the first oxygenator to be disposable, because it cost only about $5.00 (1955 dollars!) to put together. It consisted essentially of plastic tubing, which was being manufactured for a mayonnaise factory, hose clamps from a hardware store, a Tuffy sponge from the supermarket, Dow-Corning antifoam A, hypodermic needles, rubber stoppers, and a cork borer. The pump was a commercial sigmamotor pump. This apparatus, though reminiscent of Rube Goldberg, actually worked as used by C. Walton Lillehei et al.[18] It was used in the correction of atrial septal defects (including the ostium primum variety!), ventricular septal defects, and tetralogy of Fallot.

Successful open heart surgery stimulated a great deal of activity on many fronts. There were rapid developments in various diagnostic modalities such as electrocardiography, cardiac catheterization, and angiocardiography, some of which, such as ballistocardiography and phonocardiography, have become obsolete or are rarely used anymore. The occasional occurrence of surgical heart block stimulated renewed interest in the conduction system and led to the development of cardiac pacemakers, which in turn benefited from technological advances and miniaturization made possible by the invention of the transistor, the integrated circuit, and other space-age developments. Echocardiography and magnetic resonance imaging have made invasive procedures often unnecessary and have contributed to increased accuracy and much earlier diagnosis, even long before birth.

There was also renewed interest in the study of the pathology of congenital heart disease, not only among pathologists such as Maurice Lev and Jesse Edwards, but also among clinicians such as Richard van Praagh, Robert Freedom, and myself. Cardiac embryology experienced a revival that continues to this day, as is evident from the topics to be discussed in this volume. Because the bright red beating heart,

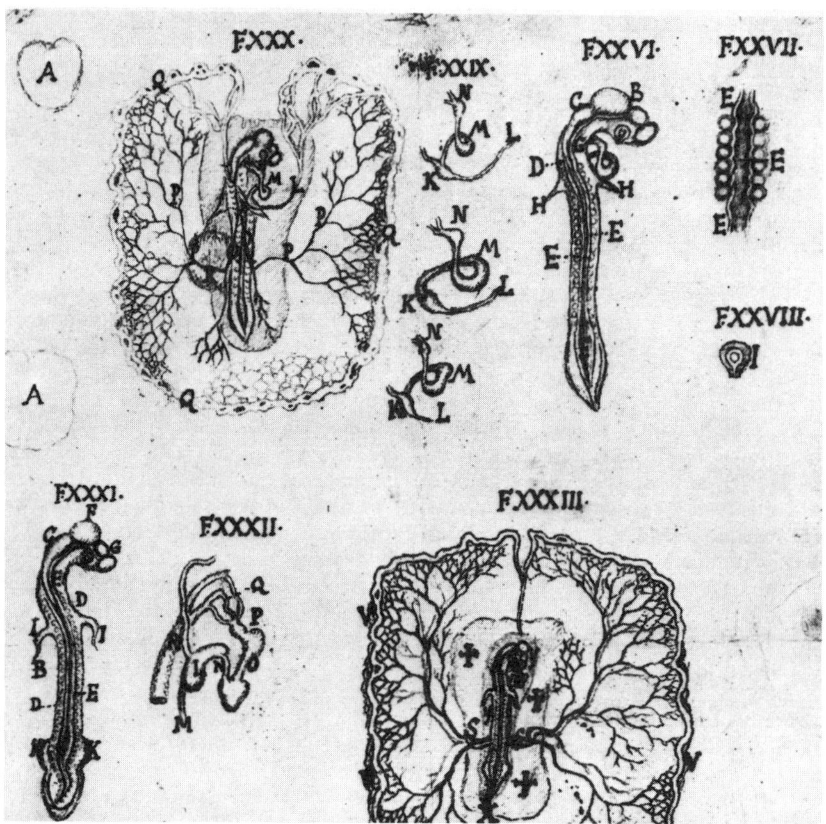

FIGURE 1. Plate IV of Malpighi's *De Ovo Incubato.*[20] Early stages of development of the chick and its cardiovascular system.

to the unaided eye, is the most conspicuous organ in an otherwise translucent early embryo, its development has received a great deal of attention for centuries. Real progress could not be made, however, until magnifying devices became available. Vesling[19] was the first to use a simple microscope to study the early embryonic heart in 1639, exactly 350 years ago. Malpighi[20] is credited with publishing the first detailed drawings of the developing chick heart some 10 years later (FIG. 1) and Von Haller[21] in 1758 produced a monograph devoted exclusively to cardiac development. During the past century our knowledge of cardiac embryology has increased markedly, and particularly in the last 30 years, the ever increasing sophistication of technology has made new avenues of study possible.

In spite of all this, we still don't know in most cases what causes congenital heart disease. The study of subjects with congenital heart disease, whether in humans or other mammals, has provided some clues. Cardiovascular defects are reasonably common as congenital anomalies go: the generally quoted prevalence is about 8/1000, although more recent studies have found an incidence of closer to 4/1000. Predominance of one sex over the other in some types of cardiac defects has long been recognized. Coarctation of the aorta, aortic valve obstruction, and transposition of the great arteries, for example, are clearly more common in males, whereas atrial septal defect, patent ductus arteriosus, and pulmonary valve stenosis are more frequent in females. Whether or not there are racial differences has been less clear. The rarity of coarctation among American Blacks reported by Hernandez *et al.*[22] was not confirmed by later studies, and Maron *et al.*[23] could find no evidence of racial difference. More recently, however, it has become quite apparent that a form of ventricular septal defect located just proximal to the arterial valves is much more common in the Far East than in western Europe or the United States. Up to 29% of all ventricular septal defects in Japan has been reported to be of the subpulmonary type, as compared to only 5-7% in Caucasians.[24] Our own studies suggest that some anomalies are more common in Caucasians, whereas others are more often seen in Blacks. More studies are needed, however, to ascertain that a bias is not introduced by differences in accessibility to health care between the two groups.

The older literature ascribes many of the cardiac anomalies to developmental errors or arrests, but also considers some, particularly those involving the valves and arteries, as being due to an intrauterine inflammatory process, for example, syphilis. An inflammatory cause was subsequently considered unlikely but was revived with the discovery that the rubella virus, and perhaps other infectious agents, could indeed produce cardiovascular defects. Our own observations on specimens with pulmonary valvar atresia and critical stenosis suggest that these may very well be caused by some kind of inflammatory process, producing first stenosis and eventually atresia of what originally may have been a normal embryonic heart. Such an etiology could also explain the rather puzzling fact that usually it is only one of the arterial valves that is stenotic, dysplastic, or both, whereas the other is perfectly normal, even though both are derived embryologically from the same endocardial cushions.

In a few anomalies there appears to be a clearly recognizable genetic factor, and some are associated with chromosomal abnormalities. In most cases, however, the etiology is not known, and it has been suggested that it may be polygenic or multifactorial, that is, due to the interaction of many genes, presumably with some contribution from environmental factors. The studies by Whittenmore *et al.*[25] and Rose *et al.*[26] have reported recurrent risks for congenital heart disease that are considerably higher than that reported by Nora *et al.*[27] and are too high to be easily explained on the basis of polygenic inheritance.

However spectacular the results of surgery for congenital heart disease have been, we must recognize that relatively few procedures will turn out to be truly curative, and late sequelae are common. As is true for other diseases, our aim should be prevention. In a few cases, for example, the cardiovascular anomalies associated with rubella syndrome, prevention is possible. These, however, represent a minuscule minority, and much more work by many investigators from many scientific disciplines remains to be done.

REFERENCES

1. OSLER, W. 1892. The Principles and Practice of Medicine. D. Appleton Co. New York.
2. HOLT, L. E. 1887. The Diseases of Infancy and Childhood. D. Appleton Co. New York.
3. PEACOCK, T. B. 1866. On Malformations of the Human Heart. 2nd Edit. J. Churchill & Sons. London.
4. ROKITANSKI, C. F. VON. 1875. Die Defecte der Scheidewände des Herzens. W. Braumüller, Vienna.
5. MÖNCKEBERG-BONN, J. G. 1924. Die Missbildungen des Herzens. *In* Handbuch der Speziellen pathologischen Anatomy und Histologie. Henke & Lubarsch, Eds. Vol. 2: 1-179. Julius Springer. Berlin.
6. ABBOTT, M. E. 1927. Congenital Cardiac Disease. *In* Osler's Modern Medicine. 3rd Edit. Vol. 3. Lea & Febiger. Philadelphia, PA.
7. SPITZER, A. 1923. Über den Bauplan der normalen und missgebildeten Herzens. Versuch einer phylogenetischen Theorie, Virch. Arch. Path. Anat. 243: 81-272.
8. GROSS, R. E. & J. P. HUBBARD. 1939. Surgical ligation of a patent ductus arteriosus. J. Am. Med. Assoc. 112: 729-731.
9. BLALOCK, A. & H. B. TAUSSIG. 1945. The surgical treatment of malformation of the heart in which there is pulmonary stenosis or pulmonary atresia. J. Am. Med. Assoc. 128: 188-202.
10. GROSS, R. E. 1945. Surgical correction for coarctation of the aorta. Surgery 18: 673-678.
11. CRAFOORD, C. & G. N. NYLIN. 1945. Congenital coarctation of the aorta and its surgical treatment. J. Thorac. Surg. 14: 347-361.
12. LANDSTEINER, K. 1900. Zur Kenntniss der antifermentativen, lytischen und agglutinierenden Wirkung des Blutserums und der Lymphe. Zentralbl. Bakteriol. 27: 357-362.
13. LANDSTEINER, K. & A. S. WIENER. 1940. An agglutinable factor in human blood recognized by immune sera for rhesus blood. Proc. Soc. Exp. Biol. Med. 24: 941-942.
14. HOWELL, W. H. & E. HOLT. 1918. Two new factors in blood coagulation: heparin and antithrombin. Am. J. Physiol. 47: 328-341.
15. MAGILL, I. W. 1930. Technique in endotracheal anesthesia. Br. Med. J. 2: 817-819.
16. FLEMING. A. 1946. History and development of penicillin. *In* Penicillin: its practical applications. Blakiston Co. Philadelphia, PA.
17. GIBBON, J. H. 1954. Application of a mechanical heart and lung apparatus to cardiac surgery. Minn. Med. 37: 171-177.
18. LILLEHEI, C. W., R. A. DEWALL, R. C. READ, H. E. WARDEN & R. L. VARCO. 1956. Direct vision intracardiac surgery in man using a simple, disposable artificial oxygenator. Dis. Chest 29: 1-8.
19. VESLING, J. 1664. Observationes anatomicae et epistolae medicae. *In* De Insolitus Partis Humani Viis Dissertatio Nova. T. Bartholin the Elder.
20. MALPIGHI, M. 1673. De Ovo Incubato. J. Martyn. London.
21. HALLER, A. VON. 1758. Sur la formation du coeur dans le poulet Lausanne.
22. HERNANDEZ, F. A., R. H. MILLER & G. L. SCHIEBLER. 1969. Rarity of coarctation of the aorta in the American Negro. J. Pediatr. 74: 623-625.
23. MARON, B. J., J. M. APPLEFIELD & L. J. KROVETZ. 1973. Racial frequencies in congenital heart disease. Circulation 47: 359-361.
24. TATSUNO, K., M. ANDO, A. TAKAO, K. HATSUNE & S. KONNO. 1975. Diagnostic importance of aortography in conal ventricular septal defect. Am. Heart J. 89: 171-177.
25. WHITTEMORE, R., J. C. HOBBINS & M. A. ENGLE. 1982. Pregnancy and its outcome in women with and without surgical treatment of congenital heart disease. Am. J. Cardiol. 50: 641-651.
26. ROSE, V., J. M. G. REYNOLD, G. LINDSAY & M. ALLEN. 1985. A possible increase in the incidence of congenital heart defects among the offspring of affected parents. J. Am. Coll. Cardiol. 6: 376-382.
27. NORA, J. J., C. W. MCGILL & D. G. MCNAMARA. 1970. Empiric recurrence risks in common and uncommon congenital heart lesions. Teratology 43: 325-330.

Inductive Interactions in Heart Development

Role of Cardiac Adherons in Cushion Tissue Formation[a]

ROGER R. MARKWALD, COREY H. MJAATVEDT,
EDWARD L. KRUG, AND ALLAN R. SINNING

Department of Anatomy and Cellular Biology
Medical College of Wisconsin
Milwaukee, Wisconsin 53226

INTRODUCTION

Heart development proceeds from a number of causally antecedent events. One of these is the formation of intracardiac mesenchyme or "endocardial cushion tissue." The significance of cushion mesenchyme is not so much its size or mass, which is relatively small compared to other cardiac tissues, but its strategic location. Cushions form protrusions in both inlet and outlet limbs of the U-shaped, primary heart tube that function as efficient, primitive valves. The eventual fusion of opposing cushion pads across the lumen of the arterioventricular (AV) canal forms a wedge of mesenchyme (the septum intermedium) that serves to "glue" and guide the union of internal muscular septa.[1,2] Accordingly, the formation of cushion tissue has important relevance to the etiology of congenital heart disease.[3]

FORMATION OF CUSHION TISSUE

Cushion mesenchyme derives from an epithelial-mesenchymal transformation that is regionally and temporally specific. The endocardial epithelium (endothelium) of the AV canal and proximal outflow track is competent to transform into the mesenchyme comprising cushion tissue (FIG. 1). Cushion mesenchyme is probably the only example of mesenchyme derived from an endothelial lineage, a fact supported

[a]This work was funded by NIH Grant K37 HL33756 and by pre- and postdoctoral support from the American Heart Association (Wisconsin affiliate).

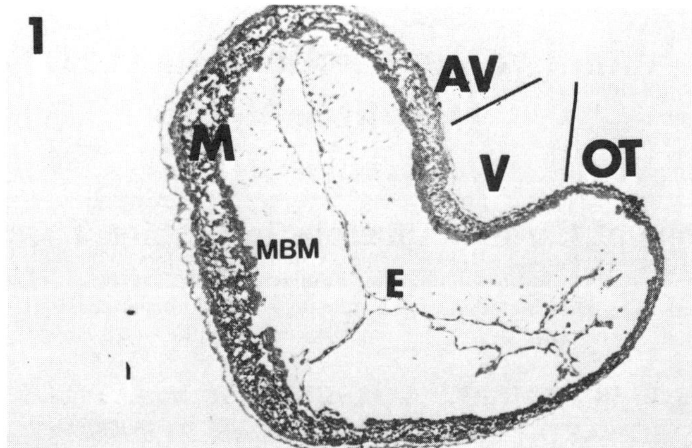

FIGURE 1. Survey micrograph of a stage 19, U-shaped chick heart, which demonstrates the regional pattern for the formation of cushion mesenchyme. Although contiguous throughout the heart, the endothelium (E) forms mesenchyme only in the atrioventricular (AV) canal and outflow track (OT) but not the ventricle (V). M, myocardium; MBM, myocardial basement membrane; $\times 50$.

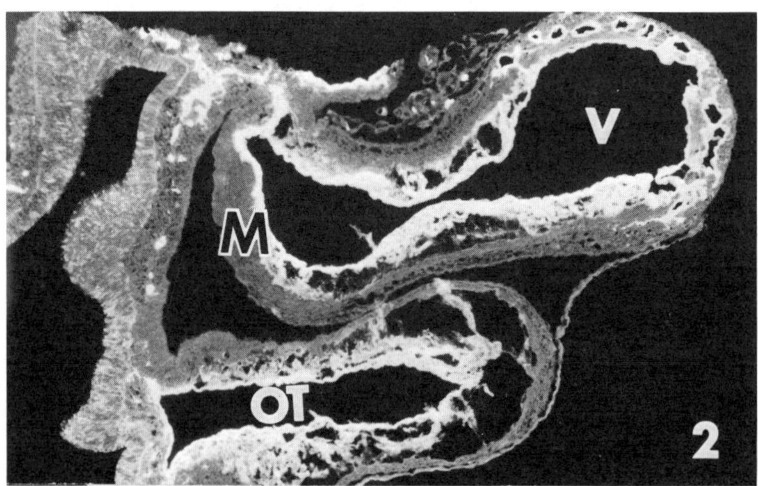

FIGURE 2. Stage 20 quail heart stained with QH1, a monoclonal antibody marker for quail endothelium. Note positively stained mesenchyme in the AV canal (also OT) indicating their endothelial origin of cushion mesenchyme; $\times 50$.

by its unique expression of the endothelial marker, QH1[4] (FIG. 2). The transformation of endothelium proceeds from a cascade of cellular dynamics that includes loss of endothelial cell:cell associations, cytoplasmic hypertrophy, and cytoskeletal rearrangements that eventuate in the formation of migratory appendages[5–7] (FIG. 3).

A major focus of our laboratory has been to determine the molecular events underlying these cellular phenomena. *In situ,* the change in endothelial cell adhesion has been found to correlate with decreased expression of neural cell adhesion molecule (N-CAM), a primary, calcium independent, adhesion molecule.[8] The characteristic hypertrophy of transforming endothelium, in turn, correlates with the increased (or sustained) expression of substrate adhesion molecules (SAM), such as proteoglycans of heparan and chondroitin sulfate[9] and fibronectin.[10] The expression of SAM may be required to initiate migration of the transformed endothelial cells into the extracellular matrix, which separates the endothelium from the myocardium.[9] Transfor-

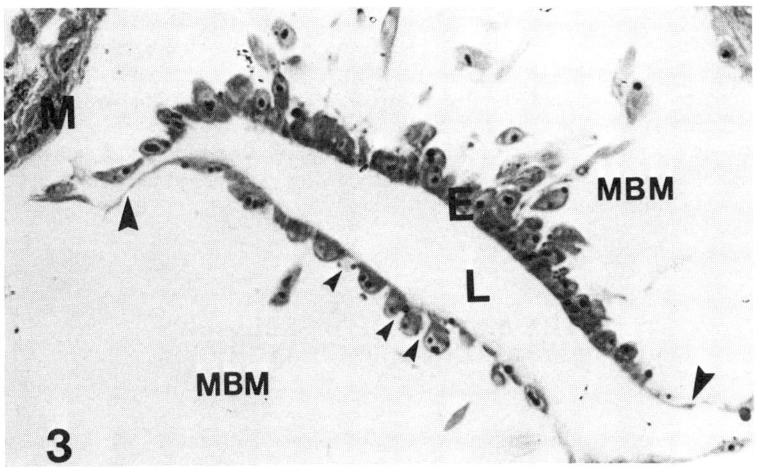

FIGURE 3. Stage 17 AV canal showing the process of endothelial transformation to mesenchyme. Note free mesenchymal cells in the myocardial basement membrane (MBM). The small arrow heads denote areas of cell:cell separation between hypertrophied endothelial cells. Large arrowheads denote unstimulated (squamous-shaped) endothelial cells; ×400.

mation of endothelium into mesenchyme also results in the expression of M38 antigen (type I procollagen), an observation that serves as a useful molecular marker in transformation bioassays.[11]

EXTRINSIC VERSUS INTRINSIC REGULATION OF THE TRANSFORMATION PROCESS

Chronologically, in both the chick and rat heart, the initiation of the transformation process is so specific as to suggest that the process might be triggered by an intrinsic "clock."[12] To test this hypothesis, we explanted segments of the AV canal onto collagen gel lattices hydrated with culture medium. In such cultures, the endothelium grew out as a monolayer on the surface of the gel, whereas, the AV myocardium formed a tight epithelial-like "myoball". When left in co-culture with the myocardium, some, but not all, AV endothelial cells transformed into mesenchyme. Conversely, ventricular endothelium remained epithelial in either the presence or absence of AV myocardium. The timing of the *in vitro* transformation process paralleled that seen *in situ,* indicating that the hypothetical intrinsic clock continued to run when AV endothelium was explanted into culture. The requirement of AV endothelium for co-culture with myocardium suggested, however, that a myocardially derived, extrinsic stimulus might be needed for the progression of the intrinsic clock.[13]

We have previously shown *in situ* that the myocardium secretes glycoconjugates—historically termed cardiac jelly—into an extracellular space that has the organization and composition of a basement membrane belonging to the myocardium.[14] Because the myocardial basement membrane/cardiac jelly (MBM/CJ) matrix directly contacts the endothelium, we proposed that the myocardium secreted into its own MBM, an inductive factor that could modify the differentiation program of a competent endothelial cell by inducing expression/suppression of genes required to transform it into mesenchyme. Support for the existence of an extrinsic signal was obtained by experiments in which the growth medium from primary cultures of myocardial cells effectively substituted for myocardial tissue in stimulating endothelial transformation to mesenchyme.[15] A diagrammatic summary of work completed to test this hypothesis is presented in FIGURE 4.

THE MYOCARDIAL CELL AS AN
EMBRYONIC STIMULATOR CELL

Intracellular protein synthesis related to contractile filaments and their assembly into sarcomeres has been the focus of most studies on the developing myocardium. Even while contractile proteins are apparently being synthesized and sarcomeres assembled, however, the myocardium secretes some 30 to 35 proteins or protein subunits[16] into the MBM/CJ space. Regional differences were noted in the myocardial secretion of extracellular proteins. Unique to the MBM/CJ of mesenchyme-forming regions were proteins corresponding to M_r of 19, 31, 46, and 104.[16] The potential significance of these differences was underscored by the important finding that the AV myocardium but not the ventricular myocardium could support transformation of AV endothelium to mesenchyme in co-culture experiments.[17] These data suggest a regionally specific, myocardial stimulus for endothelial transformation, but they tell us little about the molecular nature of the signal.

A potentially key observation for identifying this regional stimulus was the discovery of a particulate form of matrix present in the MBM/CJ of mesenchyme-forming regions. The particulates were revealed as 0.1-0.5 μm inclusions of the AV/MBM by either lectin or fibronectin antibody[17] (FIG. 5), and, as shown in FIG. 6, the particulates (especially in the AV region) were restricted to the period of cushion tissue formation and only to regions of mesenchyme formation. The particulates were extractable with EDTA but not PBS; when examined ultrastructurally, EDTA extracts were found to contain structural elements with electron dense cores measuring 30 nm in diameter from which small "arms" projected.[18] These structures were very similar

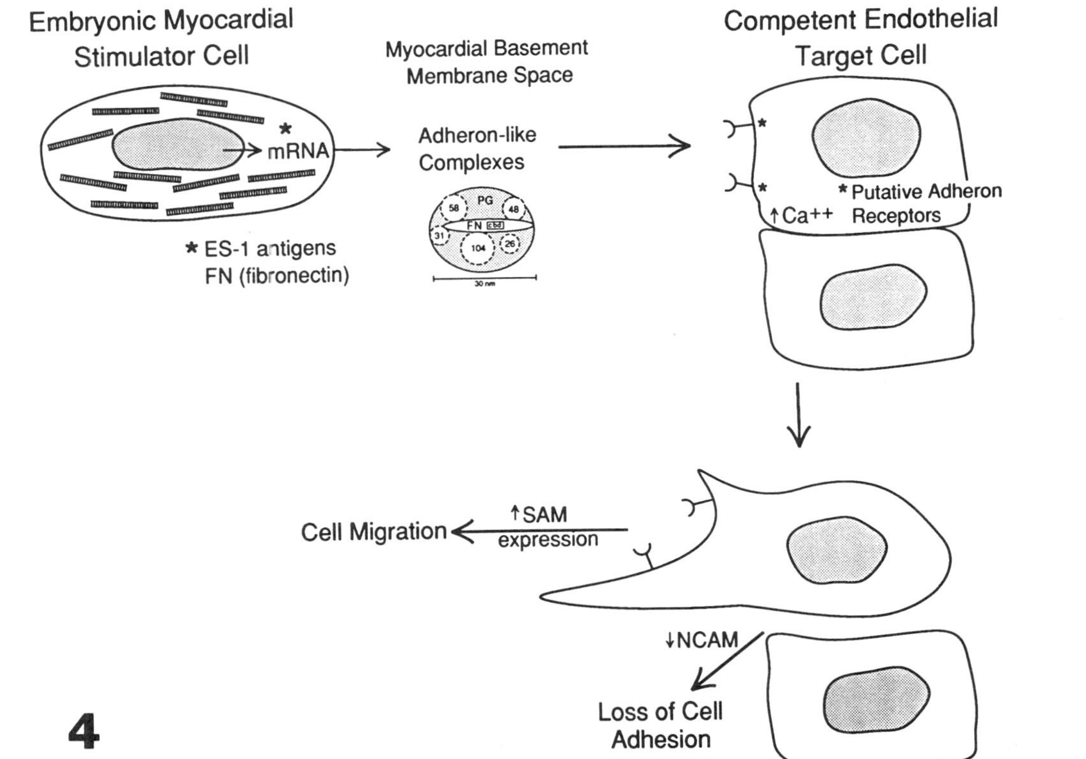

FIGURE 4. Diagrammatic summary of the inductive interaction between myocardium and endothelium that eventuates in the formation of free mesenchymal cells. The myocardial stimulator cell secretes extracellular protein complexes (adherons), into its own basement membrane, that induce competent target cells (endothelium) to decrease expression for neural cell adhesion molecules (NCAM) but to increase expression for substrate-associated molecules (SAM). Competency is hypothesized to constitute the presence of a receptor for adheron proteins that accounts for the demonstrated influx of intracellular calcium upon stimulation with myocardial conditioned medium.

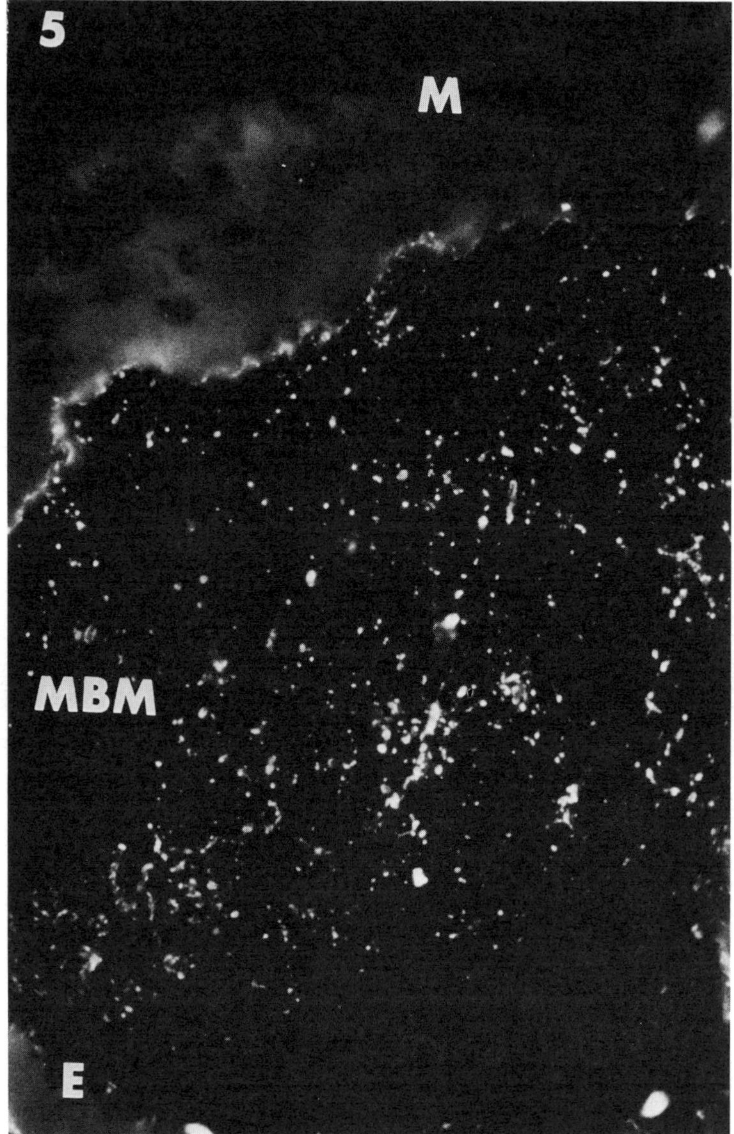

FIGURE 5. Cross-section of a stage 16 AV canal showing a portion of the myocardial basement membrane (MBM) immunostained with a polyclonal antifibronectin antibody to demonstrate the particulate form of matrix unique to presumptive mesenchyme-forming regions. (See ref. 17 for technical details, including procedure for cryopreservation). M, myocardium; E, endothelium; ×800.

FIGURE 6. Regional variation in antifibronectin antibody staining of particulate matrix in a cryopreserved, stage 20 chick heart. The region from which each section was obtained is indicated in the diagram at the bottom of this figure. Note in **A** that the particulate matrix decreases in AV regions following migration of cushion cells (F). Particulates persist only near the lamina densa (L) zone of the MBM, near the myocardium (M). Conversely, the particulate matrix is

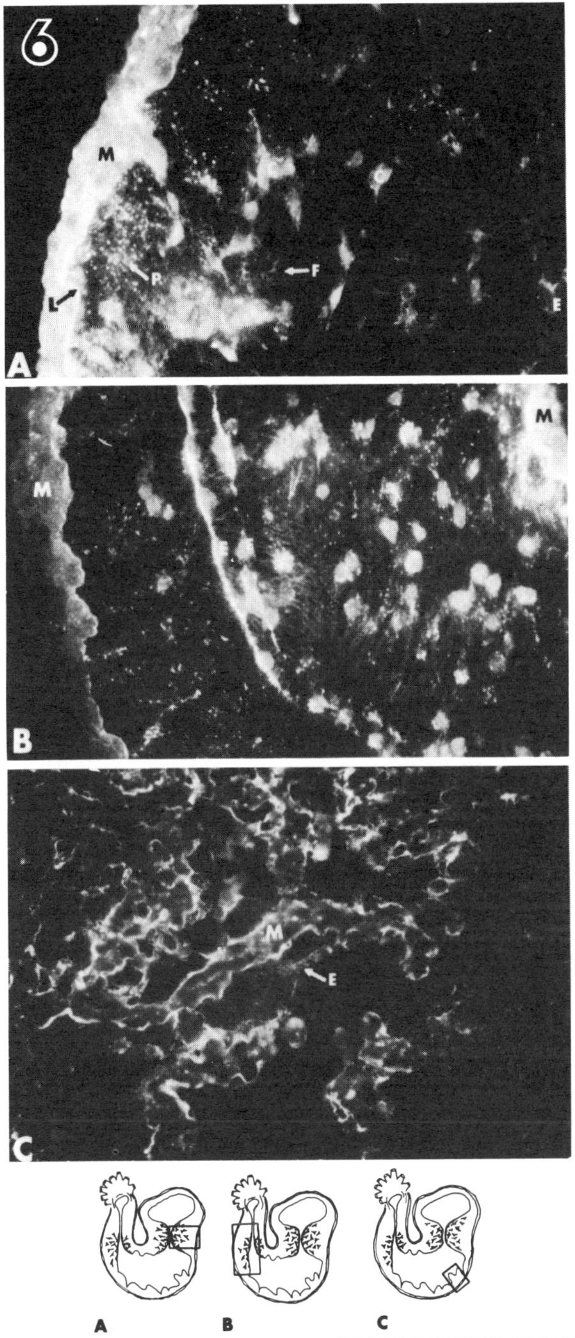

still present in the MBM of the conus region of the outflow track (**B**), whereas in the ventricle (**C**) no particulates are seen in the matrix space between the endothelium (**E**) and the positively stained lamina densa of the myocardial trabeculae. A, B, C; ×200.

to aggregates of 30 nm particles previously observed in the MBM/CJ of mesenchyme-forming areas of tissues either chemically fixed[19] or cryopreserved (FIG. 7). Accordingly, we have suggested that the particulate matrix observed by fibronectin antibody staining is composed of aggregates of a 30 nm subunit uniquely secreted by the AV myocardial cell.

Although the morphological distribution of EDTA-extractable particulates correlates with the regional specificity of the epithelial-mesenchymal transformation, these data did not prove that the 30 nm subunits contained the specific myocardial stimulatory signal. To resolve this question, EDTA extracts were centrifuged at 100,000 g and the resultant pellet and supernatant fractions tested for their inductive potential in endothelial activation assays.[20,21] The unfractionated extract and the pellet fraction both induced complete transformation of AV endothelium (but not with ventricular endothelium). Applying the pelleted extract by micropipette directly to endothelial monolayers induced the loss of N-CAM expression that was strikingly restricted to the area of treatment.[21] Conversely, the supernatant with 90% of the total protein in the unfractionated extract had no observable effects. Interestingly, electrophorectic comparisons of the supernatant versus pellet indicated that, although, several proteins were common to both fractions, the pellet fraction was highly enriched in three of the four proteins (31, 46/48, and 104 kDa) previously reported to be unique to the

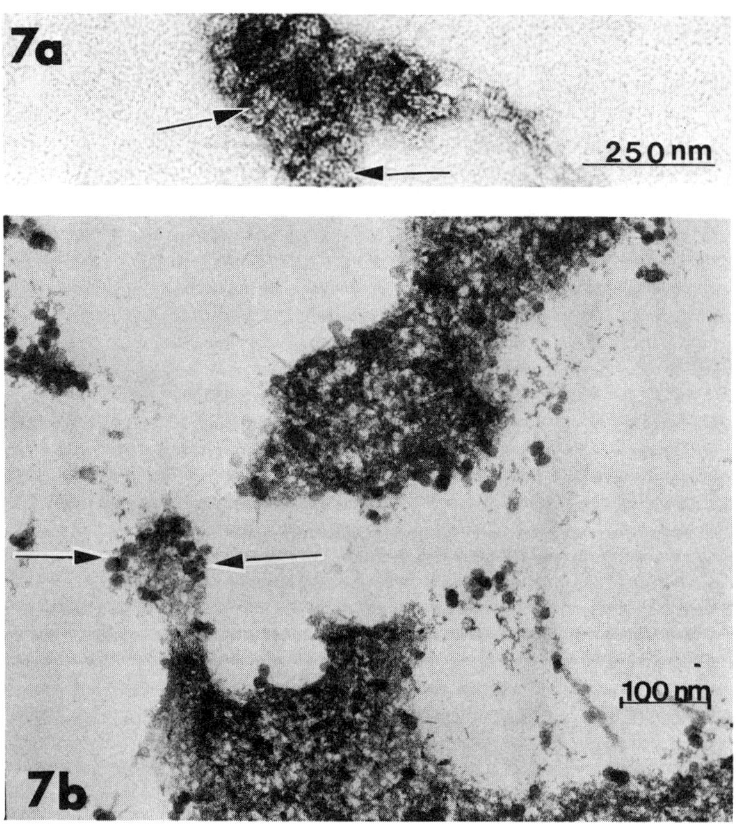

mesenchyme-forming regions of the heart.[16,21] Other bands enriched in the pellet fraction were those with M_r of 26, 28, and 58.

THE MYOCARDIAL "ADHERON"

Because the epithelial-mesenchymal transforming bioactivity of the fractionated extract was limited to the pellet fraction containing the 30 nm subunits, these multicomponent complexes appear to be the most likely candidate for a regionally specific, myocardial stimulator. In searching for a precedent for such a 30 nm structure, the closest fit appears to be glycoprotein complexes, termed adherons by Schubert and co-workers.[22-24] Adherons were initially isolated by ultracentrifugation of the growth medium of embryonic cells or embryonic cell lines such as L6 skeletal myoblasts. Compositional (*e.g.* fibronectin and several proteins under 100 kDa) and structural similarities exist between adherons and cardiac 30 nm particles. L6 adherons, however, were not active in AV endothelial activation assays.[21] Schubert has suggested that adherons are fundamental building blocks of basement membranes and play a role in

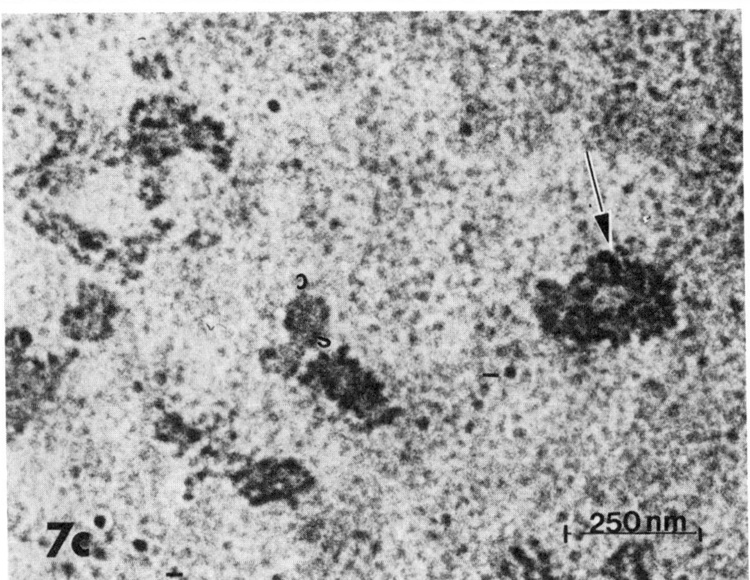

FIGURE 7. (a) Small aliquot of fresh EDTA extract air dried on a Formvar-coated grid and negatively stained with phosphotungstic acid. Note the 30-35 nm particles (arrows) that tend to aggregate in the extraction buffer. (b) Arrows denote particles similar to those in **a** that are present in the AV/MBM of a stage 16 heart fixed in glutaraldehyde containing 1% cetylpyridinium chloride (see ref. 19). Clustering of particles is commonly observed and most likely is the basis for the particulate form of matrix revealed after antifibronectin antibody staining. (c) Rapidly frozen (liquid nitrogen), cryopreserved stage 16 heart embedded in Lowicryl, sectioned through the AV/MBM and stained with uranyl acetate. Particles similar to those in **a** and **b** are observed without chemical fixation and prior to EDTA extraction.

cell-cell or cell substrate adhesion. A 21 kDa protein in adherons obtained from the conditioned medium of chick retinal epithelium also appears to have growth factor-like activities.[24] One significance of our observations is that they indicate adherons may not merely be culture phenomenology but exist *in vivo* where they may function as diffusible repositories of inductively active proteins in the myocardial basement membrane.

As shown in FIGURE 4, the cardiac adheron-like complexes contain fibronectin and several proteins mostly under 100 kDa. The actual spatial associations of these proteins is unknown. Owing to the multiple binding domains of fibronectin,[25] we have hypothesized that fibronectin may serve as a "carrier" for the other proteins of the complex. This hypothesis is supported by staining the particulate matrix with a panel of antifibronectin monoclonal antibodies directed against various regions of the molecule. Results indicate that the cell-binding region of the fibronectin molecule is free of intermolecular associations, which may represent the mechanism of adheron binding to AV endothelial cells.[21] Furthermore, passing EDTA extracts over fibronectin affinity columns removed several, nonfibronectin proteins previously shown to be associated with the pellet fraction of the extract,[26] yielding additional support for the intermolecular associations with fibronectin.

To initiate efforts to identify the specific protein(s) of the adheron-like complexes responsible for activating endothelial transformation to mesenchyme, a polyclonal serum, termed ES-1, was prepared against the particulate fraction of an EDTA extract.[15,21] On western blots, this antibody recognized two major antigens (28 and 46 kDa) and three minor antigens (58, 124, and 180 kDa). The antibody did not bind fibronectin by any analytical test. ES-1 immunostained the particulate matrix[21] as did a monoclonal antibody, HMX-1, that was also prepared against the pelleted fraction of the EDTA extract (FIG. 8). The significance of ES-1 and HMX-1 immunostaining is that they further indicate that the inductive activity of the pelleted fraction of EDTA extracts is equivalent to the *in situ* particulate matrix and that this form of matrix is a multicomponent complex.

ES-1 holds reasonable potential for ultimately resolving the specific functions of the individual proteins in the adheron-like particles or for establishing the importance of their intermolecular associations. This belief is based on the recent observation of Mjaatvedt *et al.*[21] that ES-1 is a potent reagent for blocking mesenchyme formation when added to co-culture bioassays of AV endothelium and myocardium. Purification of ES-1 antigens is in progress as is the preparation of an embryonic myocardial poly(A+) RNA/lambda gtll expression library, which will be screened with this antiserum. Isolated ES-1-positive fusion proteins and ES-1-immunopurified antigens will be used to develop monospecific polyclonal antibodies for use in endothelial bioassays. At this point, however, the precise identity of proteins in the adheron-like subunits of the particulate matrix, other than fibronectin, remains completely unknown.

THE ENDOTHELIAL TARGET CELL

As noted above, ventricular endothelium does not form mesenchyme *in situ,* nor does it respond in culture to pelleted extract (adherons). Even within transforming regions of the heart, not all endothelial cells respond to myocardial induction. Thus, as indicated in our hypothetical model (FIG. 4), adherons induce only a competent endothelial cell to transform to mesenchyme. We propose that the definition of com-

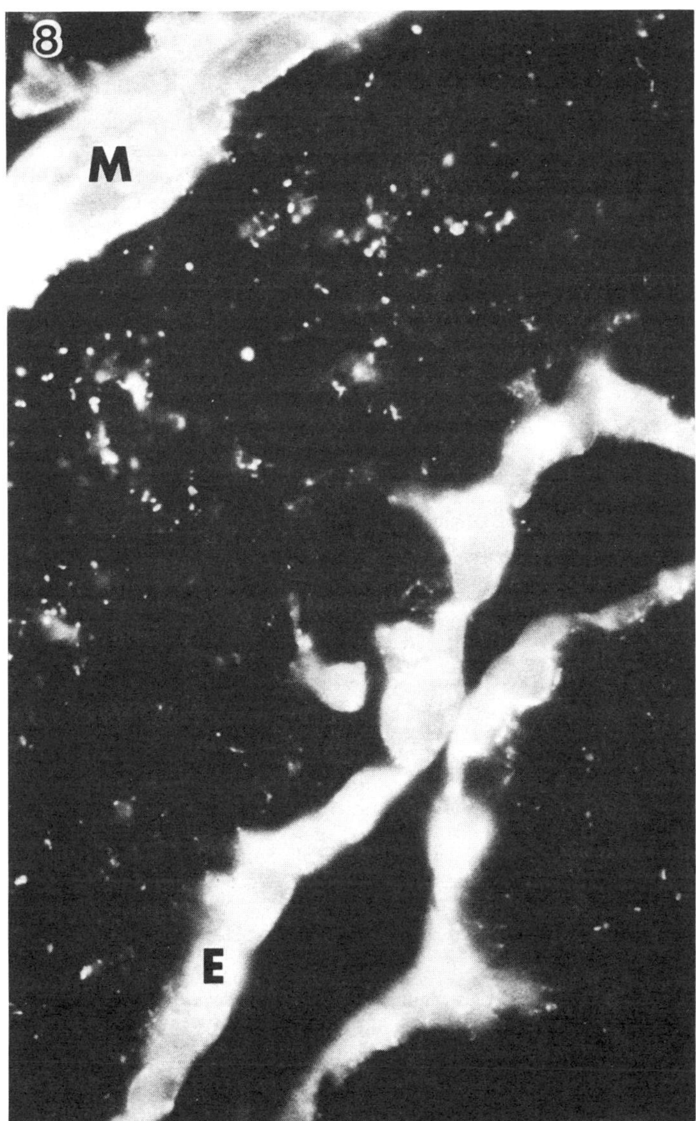

FIGURE 8. AV region of a cryopreserved, stage 16 chick heart immunostained with a monoclonal antibody, HMX-l, prepared against the pelleted fraction (100,000 g) of an EDTA extract. Note that the antibody specifically stains the particulate form of the matrix comprising the AV/MBM; ×800. Secondary antibody (rabbit anti-mouse IgG) was labeled with FITC.

petency is the possession of cell surface receptors for proteins of adherons. Due to the availability of the cell-binding domain of fibronectin, possibly an integrin family member is the receptor.[27] Whereas the identity of the putative receptor involved is unknown, the high likelihood of such a receptor has been recently indicated by the work of Runyan (see paper in this volume). The Runyan laboratory has shown that adding myocardial conditioned medium to cultures of AV but not ventricular endothelial cells triggered a rapid influx of intracellular calcium as revealed by Fura-2, a Ca^{2+}-binding fluorophore. This exciting observation indicates that in living cells myocardial secretory proteins can elicit second messenger-type activities. The actual identity of the receptor or receptors responsible for this activity, however, is likely to remain unresolved until the specific protein or proteins in the adheron particles responsible for AV endothelial transformation are identified and characterized.

REFERENCES

1. WENINK, A. C. G. & A. C. GITTENBERGER-DE GROOT. 1985. The role of atrioventricular endocardial cushions in the septation of the heart. Int. J. Cardiol. **8:** 25-44.
2. HAY, D. A. 1978. Development and fusion of the endocardial cushions. *In* Morphogenesis and malformation of the cardiovascular system. G. C. Roosenquist & D. Bergsma, Eds.: **7:** 69-90. Birth Defects: Original Article Series XIV.
3. VAN MIEROP, L. H. S. 1976. Embryology of the atrioventricular canal and pathogenesis of endocardial cushion defects. *In* Atrioventricular Canal Defects. R. H. Feldt, Ed.: 1-12. W. B. Saunders Company. Philadelphia.
4. PARDANAUD, L. C., C. ALTMAN, P. KITOS, F. DIETERLEN-LIEVRE & C. A. BUCK. 1987. Vasculogenesis in the early quail blastodisc as studied with a monoclonal antibody recognizing endothelial cells. Development **100:** 339-349.
5. MARKWALD, R. R., T. P. FITZHARRIS & W. N. ADAMS SMITH. 1975. Structural analysis of endocardial cytodifferentiation. Dev. Biol. **42:** 160-180.
6. MARKWALD, R. R., G. T. KITTEN, R. B. RUNYAN, F. M. FUNDERBURG, D. H. BERNANKE & P. R. BRAUER. 1984. Use of three-dimensional collagen gel culture to study cell:matrix interactions in heart development. *In* Role of the Extracellular Matrix in Development. Symposium of the Society of Developmental Biology. R. Trelstad, Ed.: **42:** 323-350. Academic Press. New York.
7. ICARDO, J. M. 1989. Changes in endocardial cell morphology during development of the endocardial cushions. Anat. Embryol. **179:** 443-448.
8. MARKWALD, R. R. & R. C. LEPERA. 1987. The temporal and site restricted expression of cell adhesion and substrate associated molecules during endothelial transformation to mesenchyme in the embryonic chick heart. Anat. Rec. **218:** 87A.
9. FUNDERBURG, F. M. & R. R. MARKWALD. 1986. Conditioning of native substrates by chondroitin sulfate proteoglycan during cardiac mesenchymal cell migration. J. Cell Biol. **103:** 2475-2488.
10. FFRENCH-CONSTANT, C. & R. O. HYNES. 1988. Patterns of fibronectin gene expression and splicing during cell migration in chicken embryos. Development **104:** 369-382.
11. SINNING, A. R., R. C. LEPERA & R. R. MARKWALD. 1988. Initial expression of type I procollagen in chick cardiac mesenchyme is dependent upon myocardial stimulation. Dev. Biol. **130:** 167-174.
12. BERNANKE, D. H. & R. R. MARKWALD. 1982. Cardiac cushion morphogenetic events in a three-dimensional collagen lattice culture model. Dev. Biol. **92:** 235-245.
13. RUNYAN, R. B. & R. R. MARKWALD. 1983. Invasion of mesenchyme into three-dimensional collagen gels: A regional and temporal analysis of interaction in embryonic heart tissue. Dev. Biol. **95:** 108-114.
14. KITTEN, G. T., R. R. MARKWALD & D. L. BOLENDER. 1987. The distribution of basement membrane antigens in cryopreserved early embryonic hearts. Anat. Rec. **217:** 379-390.

15. KRUG, E. L., C. H. MJAATVEDT & R. R. MARKWALD. 1987. Induction of embryonic cardiac endothelial differentiation into mesenchyme by myocardially-derived extracellular proteins. Dev. Biol. **120:** 348-355.
16. KRUG, E. L., R. B. RUNYAN & R. R. MARKWALD. 1985. Protein extracts from early embryonic hearts initiate endothelial cytodifferentiation. Dev. Biol. **112:** 414-426.
17. MJAATVEDT, C. H., R. C. LEPERA & R. R. MARKWALD. 1987. Myocardial specificity for initiating endothelial-mesenchymal cell transition in embryonic heart correlates with a particulate distribution of fibronectin. Dev. Biol. **119:** 59-67.
18. MJAATVEDT, C. H. & R. R. MARKWALD. 1989. Induction of an epithelial-mesenchymal transition by an *in vivo* adheron-like complex. Dev. Biol. **136:** 118-128.
19. MARKWALD, R. R., T. P. FITZHARRIS, H. BANK & D. H. BERNANKE. 1978. Structural analyses on the matrical organization of glycosaminoglycans in developing endocardial cushions. Dev. Biol. **62:** 292-316.
20. KRUG, E. L. & R. R. MARKWALD. 1985. Extracellular cardiac proteins activate chick endothelial transition to mesenchyme. *In* Progress in Developmental Biology Part IB. H. Slavkin, Ed.: 195-198. Alan R. Liss. New york.
21. MJAATVEDT, C. H., E. L. KRUG & R. R. MARKWALD. 1989. Early cardiac mesenchyme formation is inhibited by an antibody (ESl) against an adheron-like fraction of myocardial basement membrane. Submitted for publication.
22. SCHUBERT, D. & M. LACORBIERE. 1980. The role of a 16S glycoprotein complex in cellular adhesion. Proc. Natl. Acad. Sci. USA **77:** 4137-4141.
23. SCHUBERT, D., M. LACORBIERE, F. G. KLIER & C. BIRDWELL. 1983. The structure and function of myoblast adherons. Cold Spring Harbor Symp. Quant. Biol. **48:** 539-549.
24. BERMAN, P., P. GRAY, E. CHEN, K. KEYSER, D. EHRICH, H. KARTEN, M. LACORBIERE, F. ESCH & D. SCHUBERT. 1987. Sequence analysis, cellular localization, and expression of a neuroretina adhesion and cell survival molecule. Cell **51:** 135-142.
25. HYNES, R. O. 1985. Molecular biology of fibronection. Annu. Rev. Cell Biol. **1:** 67-90.
26. SINNING, A. R., E. L. KRUG & R. R. MARKWALD. 1989. A lectin positive, adheron-like particle associated with the EDTA soluble fraction of the myocardial basement membrane during early cardiac morphogenesis. Submitted for publication.
27. HYNES, R. O. 1987. Integrins: a family of cell surface receptors. Cell **48:** 549-554.

Development of the Outflow Tract

A Study in Hearts with Situs Solitus and Situs Inversus[a]

JOSE M. ICARDO

Department of Anatomy and Cell Biology
Faculty of Medicine
University of Cantabria
39011-Santander, Spain

INTRODUCTION

One of the points that has aroused much controversy among heart researchers through the years is the development of the outflow tract. This conflict stems from several areas. First, there is not a widely accepted terminology that can identify similar structures with identical names. This is not simply a semantic question: it originates, at least in part, from profound differences in the understanding of the fate of the different parts of the heart tube. Another major obstacle to the unification of concepts on outflow tract development is the use of different species to complement partial observations. Although cellular and subcellular mechanisms may be similar in different species, the contribution of the different structures to the definitive heart shape may not be identical. Another difficulty is the identification of changing structures (and their external and internal limits) as they progress through the different developmental stages. Finally, the task is complicated by the involvement of the different structures that have to join together in the course of normal morphogenesis.

Formation of the outflow tract results from coordinated development in three different regions of the embryonic heart. It involves formation of the aorticopulmonary (A-P) septum, septation of the bulbus cordis, and formation of the aortic vestibulum. As a result of the coordination of these three developmental events, the ventricles attain independent arterial connections. In this presentation, I shall attempt to describe the development of the outflow tract and to discuss possible morphogenetic mechanisms. The terminology employed here is similar to the one used in the past,[1,2] and it is basically that of previous authors.[3–5] The study focuses on two different species, chick and mouse. The inbred strain of mice, *iv/iv*, is used, which presents situs inversus in 50% of the cases.[6,7]

[a] This work was supported by Grants 257UC and 332UC from the Universidad de Cantabria-Caja Cantabria.

BULBUS CORDIS

The term *bulbus cordis*, as used here, refers to the most distal part of the heart. It extends from the bulboventricular sulcus to the origin of the aortic arches, and represents the truncoconal portion of the heart (FIG. 1). Septation of the bulbus cordis in the chick takes place by formation of two sets of opposite cardiac jelly mounds.[1-4,8-10] These are the dextrodorsal and sinistroventral conal and truncal cushions. The dextrodorsal conal cushion is located dorsally and to the right. It develops following a spiraling course ventral and to the left, eventually becoming continuous with the sinistroventral truncal cushion. Similarly, the sinistroventral conal cushion develops dorsal and to the right to become continuous with the dextrodorsal truncal cushion. Thus, two spiraling ridges of cushion tissue develop along the entire length of the bulbus. The two systems cross each other at the truncoconal junction. The presence of these ridges separates the still undivided bulbus into aortic and pulmonic channels. Whereas the pulmonic channel appears in a ventral position, the aortic one is located dorsally and appears directed toward the interventricular foramen.

In the chick, the conal cushions are separated from their truncal counterparts from deep indentations. These indentations disappear when the cushions become continuous, just before septation. The development of the bulbar cushions in the mouse appears to be slightly different from that in the chick. In the mouse, no conotruncal cushions appear to develop separately (FIG. 2). Rather, two sets of spiraling ridges develop simultaneously with no separation between the conal and truncal components. The two ridges follow a spiraling course from the beginning, and only a small indentation appears to indicate the division between the truncal and conal portions (FIGURES 2 and 3).

THE AORTICOPULMONARY SEPTUM

While these changes are taking place in the bulbus, the part of the heart connected to the aortic arches enlarges to become a distinct region, the truncoaortic sac. The wall of the truncoaortic sac is formed of endothelium surrounded by mesenchyme and contains neither myocardium nor cushion tissue. As the truncoaortic sac is enlarging, a wedge of mesenchymal tissue, the aorticopulmonary septum (A-P), appears between the fourth and sixth aortic arches. The A-P septum is made up of condensed mesenchyme, most of which originates in the mesenchyme that surrounds the fourth aortic arch.[11] These cells appear to be primarily of neural crest origin.[11,12] The A-P septum continues downwards into two limbs or prongs of condensed mesenchyme. The prongs of the A-P septum penetrate into the truncal cushions where they extend down to the semilunar valve level.

Division of the truncus takes place in a caudal direction. The two prongs of the A-P septum fuse caudally dividing the truncus into two separate channels (FIGURES 4-6). These are the prospective proximal parts of the aorta and the pulmonary artery. The A-P prongs are first observed beneath the myocardium. As fusion progresses caudally, however, the truncal cushions become apposed to each other, and the two prongs appear subjacent to the endocardial surface. Then, the endocardial lining disappears, and the two prongs fuse and become continuous, forming a single central focus of cells between the two emerging lumens (FIG. 4). At the same time, the

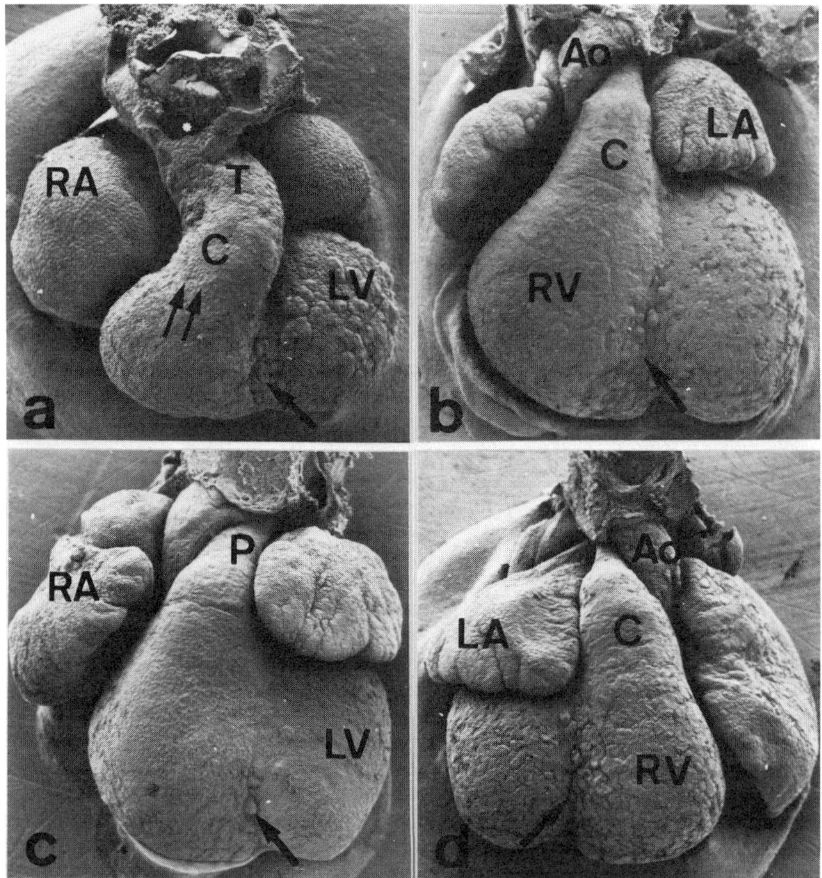

FIGURE 1. Scanning electron micrographs (SEM) showing the external modifications undergone by the heart during truncoconal septation. *iv* mouse. **a, b,** and **c,** situs solitus; **d,** situs inversus. Ao, aorta; P, pulmonary artery; RA, right atrium; RV, right ventricle; LA, left atrium; LV, left ventricle; T, truncus; C, conus. Arrow indicates the interventricular sulcus. **a:** The bulbus cordis extends between the bulboventricular sulcus (double arrow) and the origin of the aortic arches (*). The ventral bending of this region marks the separation between truncus and conus; 11.5 days; × 72. **b:** At a later stage the truncus appears divided into the proximal parts of the aorta and the pulmonary artery. The conus is still undivided; 12.5 days; × 65. **c:** Later, the external changes are not very apparent. Bulbar septation, however, has been completed; 15.5 days; × 54. **d:** This micrograph shows a situs inversus of the same developmental age as that shown in **b.** The heart appears normal except for the left-sided position of the normally right-sided structures; 12.5 days; × 57.

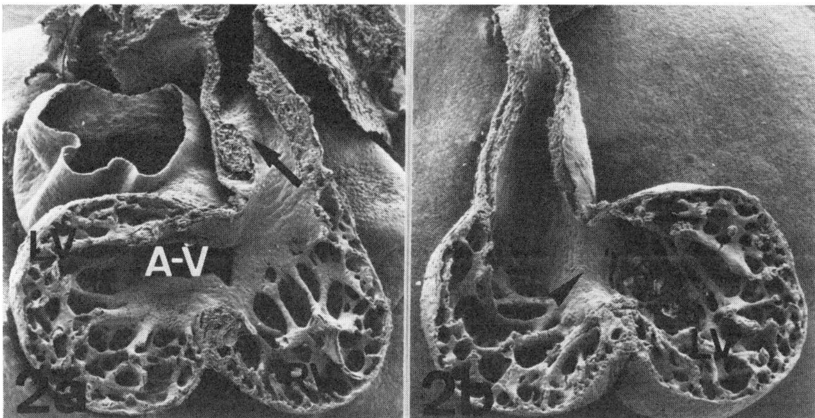

FIGURE 2. SEM showing the internal appearance of the bulbus cordis. *iv* mouse, situs inversus; 11.5 days. The bulbus cordis is open throughout its entire length, and the two halves are presented: **a:** dorsal half; **b:** ventral half. The spiral development of the bulbar ridges (arrow) can clearly be observed in **a**. The free border of the interventricular septum is indicated (arrowhead). The atrioventricular (A-V) canal communicates the atrial and the ventricular regions; note the presence of the developing dorsal and ventral endocardial cushions. The right ventricle (RV) and the bulbus are left-sided. LV, left ventricle. × 72.

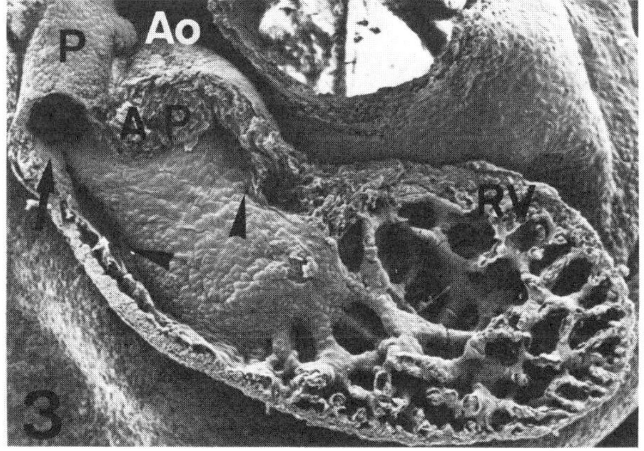

FIGURE 3. SEM of the bulbus cordis at a later stage than that shown in FIG. 2. *iv* mouse, situs solitus; 12,5 days. The heart has been dissected through the bulbus. Right side of the specimen: the truncoaortic sac has been divided. Ao, aorta; P, pulmonary artery. The aortico-pulmonary septum (A-P) is dividing the truncus. A small indentation (arrowheads) separates the truncal and conal portions of the bulbar ridge. Note the anlage of the semilunar valves (arrow) on the pulmonary side; × 123.

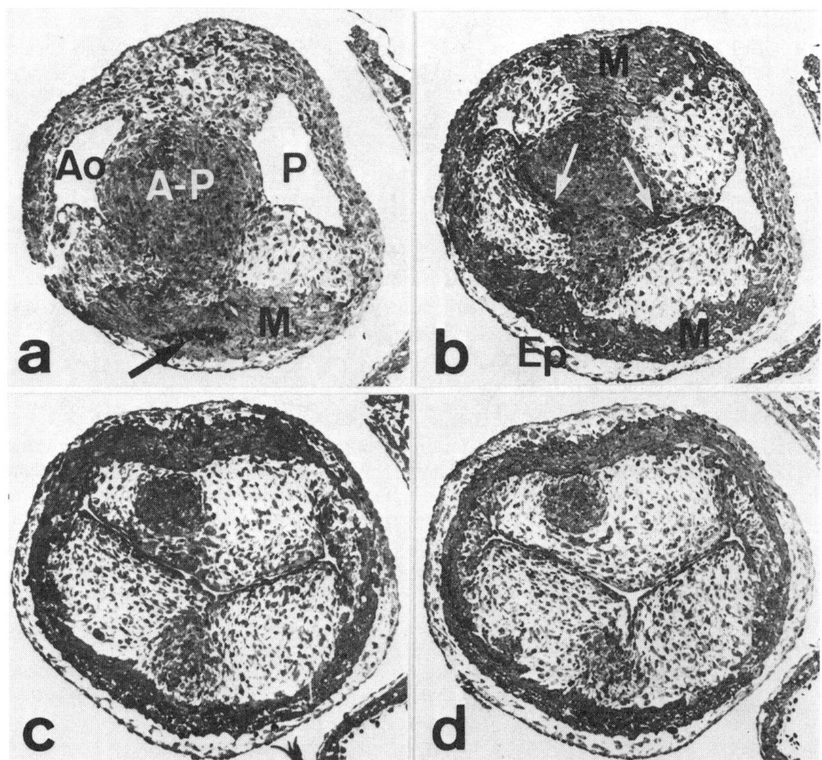

FIGURE 4. Light micrographs from selected transverse semithin sections of a 5-day-old chicken embryo. This craniocaudal sequence illustrates the development of the aorticopulmonary (A-P) septum. In **a,** fusion has been completed. A tongue of myocardium (M) is observed on the left posterior side of the truncus. An area of death (arrows) appears in the myocardium. In **b,** the truncal cushions are apposed to each other, and the two prongs of the A-P septum are becoming continuous. The limits of the still unfused endocardium are indicated (arrows). Note the irregular margins of the myocardium (M) and epicardium (Ep). In **c,** the two A-P prongs appear subjacent to the myocardium. Mesenchymal cells located between the prongs and the endocardium change their appearance; they appear to be recruited to participate in truncal septation (compare with **b**). In **d,** at the valve level, the left-sided prong becomes disorganized. Then cell death appears in the mesenchymal tissue; × 33.

myocardium recedes or disappears from the same plane as the advancing septum. Contrary to what has previously been asserted, however, the myocardium and the A-P septum can be found at the same histologic level. During the fifth day of incubation, the two structures are seen together along a short segment. During the sixth day of incubation, a tongue of myocardial tissue can still be observed on the dorsal aspect of the two main vessels, up to the original bifurcation of the pulmonary artery (FIG. 6). The shortness of this segment, together with the uneven disappearance of the myocardium, may be the reason why this fact has been disregarded or misinterpreted previously (and I include myself).

Another fact that has not been emphasized is the existence of clear differences between the two prongs. The right-sided prong is more rounded and presents clearer limits than the left-sided one. Furthermore, only the right-sided prong is distinctly observed below the semilunar valve level.[13] The left-sided prong appears to disintegrate around and below the bifurcation cleft between the developing semilunar valves. It is curious that intense cell death occurs in the cushion mesenchyme below this level. Cell death cannot be observed, however, in the mesenchyme near the right-sided prong. Although the presence of cell death in the cushion mesenchyme has not previously been related to the presence or absence of the A-P prongs, differences similar to the ones observed here have also been shown to occur in mice[14] and humans.[15] It could be suggested that the left-sided prong becomes disorganized below the valve level and that the cells that form it are destined to die. Many (or all) of these cells are of neural crest origin.[12] In fact, death may be the ultimate fate of many of the cardiac neural crest cells. Cell death also occurs in the A-P septum and the surrounding mesenchyme (FIG. 6) after the establishment of the arterial lumens,[16,17] and after valve formation.[15,17,18]

The direction followed by the A-P septum accounts for much of the spiraling trajectory of the aorta and the pulmonary artery. The contribution to this trajectory in the chick, however, appears to be different from that in the mouse. The twisting of the two arteries around each other is more intense in the mouse than in the chick. Also, the spiraling of the bulbar cushions in the chick appears to be more intense than in the mouse.

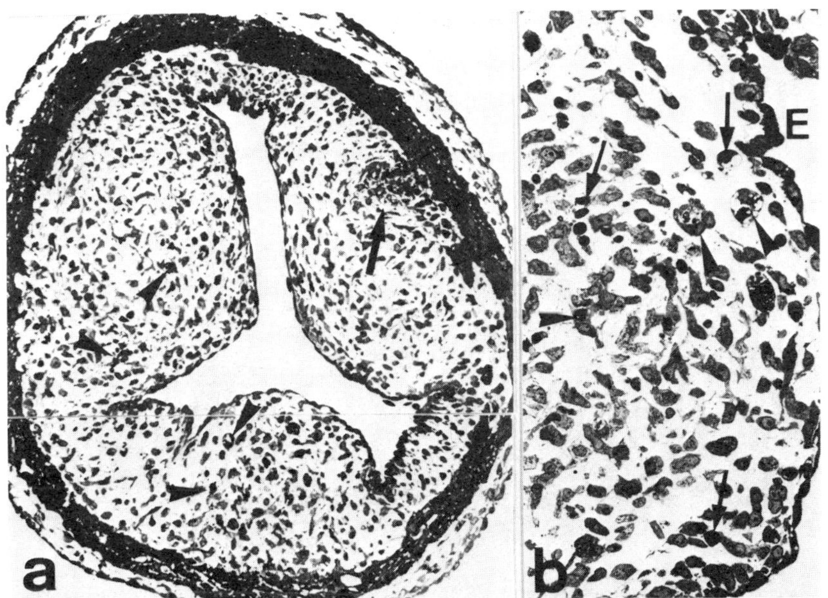

FIGURE 5. Light micrographs from the same chick embryo as that shown in FIG. 4. **a:** Below the valve level only the right-sided prong (arrow) is visible. Intense cell death can be observed in the cushion mesenchyme, except around the remaining prong. Cell debris and phagocytes are indicated (arrowheads); × 81. **b:** This micrograph shows a detailed view of a consecutive section of the cushion area located at the bottom of **a**. Note the conspicuous presence of cell debris (arrows) and phagocytes (arrowheads). E, endocardial lumen. × 121.

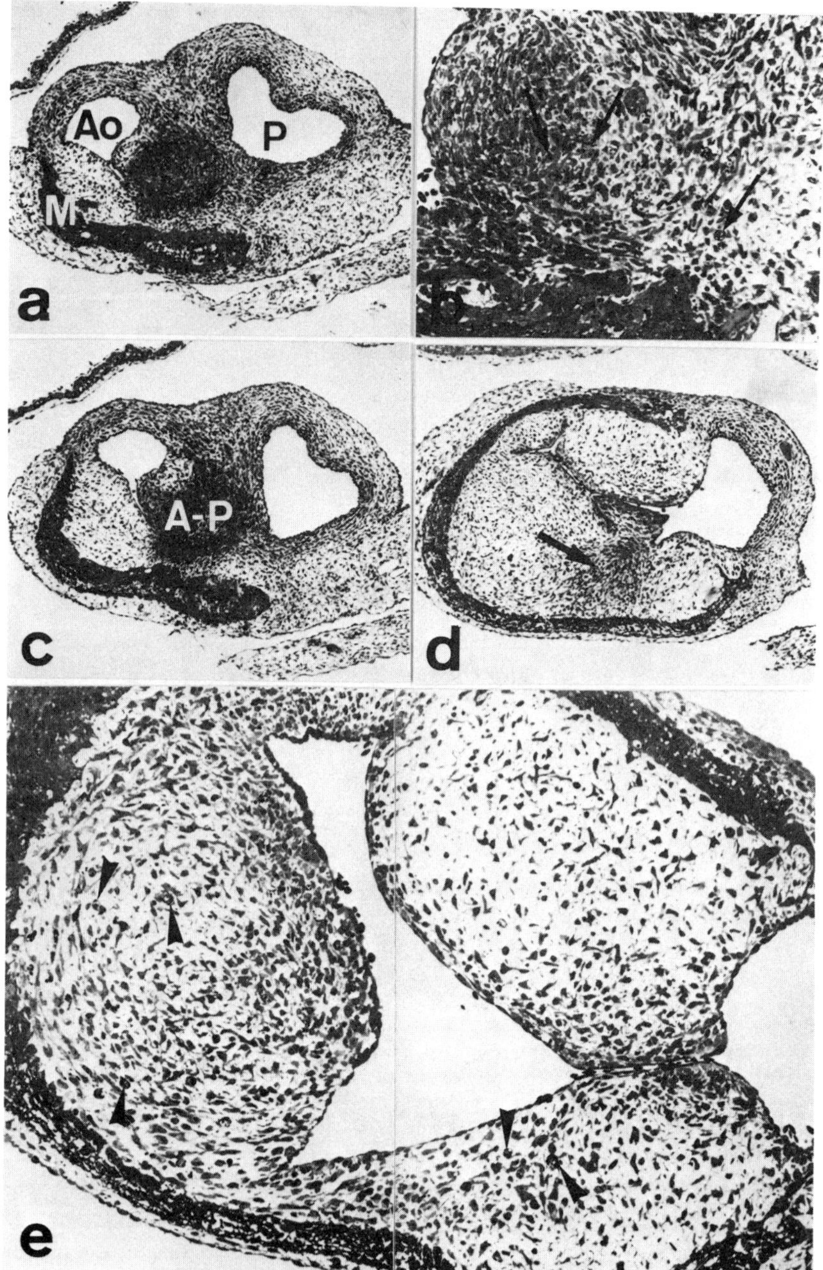

FIGURE 6. Light micrographs from selected transverse semithin sections of a 6-day-old chicken embryo. Craniocaudal sequence. **a:** The aorticopulmonary septum is observed between the aorta (Ao) and the primitive division of the pulmonary artery (P). Note the presence of a tongue of myocardial tissue (M). Whereas the pulmonary side shows the tissues with an arterial structure,

It is possible that some of the differences in the development of truncal septation reported in the literature may be species-related. For example, the A-P prongs in the chick appear to be more conspicuous than in mice and humans. Also, cell death occurs in the chick myocardium but not in mice.[14]

While these changes are taking place, some mesenchymal cells begin to organize around the two emerging vessels to form the arterial tunica media.[13,19,20] Normal development of the A-P septum and of the tunica media of the great arteries involves extensive cell rearrangement and the establishment of appropriate relationships between cells and their extracellular microenvironment. These relationships have been attracting a great deal of interest. Condensed cells in the A-P septum are intensely fluorescent for fibronectin (FN).[13] This makes them easily distinguishable from the surrounding mesenchyme.[13,21] These cells are also positive for desmin,[22] for elastin precursors,[23] and for F-actin.[24] While FN may be primarily involved in cell movement and rearrangement, the later characteristics suggest that A-P cells are precursor muscle cells. Staining for FN, desmin, and elastin precursors, however, declines rapidly in the A-P septum after fusion of the A-P prongs and division of the truncal lumen. Thus, the relationship between A-P cells and those involved in tunica media formation are unclear.

The differences in the reactivity for desmin between A-P cells and tunica media cells have been interpreted as indicating that the two systems have different origins.[22] The decline in the staining for elastin precursors in the A-P septum would appear to sustain this suggestion. Furthermore, reactivity for elastin precursors is very intense only around the definitive aortic and pulmonary lumens.[23] It may be erroneous, however, to interpret the above facts as indicative of different origin. Instead, they could indicate that most cells are primarily ectomesenchyme, but that they follow divergent paths. Cells in the A-P septum may be precursor muscle cells but with low levels of phenotypic expression. It has been suggested that these cells are relatively undifferentiated.[25] The lack of reactivity of these cells at later stages may only indicate loss of their differentiative ability and their transformation into loose undifferentiated mesenchyme. This loose mesenchyme will probably form the arterial adventitia. The ultimate fate of the A-P cells, however, is unclear as yet. Whereas some appear to die (see above), others could be incorporated into the developing tunica media to become overt smooth muscle. If so, they would be indistinguishable from the original muscle cells. Intermingling of A-P cells and of tunica media cells can be observed at many points (FIG. 6).

The relationships established between the cells involved in septation of the truncus and the surrounding extracellular matrix are also unclear. A-P cells invade the truncus where they are surrounded by a matrix rich in type-I collagen and glycosaminoglycan aggregates. These cells, however, selectively exclude most of the alcian blue stain.[14] Similarly, the extracellular matrix that surrounds the cells involved in formation of

---

the aortic side presents a myocardium-cushion tissue structure; × 20. **b:** A detailed view of a similar level to that shown in **a**. Cell death (arrows) appears in the A-P septum and in the surrounding mesenchyme; × 50. **c:** This section at a lower level shows the same differences in structure as those observed in **a**. Note, on the aortic side, the structural continuity of the developing tunica media with the myocardium and with the A-P septum. Also note in **a** and **c** that the laminarity typical of tunica media starts to develop far from the arterial endothelium; × 20. **d:** At a lower level, the right-sided prong (arrow) becomes disorganized. The differences in structure between the aortic and pulmonic side persist; × 20. **e:** Cell death (arrowheads) appears in the cushion areas where the remaining A-P prong has become disorganized. Note the absence of cell death in the opposite cushion area; × 49.

the tunica media is rich in FN[13] and type-I collagen,[19] but it also excludes proteoglycan aggregates.[19] It is only later, when definitive muscle cells begin to organize around the emerging arterial lumens, that the amount of FN diminishes and the fibrils associated with elastogenesis appear.[26] It is also at this time that the staining for elastin precursors becomes very intense.[23] It has been suggested that FN may interact with the collagen microfibrils in order for the cells to acquire the laminarity typical of tunica media.[13] The decrease in the amount of FN has been related to the acquisition by these cells of a mature phenotype. A-P cells, as well as tunica media cells, also express specific fucosylated glycoconjugates,[27] but the significance of this fact is unknown as yet.

FORMATION OF THE AORTIC VESTIBULUM

After completion of aorticopulmonary septation, the conal ridges fuse caudally forming a septum that is continuous with the A-P septum. Thus, after the truncus has been divided into the proximal parts of the aorta and the pulmonary artery, the conus is separated into an aortic and a pulmonic channel (FIGURES 7, 8). The inferior orifice of the dividing conus resembles a double-barreled tunnel that opens ventrally to the atrioventricular canal and to the right of the developing interventricular septum (FIG. 7). Then, enlargement to the right of the atrioventricular canal, together with recession of the bulboventricular edge, brings the aortic conus above the interventricular foramen. With further development the right side of the conus septum becomes continuous with the anterior border of the interventricular septum; at the same time, its left side becomes continuous with the right margin of the atrioventricular canal (FIGURES 7, 8). Thus, the aorta gains independent access to the left ventricle. Definitive closure of the aortic vestibulum takes place by growing and blending of tissue derived from nearby mesenchyme (the atrioventricular cushion septum, the conal septum, and the interventricular septum).[1–5,8–10]

GENERAL DISCUSSION

The developmental features described here will probably be accepted, at least at the morphologic level, by most authors. It is the interpretation of these events, however, that has led to a great deal of controversy. There are currently two main ways of looking at outflow tract development. The first is similar to the one described here. Basically, it assumes that truncoconal septation takes place by fusion of two spiraling ridges, with longitudinal growth but little or no rotatory displacement. The transformation of the truncus into the proximal part of the aorta and the pulmonary artery would occur through disintegration of the myocardium,[7] cell death,[28] or dedifferentiation.[29] Some of these processes are not mutually exclusive. The temporospatial changes that occur in the different structures may be the result of differential growth and tissue remodeling. The second theory interprets those temporospatial changes as the result of rotation of truncal structures and absorption (or uneven growth) of part of the conus. In this way, proper connections would be established between the two ventricles and the two main vessels. Recently, the existence of a structural complex

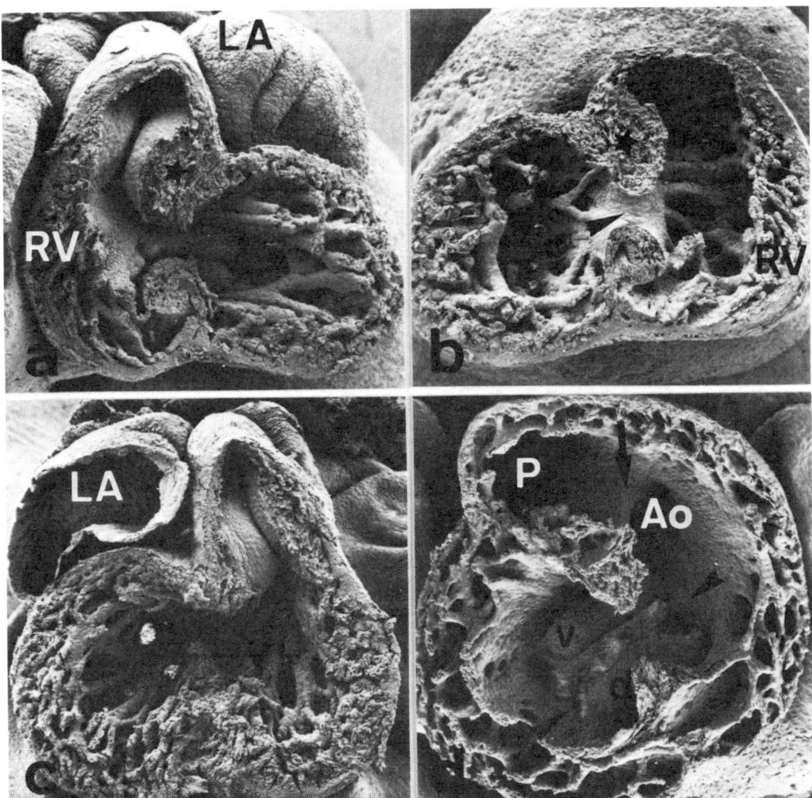

FIGURE 7. SEM illustrating several aspects of truncoconal septation in the *iv* mouse. **a** and **b** show the two halves of the same heart, 12.5 days; situs solitus, frontal dissection. **a**, dorsal side; **b**, ventral side. In **a**, the conal ridges are still unfused. The inferior border of the left ridge (sinistroventral conal cushion) is continuous with the anterior horn of the interventricular septum (stars in **a** and **b**). The conus opens to the right of the atrioventricular canal; LA, left atrium. The interventricular septum grows toward the right side of the atrioventricular canal. The free border of the interventricular septum is indicated (arrowhead) in **b**; × 100. **c:** This micrograph shows a similar stage of development as that shown in **a**, situs inversus, 12.5 days. The LA is right-sided; compare with a; × 86. **d:** Transversal section of an *iv* mouse heart at 13.5 days, situs inversus. The conus has been divided. Ao and P represent the aortic and pulmonic conus. The inferior border of the conus septum (arrow) is continuous with the anterior border of the interventricular septum. The anterior and posterior horns of the developing interventricular septum can be observed in the center of the picture. The atrioventricular canal is bordered by the ventral (v) and dorsal (d) endocardial cushions and by the lateral cushions (arrowheads); × 98.

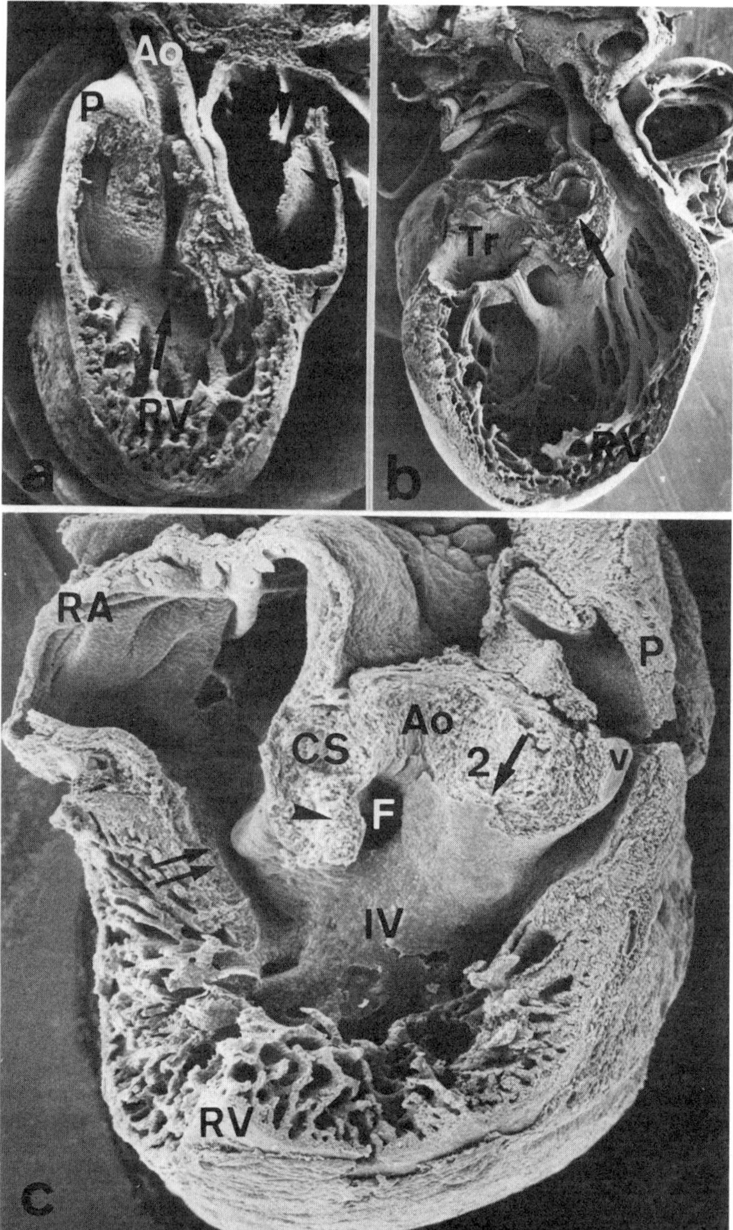

FIGURE 8. SEM illustrating several aspects of the closure of the aortic vestibulum. **a:** *iv* mouse, situs inversus, 12.5 days. The heart has been opened through the (left-sided) right ventricle (RV), right side of the specimen. The conal cushions are in the process of fusion; the zone of blending is exposed. Note the development of the semilunar valves in the longitudinally dissected aorta (Ao). P, pulmonary artery. The free border of the interventricular septum and the inter-

formed of the truncal myocardium, the condensed mesenchyme of the A-P septum, and the bifurcation of the vascular lumen[18,20] has been described. This septation complex would work as a single, structural unit that retracts toward the ventricles at the same time that it rotates about the long axis of the truncus to accommodate the spiraling arteries of the two ventricles. The different parts of the septation complex would move in tandem to anchor the developing semilunar valves to the ventricles.

I must stress at this point that there is no real and incontrovertible evidence to definitively support either of the two viewpoints. Indeed, the same schematic representation of the different structures involved in truncal septation can be used alternatively to illustrate either one of the two models.[30] It is not my intention at this time to propose a third perspective. Let us simply discuss the evidence reported so far.

As for the first model, it is very easy to understand. It relies, however, almost completely on descriptive studies, and the cellular mechanisms underlying the events related above are yet to be clarified.[30] Although some experimental evidence would appear to confirm this interpretation,[31,32] terms like differential growth and tissue remodeling are quite ambiguous and seem more indicative of what is unknown than of what we really understand.

The second model involves gross tissue movement during the preseptation and septation stages. Whether and how these tissue movements really occur, however, is still a matter of discussion. Several types of marking techniques have been devised to evidence tissue displacements: carbon particles,[31,32] electrocautery wounds,[33] and radiolabeled tattoos[34] have been employed. Some of these markers have demonstrated movements along the longitudinal axis of the truncus;[31,32] others have shown only rotation,[33] or both.[34] Thus, even from an experimental vantage point, there is not consensus on the exact nature of these displacements. Furthermore, marking experiments present specific problems depending upon the type of marking used, as well as the general problems inherent in tissue manipulation. All these problems have recently been reviewed.[34]

Let us admit that active truncal rotation does exist. Rotation is just a mechanical phenomenon evidenced by spatial changes (absolute or relative) between different parts of the heart. The question, then, is, What are the mechanisms underlying rotation?

---

ventricular foramen are indicated (big arrow). Two valve leaflets (arrowheads) guard the opening of the superior vena cava into the right atrium. Coronary vessels in the atrioventricular sulcus are indicated (small arrow); × 62. **b:** *iv* mouse, situs solitus, 18.5 days of incubation. The heart has been dissected through the pulmonary artery (P), the right ventricle (RV), and the right atrioventricular orifice. The tricuspid valve (Tr) with its valve leaflets and associated chordae tendinae has been exposed. The base of the aorta with its sigmoid valves is indicated (arrow). The aorta has been transferred to the left ventricle, and no communication between the two ventricles remains; × 46. **c:** Chicken embryo, 5.5 days of incubation. The heart has been dissected through the pulmonary artery (P), the right ventricle (RV), the right atrioventricular orifice (double arrow), and the right atrium (RA). This stage of development is intermediate between **a** and **b**, but closer to **a**. In front of the interventricular foramen (F) the fusion of the conal ridges is taking place, but the inferior part of the sinistroventral conal ridge (2) is still unfused. The dextrodorsal conal ridge (left out of the dissection) blends with the cushion septum (CS). The line of fracture passes through the zone of blending (arrowhead). The continued fusion of the conal ridges in a downward direction (arrow) together with the growth of the right side of the cushion septum along the top of the interventricular foramen (direction of growth marked by arrowhead) isolate the ventricular foramen from the right ventricle. Then, the interventricular foramen becomes part of the aortic vestibulum. Ao indicates the position of the aortic outflow tract (most of it has been removed). v, semilunar valve cushions; × 55. (8c from J. M. Icardo.[1] With permission from Raven Press.)

That is, what are the cellular and subcellular activities that produce the mechanical tension necessary to induce rotatory displacements? This question has been avoided in the past. Only recently has a search for these mechanisms been undertaken. The elongation of cells along the A-P prongs and the deformation of the myocardial rim has been taken as indicative of the existence of tensile patterns along the truncus. Differences in the rate of growth between adjacent tissues could originate this tension.[34,35] Furthermore, it has been suggested that there is some kind of kinetic relationship between the truncal myocardium and the A-P prongs.[18,25] The existence of aldehyde-rich fibers, radially oriented between the myocardium and the A-P prongs,[23] may serve to anchor the mesenchymal condensations to the myocardium. The presence of aligned bundles of microfilaments within the A-P cells[18] may indeed reflect the existence of tensile stress in the truncus. It is difficult, however, to see how these fibrillar systems could drive complex tissue displacements. On the other hand, oriented systems of extracellular fibers, extending between the epithelium and the condensed mesenchyme, have also been demonstrated during the development of organs that do not undergo torsion.[36,37]

Although doubts remain as to whether the truncus undergoes torsion, there are still some other points that deserve comment. The exact role played by the A-P prongs during truncal septation remains obscure. The prongs could align the truncal cushions, guiding the process of fusion. The relationships established between the cells of the A-P prongs and the rest of the cushion mesenchyme are unclear at this time. Some of the mesenchymal cells located between the A-P prongs and the endocardial cushion appear to be recruited to participate in truncal septation. The size of the A-P septum during the process of fusion appears to be larger than what would result from the mere fusion of the two prongs. Also, cells that appear to be transitional are observed around the A-P prongs along the truncus. This could be interpreted as indicative of either mesenchymal recruitment or of loosening of cells from the prongs and subsequent cell seeding. If the latter is true, the role of these cells remains to be investigated. The use of neural crest cell markers may help us to clarify some of these issues. It has been stated above that many of the cardiac neural crest cells are destined to die. In light of the present observations, this seems to be quite a logical assumption. The opposite explanation, however, is also plausible. That is, these cells may play a regulatory role in cushion cell population, retarding or controlling the appearance of cell death. Removal of the neural crest has been shown to delay the disappearance of arch arteries one and two.[38] Clearly, further investigation and concept reappraisal are needed to fully understand the development of this complex region of the heart.

ACKNOWLEDGMENTS

The author wishes to thank Dr. William Layton, Dartmouth Medical School, Hanover, New Hampshire, for the kind gift of the *iv/iv* mice. Thanks are also due to M.-J. Sanchez for her invaluable help with the mouse colony.

REFERENCES

1. ICARDO, J. M. 1984. *In* Growth of the Heart in Health and Disease. R. Zak, Ed.: 41–80. Raven Press, Inc. New York.

2. MANASEK, F. J., J. M. ICARDO, A. NAKAMURA & L. J. SWEENEY. 1986. *In* The Heart and Cardiovascular System. H. A. Fozzard, E. Haber, R. B. Jennings, A. M. Katz & H. E. Morgan, Eds.: 965-986. Raven Press, Inc. New York.

3. DE VRIES, P. A. & J. B. DE C. M. SAUNDERS. 1962. Carnegie Inst. Washington Contrib. Embryol. **37:** 87-114.

4. VAN MIEROP, L. H. S., R. D. ALLEY, H. W. KAUSEL & A. STRANAHAN. 1963. J. Thorac. Cardiovasc. Surg. **43:** 71-83.

5. LAYTON, W. M., JR. 1978. *In* Morphogenesis and Malformations of the Cardiovascular System. G. C. Rosenquist & D. Bergsma, Eds.: 277-293. Alan R Liss. New York.

6. LAYTON, W. M., JR. & F. J. MANASEK. 1980. *In* Etiology and Morphogenesis of Congenital Heart Disease. R. van Praagh & A. Takao, Eds.: 109-126. Futura Publishing Co. Mt. Kisco, New York.

7. KRAMER, T. C. 1942. Am. J. Anat. **71:** 343-370.

8. VAN MIEROP, L. H. S. & F. H. NETTER. 1962. *In* CIBA Journal, Vol. 5, The Heart. F. H. Netter, Ed.: 112-126. Ciba. Summit, NJ.

9. PEXIEDER, T. 1978. *In* Morphogenesis and Malformations of the Cardiovascular System. G. C. Rosenquist & D. Bergsma, Eds.: 29-68. Alan R Liss, Inc. New York.

10. STEDING, G. & E. SEIDL. 1980. J. Thorac. Cardiovasc. Surg. **28:** 386-409.

11. PHILLIPS, M. T., M. L. KIRBY & G. FORBES. 1987. Circ. Res. **60:** 27-30.

12. KIRBY, M. L., T. F. GALE & D. STEWART. 1983. Science **220:** 1059-1061.

13. ICARDO, J. M. 1985. Anat. Embryol. **171:** 193-200.

14. BLANCO, M., E. COLVEE & J. M. HURLE. 1981. An. Desarrollo **25-27:** 51-57.

15. OKAMOTO, N., N. AKIMOTO, Y. SATOW, N. HIDAKA & S. MIYABARA. 1981. *In* Mechanisms of Cardiac Morphogenesis and Teratogenesis. T. Pexieder, Ed.: 127-137. Raven Press, Inc. New York.

16. MENKES, B., C. ALEXANDRU, A. PAVKOV & O. MIRKOV 1965. Rev. Roum. Embryol. Cytol. Ser. Embryol. **2:** 79-91.

17. PEXIEDER, T. 1975. Adv. Anat. Embryol. Cell Biol. **51:** 1-100.

18. THOMPSON, R. P., H. SUMIDA, V. ABERCROMBIE, Y. SATOW, T. P. FITZHARRIS & N. OKAMOTO. 1985. Anat. Rec. **213:** 578-586.

19. FITZHARRIS, T. P., R. P. THOMPSON & R. R. MARKWALD. 1979. Tex. Rep. Biol. Med. **39:** 287-304.

20. THOMPSON, R. P. & T. P. FITZHARRIS. 1979. Am. J. Anat. **156:** 251-264.

21. ICARDO, J. M. & F. J. MANASEK. 1984. Dev. Biol. **101:** 336-345.

22. SUMIDA, H., H. NAKAMURA, N. AKIMOTO, N. OKAMOTO & Y. SATOW. 1987. Arch. Histol. Jpn. **50:** 525-531.

23. ROSENQUIST, T. H., J. R. McCOY, K. L. WALDO & M. L. KIRBY. 1988. Anat. Rec. **221:** 860-871.

24. SUMIDA, H., R. A. ASHCRAFT, JR. & R. P. THOMPSON. 1989. Anat. Rec. **223:** 82-89.

25. THOMPSON, R. P. & T. P. FITZHARRIS. 1979. Am. J. Anat. **154:** 545-556.

26. KADAR, A., D. L. GARDNER & V. BUSH. 1972. J. Pathol. **108:** 275-280.

27. FAZEL, A. R., H. SUMIDA, B. A. SCHULTE & R. P. THOMPSON. 1989. Am. J. Anat. **184:** 76-84.

28. HURLE, J. M., M. LAFARGA & J. L. OJEDA. 1977. J. Embryol. Exp. Morphol. **41:** 161-170.

29. ARGUELLO, C., M. V. DE LA CRUZ & C. SANCHEZ. 1978. J. Mol. Cell. Cardiol. **10:** 307-315.

30. THOMPSON, R. P. & T. P. FITZHARRIS. 1985. *In* Cardiac Morphogenesis. V. J. Ferrans, G. C. Rosenquist & C. Weinstein, Eds.: 169-180. Elsevier. New York.

31. DE LA CRUZ, M. V., C. SANCHEZ, M. M. ARTEAGA & C. ARGUELLO. 1977. J. Anat. **123:** 661-686.

32. RYCHTER, Z. 1978. *In* Morphogenesis and Malformations of the Cardiovascular System. G. C. Rosenquist & D. Bergsma, Eds.: 443-448. Alan R Liss, Inc. New York.

33. DOR, X. & P. CORONE. 1983. Arch. Mal. Coeur Vaiss. **5:** 513-523.

34. THOMPSON, R. P., V. ABERCROMBIE & M. WONG. 1987. Anat. Rec. **218:** 434-440.

35. VAN PRAAGH, R., W. L. LAYTON & S. VAN PRAAGH. 1980. *In* Etiology and Morphogenesis of Congenital Heart Disease. R. Van Praagh & A. Takao, Ed.: 271-316. Futura Publishing Co. Mt. Kisco, New York.

36. HAAKE, A. R. & R. SAWYER. 1982. J. Exp. Zool. **221:** 119-123.
37. HURLE, J. M., J. R. HINCHLIFFE, M. A. ROS & J. M. GENIS-GALVEZ. 1989. Development **27:** 103-120.
38. BOCKMAN, D. E., M. E. REDMOND, K. WALDO, H. DAVIS & M. L. KIRBY. 1987. Am. J. Anat. **180:** 332-341.

Hemodynamics of the Developing Cardiovascular System

EDWARD B. CLARK AND NORMAN HU

The Cook Research Laboratory
Division of Pediatric Cardiology
Department of Pediatrics
University of Rochester School of Medicine and Dentistry
Rochester, New York 14642

The development of the heart represents an intriguing, yet poorly understood inter-relationship of function and form. Early in development, the heart is a pulsatile muscle-wrapped tube that transforms through morphogenesis into a four-chambered, four-valved pump with separate systemic and pulmonary circulations. The cellular processes involved in morphogenesis are an intriguing aspect of cardiac development. The eventual shape and function of the heart is a complex interrelationship of genetics and epigenetics. The biochemical forces generated by the embryonic heart participate in the ultimate shape through modulation of the developmental process.

Our research team has spent the last decade studying the interrelationship of function and form in cardiac development. This chapter summarizes our extensive studies of normal hemodynamic function and new work that links work load and heart growth. We have chosen the chick embryo model for several reasons. First, this is a widely accepted model of vertebrate heart development. Second, many laboratories are studying cellular and molecular biology of normal cardiac development. Third, the access to the chick embryo, although complicated, is not as difficult as a mammalian model.

Accurate physiologic measurement required the adaptation of a variety of techniques to measure pressure and flow in the embryonic heart. We measured blood flow with a 20 MHz pulse Doppler velocity system and piezoelectric crystals between 0.5 and 0.75 mm in diameter.[1] Pressure measurements were made with a servo-null micropressure system from 5 micron diameter probes inserted into the various portions of the cardiovascular system.[1] These techniques have been detailed in our previous publications and are now used by other laboratories in their own studies of cardiovascular development.[2,3]

The period of initial heart formation is characterized by morphogenesis of the heart and by rapid growth of the embryo and the extraembryonic vascular bed. The primary function of the cardiovascular system is to meet the metabolic demands of the body, delivering nutrients and removing metabolic waste products from areas of rapid growth. Remarkably, the heart continues these roles during the process of heart formation and adaptation of marked hemodynamic demands.

Growth of the embryo and the extraembryonic bed is extremely rapid. From stage 12 to 29,[4] there is nearly a 120-fold increase in embryo mass (FIG. 1). During this time, the extraembryonic vascular bed responsible for gas exchange and nutrient delivered from the yolk sac increases only 30-fold. The relative weight of the ventricle

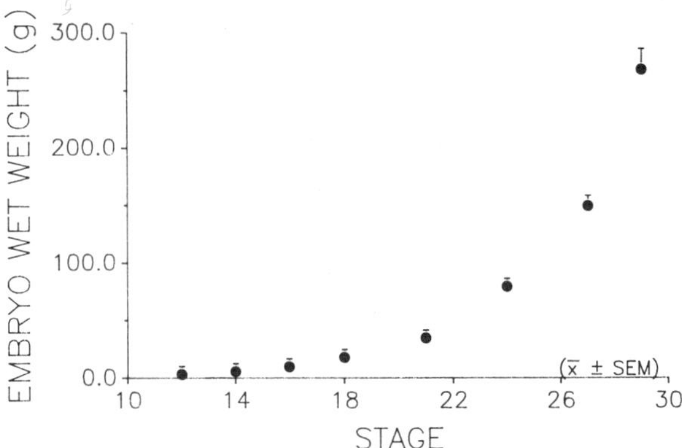

FIGURE 1. Embryo wet weight of chick embryos from stages 12, 14, 16, 18, 21, 24, 27, and 29, with an approximate twofold increase between the mentioned stages (N ≥ 25 at each stage).

actually decreases during this time (FIG. 2). At stage 12 the ventricle accounts for 4.5 percent of the total embryo weight. By stage 29 it is only 1 percent. The change in relative weight suggests an increase in effectiveness of the embryonic cardiovascular system, a suggestion that is supported by hemodynamic studies.

Heart rate in the embryo gradually increases with development. In mature animals, there is a reciprocal relationship among animal size, body size, and heart rate. In the embryo, the heart begins at a baseline rate of 100 beats per minute and rises gradually during these developmental stages to more than 200 beats per minute (FIG. 3). This poorly understood paradox may be dependent on coupling between the ventricle and vascular bed.[5] Heart rate markedly alters the filling characteristics of the embryonic heart. As heart rate increases, diastolic time decreases while the systolic ejection time remains relatively constant.[5]

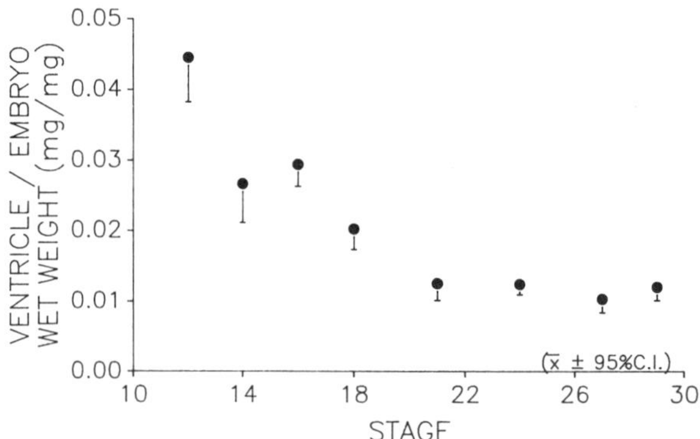

FIGURE 2. Ratio of ventricular wet weight normalized with embryo wet weight (N ≥ 9 at each stage).

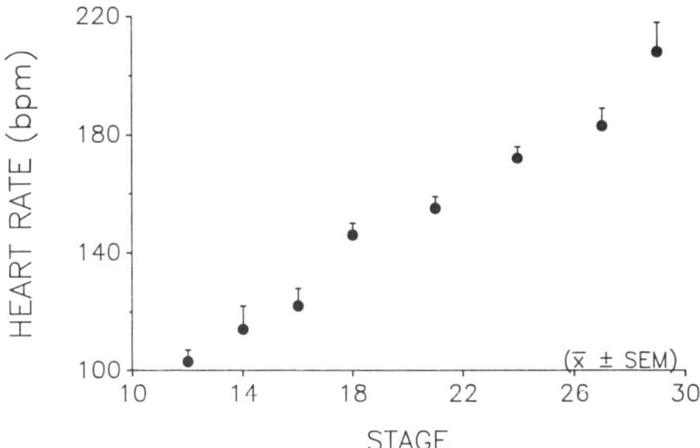

FIGURE 3. Linear increase of heart rate of chick embryos in stages 12 to 29 (N ≥ 20 at each stage).

Accompanying development is a proportional increase in stroke volume (FIG. 4). Hypothermia is the environmental risk factor for the developing heart. With a wide range of temperature-induced heart rate, stroke volume remains constant.[6,7] Thus, regulation of heart rate is one mechanism for the control of the preinnervated cardiovascular system.

We found that cardiac output-measured mean dorsal aortic blood flow matches embryonic growth (FIG. 5). Across the 120-fold change in embryo weight, blood flow per milligram embryo weight remains constant when related to total embryo weight and decreases when compared to the embryo and the extraembryonic vascular bed (FIG. 6). A yet undefined mechanism matches metabolic demands and blood flow. Circulation is driven by the pressure differences across a vascular bed. The first pulsations appear before the establishment of blood flow. Thus, ventricular pressure precedes flow.

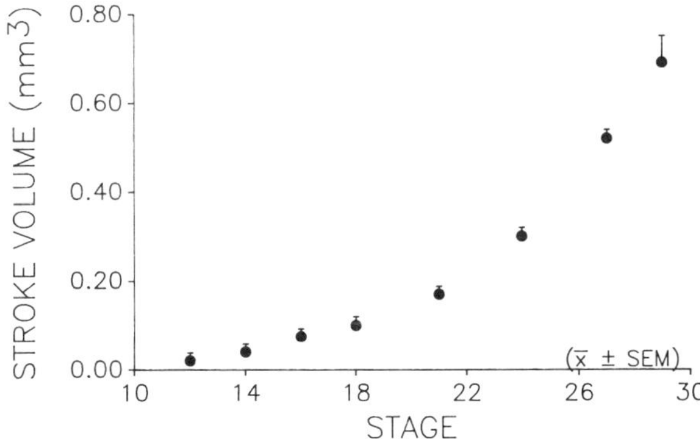

FIGURE 4. Quotient of stroke volume index derived from mean dorsal aortic blood flow and heart rate (N ≥ 20 at each stage).

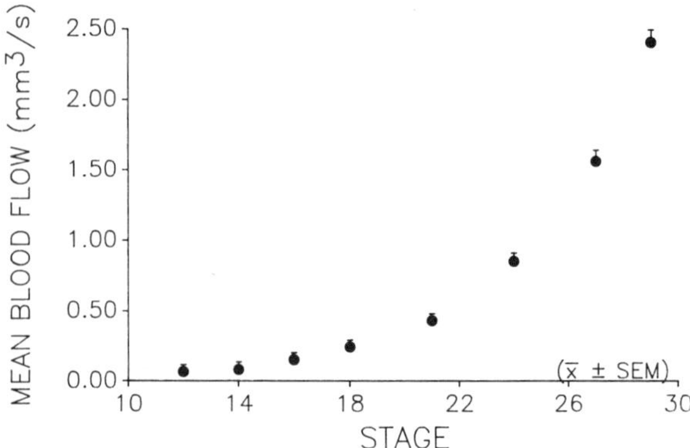

FIGURE 5. Mean dorsal aortic blood flow of chick embryos in stages 12 to 29 (N $\geq$ 20 at each stage).

The wave forms of the pressure curves in the embryo are similar to those of mature animals. In the ventricle, the diastole has a passive and active filling phase, the latter reflected in atrial systole. There is an early pressure rise, plateau pressure, and a late systolic pressure decrease. Peak systolic pressure increases gradually across the stage range in the ventricle. There is a pressure gradient between ventricular and vitelline artery pressure. Part of this pressure drop is across the aortic arches and is likely a mechanism for aortic arch selection.[8]

Ventricular end-diastolic pressure increases gradually. Even at early stages, vitelline arterial diastolic pressure and ventricular end-diastolic pressure are different, indicating valve-like function of the conotruncal cushions.[9] The pre-ejection measure of ventricular function, dP/dt, gradually increases (FIG. 7).

Reciprocal changes in vascular resistance and cardiac work accompany the dramatic changes in vascular pressure and cardiac output. At the early stages, the vascular resistance is extremely high and decreases rapidly with the expansion of the vascular

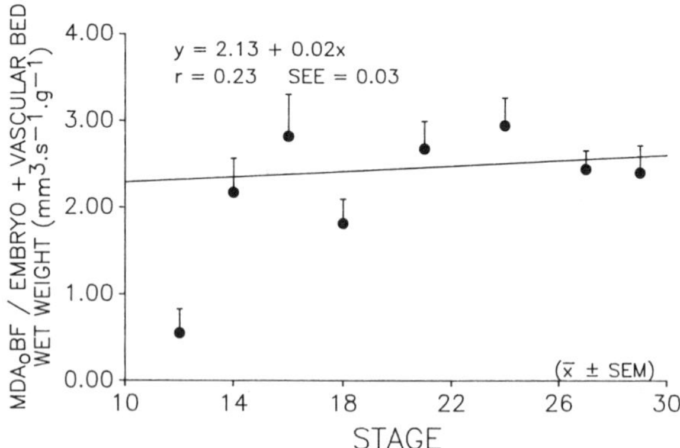

FIGURE 6. Mean dorsal aortic blood flow normalized with embryo and extraembryonic vascular bed wet weight across stages (N $\geq$ 16 at each stage).

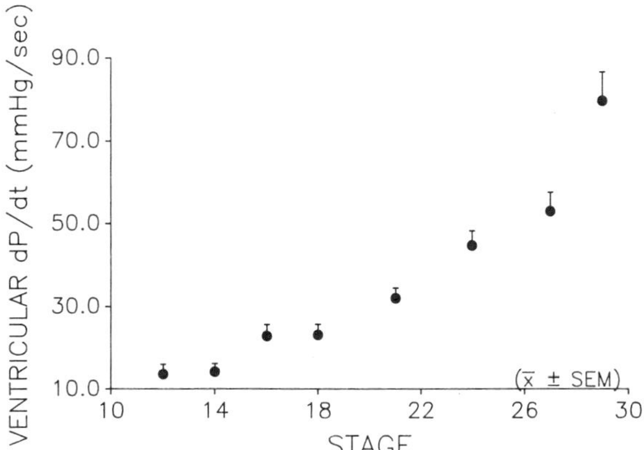

FIGURE 7. Ventricular dP/dt derived from electrically integrated ventricular pressure (N ≥ 19 at each stage).

bed (FIG. 8). The vitelline vascular bed is the sole contributing vascular bed with most embryonic vascular bed being accounted for by the large veins and arteries. With rapid embryo growth, the vitelline membrane vascular bed expands and the chorioallantoic membrane vascular bed develops. The addition of new resistance units is one factor accounting for the geometric decrease in vascular resistance.

There are other factors that influence the afterload to the embryonic system. One is the dynamic characteristic of the vascular bed. Our studies of dorsal aortic impedance show that in addition to the zero of the modulus and steady state resistance, there are parallel changes in the first-, second-, and third-order moduli, indicating changes in wave reflection and compliance of vessel walls down stream from the dorsal aorta.[10]

The steady state of cardiac work increases nearly 350-fold. With the change in cardiac work, there is a marked increase in the amount of energy required for pulsatile flow. At stage 18, about one-third of total energy is expended in pulsatile flow. By stage 29, nearly two-thirds of the energy is required for pulsatile flow (FIG. 9).

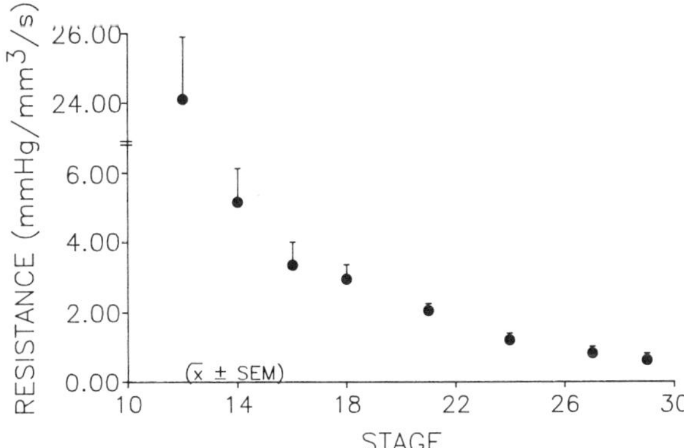

FIGURE 8. Peripherial vascular resistance computed from the ratio of stroke volume and vitelline artery pressure (N ≥ 19 at each stage).

Changes in the cardiovascular function and ventricular growth are integrated. We found that ventricular pressure is directly related to the mass of the heart. Following banding of the outflow tract, ventricular pressure increased with the rate of growth of the ventricle (FIG. 10). While ventricular mass increased, there were no changes in morphogenesis. The morphologic features of the ventricle are similar to the degree of atrioventricular septation and ventricular septal formation in control and experimental embryos.[11]

We found a similar relationship with a decrease in ventricular pressure and a slowing of the rate of ventricular growth. We have, however, not yet evaluated the effects on the extraembryonic vascular bed, that is, structural or steady state and dynamic characteristics.

From these studies of hemodynamic function, embryo growth, and ventricular morphogenesis, we are developing a hypothesis that leads to the complex interrelationship of function and form during development. These studies would suggest that morphogenesis has a primary genetic determination, but growth including the laying down of the ventricular mass, is related to epigenetic factors.

A fundamental characteristic of the mature heart is the adjustment of myocardial mass to meet functional loan. This ability is likely expressed early in development and is a fundamental mechanism to match embryo growth and heart development. These observations shed new light on the dynamics of heart development and have implications for investigators studying cell biology and molecular expression on control of the cardiovascular system. Defining the mechanisms of normal cardiovascular development is an integral step in understanding abnormalities of cardiovascular morphogenesis. It is not simply enough to know the gene, but one must also understand the mechanism of the expression of genetic information in the progression from protein strands to the complex three-dimensional shape of the heart.

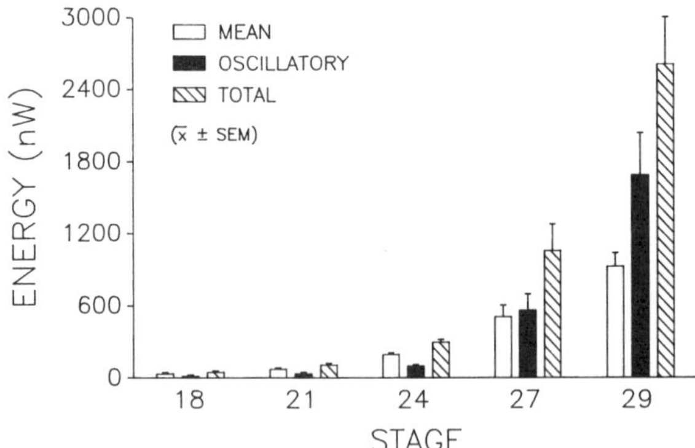

FIGURE 9. Mean, oscillatory, total energy across chick embryos in stages 18 to 29 (N ≥ 6 at each stage).

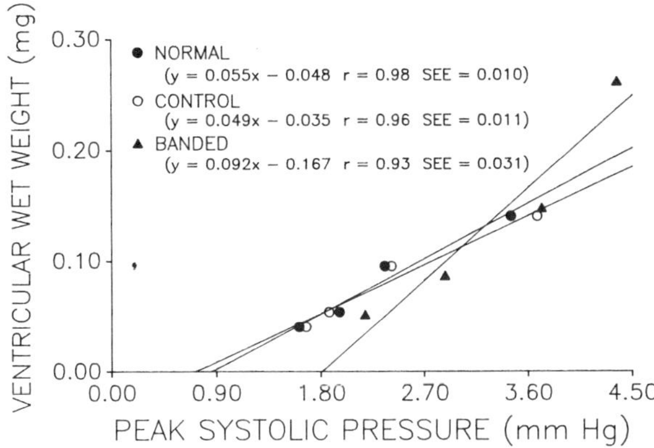

FIGURE 10. Regression plot of normal, sham-operated, and banded embryos of chicks in stages 21 to 29.

REFERENCES

1. CLARK, E. B. & N. HU. 1982. Developmental hemodynamic changes in the chick embryo stages 18 to 27. Circ. Res. **51:** 810-815.
2. STEWART, D. E., M. L. KIRBY & K. K. SULIK. 1986. Hemodynamic changes in chick embryos precede heart defects after cardiac neural crest ablation. Circ. Res. **59:** 545-550.
3. NAKAZAWA, M., S. MIYAGAWA, T. OHNO, S. MIURA & A. TAKAO. 1988. Developmental hemodynamic changes in rat embryos at 11 to 15 days of gestation: Normal data of blood pressure and the effect of caffeine compared to data from chick embryo. Pediatr. Res. **23:**(2): 200-205.
4. HAMBURGER, V. & H. L. HAMILTON. 1951. A series of normal stages in the development of the chick embryo. J. Morphol. **88:** 49-92.
5. DUNNIGAN, A., N. HU, D. W. BENSON, JR. & E. B. CLARK. 1987. Effect of heart rate increase on dorsal aortic flow in the stage 24 chick embryo. Pediatr. Res. **22**(4): 442-444.
6. WISPE, J., N. HU & E. B. CLARK. 1983. Effect of environmental hypothermia on dorsal aortic blood flow in the chick embryo, stages 18 to 24. Pediatr. Res. **17**(12): 945-948.
7. NAKAZAWA, M., E. B. CLARK, N. HU & J. WISPE. 1985. Effect of environmental hypothermia on vitelline artery blood pressure and vascular resistance in the stage 18, 21, and 24 chick embryo. Pediatr. Res. **19:** 651-654.
8. CLARK, E. B. 1989. Growth, morphogenesis and function: The dynamics of cardiac development. *In* Fetal, neonatal and infant heart disease. J. H. Moller, W. Neal & J. Lock, Eds.: 1-17. Appleton-Century-Crofts. New York.
9. PATTEN, B. M., T. C. KRAMER & A. BARRY. 1948. Valvular action in the embryonic chick heart by localized apposition of endocardial masses. Anat. Rec. **102:** 299-311.
10. ZAHKA, K. G., N. HU, K. P. BRIN, F. C. P. YIN & E. B. CLARK. 1989. Aortic impedance and hydraulic power in the stage 18 to 29 chick embryo. Circ. Res. **64:** 1091-1095.
11. CLARK, E. B., N. HU, P. FROMMELT, G. K. VANDEKIEFT, J. L. DUMMETT & R. J. TOMANEK. 1989. Effect of increased pressure on ventricular growth in the stage 21 chick embryo. Am. J. Physiol. **257** (Heart Circ. Physiol. 26): H55-H61.

A Potential Role for Mechanical Stimulation in Cardiac Development[a]

LOUIS TERRACIO,[b] ANDERS TINGSTRÖM,[c]
WALTER H. PETERS III,[d] AND THOMAS K. BORG[e]

[b]*Department of Anatomy*
[d]*Department of Mechanical Engineering*
[e]*Department of Pathology*
School of Medicine
University of South Carolina
Columbia, South Carolina 29208

[c]*Department of Medical and Physiological Chemistry*
Box 575 Biomedical Center
S-751 23 Uppsala, Sweden

INTRODUCTION

The role of mechanical stimulation in embryonic development has been difficult to investigate due to methodological problems preventing a logical and systematic approach to the isolation of the mechanical stimulation. Because both chemical and physical factors are known to affect cell behavior during development, it has been difficult to separate the effects of mechanical stimulation from other stimuli. Therefore, it is important to develop *in vitro* models to isolate and investigate the role of mechanical stimulation in embryonic development.[1]

Mechanical stimulation is of particular importance in the cardiovascular system in a variety of developmental and disease conditions. During development and in the adult, the cells and tissues are continually subjected to physical forces. A primary developmental force in the heart is mechanical stimulation resulting from contractile force as well as increased pressure and volume. In addition to the mechanical stimulation induced by the developing vascular tree, passive traction forces generated by fibroblasts may also play a significant role in the morphogenesis of the heart during the latter stages of fetal development.

Investigations by Harris[1] have suggested that these forces could be important in morphogenesis. Passive traction force can be demonstrated by the ability of fibroblasts to contract collagen gels. Mechanical forces are especially critical during late embryonic and early neonatal development where they could influence myofibrillogenesis, fiber pattern, and the final geometry of the heart.[2,3] Only recently has there been a clear

[a]This work was supported in part by NIH Grants HL40424, HL42249, HL37669, and HL24935. This work was presented in part at the Society for Mechanical Engineering Meetings in May 1989, in Cambridge, MA.

demonstration that mechanical stimulation *in vitro* can alter such fundamental components and cause cellular hypertrophy.[4-6] These investigations have shown that it is possible to alter the cytoskeletal and contractile myofibrillar pattern of the cellular components of the heart by the duration and strength of mechanical stimulation. Mechanical stimulation also causes an increase in protein and RNA synthesis as indicated by an increase in [14C]tyrosine and [3H]uridine incorporation and an increase in cell size.[6] The formation of specific contractile fiber patterns of the myocytes in the mature heart may be in response to mechanical stimulation either alone or in combination with chemical factors such as components of the extracellular matrix (ECM). As the ECM begins to influence the formation of new myofibrils, a resultant increase in contractile force is seen.[7] In order to direct this increased force, the connective tissue network forms between adjacent myocytes and between myocytes and capillaries.[8] The resultant increase in pressure is associated with increased blood flow as well as the mechanical stimulation from the turbulence generated by this increased flow.

Our hypothesis is that following the initial events of migration and adhesion of cardiac myocytes, the major factors that influence the mature form of the heart are (1) mechanical forces, both active and passive, that regulate the contractile fiber pattern in the myocardium as well as the overall shape of the ventricles and valves; (2) ECM components and their receptors, which are essential in the formation of the stress-tolerant network that directs the mechanical energy and makes an efficient pump; and (3) growth factors that are intimately associated with these processes by regulating cell division, especially of fibroblasts, synthesis of ECM components, and the expression of receptors for the specific ECM components.

We therefore have developed the *in vitro* models presented herein to test the effect of mechanical stimulation on cardiac development using primary cell cultures isolated from the developing and adult rat heart as our test system.

MATERIAL AND METHODS

Isolation and Culture of Cells

Cardiac myocytes, fibroblasts, and endothelial cells were isolated from developing[9] and adult rat hearts[10] as described. Myocytes were cultured on laminin-coated Silastic® membranes as described[11] and used in the apparatus for inducing linear cyclical stretch (FIG. 1). Fibroblasts and endothelial cells were subcultured and maintained in Dulbecco's Modified Eagle's Medium (DMEM) supplemented with 10% newborn bovine serum and 5% fetal bovine serum and used in all three test systems.

System for Induction of Linear Cyclical Mechanical Stimulation on Silastic Substrates

An integral part of the *in vitro* system for exerting mechanical tension on cells was finding an appropriately distensible membrane. We found that commercially

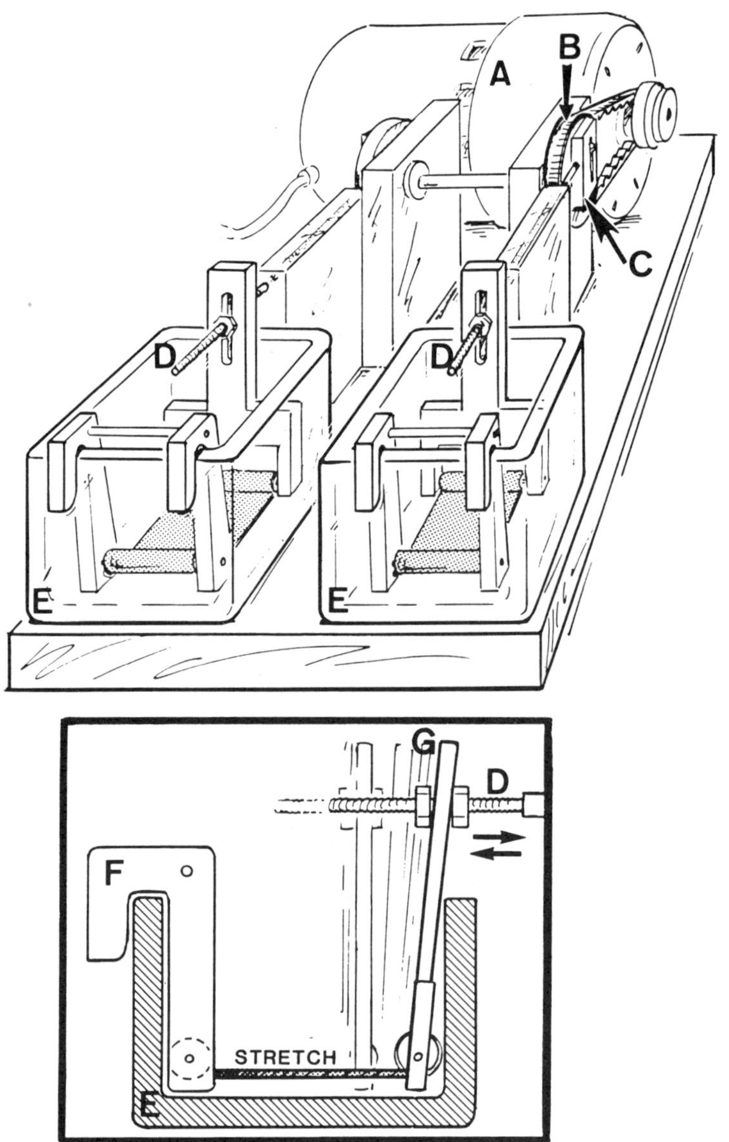

FIGURE 1. Apparatus designed for induction of calibrated linear cyclic mechanical tension. It is composed of a variable speed AC gear reduction motor (A). The motor drive is connected to a reduction pulley (B). The pulley drives a "Scotch-Yoke" (C) that adjusts the main push rods (D). Each apparatus holds two frames that are housed in a pyrex glass reservoir (E) containing tissue culture medium. The frame is firmly anchored in the media reservoir. The Silastic® membrane is attached at one end of the frame to a fixed cross member (F) and at the other end to a cross member that can easily move (G) and is attached to the push rod. Thus, when the motor is engaged, the Silastic® membrane is stretched and relaxed cyclically.

available Silastic® sheets 0.0127 cm and 0.0254 cm in thickness are available from Dow Corning (Midland, MI). These are readily distensible, nondeformable, nontoxic, autoclavable, and not autofluorescent. These membranes are not optically clear but are translucent and allow for enough light transmission to permit observation of the cultures by phase contrast microscopy.

Apparatus for Induction of Mechanical Stretch

The apparatus for induction of calibrated mechanical tension is shown in FIGURE 1. It is composed of a variable speed AC gear reduction motor (A) that allows for accurate and reproducible changes in the rate of stretch. The motor is connected to a reduction pulley (B) in order to obtain a sufficiently slow rate that is without hesitation. It was necessary that each cycle of stretch and relaxation be free of vibrations and hesitation. A belt-driven pulley instead of gears was chosen because they can be made vibration-free more economically and easier than gears. The pulley drives a "Scotch-Yoke" (C), which is used to coarsely adjust the range of motion of the main push rods (D). The push rods are attached to the frames that hold the Silastic® membranes with attached cells. Fine regulation of the degree of stretch is achieved by placing calibrated spacers between the attachment upright of the sled and the main push rods. Each apparatus holds two frames that are housed in a Pyrex glass reservoir (E). The Silastic® membrane is attached at one end of the frame to a fixed cross member (F) and at the other end to a cross member that can easily move (G) and is attached to the push rod (see side view in FIG. 1).

System for Studying Traction Forces in a Three-Dimentional Collagen Gel

Cells grown in a three-dimentional matrix such as a collagen gel have been shown to develop a cellular morphology similar to that seen *in vivo.*[12] Furthermore, fibroblasts grown in collagen gels are capable of reorganizing the collagen fibers and contracting the gel into a dense tissue-like structure.[13] This is thought to resemble normal processes such as wound repair or morphogenic migration. This system is ideal for studying the traction forces exerted by cells on the surrounding collagen matrix; however, the measurement of these forces has not been performed.

Isolated cells were cultured in collagen gels made by the following procedure: 1 mL of 10 × DMEM was mixed with 1 mL of 0.2 M HEPES, pH 9.0, and 8 mL of Vitrogen-100 (Collagen Corp, Paolo Alto, CA) or Vitrogen-100 mixed with purified collagen type III. The gel solution was kept on ice and quickly combined (1:1) with a DMEM cell suspension to yield concentrations from 5×10^4 to 5×10^5. The collagen, cells, and culture medium were vortexed and plated into culture dishes that had been coated with 2% sterile BSA in PBS at 37° C for at least 2 hours. One hour after the gels formed, culture medium containing fetal bovine serum or various concentrations of platelet-derived growth factor (PDGF) on transforming growth factor-β (TGF-β) were added. For contraction studies, 24-well plates (16 mm wells from NUNC) were used. For force measurement studies, a gel was poured in the trough formed by a 35 mm dish solvent welded into the center of a 60 mm dish. This doughnut-shaped gel was then attached to a strain gauge (Grass Instruments) and allowed to contract. The force generated by the contracting gel was divided by the number of cells in the gel to yield force per cell.

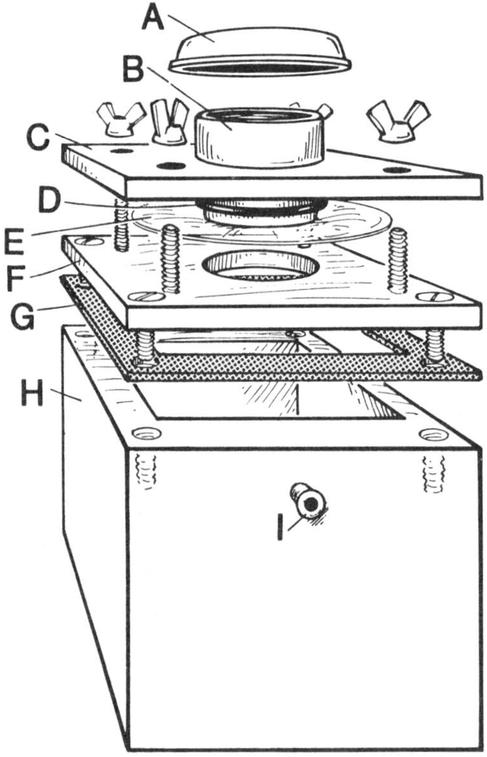

FIGURE 2. Apparatus designed to generate radial stretch of cultured cells. Cells are cultured on Silastic® membranes or in collagen gels (E) sealed between two stainless steel plates (C and F) with 35 mm diameter holes. The upper plate (C) possesses a nylon sleeve (B) that forms a culture well and is sealed to the culture membrane by an O-ring (D). The stainless steel plates are firmly sealed to a Plexiglas reservoir (H) by a gasket (G). Once assembled the reservoir (H) and the nylon sleeve (B) are filled with culture medium for collagen gels or sterile fluid for stretching the Silastic® membrane. The port (I) in the reservoir is connected to a hydraulic pump that can accurately alter the fluid volume of the reservoir causing the membrane to bulge into the culture well formed by the nylon sleeve (B). The apparatus can be autoclaved, and a sterile 35 mm petri dish lid (A) can be used to maintain the sterile environment.

System to Examine Radial Stretch

We have developed a system to radially stretch cells (FIG. 2). Although our experiments are still preliminary, we feel that this system will better mimic the *in vitro* condition and can be used for cells grown on Silastic® and/or in three-dimensional collagen gels. This system will allow for the examination of continual stretch of cells and the analysis of strain on the cells and substrates.

Analysis of the Influence of Mechanical Stimulation on Cells in Culture

Precision digital image correlation (PDIC) has been used for further analysis of mechanical stimulus in a variety of biological systems. PDIC methodology has been used to study a variety of deformation problems in fluid and solid mechanics including problems in fracture mechanics and composite materials. In addition, this methodology has been used to quantify the deformation (displacement and strain) in bovine retina *in vitro* subjected to uniform tensile stretch.[14–17] The digital image correlation techniques involve two digitized images. The first is the nondeformed image, and the second is the deformed image of the object.

The correlation is performed between a subset of the nondeformed image and a subset from the deformed image that has been fitted using a bilinear function. The subset x is mapped to a new position, x*, where x* is related to x by the local deformation. This technology has been previously described in detail by Peters *et al.*[14–18]

RESULTS

Integral to these investigations was the ability of the Silastic® membrane to support cell growth. All three cell types could be cultured on the membranes with and without ECM components; however, plating efficiency and the ability to stay attached during mechanical stimulation was dramatically improved if the cells were plated on ECM-coated Silastic®.

Consistent alterations in morphology were observed in all three cell types under moderate to low levels of cyclic stretch (*i.e.,* 5-10% at a rate of 10 cycles/minute) for 24 to 72 hours. The cells and their cytoskeleton oriented themselves perpendicular to the direction of stretch (FIG. 3). Cell density affected the reorientation process for myocytes (FIG. 3). At low cell density, where cells did not make contact with each other, the myocytes oriented themselves perpendicular to the direction of stretch (FIG. 3b). When cells were grown at high density, however, the orientation of the cells and their myofibrils were not always perpendicular to the direction of stretch (FIGURES 3c and d). This may be due to the force of contraction of the adjacently attached myocytes being transmitted by way of cell junctions and partly overriding the influence of the stretching substrate. This change in cell orientation was a gradual process taking place over about a 24-hour time period.[5] The use of PDIC should allow us to determine the minimal physical signal necessary to evoke this potentially important morphogenic signal.

Fibroblasts grown in collagen gels contract the collagen lattice and thereby decrease the size of the gels with a concomitant increase in density (FIGURES 4-6). This is thought to be the result of traction forces exerted by migrating cells. The greater the number of cells present in the gel, the greater rate and degree of contraction of the gel (FIGURES 4 and 5). Also the composition of collagen can affect the rate and degree of contraction (FIG. 6). Gels made of collagen type I are stiffer and contract more slowly than gels made of a mixture of collagen types I and III (FIG. 6). Collagen type III is considerably less stiff than collagen type I. Thus, gels made predominantly of collagen type III would be expected to contract faster and to a greater degree.

Preliminary results on the force generated by neonatal heart fibroblasts contracting a collagen type I gel (FIG. 7) indicate that the force generated ranges between 2.6

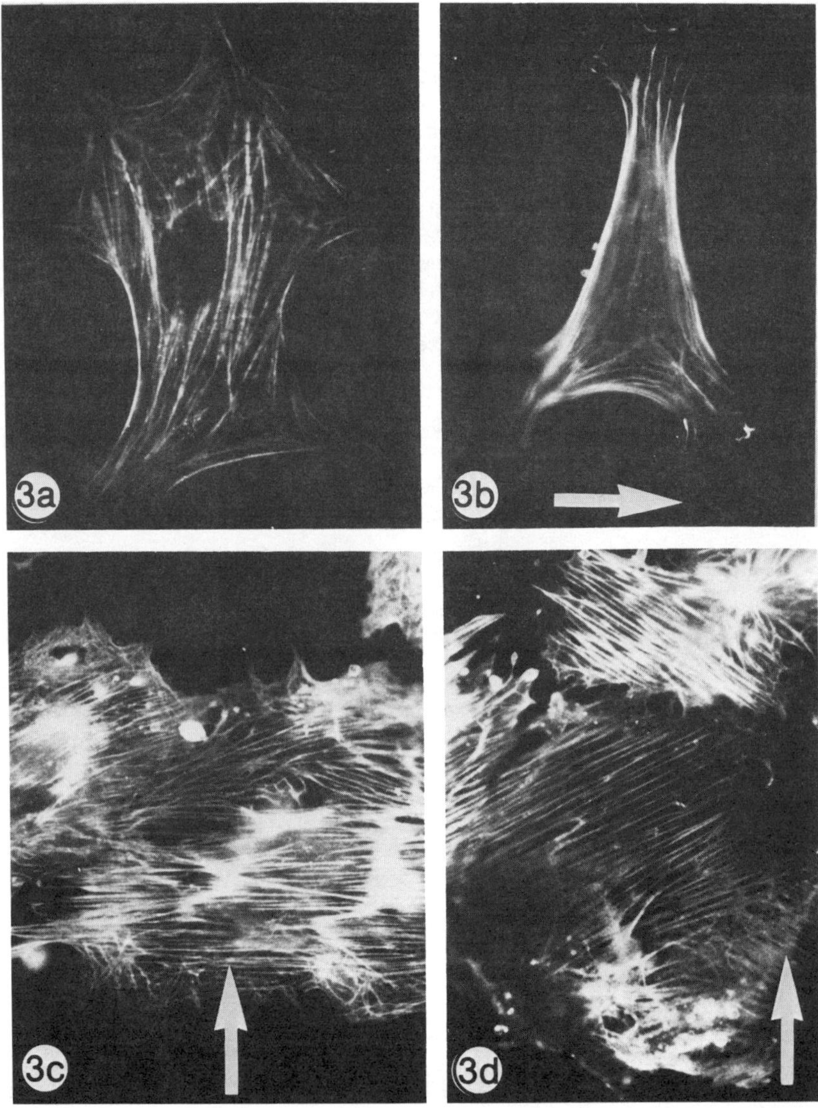

FIGURE 3. Photomicrographs of rhodamine phalloidin-stained neonatal myocytes grown on Silastic® membranes. (**a**) Control cell showing a random orientation of myofibrils and cell processes. (**b**) A cell grown at low density and exposed to cyclical linear stretch. The cell and its myofibrils are oriented perpendicular to the direction of stretch. (Arrow indicates direction of stretch in all figures). (**c** and **d**) Cells grown at high density and exposed to cyclical linear stretch. Note that the cells and fibrils are not uniformly oriented perpendicular to the direction of stretch. This may be due to the force of contraction of the adjacent cells being transmitted by the cell junction, which overrides the influence of the stretching substrate.

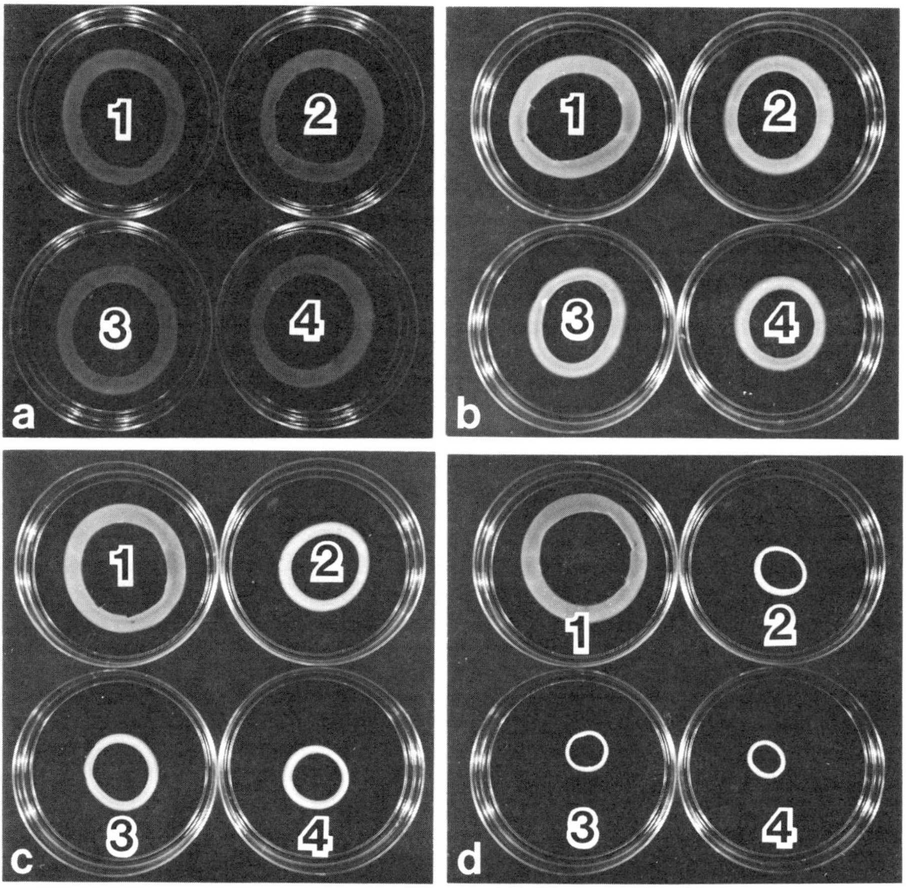

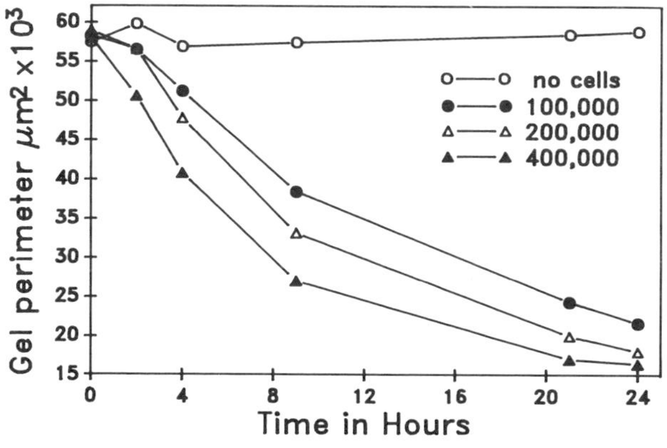

FIGURE 4. Collagen gels, made with collagen type I, containing varying numbers of cells. (1) No cells, (2) 100,000 cells/mL (3) 200,000 cells/mL (4) 400,000 cells/mL. (**a**) 0 time in culture; (**b**) 4 h in culture; (**c**) 8 h in culture; (**d**) 24 h in culture.

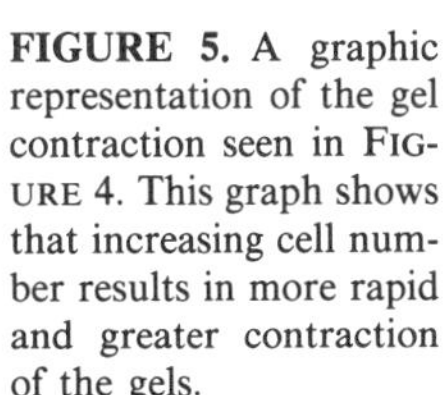

FIGURE 5. A graphic representation of the gel contraction seen in FIGURE 4. This graph shows that increasing cell number results in more rapid and greater contraction of the gels.

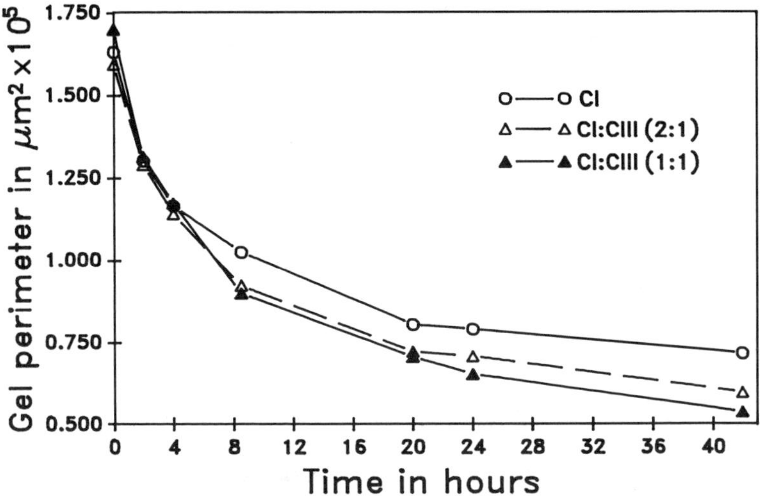

FIGURE 6. A graphic representation of gel size at various time periods. The number of cells was constant (60,000/mL); however, the composition of collagen was changed. When the gels contained more collagen type III, which is less stiff than collagen type I, the gel contraction was greater.

and 5.3×10^{-5} mg/cell. The variability seen to date may be due to measuring forces at the limit of current transducer sensitivity, or may reflect biological variability in cell populations. FIGURE 8 shows that the contraction of the collagen gels can be inhibited by antibodies against the B_1-integrin chain that has specificity for collagen.[19] Immunogold localization indicates that there is specific labeling on the cell surface in association with collagen (FIG. 9), thus indicating that the cells attach to the collagen by way of the β_1-integrin receptor. This interaction is necessary for the cells to migrate and contract the gel. Expression of the collagen integrin receptor *in vitro* can be modulated by using serum, PDGF or TGF-β (FIG. 10). In serum-free cultures both PDGF and TGF-β can stimulate gel contraction (FIG. 10) that can be blocked by the antiserum against the collagen integrin.

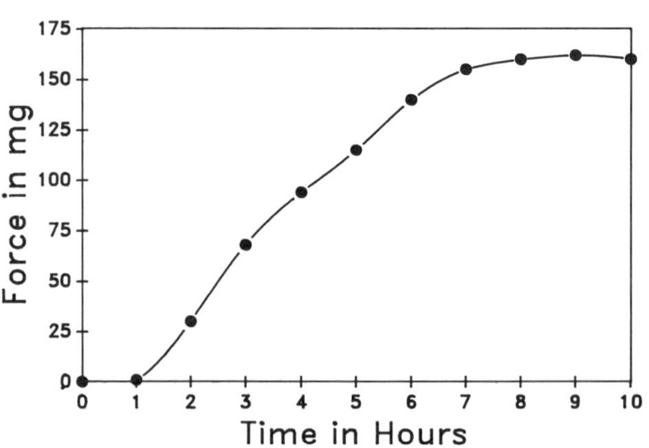

FIGURE 7. A representative experiment of the force generated by a 9 mL doughnut-shaped gel containing 500,000 cells/mL. The peak force generated was approximately 160 mg or 5.3×10^{-5} mg/cell.

DISCUSSION

The overall goal of this study is to determine if mechanical stimulation serves as a morphogenic signal during cardiovascular development. In order to do this we have developed the three apparatuses presented herein. Mechanical stimulation can be arbitrarily divided into three possible modes: (1) linear stretch of a surface such as occurs in skin or skeletal muscle; (2) traction forces generated by the contraction or pulling of tissues by cells to cause alteration of shapes, especially those associated with embryological growth as well as surgical closure of wounds; and (3) the pulsatile, radial force such as observed within the heart or vasculature.

Initially it is necessary to determine the minimal signal necessary to cause a biological response by the cell. In the first apparatus where degree of stretch can be

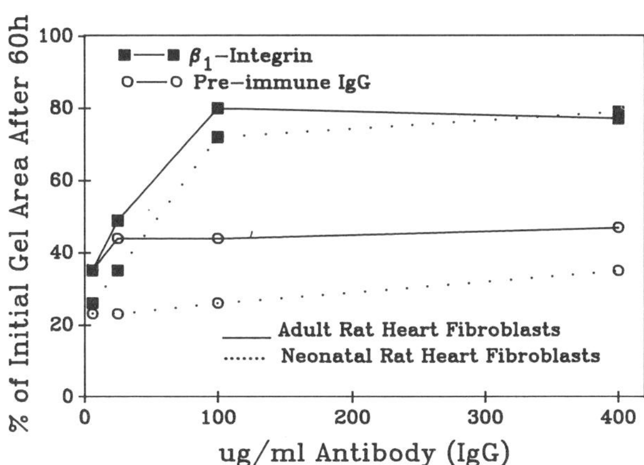

FIGURE 8. Collagen gel contraction by neonatal and adult heart fibroblasts showing that antibodies against the β_1-integrin receptor with specificity for collagen inhibits gel contraction.

critically varied and measured, experiments can be executed where minute mechanical stimuli in a linear mode can be measured using the PDIC methodology. Once the minimum signal has been determined, it becomes necessary to determine if force of sufficient magnitude occurs during development and disease. Contractile forces developed by myocyte contraction, blood pressure, and volume changes have been studied, and the force generated can hopefully be determined from published literature. In addition PDIC can be used to determine the force of contraction of myocytes grown *in vitro* on very thin Silastic® membranes. No data exist, however, on the traction forces exerted by cells *in vivo* or *in vitro*. Thus, the second apparatus will be used for determining the force exerted by varying numbers of cells during gel contraction to provide the fundamental new data necessary for determining the role of mechanical stimulation during development. This process is also thought to be important in wound healing and scar formation. This system will also allow us to study the effects of growth factors, ECM, and their receptors on gel contraction.

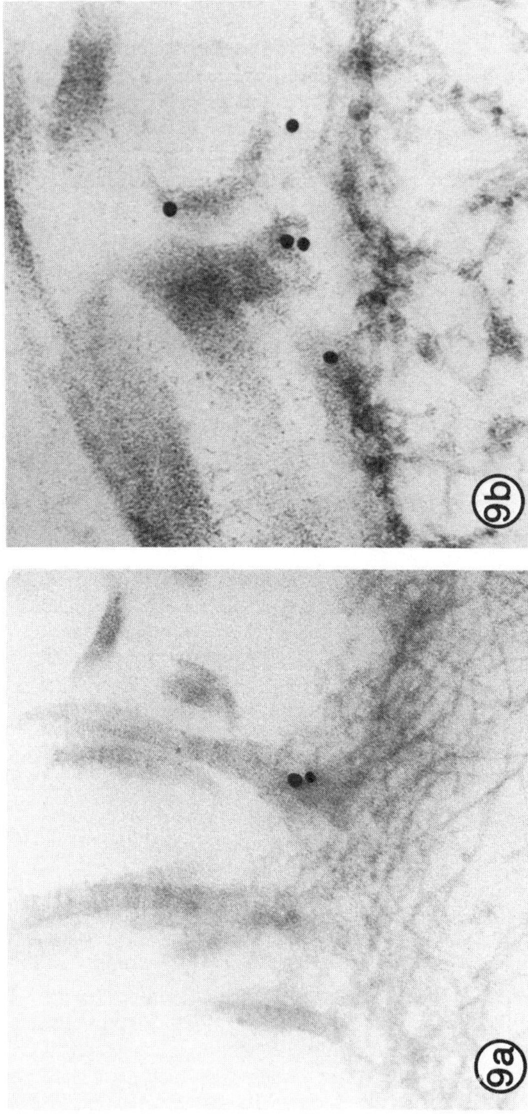

FIGURE 9. Electron micrographs of a 9 h culture of neonatal cardiac fibroblasts grown in a collagen gel containing 50 ng/mL of PDGF. Thin sections of the cultures were incubated with the anti-β_1-integrin antiserum and protein-A conjugated gold (15 nm). The gold particles can be seen at or near the cell surface associated with collagen fibrils. Although not all points of contact between collagen and the cells are labeled (**a**), what appears to be a specific labeling can be seen on the surface of the cells. **a:** $\times 77,000$; **b:** $\times 100,000$.

The third apparatus offers a method of analyzing the effects of radial stimulation to the cell surface. It will be possible with this type of apparatus to provide mechanical stimulation to the cells grown on the substrate as well as those grown in a collagen gel. This apparatus is designed to mimic radial stretch because it is a close approximation of the mechanical stimulation seen in the wall of a pulsing blood vessel or the heart. These studies are necessary inasmuch as it is imperative to obtain a model system that mimics the three-dimensional *in vivo* environment, but is still able to be quantitated using the PDIC methodology.

Once all of the models have been examined and data have been collected, we plan to use this information in conjunction with finite element modeling to determine if mechanical stimulation can account for structural changes seen in the heart during development. Expanding this work to use a wide variety of cells combined with the

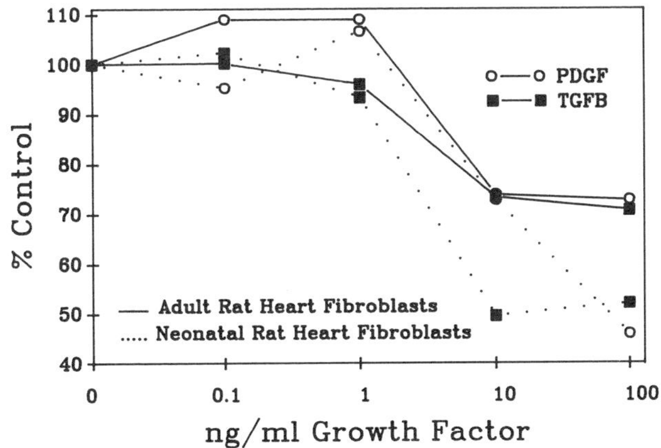

FIGURE 10. Collagen gel contraction by neonatal and adult heart fibroblasts showing that PDGF and TGF-β stimulate serum-free gel contraction. Neonatal cells show a greater response to the growth factor than the adult cells, possibly indicating a developmental difference.

ability to make measurements of biomechanical alterations will provide new data and aid in our understanding of the influence of mechanical stimulation on cellular structure and function especially as it applies to heart development.

ACKNOWLEDGMENTS

The authors would like to thank Art Dewey, Marge Terracio, Nancy Vinson, and Scott Berry for technical assistance; Mike Gore for constructing the stretch apparatus; and Judy Lawrence for typing this paper.

REFERENCES

1. HARRIS, A. K. 1987. Cell motility and the problem of anatomical homeostatsis. J. Cell Sci. Suppl. **8:** 121-140.
2. NAKAMURA, A., R. R. KULIKOWSKI, J. W. LACKTIS & F. J. MANASEK. 1980. Heart looping: a regulated response to deforming forces. *In* Etiology and Morphogenesis of Congenital Heart Disease. R. Van Praagh & A. Takao, Eds.: 81-98. Futura Publishing Co. Mount Kisco, NY.
3. STREETER, D. D. 1979. Gross morphology and fiber geometry of the heart. *In* Handbook of Physiology. R. M. Berne, Ed. Vol. **1:** 61-112. American Physiological Society. Bethesda, MD.
4. HATFALUDY, S., J. SHANSKY & H. H. VANDENBURGH. 1989. Metabolic alterations induced in cultured skeletal muscle by stretch/relaxation activity. Am. J. Physiol. In press.
5. TERRACIO, L., B. MILLER & T. K. BORG. 1988. Effects of cyclic mechanical stimulation of the cellular components of the heart: *in vitro.* 1988. In Vitro **24:** 53-58.
6. TERRACIO, L., W. PETERS, B. DURIG et al. 1988. Cellular hypertrophy can be induced by cyclical mechanical stretch *in vitro. In* Tissue Engineering. R. Skalak & C. F. Fox, Eds.: 51-56. Alan R. Liss. New York.
7. BORG, T. K. & J. B. CAULFIELD. 1979. Collagen in the heart. Tex. Rep. Biol. Med. **39:** 321-333.
8. TERRACIO, L. & T. K. BORG. 1988. Factors affecting cardiac cell shape. Heart Failure **4:** 114-124.
9. BORG, T. K., K. RUBIN, E. LUNDGREN, K. BORG & B. OBRINK. 1984. Recognition of extracellular matrix components by neonatal and adult cardiac myocytes. Dev. Biol. **104:** 86-96.
10. LUNDGREN, E., T. K. BORG & S. MARDH. 1984. Isolation, characterization and adhesion of calcium tolerant myocytes from adult rat heart. J. Mol. Cell. Cardiol. **16:** 355-365.
11. LUNDGREN, E., L. TERRACIO, S. MARDH & T. K. BORG. 1985. Extracellular matrix components influence the survival of adult cardiac myocytes *in vitro.* Exp. Cell Res. **158:** 371-381.
12. TOMASEK, J. J. & E. D. HAY. 1984. Analysis of the role of microfilaments and microtubules in acquisition of bipolarity and elongation of fibroblasts in hydrated collagen gels. J. Cell. Biol. **99:** 536-549.
13. GRINNEL, F. & C. R. LAMKE. 1984. Reorganization of hydrated collagen lattices by human skin fibroblasts. J. Cell. Sci. **66:** 51-63.
14. DURIG, B. R., W. H. PETERS, L. TERRACIO & T. K. BORG. 1988. Mechanical testing of soft tissue. In Proceedings of the VI International Congress on Experimental Mechanics. **2:** 390-397. The Society for Experimental Mechanics. Bethel, CN.
15. CHU, T. C., W. F. RANSON, M. A. SUTTON & W. H. PETERS. 1985. Application of digital image correlation techniques to experimental mechanics. Exp. Mechanics **25(3):** 232-244.
16. LEE, C., W. H. PETERS, Y. J. CHAO & M. A. SUTTON. 1986. An improved digital image processing technique to investigate plastic zone formation in steel. Image Vision Computing **4:** 203-207.
17. PETERS, W. H. 1987. Basic mechanical properties of retina in simple elongation. J. Biomech. Eng. **109:** 65-67.
18. RANSON, W. F., M. A. SUTTON & W. H. PETERS. 1985. Digital image correlation of white light speckle including the effect of image distortion. In Proceedings of the International Conference on Speckle. San Diego. Vol. **556:** 160-167. The International Society for Optical Engineering. Bellingham, WA.
19. GULLBERG, D., L. TERRACIO, T. K. BORG & K. RUBIN. 1989. Identification of integrin-like matrix receptors with affinity for interstitial collagens. J. Biol. Chem. **264:** 12686-12694.

The Role of Basement Membranes in Vascular Development

DERRICK S. GRANT, HYNDA K. KLEINMAN, AND
GEORGE R. MARTIN [a]

Laboratory of Developmental Biology and Anomalies
National Institute of Dental Research
National Institutes of Health
Bethesda, Maryland 20892

[a]Gerontology Research Center
National Institute on Aging
Baltimore, Maryland 21224

INTRODUCTION

Basement membranes are extracellular substrata that lie along the basal surface of endothelial cells throughout the entire vascular system. These matrices are also closely adherent to epithelia, smooth and skeletal muscle, and the nervous system. In electron micrographs, basement membranes appear as an electron dense layer (80-100 nm thick) closely opposed to the surface of cells (FIG. 1). In the case of capillaries, arteriole and venule, basement membranes form a sleeve around the endothelium, supporting the vascular architecture. This important extracellular matrix maintains cell polarity of the vessel and regulates many processes including endothelial cell adhesion, differentiation and proliferation.[1-4] Although endothelial cells tend to appear to flatten against the basement membrane in cross sections of vessels, the cells still maintain a highly polarized cytoplasm, and the luminal cell membrane contains different membrane proteins than the membrane on the basal-lateral surface.[5-7] Endothelial cells also sort and secrete the intracellular proteins to either the basal-lateral or luminal plasmalemma.[8] In the adult, blood vessels are fairly stable structures due mainly to the presence of a basement membrane. Blood vessels are modified primarily only in response to injury[9,10] or cyclic changes such as those observed in the endometrium of the uterus. The initiation of new vascular branches, angiogenesis, is usually accompanied by the presence of stimulatory factors secreted by various distal target cells.[1,2,11]

The basement membrane underlying the endothelial cell layer has been implicated as a regulator of endothelial cell behavior.[1,3,12,13] Endothelial cells synthesize various matrix proteins and are found to attach and migrate on these endogenously produced proteins.[14-16] It is believed that the basement membrane produced by the endothelial cells themselves maintains the polarity of these cells and sustains their well-differentiated state. Furthermore, receptors to some of the basement membrane components have been identified on epithelial as well as on endothelial cell surfaces. *In vitro,*

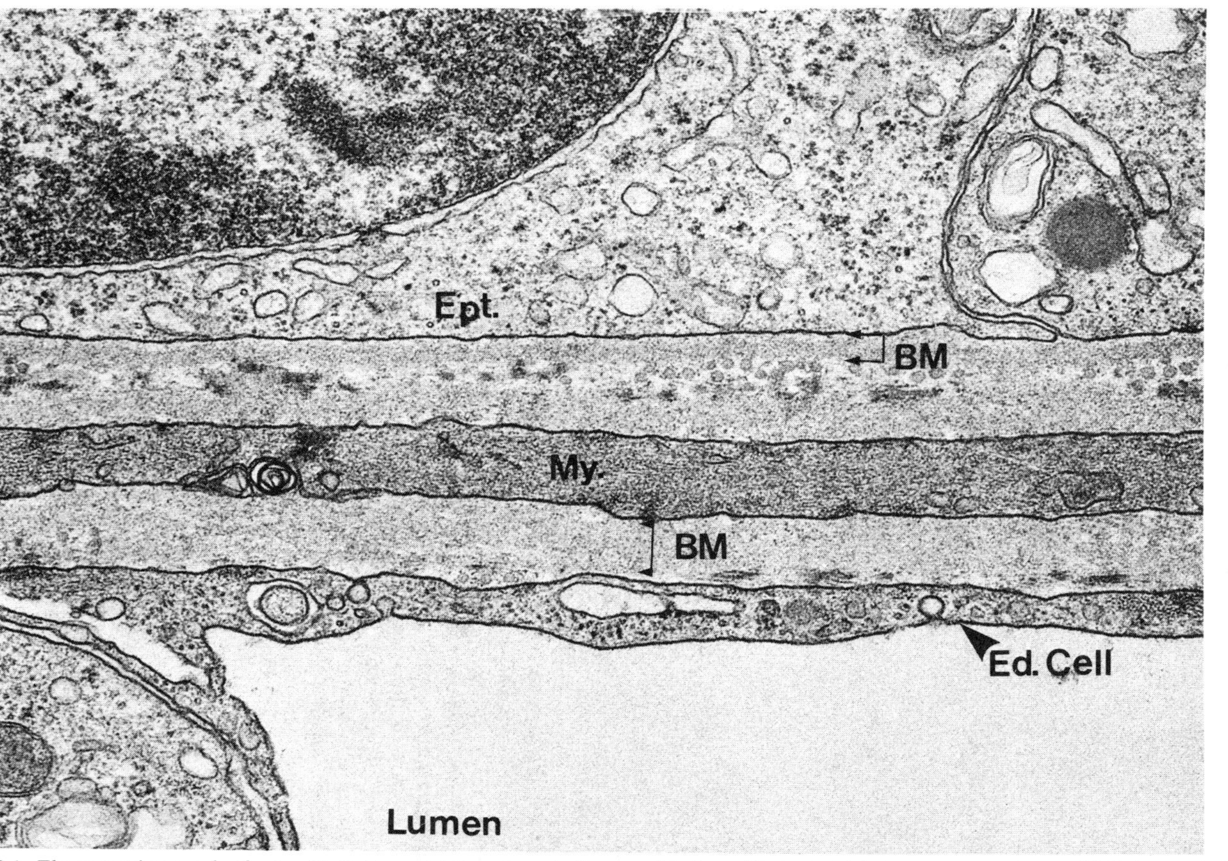

FIGURE 1. Electron micrograph of subepithelial layer of the rat seminiferous epithelium (Ept). A thick basement membrane (BM) is seen below the epithelium under which lies another basement membrane belonging to a muscle-like (My) cell. A capillary endothelial cell is directly beneath, contributing to this latter basement membrane. (Photograph courtesy of Martin Dym).

endothelial cells on tissue culture plastic show a cobblestone morphology and are contact-inhibited, similar to the *in vivo* situation. The culture of these cells on other substrata, such as collagen I or fibronectin, increases their proliferation, whereas a laminin substratum promotes the differentiation of the endothelial cells into capillary-like structures.[17,18] Tumor cells also bind to the basement membrane but immediately degrade it, as this is an initial step in invasion and tumor metastasis.[19–22] The properties mentioned above are exhibited by endothelial cells from both large and small blood vessels. Thus, Folkman and Haudenschild[23] concluded that endothelial cells express all the attributes necessary in forming capillary-like structures *in vitro,* and their differentiation state is dependant on the substratum on which they are cultured.

TABLE 1. Basement Membrane Components and Endothelial Cells

Components	Shape	MW	Receptor	Major Role
Laminin		800,00	Integrins LBP 32/67 Sulfatides	attachment differentiation migration
Collagen IV		540,000	Integrin	attachment differentiation
Heparan sulfate proteoglycan		750,000	38/36 kDa[a] 26 kDa	filtration attachment[a]
Nidogen/Entactin		150,000	?	adhesion ?
Fibronectin		440,000	Integrin family	attachment proliferation

[a] As determined for rat hepatocytes.

BASEMENT MEMBRANE COMPOSITION

Basement membranes contain several specific and constant components including collagen IV, the glycoproteins laminin and entactin/nidogen, and a heparan sulfate proteoglycan (TABLE 1).[24] Collagen IV ($M_r = 540,000$) is a triple-helical molecule arranged in a highly cross-linked network. It is the major structural component of the basement membrane and binds the other components. Collagen IV has been shown to promote cell attachment and differentiation primarily through a specific family of cell surface receptor proteins known as integrins.[4,12,25] Laminin ($M_r = 800,000$) is a large noncollagenous glycoprotein consisting of at least three separate polypeptide chains (A, B1, and B2) held together by disulfide bonds.[26,27] Laminin has multiple domains as seen by rotary shadowing (TABLE 1). Its cross-like shape consists of one long and three short arms,[28–30] with globules at the ends of the short and the long arm (FIG. 2). Each chain forms a short arm and a triple-helical coiled-coil long arm. The A chain also has a large globule at the end of the long arm. Laminin is biologically active promoting cell attachment, migration, differentiation, and cell-growth; it also stimulates neurite outgrowth (TABLE 1).[26,29–33] The three chains of laminin have been cloned and sequenced.[27,34] Cell binding sites corresponding to sequences identified on the A and B1 chains have been prepared, and the synthetic peptides from these different sites on the molecule were used in cell attachment assays.[30,31,33,35] Two peptides had significant activity. One with the amino acid sequence YIGSR, promoted cell adhesion through a laminin-binding protein (LBP 32/67) and inhibited tumor metastasis to the lung.[29–31,35] Second, an active RGD peptide was identified in a site in the laminin A chain that promoted cell attachment.[33,34] The RGD site is thought to bind to a receptor related to integrins present on the surface of endothelial cells.[18] Entactin/nidogen is a sulfated glycoprotein ($M_r = 150,000$) that is tightly bound to laminin by noncovalent bonds.[36,37] It has been cloned and sequenced and characterized by physical techniques. These studies show that it has a dumbbell shape and is associated with the short arms of laminin. Its role in cell attachment and regulation is still unclear, but it may modify cell binding activity on laminin. Basement membranes also contain a large heparan sulfate proteoglycan that is unique to this matrix.[38] The

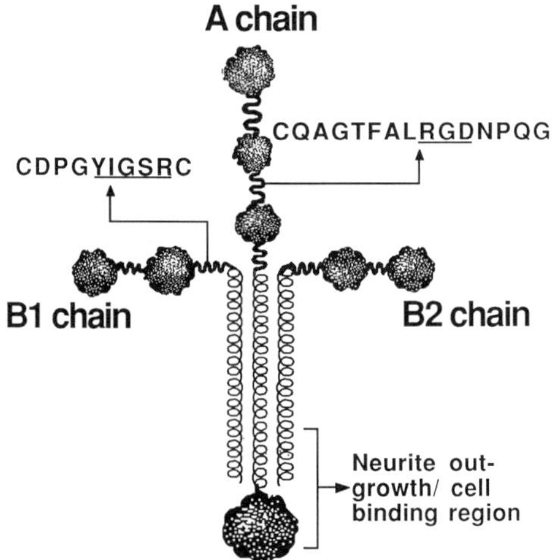

FIGURE 2. Schematic model of laminin. Laminin is composed of the three chains with the eight globular domains and seven EGF-like repeating domains. The locations of the YIGSR site in the B1 chain and of the RGD site in the A chain are shown.

heparan sulfate chains of this proteoglycan form an anionic shield in basement membranes that prevent the passage of macromolecules.[39–41] Heparan sulfate appears to be the major glycosaminoglycan in basement membranes, although some chrondroitin sulfate has been detected.[42]

THE ROLE OF THE EXTRACELLULAR MATRIX IN EMBRYOLOGICAL BLOOD VESSEL DEVELOPMENT

Vasculogenesis begins early in development by the formation of blood islands in the yolk sac.[43] These blood vessels grow toward various tissues in a directed way, presumably guided by factors secreted by target cells. These factors may be growth factors such as fibroblast growth factor[43-45,46] or components of the extracellular matrix that comprise the embryonic mesoderm. These substances may guide migration and mediate important events in endothelial cell differentiation. For example, fibronectin (TABLE 1) appears to function in cell adhesion and motility.[43,46] Fibronectin has been shown to contain an RGD site that binds to cells through the integrin receptor(s).[25,47] Using antibodies to fibronectin and to laminin, the mobile intraembryonic capillaries of the 6-day-old chick embryo were found associated with fibronectin but not laminin until days 8 to 10, when an "adult-like" distribution of laminin was observed. This time course corresponded to the completion of the central aorta of the chick, and thus suggests that fibronectin promoted migratory and proliferative behavior while the cells were distributing themselves to form blood vessels. Subsequently, the cells switch to laminin secretion, and thus initiate differentiation of the primordial vessels. This pattern was also observed in sprouts of endothelial cells originating from pre-existing blood vessels.[43]

EXTRACELLULAR MATRIX EFFECTS ON ENDOTHELIAL CELLS
IN VITRO

In culture, endothelial cells attach well to laminin, fibronectin, and various collagens.[1,4,10,15] When rat microvascular cells are cultured on interstitial collagens I and III or on fibronectin, their proliferation is greatly enhanced over differentiation.[14,48] By contrast, cells on laminin or collagen IV attach and proliferation is suppressed.

When endothelial cells are cultured on plastic to a postconfluent state, the formation of capillary-like tubes occurs spontaneously.[2] This phenomenon can also be observed when the cells are incubated either in three-dimensional collagen gels[49] or in the presence of tumor-conditioned media,[23] or after the 4–5 week withdrawal of endothelial cell growth factors.[44,50] When microvascular and large vessel (from the human umbilical vein) endothelial cells are cultured on a gel of reconstituted basement membrane components (Matrigel), tube formation is induced within 18 hours (FIG. 3). The endothelial cells in the form of tubes on Matrigel remained positive for factor VIII.[17] In this latter system, the cells initially attached to the matrix (within 1 hour), began to line up in 2 hours, and by 18 hours formed tube-like structures in which a lumen was present.[17] At low power, an extensive network of interconnected tubes is observed (FIG. 3). When examined in the scanning electron microscope, the tubes are on the surface of the Matrigel (FIG. 3, center panel). This is different from endothelial cells cultured on collagen I gels, which tend to grow inside the gel.[49] At a higher magnification, the cells are seen to be in close contact with one another (FIG. 3, bottom panel). Each "vessel" in cross section is observed to contain one to three cells, and junctional complexes are present between the cells (not shown). A few microvilli are seen on the surface of the tube as on the endothelial cells themselves. These microvilli are eventually lost after 24 to 36 hours of incubation on Matrigel.

We have used the model system of human umbilical vein endothelia cells (HUVEC) on Matrigel to examine the components present in the reconstituted matrix that is responsible for the formation of capillary-like tubes. Antiserum to some of the components known to be present in the matrix were tested for their effect on the formation of tubes (FIG. 4). The antiserum to the basement membrane components, collagen IV, laminin, and entactin, were first incubated with the matrix, and then the cells

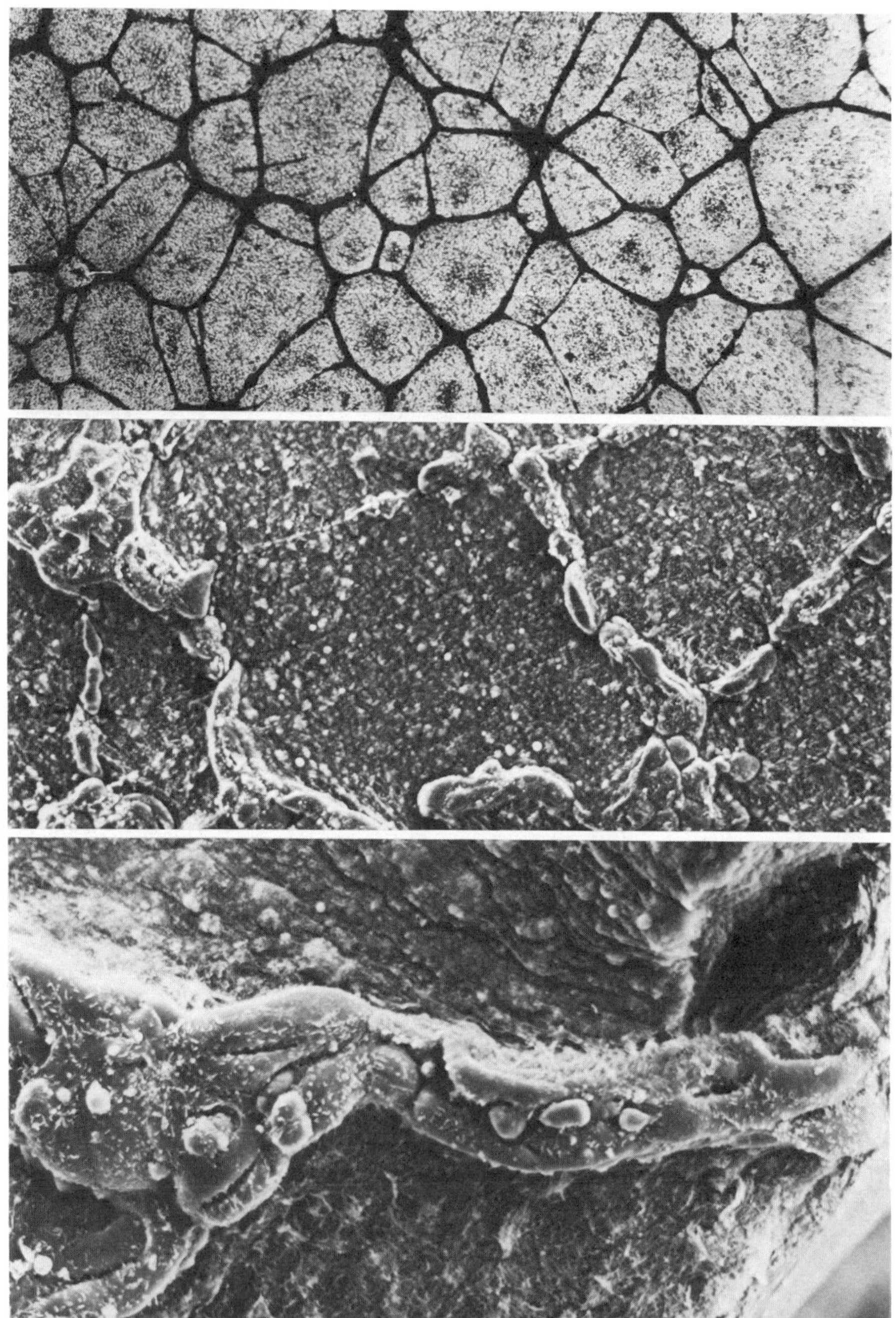

FIGURE 3. Appearance of endothelial cells on Matrigel in light and in scanning electron microscopy. Upper panel shows the interconnecting network of tube-like structures at low power

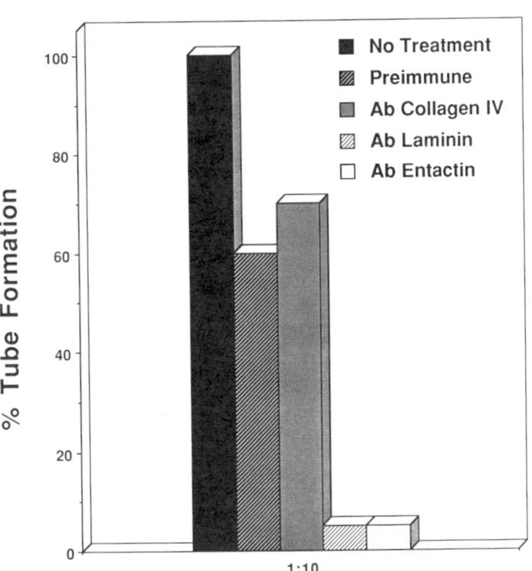

FIGURE 4. Effect of antibodies to basement membrane components on tube formation. The graph shows the percent tube formation/control after the solidified Matrigel as exposed to antiserum to collagen IV, laminin, and entactin, or to preimmune rabbit serum at dilutions of 1:10.

were added to the Matrigel. The ability of the matrix to induce subsequent tube formation was assessed by measuring the total areas of tubes formed (FIG. 4). Preimmune serum and anticollagen IV had little effect on tube formation, whereas antibodies to laminin and to entactin blocked tube formation (FIG. 4). The amount of collagen IV in the Matrigel is low, therefore its effect may not be detectable in this model system. In addition, we have added anticollagen IV antiserum to the assay 1 h after the cells were added and found that tube formation could be inhibited. Because the titer of the antibodies was not controlled, no conclusions can be made about the relative effect of these components. It can be concluded, however, from the data that multiple cellular interactions with extracellular matrix components are needed to produce the tubes.

MOLECULAR BASIS OF TUBE FORMATION INDUCED BY LAMININ

Inasmuch as laminin is known to contain different activities in separate regions of the molecule, we have sought to identify the actual site(s) on laminin that are involved in vessel formation. Using synthetic peptides and their corresponding antibodies, a major active site on the BI chain, which contains Tyr-IIe-Gly-Ser-Arg

---

in the light microscope. The middle panel shows the alignment of the cells prior to final differentiation at the electron microscopic level. The bottom panel shows the appearance of the cells at the terminal stages of tube formation on Matrigel. Note that the cells are on top of the Matrigel.

TABLE 2. Activities of the Peptides

Peptides	HUVEC Attachment	Inhibition of Tube Formation
B1 Chain peptides		
CDPGYIGSR	+++	+
CYC-YIGSR	+++	+++
Control peptide		
YIGSK	−	−
A chain peptide		
CQAGTFALRGDNPQG	++++	++
CTFALRGDNPQ	++++	++++
Fibronectin peptide		
CGRGDSP	++	++

(YIGSR), was identified (FIG. 2), which is contained within a major active proteolytic fragment. YIGSR promotes cell adhesion, migration, and inhibits melanoma colonization of murine lungs *in vivo*.[30,35] The cloning and sequencing also revealed an Arg-Gly-Asp (RGD) sequence in the A chain in the cross region as well (FIG. 2). This sequence is an active adhesion site first identified on fibronectin and subsequently found in many adhesion proteins.[25]

We assessed the roles of two sites in laminin using synthetic peptides. The peptides were used to coat plastic tissue culture-clustered plates (0-200 μg/16 mm). Cells were then added, and their binding was assessed. Both peptides promoted and increased attachment.[18,33] When compared to laminin, the RGD peptide had the strongest binding activity (TABLE 2). Then peptides were added at the time of plating endothelial cells onto the Matrigel, and the formation of tubes was assessed 18 hours later. Both peptides blocked the formation of the tubes but probably at different steps (TABLE 2). The RGD-containing peptide blocked cell adhesion to Matrigel, and many cells were found floating in medium in the presence of the RGD peptide (FIG. 5). By

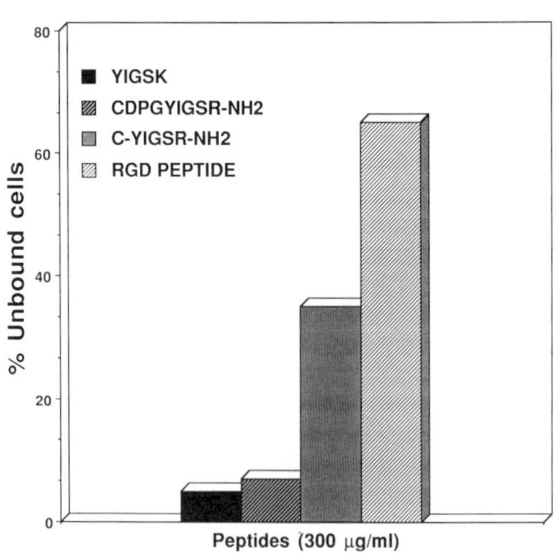

FIGURE 5. Effect of synthetic laminin peptides on endothelial cell attachment to Matrigel. The FIGURE shows the number of cells floating in the medium following the 18 h incubation of the endothelial cells on Matrigel in the presence of peptides at 300 μg/mL.

contrast, the cells in the presence of the YIGSR peptide remained well-attached to Matrigel (FIG. 5) and aligned, but were unable to form tubes due to inhibition of cell-cell interactions (TABLE 2). We conclude that the RGD site on laminin is involved in cell to substratum adhesion, whereas the YIGSR site is involved in cell to cell adhesion. YIGSR-containing peptides were most active in the cyclized form (TABLE 2). Substitution of the terminal arginine with lysine resulted in a complete loss of activity as previously reported for HT-10 80 fibrosarcoma cell adhesion.[30,31]

SUMMARY

Endothelial cells produce and bind to multiple basement membrane components. Fibronectin and interstitial collagens seem to promote migration and proliferation, whereas basement membrane collagen and laminin stimulate attachment and differentiation. Human umbilical vein endothelial cells will rapidly form capillary-like

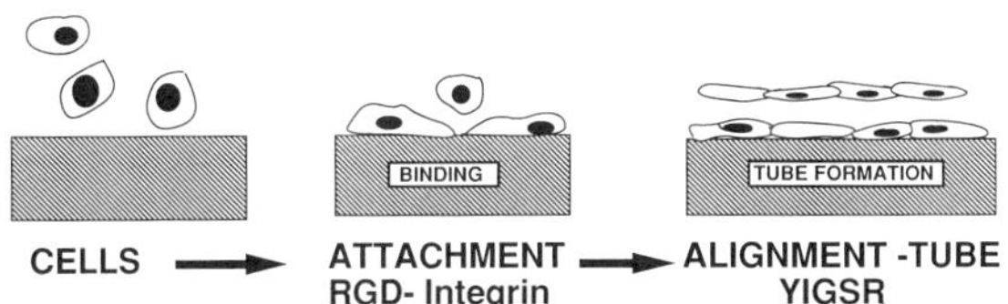

FIGURE 6. Differentiation of endothelial cells into tubes. Diagrammatic illustration of the mechanistic steps involved in endothelial cell tube formation on matrigel. The first attachment is promoted by the RGD site in laminin through the integrin receptors on the cells; then the YIGSR site on laminin promotes cell alignment and subsequent tube formation.

structures when plated on a reconstituted basement membrane gel. This morphological differentiation involves the alignment of the cells followed by their close association with one another and the formation of a central lumen. Using antibodies to basement membrane components, we find that the formation of these vessels is a complex process involving multiple interactions with several matrix components (FIG. 6). Synthetic peptides to active sequences in laminin have demonstrated that at least two sites in laminin participate in tube formation (FIG 6). An RGD-containing site on the A chain appears to mediate cell to matrix adhesion, and synthetic RGD-containing peptides block cell to matrix adhesion during tube formation. A YIGSR-containing site on the B1 chain appears to mediate cell to cell adhesion and promote tube formation because synthetic peptides block the strong cell interactions involved in tube formation. Our data with laminin peptides show that for at least one protein, multiple sites are recognized. Such data would also suggest that several cellular receptors are involved in a concerted process in laminin-induced differentiation of endothelial cells. We conclude that vessel formation is a complex, multistep process. Identification of active sites that block this process may have potential use in blocking angiogenesis in diseases such as diabetic retinopathy and Kaposi's sarcoma.

REFERENCES

1. FURCHT, L. T. 1986. Critical factors controlling angiogenesis: cell products, cell matrix, and growth factors. Lab. Invest. **55:** 505-509.
2. FOLKMAN, J. & M. KLAGSBURN. 1987. Angiogenic factors. Science **235:** 442-447.
3. MADRI, J. A., B. M. PRATT & A. M. TUCKER. 1988. Phenotypic modulation of endothelial cells by transforming growth factor-β depends upon the composition and organization of the extracellular matrix. J. Cell Biol. **106:** 1375-1384.
4. HERBST, T. J., J. B. MCCARTHY, E. C. TSILIBARY & L. T. FURCHT. 1988. Differential effects of laminin, intact type IV collagen, and specific domains of the type IV collagen on endothelial cell adhesion and migration. J. Cell Biol. **106:** 1365-1373.
5. PALADE, G. 1960. Transport in quanta across the endothelium of blood capillaries. Anat. Rec. **136:** 254-263.
6. SIMIONESCU, N., M. SIMIONESCU & G. E. PALADE. 1981. Differentiated microdomains on the luminal surface of the capillary endothelium. I. Preferential distribution of anionic sites. J. Cell Biol. **90:** 605-613.
7. NAKACHE, M, A. B. SCHREIBER, H. GAUB & H. M. MCCONNELL. 1985. Heterogeneity of membrane phospholipid mobility in endothelial cells depends on cell substrate. Nature **317:** 75-77.
8. SPORN, L. A., V. J. MARDEN & D. D. WAGNER. 1989. Differing polarity of the constitutive and regulated secretory pathways for von Willebrand factor in endothelial cells. **108:** 1283-1289.
9. WONG, M. K. & A. I. GOTLIEB. 1988. The reorganization of microfilaments, centromeres, and microtubules during in vitro small wound reendothelialization. J. Cell Biol. **107:** 177-1783.
10. MADRI, J. A. & B. M. PRATT. 1988. Angiogenesis. In The molecular and cellular biology of wound repair. R.A.E. Clark & P.M. Henson, Eds: **94:** 337-371 Plenum Publishing Corp. New York.
11. GOSPODAROWICZ, D., K. D. BROWN, C. R. BIRDWELL & B. R. ZETTER. 1978. Control of proliferation of human vascular endothelial cells. J. Cell Biol. **77:** 774-788.
12. DEJANA, E., S. COLELLA, G. CONFORTI, M. ABBADINI, M. GABOLI & P. C. MARCHISIO. 1988. Fibronectin and vitronectin regulate the organization of their respective Arg-Gly-Asp adhesion receptors in cultured human endothelial cells. J. Cell Biol. **107:** 1215-1223.
13. KRAMER, R. H., G. M. FUH & M. A. KARASEK. 1985. Type IV collagen synthesis by cultured human microvascular endothelial cells and its deposition into the subendothelial basement membrane. Biochemistry **24:** 7423-7430.
14. MADRI, J. A., S. K. WILLIAMS, T. WYATT & C. MEZZIO. 1983. Capillary endothelial cell cultures: phenotypic modulation by matrix components. J. Cell Biol. **97:** 153-165.
15. CARLEY, W. W., A. J. MILICI & J. A. MADRI. 1988. Extracellular matrix specificity for the differentiation of capillary endothelial cells. Exp. Cell Res. **178:** 426-434.
16. KRAMER, R. H., K. G. BENSCH, P. M. DAVISON & M. A. KARASEK. 1984. Basal lamina formation by cultured microvascular endothelial cells. J. Cell Biol. **99:** 692-698.
17. KUBOTA, Y., H. K. KLEINMAN, G. R. MARTIN & T. J. LAWLEY. 1988. Role of laminin and basement membrane in the morphological differentiation of human endothelial cells into capillary-like structures. J. Cell Biol. **107:** 1589-1598.
18. GRANT, D. S., K. TASHIRO, B. SEGUI-REAL, Y. YAMADA, G. R. MARTIN & H. K. KLEINMAN. 1989. Two different laminin domains mediate the differentiation of human endothelial cells into capillary-like structures in vitro. Cell **58:** 933-943.
19. VLODAVSKY, I., Z. FUKS & V. SCHIRRMACHER. 1983. In vitro studies on tumor cell interaction with the vascular endothelium and the subendothelium basal lamina; relationship to tumor cell metastasis in the endothelial cell—a pluripotent cell of the vessel wall. D.G.S. Thilo-Korner, Giesson & R. I. Freshney, Eds.: 126-157. Glasgow Publishers: S. Karger. Basel, Switzerland.
20. LIOTTA, L. A., S. ABE, P. GEHRON-ROBEY & G. R. MARTIN. 1979. Preferential digestion of a basement membrane collagen by an enzyme derived from a metastatic murine tumor. Proc. Natl. Acad. Sci. USA **76:** 2268-72.

21. KRAMER, R. H. & K. G. VOGEL. 1980. Solubilization and degradation of subendothelial matrix glycoproteins and proteoglycans by metastatic tumor cells. J. Biol. Chem. **257:** 2678-2686.

22. MULLINS, D. E. & D. B. RIFKIN. 1984. Stimulation of motility in cultured bovine capillary endothelial cells by angiogenic preparations. J. Cell Physiol. **119:** 247-54.

23. FOLKMAN, J. & C. HAUDENSCHILD. 1980. Angiogenesis *in vitro.* Nature **228:** 551-556.

24. MARTIN, G. R. & R. TIMPL. 1987. Laminin and other basement membrane components. Annu. Rev. Cell Biol. **3:** 57-85.

25. RUOSLAHTI, E. & M. D. Pierschbacher. 1987. New perspectives in cell adhesion: RGD and integrins. Science **238:** 491-497.

26. KLEINMAN, H. K., F. B. CANNON, G. W. LAURIE, J. R. HASSELL, M. AUMAILLEY, V. P. TERRANOVA, G. R. MARTIN & M. DUBOIS-DALCQ. 1985. Biological activities of laminin. J. Cell Biol. **27:** 317-325.

27. YAMADA, Y., A. ALBINI, I. EBIHARA, J. GRAF, S. KATO, P. KILLEN, H. K. KLEINMAN, K. KOHNO, G. R. MARTIN, C. RHODES, F. A. ROBEY & M. SASAKI. 1987. Structure, expression and function of mouse laminin. *In* Mesenchymal-epithelial interactions in neural development. J. R. Wolf *et al.,* Eds.: 31-43. Springer-Verleg. Berlin, Heidelberg.

28. ENGEL, J., E. ODERMATT, A. ENGEL, J. A. MADRI, H. FURTHMAYR, H. ROHDE & R. TIMPL. 1981. Shapes, domain organizations and flexibility of laminin and fibronectin, two multifunctional proteins of the extracellular matrix. J. Mol. Biol. **150:** 97-120.

29. TIMPL, R., J. ENGEL & G. R. MARTIN. 1983. Laminin—a multifunctional protein of basement membranes. Trends Biochem. Sci. **8:** 207-209.

30. GRAF, J., Y. IWAMOTO, M. SASAKI, G. R. MARTIN, H. K. KLEINMAN, F. A. ROBEY & Y. YAMADA. 1987. Identification of an amino acid sequence in laminin mediating cell attachment, chemotaxis and receptor binding. Cell **48:** 989-996.

31. GRAF, J., R. C. OGLE, F. A. ROBEY, M. SASAKI, G. R. MARTIN, Y. YAMADA & H. K. KLEINMAN. 1987. A pentapeptide from the laminin B1 chain mediates cell adhesion and binds the 67000 laminin receptor. Biochemistry **26:** 6896-6900.

32. BARON VAN EVERCOOVEN, A., H. K. KLEINMAN, S. OHNO, P. MARANGOS, J. P. SCHWARTZ & M. DUBOIS-DALCQ. 1982. J. Neurosci. Res. **8:** 179-193.

33. TASHIRO, K., G. C. SEPEHL, D. GREATOREX, M. SASAKI, G. R. MARTIN, H. K. KLEINMAN & Y. YAMADA. 1990. The RGD containing site of the mouse laminin A chain is active for cell attachment, spreading, migration, and neurite outgrowth. Submitted to J. Cell Biol.

34. SASAKI, M., H. K. KLEINMAN, H. HUBER, R. DEUTZMAN & Y. YAMADA. 1988. Laminin, a multi-domain protein: The A chain has a unique globular domain and is homologous with the basement membrane heparan proteoglycan and the laminin B chains. J. Biol. Chem. **263:** 16536-16554.

35. IWAMOTO, Y., F. A. ROBEY, J. GRAF, M. SASAKI, H. K. KLEINMAN, Y. YAMADA & G. R. MARTIN. 1987. YIGSR, a synthetic pentapeptide, inhibits experimental metastasis formation. Science **238:** 1132-1134.

36. TIMPL, R., M. DZIADEK, S. FUJIWARA, H. NOWACK & G. WICK. 1983. Nidogen: a new self-aggregating basement membrane protein. Eur. J. Biochem. **137:** 455-465.

37. CARLIN, B., R. JAFFE, B. BENDER & A. E. CHUNG. 1981. J. Biol. Chem. **256:** 5209-5214.

38. HASSELL, J. R., P. GEHRON-ROBEY, H. J. BARRACH, J. WILCZEK, S. I. RENNARD & G. R. MARTIN. 1980. A basement membrane proteoglycan isolated from the EHS sarcoma. Proc. Natl. Acad. Sci. USA **77:** 4494-4498.

39. KANWAR, Y. S., V. C. HASCALL & M. G. FARQUHAR. 1981. Partial characterization of newly synthesized proteoglycans isolated from the glomerular basement membrane. J. Cell Biol. **90:** 527-532.

40. KANWAR, Y. S. & L. J. ROSENZWEIG. 1983. Distribution of sulfated glycosaminoglycans in the glomerular basement membrane and mesangial matrix. Eur. J. Cell Biol. **31:** 290-295.

41. LEDBETTER, S. R., L. W. FISHER & J. R. HASSELL. 1987. Domain structure of the basement membrane heparan sulfate proteoglycan. Biochemistry **26:** 988-995.

42. IOZZO, R. V. & C. C. CLARK. 1986. Biosynthesis of proteoglycans by rat embryo parietal yolk sacs in organ cultures. J. Biol. Chem. **261:** 6658-6669.

43. RISAU, W & V. LEMMON. 1988. Changes in the vascular extracellular matrix during embryonic vasculogenesis and angiogenesis. Dev. Biol. **125:** 441-450.
44. MACIAG, T. & W. H. BURGESS. 1986. Endothelial cell growth factor. Prog. Clin. Biol. Res. **226:** 361-369.
45. BURGESS, W. H., T. MEHLMANN, D. R. MARSHAK, B. A. FRASER & T. MACIAG. 1986. Structural evidence that endothelial cell growth factor beta is the precursor of both endothelial cell growth factor alpha and acidic fibroblast growth factor. Proc. Natl. Acad. Sci. USA **83:** 7216-7220.
46. SAKSELA, O., D. MOSCATELLI & D. B. RIFKIN. 1987. The opposing effects of basic fibroblast growth factor and transforming growth factor beta on the regulation of plasminogen activator activity in capillary endothelial cells. J. Cell Biol. **105:** 957-963.
47. HAYNES, R. O. 1986. Fibronectins. Sci. Am. **254:** 42-51.
48. FUKUDA, K., Y. KOSHIHARA, H. ODA, M. OHYAMA & T. OOYAMA. 1988. Type V collagen selectively inhibits human endothelial cell proliferation. Biochem. Biophys. Res. Comm. **151:** 1060-1068.
49. MONTESANO, R., L. ORCI & P. VASSALLI. 1983. *In vitro* rapid organization of endothelial cells into capillary-like networks is promoted by collagen matrices. J. Cell Biol. **97:** 1648-1652.
50. MACIAG, T., J. KADISH, L. WILKINS, M. B. STEMERMAN & R. WEINSTEIN. 1982. Organizational behavior of human umbilical vein endothelial cells. J. Cell Biol. **94:** 511-520.

Expression and Function of Cell Adhesion Molecules during the Early Development of the Heart[a]

STANLEY HOFFMAN, KATHRYN L. CROSSIN,
ELLEN A. PREDIGER, BRUCE A. CUNNINGHAM,
AND GERALD M. EDELMAN

*The Rockefeller University
New York, New York 10021*

INTRODUCTION

The functioning of the heart is dependent upon the proper development and organization of its complex structures: the muscle, the conduction system, and the fibrous skeleton that forms the chambers and valves of the heart. These structures arise through a series of dynamic remodelings of tissues during development,[1-3] utilizing the primary processes of cell adhesion, cell migration, cell proliferation, programmed cell death, and differentiation.[4] Failures in these processes, particularly during the septation of the heart, can result in anomalies some of which are seen in human patients.[3]

To determine at the molecular level how cell adhesion affects other primary processes, we have focused on a cell-cell adhesion molecule, N-CAM, and two cell-substrate adhesion molecules (SAMs), cytotactin and cytotactin-binding (CTB) proteoglycan. The data suggest that all three of these molecules play important roles in heart development. N-CAM mediates cell-cell adhesion in the myocardium, and at least some N-CAM molecules in the heart contain a novel insert not found in brain or gizzard N-CAM. The distributions of cytotactin and CTB proteoglycan and their roles in cell-substrate adhesion and cell migration suggest that these molecules are involved in the formation of the endocardial cushion tissue, the developmental precursor of most of the septation in the heart.

[a] This work was supported by U.S. Public Health Service Grants HL 37641, HD16550, DK 04256, and HD 09635 and a Senator Jacob Javits Center of Excellence in Neuroscience Grant (NS 22789).

STRUCTURES OF ADHESION MOLECULES

N-CAM

N-CAM was first characterized using protein and cDNAs isolated from chicken brain.[5,6] Three N-CAM polypeptides from brain were described: the large cytoplasmic domain (ld) polypeptide of 180 kDa, the small cytoplasmic domain (sd) polypeptide of 140 kDa, and the small surface domain (ssd) polypeptide of 120 kDa.[7] These variants are generated by alternative mRNA splicing[8] of the 19 exons initially identified within the greater than 50 kb of the N-CAM gene. The ld and sd forms are transmembrane proteins that differ only in the size of their cytoplasmic domains.[9] The ssd form is linked to the membrane through a phospholipase C-sensitive bond.[10] In contrast to their distinct membrane-associated regions, these three forms of N-CAM are all essentially identical in their extracellular domains. This common region contains five immunoglobulin-like loops in the amino-terminal portion of the molecule and a region that is similar to two consecutive fibronectin type III repeats. The portion of N-CAM that mediates cell-cell adhesion by a homophilic molecular mechanism, that is, N-CAM to N-CAM,[11] is located within the region of immunoglobulin homology.[7]

In heart tissue, N-CAM polypeptides different from those in brain are seen;[12] the heart N-CAM polypeptides have apparent molecular masses of 150, 140, and 130 kDa. The 150 and 140 kDa polypeptides arise early during heart development and are integral membrane proteins, whereas the 130 kDa polypeptide does not appear until embryonic day 8 but persists in adult chickens when the other forms are no longer expressed (FIG. 1). Like the ssd form of neural N-CAM, the 130 kDa form

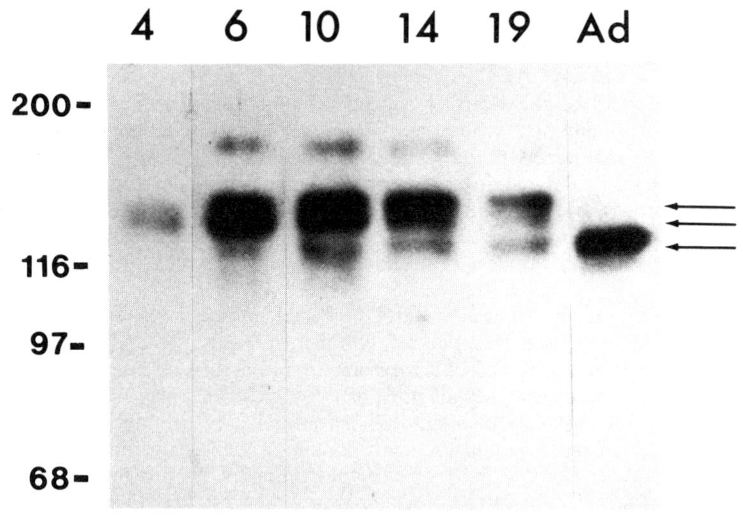

FIGURE 1. Expression time course of heart N-CAM. N-CAM was purified from NP-40 extracts of embryonic (E) and adult (Ad) heart by immunoaffinity chromatography. Following neuraminidase digestion, aliquots were resolved by SDS-PAGE and immunoblotted using polyclonal anti-N-CAM antibodies and [^{125}I]protein A. The three forms of heart N-CAM are marked by arrows on the right; the migration of standard proteins is indicated on the left by their molecular weights $\times$ 10^{-3}.

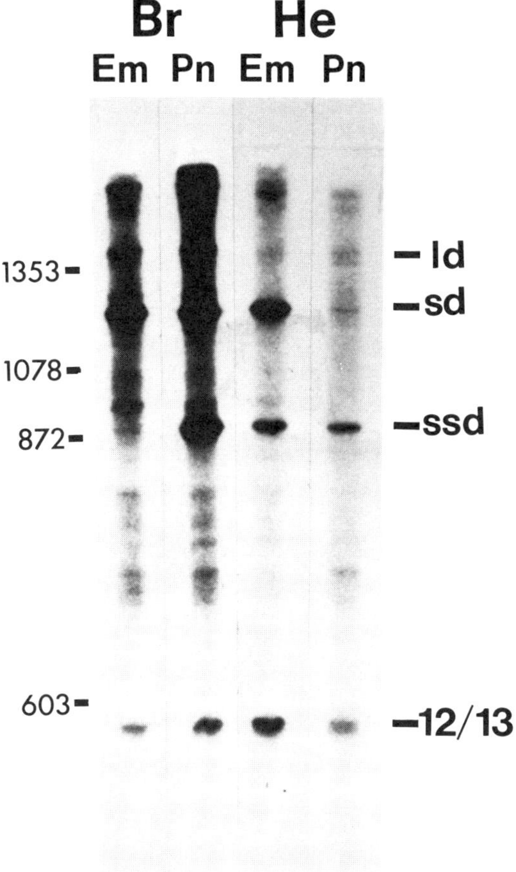

FIGURE 2. S1 nuclease mapping of brain and heart N-CAM. A 6.4 kb *Hind* III fragment of pEC208, beginning at the nucleotides encoding amino acid 389 of the ld form of N-CAM, was hybridized to 10-day embryonic (Em) or 3-day postnatal (Pn) brain (Br) or heart (He) RNA. S1 nuclease-resistant RNA was separated on an 8% polyacrylamide-urea gel. The products, representing the three major forms of N-CAM (ld, sd, and ssd) and a novel form diverging from these at the 12/13 junction (12/13), are marked on the right. The migration of molecular weight markers of the indicated size in base pairs is shown on the left.

is linked to the membrane by a phospholipase C-sensitive bond.[12] Experiments with endoglycosidases indicate that neither the differences in molecular weight among the components of heart N-CAM nor the difference in apparent molecular weight between neural and cardiac N-CAM can be accounted for by variations in glycosylation alone.[12] Nevertheless, glycosylation of heart N-CAM differs from that of neural N-CAM in that monoclonal antibody HNK-1, which recognizes a carbohydrate epitope, binds to neural N-CAM but not to heart N-CAM (unpublished observations).

S1 nuclease analyses suggested that both brain and heart N-CAM contain novel inserts in the extracellular portion of the molecule (FIG. 2) in the region between the two fibronectin repeats and involving genomic elements that map between exons 12 and 13 of the N-CAM gene. To identify sequences specific for heart N-CAM, cDNA clones coding for N-CAM were isolated from a heart cDNA library. One of these clones (λN101B) contained a 93-base pair insert at the exon 12-13 junction.[12]

Clone λN101B contained no sequences encoding the transmembrane or cytoplasmic regions of N-CAM but included sequences encoding a phosphatidylinositol addition signal. Therefore, λN101B appears to encode the phospholipase C-releasable 130 kDa component of heart N-CAM.[12] All or part of the 93-base pair insert in λN101B may also be present in mRNAs that code for other forms of heart N-CAM. RNA transfer blots probed with sequences from the insert recognized three N-CAM mRNA species in heart and skeletal muscle, but none in brain, gizzard, or liver.[12] Alternatively these mRNAs may all code for the same polypeptide but vary in the lengths of their 3' untranslated regions.

To determine the genomic structure of the 93-base pair insert in λN101B, a 25 kb genomic clone containing this portion of the N-CAM gene[12] was characterized. The 93-base pair insert was derived from four separate small exons, called 12A-D, that were distributed in the large space in the N-CAM gene between exons 12 and 13. Brain N-CAM mRNA does not hybridize to two probes that constitute most of the λN101B insert, but brain N-CAM does contain inserts at the exon 12-13 junction (FIG. 2), suggesting that other small exons may exist between exons 12 and 13. Alternatively brain N-CAM may contain only exon 12D, a 3-base insert that was not included in the probes.

At present, no functions have been identified for the portion of N-CAM encoded by the insert in λN101B. An insert (MSD-1) of similar size and location has been found in N-CAM from human muscle cell cultures.[13] The amino acid sequences encoded by the inserts in λN101B and MSD-1 were similar in their 3' halves, but were very different in their 5' halves.[12] These results suggest that the 3' halves of the insert in λN101B and MSD-1 represent the same sequence with variance due to species divergence, whereas their distinct 5' halves result from alternative mRNA splicing, supporting the notion that there are still other exons between exons 12 and 13. Recent studies suggest that the MSD-1 sequence, including the region similar to λN101B, may provide targets for O-glycosylation.[14] We have as yet found no evidence for O-glycosylation of heart N-CAM, but such a modification could modulate N-CAM structure and activity. Because the 93-base pair insert occurs between the two consecutive fibronectin type III repeats,[7,12] it (with or without glycosylation) may affect the flexibility of the N-CAM molecule and thereby alter its adhesive function and its effects on cell behavior.

Cytotactin

Cytotactin (also known as tenascin[15]) appears in EM images as a six-armed figure (designated a hexabrachion) with a central core.[16,17] Biochemical analyses indicate that the hexabrachion is a disulfide-linked hexamer with a single polypeptide chain forming each arm of the molecule. Cytotactin polypeptides of different molecular weights have been identified in various tissues. In embryonic brain two major polypeptides of 220 kDa and 200 kDa are seen,[18] along with a larger 250-kDa form containing covalently attached chondroitin sulfate.[17] In gizzard, polypeptides of 240 kDa and 200 kDa are found.[19] In heart, the two major components of cytotactin comigrate with the major components (220 and 200 kDa) of brain cytotactin, but additional polypeptides, both larger and smaller, are detected (FIG. 3).

Cytotactin isolated from neural tissue is recognized by monoclonal antibody HNK-1, but cytotactin from other tissues, including heart, lacks the carbohydrate epitope recognized by this monoclonal antibody. The HNK-1 carbohydrate does not appear to be involved in any of the known functions of cytotactin; molecules lacking the epitope are comparable to molecules expressing the epitope in their abilities to bind to cells, to CTB proteoglycan, or to fibronectin.[17]

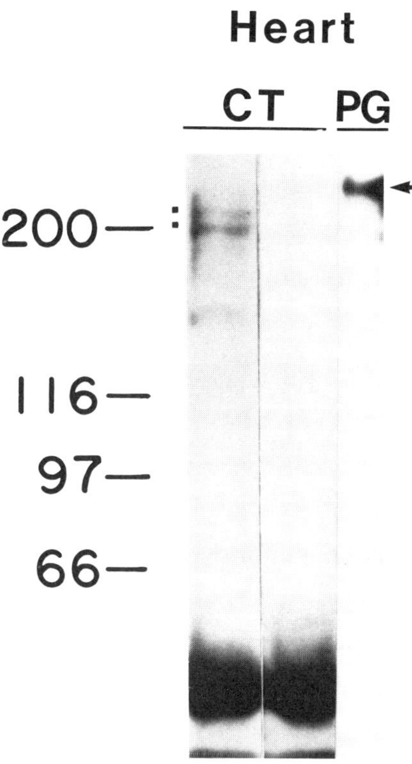

FIGURE 3. Heart cytotactin and CTB proteoglycan. Proteins immunoprecipitated from 14-day chicken embryo heart extracts with anticytotactin antibodies (left lane under CT) and antibodies from an unimmunized rabbit (right lane under CT) were immunoblotted with anticytotactin antibodies. Dots indicate the components of heart cytotactin that comigrate with components of brain cytotactin. The 50 kDa protein detected in both lanes is the IgG heavy chain. CTB proteoglycan was purified from 14-day chicken embryo heart,[17] treated with chondroitin ABC lyase prior to electrophoresis and detected by immunoblotting with anti-CTB proteoglycan antibodies (PG). The migration of chondroitinase-treated CTB proteoglycan from brain is indicated with an arrow. The migration of standard proteins is indicated by their molecular weights $\times$ 10^{-3}.

Recently, a molecular model of cytotactin was proposed based on the sequence of cDNAs encoding the two major polypeptides in embryonic chicken brain and on binding experiments with fragments of the molecule. The two polypeptides appear to be identical except for a 273 amino acid insert in the center of the larger species.[20] At their amino termini, both polypeptides contain a cysteine-rich segment that probably includes those residues that link monomers into hexamers; two potential sites for the covalent attachment of glycosaminoglycans[21] are also located in this region of the molecule. The next segment consists of 13 epidermal growth factor (EGF)-like repeats[22] that are each 31 amino acids long and are very similar to each other; 80% of the residues in each repeat match a consensus sequence derived from the 13 EGF-like repeats. Next, the two polypeptides contain consecutive segments that each resemble the type III repeats found in fibronectin;[23] the smaller polypeptide contains eight such units and the larger eleven. The additional sequence in the larger polypeptide is inserted after the fifth repeat and includes three complete repeats. The carboxyl terminal regions of the polypeptides are similar to the β and γ chains of fibrinogen and include a potential calcium-binding segment.[24] Sites in the molecule that are involved in its interactions with cell surface receptors, with CTB proteoglycan, and with fibronectin appear to be located in the distal portion of the arms of the hexabrachion,[25,26] either in one of more of the type III repeats or in the region that is similar to fibrinogen.

CTB Proteoglycan

CTB proteoglycan is a large chondroitin sulfate proteoglycan.[27] It is functionally distinct from the large cartilage chondroitin sulfate proteoglycan in that it does not bind to hyaluronic acid. Like other proteoglycans, it is predominantly carbohydrate ($>60\%$), and is too large and heterogeneous to enter an SDS gel containing 6% polyacrylamide. Following enzymatic removal of the chondroitin sulfate, the core protein of CTB proteoglycan is a single 280 kDa component in both brain[27] and heart (FIG. 3). Although brain CTB proteoglycan is the first proteoglycan to be identified whose core protein bears the HNK-1 carbohydrate epitope,[27] CTB proteoglycan from heart and other nonneural sources lacks the epitope.[17]

DISTRIBUTIONS OF CAMS AND SAMS DURING HEART DEVELOPMENT

Previous studies showed that the patterns of expression of adhesion molecules correlated with specific events in morphogenesis and histogenesis.[28] In extending this analysis in the heart, we found that both the sites of tissue borders and patterns of cell migration were related to patterns of CAM and SAM expression.

Early Development

The primitive heart appears as paired primordia, which arise from the splanchnic mesoderm. Each primordia contains an outer layer, myocardium, and an inner layer, endocardium. The splanchnic mesoderm (FIG. 4) and the myocardium express N-CAM, but not L-CAM. Cytotactin is strongly expressed in the endocardium, but not in the myocardium.[29] When the paired primordia fuse to form one double-layered tube, both the myocardium and the endocardium forming this tube express N-CAM, whereas the middle, acellular region known as the cardiac jelly does not (FIG. 5). The location of N-CAM on the outer surface of each primordium and the fact that it binds by a homophilic mechanism[11] suggest that N-CAM-mediated cell-cell adhesion may be an important step in the fusion process.

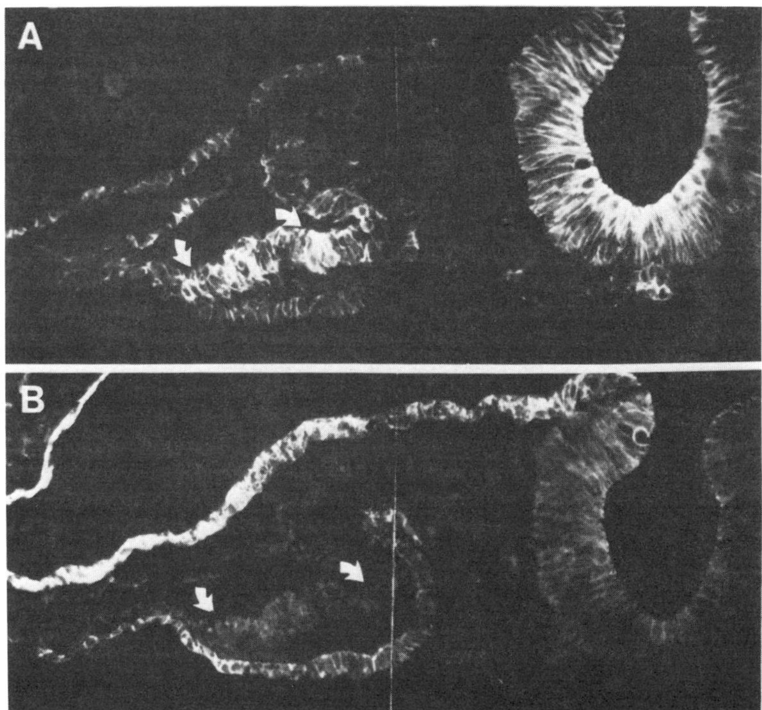

FIGURE 4. N-CAM and L-CAM expression in the cardiac primordium. In a stage 8 embryo, N-CAM (**A**) is strongly expressed on the neural tube but is diminishing in the somatic ectoderm and endoderm. N-CAM is expressed on the somatic mesoderm but is highly concentrated in the splanchnic mesoderm in the region of the heart primordium (area between arrows). By contrast, L-CAM (**B**) is diminishing in the neural epithelium and is absent from mesodermal derivatives at this stage, but is strongly expressed in somatic ectoderm and endoderm.

Septation of the Heart

The transformation of the heart from a simple tube to a four-chambered structure containing valves and the appropriate connections to the rest of the circulatory system is primarily the result of the growth of the endocardial cushion tissue (ECT). This tissue is the developmental precursor of the mitral and tricuspid valves, and participates in the formation of the interventricular septum, interatrial septum, aorticopulmonary septum, and conotruncal septum. The ECT arises from cells of the endocardial epi-

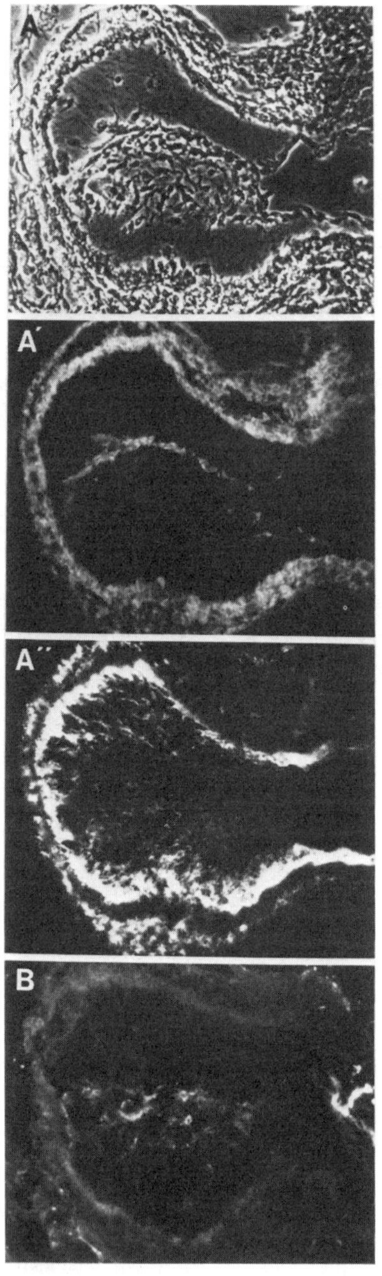

FIGURE 5. See legend on opposite page.

thelium that lose their surface N-CAM as they are converted into mesenchymal cells (FIG. 5). They then migrate into the cardiac jelly as single cells.

At stage 18, both cytotactin and migrating ECT cells are present in the outflow tract in a zone adjacent to the endocardial epithelium (FIG. 5), whereas CTB proteoglycan is present at its highest levels in and adjacent to the myocardium, and fibronectin is present throughout the cardiac jelly.[30] These results suggest that, at this stage of development, ECT cells or cells of the endocardial epithelium synthesize cytotactin, whereas myocardial cells synthesize CTB proteoglycan.

Later in development (stage 26), when the cardiac jelly has been filled with migrating cells, cytotactin, like CTB proteoglycan, is preferentially localized in the region of the ECT adjacent to the myocardium, whereas fibronectin is present throughout the ECT (FIG. 6). At this stage, multipolar mesenchymal cells are ceasing their migration and becoming bipolar fibroblastic cells organized into tendon-like strata.[31] This developmental change in cell behavior and shape may be related to the changes in the SAMs that the cells encounter (see below). Cytotactin remains in endocardial derivatives even after differentiation has occurred; its localization in the valves of a 13-day embryo but not in surrounding muscle suggests that the molecule plays a continuing role in the function of this tissue.[29]

Cardiac Muscle

The expression of particular CAMs and SAMs varies between the myocardium, skeletal muscle, vascular smooth muscle, and endocardial derivatives. High levels of N-CAM are expressed on cardiac muscle cells throughout development; N-CAM remains on these cells in adult animals,[28] in contrast to skeletal muscle where it becomes localized to the region of the neuromuscular junction.[32] N-CAM is also expressed on vascular smooth muscle cells throughout embryonic development.[28]

Little or no cytotactin is expressed in the myocardium, whereas the molecule is expressed at high levels in vascular smooth muscle,[17] providing a sharp border between these contiguous tissues. Nevertheless, the myocardium contains high levels of fibronectin, CTB proteoglycan, and other SAMs (FIG. 6 and references 30 and 33). Therefore, cytotactin is the only known SAM present in endocardial derivatives but not in the myocardium.

TABLE 1 summarizes several aspects of the expression patterns of N-CAM, cytotactin, CTB proteoglycan, and fibronectin that suggest their importance in cardiac morphogenesis. The functions of these proteins in heart cell behavior have also been analyzed in cell biological studies.

 FIGURE 5. Expression of N-CAM, CTB proteoglycan, and cytotactin in the outflow tract of the stage 18 heart. Panel **A** is a phase micrograph of a transverse section. Cells can be seen delaminating from the endocardium and migrating into the cardiac jelly (clear area). This section was double-stained for N-CAM (**A′**) and CTB proteoglycan (**A″**). N-CAM is present in both the myocardium and endocardium. Cells that have migrated from the endocardium no longer express N-CAM. The highest expression of CTB proteoglycan is at the periphery of the cardiac jelly, near the border of the myocardium; it diminishes toward the endocardium and is expressed in the outer layers of the myocardium. Cytotactin staining (**B**) is shown in an adjacent section. Staining is low everywhere, except around the cells migrating away from the endocardium.

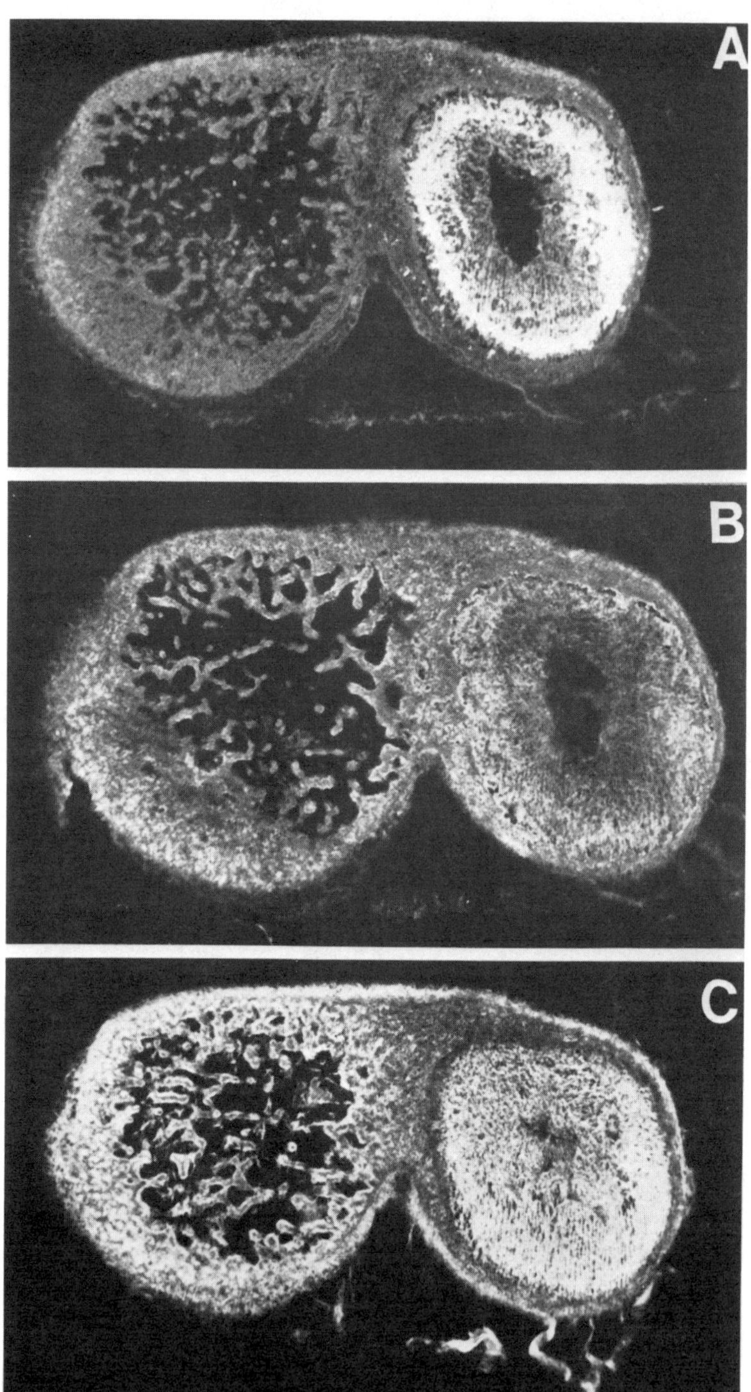

A
B
C

TABLE 1. Adhesion Molecules in the Developing Heart

N-CAM
  Present in myocardium throughout development
  Present in endocardial epithelium
  Absent from migrating cells derived from endocardial epithelium
  Heart-specific form
Cytotactin
  Colocalized with early migrating cells in cardiac jelly adjacent to endocardial epithelium
  Absent from myocardium but present in vascular smooth muscle
CTB Proteoglycan
  Present in myocardium and in cardiac jelly adjacent to myocardium
Fibronectin
  Present in myocardium and cardiac jelly

FUNCTIONS OF CAMS AND SAMS IN HEART CELL ADHESION AND MIGRATION

Cell-Cell Adhesion

N-CAM mediates neuron-neuron and neuron-muscle cell adhesion through a homophilic mechanism, that is, N-CAM molecules on one cell bind to N-CAM molecules on an apposing cell.[11] N-CAM also appears to be involved in myocardial cell adhesion, because monovalent Fab' fragments of anti-N-CAM antibodies strongly inhibit the aggregation of membrane vesicles prepared from these cells (TABLE 2).

As indicated above, the polypeptides in heart N-CAM are distinct from those in neural N-CAM,[12] and the carbohydrate epitope recognized by monoclonal antibody HNK-1 is absent from heart N-CAM, although it is present in neural N-CAM and

TABLE 2. Myocardial Membrane Vesicle Aggregation[a]

Antibody	Relative Aggregation
Nonimmune	100
Anti-N-CAM	17

[a] Membrane vesicles were prepared from 14-day embryonic chicken heart myocardial tissue, were filtered through a 0.6 μm Uni-Pore filter to break up aggregates, and were incubated 30 minutes, 37°C, at 70 rpm. The formation of aggregates was quantitated using a particle counter as previously described.[11] In this experiment, the relative level of aggregation obtained in the presence of anti-N-CAM Fab' fragments was normalized against the level of aggregation obtained in the presence of Fab' fragments prepared from nonimmune serum.

◄—FIGURE 6. Cytotactin, CTB proteoglycan, and fibronectin expression in the stage 26 heart. Cytotactin (**A**) is heavily localized in the portion of the endocardial cushion tissue adjacent to the myocardium but is absent from the myocardium itself. Whereas CTB proteoglycan (**B**) is also preferentially expressed in the portion of the ECT adjacent to the myocardium, it is also present in the inner portion of the ECT and in the myocardium. Fibronectin (**C**) is uniformly expressed throughout the ECT and is also present in the myocardium.

has been proposed to be a ligand in cell adhesion.[34] Thus, despite their differences, N-CAM polypeptides in both brain and heart mediate cell adhesion, and this adhesion in the heart does not require HNK-1 epitopes.

Cell-Substrate Adhesion and Cell Migration

Extracellular matrix proteins that mediate cell-substrate adhesion *in vitro* are likely to be involved in the control of cell migration *in vivo* because these molecules are present along migration pathways.[29,35] Cell migration is particularly important in heart development because the ECT, which forms most of the septation of the heart, develops from cells that migrate into the previously acellular cardiac jelly. As described above, the cardiac jelly contains fibronectin in a relatively uniform distribution and cytotactin and CTB proteoglycan in dynamically changing distributions.

TABLE 3. Endocardial Cushion Tissue Cell Adhesion

Molecule(s) on Substrate[a]	Total Bound Cells[b]	Spread Cells[b]
Fibronectin	143	111
Cytotactin	74	0
CTB Proteoglycan	0	0
Fibronectin plus cytotactin	65	2
Fibronectin plus CTB proteoglycan	21	0
Fibronectin plus BSA	136	109

[a] When present in solutions used to coat substrates, proteins were at the following concentrations: fibronectin, 10 μg/mL; cytotactin, 20 μg/mL; CTB proteoglycan, 20 μg/mL; BSA, 200 μg/mL.

[b] Small drops of each coating solution were placed at marked positions in the same 35 mm culture dish. After coating and blocking of the substrate with 10 mg/mL BSA, 5×10^5 ECT cells in medium were incubated in the dish for 50 minutes at 37°C, unbound cells were removed, and the number of bound or bound and spread cells were counted on 0.38 mm^2 of each substrate.

When ECT cells are plated on fibronectin-coated substrates, they bind and spread; by contrast, although ECT cells also bind to cytotactin-coated substrates, the bound cells remain round (TABLE 3). When ECT cells are incubated on a mixture of fibronectin and cytotactin, fewer cells bind than on fibronectin alone, and the bound cells remain round. This effect is not due to a lack of fibronectin on the substrate because even when substrates were coated in the presence of larger doses of BSA, fibronectin promoted both binding and spreading (TABLE 3).

Although intact CTB proteoglycan by itself does not support cell binding, when mixed with fibronectin it also inhibits cell binding and cell spreading (TABLE 3). This effect does not appear to be due to the presence of highly charged proteoglycan molecules on the substrate. Binding to fibronectin is still inhibited when most of the glycosaminoglycan side chains are removed from CTB proteoglycan, but is not inhibited by a heparan sulfate proteoglycan from Engelbreth-Holm-Swarm tumor cells. The combined results indicate that the binding of cells to different substrates can alter their subsequent behavior and that the behavior of cells on mixed substrates is not simply the sum of their behavior on each component of the substrate.

The influence of cytotactin and CTB proteoglycan on cell binding to fibronectin may be mediated by a combination of direct interactions between SAMs[17,27] and interactions between SAMs and cell-surface proteins.[25] Cytotactin binds to fibronectin, and this interaction may inhibit the ability of fibronectin to bind to cells.[17] CTB proteoglycan does not interact with fibronectin, but it is even more effective than cytotactin in blocking fibronectin binding to cells (reference 17 and TABLE 3). Both cytotactin and CTB proteoglycan may also inhibit cell spreading through their interactions with cell surface receptors. The resulting round cells would contact a two-dimensional substrate over a smaller area than cells that are spreading, allowing fewer fibronectin molecules to bind to each cell and causing a net inhibition of cell binding.

The effects of cytotactin and CTB proteoglycan on cell shape may affect cell migration as well as cell-substrate adhesion. *In vitro,* neural crest cells spread and migrate readily on fibronectin-coated substrates,[36] but these same cells round up and will not migrate onto cytotactin- or CTB proteoglycan-coated substrates.[37] Mixtures of fibronectin and cytotactin, or fibronectin and CTB proteoglycan inhibit migration as compared to fibronectin alone.[37] *In vivo,* cytotactin and neural crest cells both become localized in the rostral half-sclerotome, whereas CTB proteoglycan is localized in the caudal half-sclerotome[37] and fibronectin is present in a uniform distribution.[35] These observations raise the possibility that the dynamic expression of cytotactin and CTB proteoglycan in neural crest and ECT cell migration pathways influences pattern formation by inhibiting the migration of cells on an otherwise permissive and ubiquitous fibronectin substrate.

PERSPECTIVES

The studies summarized here on the structures, functions, and distributions of the adhesion molecules N-CAM, cytotactin, and CTB proteoglycan suggest strongly that these proteins play roles in heart development. Major questions to be answered in future experiments include: What is the distribution and function of the form of N-CAM containing the heart-specific insert? What are the roles of each of these proteins in the control of the known primary cellular processes of development (cell migration, cell proliferation, differentiation) in the heart? What are the molecular mechanisms through which these effects on cell behavior are mediated? The answers to these questions will be of fundamental importance to our understanding of normal and aberrant morphogenesis in the heart.

REFERENCES

1. CARLSON, B. M. 1981. Patten's Foundations of Embryology. McGraw-Hill, Inc., New York.
2. ROMANOFF, A. L. 1960. The Avian Embryo: Structural and Functional Development. MacMillan Co., New York.
3. VAN MIEROP, L. H. S. & L. M. KUTSCHE. 1982. The Heart, Arteries, and Veins. J. W. Hurst, Ed.: 7-22. McGraw-Hill Book Co., New York.
4. EDELMAN, G. M. 1988. Topobiology: An Introduction to Molecular Embryology. Basic Books. New York.
5. HOFFMAN, S., B. C. SORKIN, P. C. WHITE, R. BRACKENBURY, R. MAILHAMMER, U.

RUTISHAUSER, B. A. CUNNINGHAM & G. M. EDELMAN. 1982. J. Biol. Chem. **257:** 7720-7729.

6. MURRAY, B. A., J. J. HEMPERLY, W. J. GALLIN, J. S. MACGREGOR & G. M. EDELMAN. 1984. Proc. Natl. Acad. Sci. USA **81:** 5584-5588.

7. CUNNINGHAM, B. A., J. J. HEMPERLY, B. A. MURRAY, E. A. PREDIGER, R. BRACKENBURY & G. M. EDELMAN. 1987. Science **236:** 799-806.

8. OWENS, G. C., G. M. EDELMAN & B. A. CUNNINGHAM. 1987. Proc. Natl Acad. Sci. USA **84:** 294-298.

9. MURRAY, B. A., J. J. HEMPERLY, E. A. PREDIGER, G. M. EDELMAN & B. A. CUNNINGHAM. 1986. J. Cell Biol. **102:** 189-193.

10. HEMPERLY, J. J., G. M. EDELMAN & B. A. CUNNINGHAM. 1986. Proc. Natl. Acad. Sci. USA **83:** 9822-9826.

11. HOFFMAN, S. & G. M. EDELMAN. 1983. Proc. Natl. Acad. Sci USA **80:** 5762-5766.

12. PREDIGER, E. A., S. HOFFMAN, G. M. EDELMAN & B. A. CUNNINGHAM. 1988. Proc. Natl. Acad. Sci. USA **85:** 9616-9620.

13. DICKSON, G., H. J. GOWER, C. H. BARTON, H. M. PRENTICE, V. L. ELSOM, S. E. MOORE, R. D. COX, C. QUINN, W. PUTT & F. S. WALSH. 1987. Cell **50:** 1119-1130.

14. WALSH, R. E. 1988. Neurochem. Int. **12:** 262-267.

15. CHIQUET-EHRISMANN, R., E. J. MACKIE, C. A. PERSON & T. SAKAKURA. 1986. Cell **47:** 131-139.

16. ERICKSON, H. P. & J. L. IGLESIAS. 1984. Nature **311:** 267-269.

17. HOFFMAN, S., K. L. CROSSIN & G. M. EDELMAN. 1988. J. Cell Biol. **106:** 519-532.

18. GRUMET, M., S. HOFFMAN, K. L. CROSSIN & G. M. EDELMAN. 1985. Proc. Natl. Acad. Sci. USA **82:** 8075-8079.

19. JONES, F. S., M. P. BURGOON, S. HOFFMAN, K. L. CROSSIN, B. A. CUNNINGHAM & G. M. EDELMAN. 1988. Proc. Natl. Acad. Sci. USA **85:** 2186-2190.

20. JONES, F. S., S. HOFFMAN, B. A. CUNNINGHAM & G. M. EDELMAN. 1989 Proc. Natl. Acad. Sci. USA **86:** 1905-1909.

21. BOURDON, M. A., T. KRUSIUS, S. CAMPBELL, N. B. SCHWARTZ & E. RUOSLAHTI. 1987. Proc. Natl. Acad. Sci. USA **84:** 3194-3198.

22. COOKE, R. M., A. J. WILKINSON, M. BARON, A. PASTORE, M. J. TAPPIN, I. D. CAMPBELL, H. GREGORY & B. SHEARD. 1987. Nature **327:** 339-341.

23. KORNBLIHTT, A. R., K. VIBE-PEDERSEN & F. E. BARALLE. 1984. EMBO. J. **3:** 221-226.

24. DANG, C. V., R. F. EBERT & W. R. BELL. 1985. J. Biol. Chem. **260:** 9713-9719.

25. FRIEDLANDER, D. R., S. HOFFMAN & G. M. EDELMAN. 1988. J. Cell Biol. **107:** 2329-2340.

26. CHIQUET-EHRISMANN, R., P. KALLA, C. A. PEARSON, K. BECK & M. CHIQUET. 1988. Cell **53:** 383-390.

27. HOFFMAN, S. & G. M. EDELMAN. 1987. Proc. Natl. Acad. Sci. USA **84:** 2523-2527.

28. CROSSIN, K. L., C.-M. CHUONG & G. M. EDELMAN. 1985. Proc. Natl. Acad. Sci. USA **82:** 6942-6946.

29. CROSSIN, K. L., S. HOFFMAN, M. GRUMET, J.-P. THIERY & G. M. EDELMAN. 1986. J. Cell Biol. **102:** 1917-1930.

30. KITTEN, G. T., R. R. MARKWALD & D. L. BOLENDER. 1987. Anat. Rec. **217:** 379-390.

31. MARKWALD, R. R., R. B. RUNYAN, G. T. KITTEN, F. M. FUNDERBERG, D. H. BERNANKE & P. R. BRAUER. 1984. *In* The Role of the Extracellular Matrix in Development. 323-350. Alan R. Liss. New York.

32. RIEGER, F., M. GRUMET & G. M. EDELMAN. 1985. J. Cell Biol. **101:** 285-293.

33. LITTLE, C. D., D. M. PIQUET, L. A. DAVIS & C. V. DRAKE. 1989. Anat. Rec. **224:** 417-425.

34. KRUSE, J., R. MAILHAMMER, H. WERNECKE, A. FAISSNER, I. SOMMER, C. GORIDIS & M. SCHACHNER. 1984. Nature **311:** 155-157.

35. DUBAND, J.-L., S. DUFOUR, K. HATTA, M. TAKEICHI, G. M. EDELMAN & J.-P. THIERY. 1987. J. Cell Biol. **104:** 1361-1374.

36. ROVASIO, R. A., A. DELOUVÉE, K. M. YAMADA, R. TIMPL & J.-P. THIERY. 1983. J. Cell Biol. **96:** 462-473.

37. TAN, S.-S., K. L. CROSSIN, S. HOFFMAN & G. M. EDELMAN. 1987. Proc. Natl. Acad. Sci. USA **84:** 7977-7981.

Potential Role of the Extracellular Matrix in Postseptation Development of the Heart[a]

THOMAS K. BORG,[b] DOMINIC S. RASO,[c] AND
LOUIS TERRACIO[c]

[b]Department of Pathology
[c]Department of Anatomy
University of South Carolina
Columbia, South Carolina 29208

INTRODUCTION

The components of the extracellular matrix (ECM) have been shown to influence numerous phenotypic and genetic changes in the maturation of several tissues and organs.[1-3] There have been relatively few investigations, however, on the role of various ECM components on the development of the heart. Most of the recent experimentation on the potential role of ECM components has been focused on the early stages during the formation of the heart where the ECM may be responsible for the signaling of migration, cell sorting, and adhesion.[4,5] But equally important is the stimulation provided by the ECM in the late fetal and early neonatal stages in the development of the heart. The responses during these later stages of fetal development are similar to those expressed by the mature heart in response to physiological stimuli present in disease and/or stress situations.[6]

ECM components present in the heart during development are quantitatively but not qualitatively similar to the adult.[7-9] The ECM consists of three basic components: collagens; glycoproteins; and proteoglycans and glycosaminoglycans.[10,11] The collagens are primarily the interstitial types I and III with type IV present in the basement membranes surrounding individual myocytes. The presence of collagen type V has been reported by some investigators and not by others.[8,12] Several glycoproteins of the ECM are present at various times of development, including fibronectin, laminin, merosin, entactin (nidogen) and others.[4,13,14] The presence of various proteoglycans and glycosaminoglycans has clearly shown the presence of dermatan sulfate, chondrotin sulfate, and hyaluronic acid.[15-19]

Recent investigations have demonstrated that the qualitative arrangement of the ECM components is in part dictated by the presence of specific receptors for the individual components.[7] These receptors belong to the superfamily of integrins and are involved in the recognition of several ECM components, including collagen, fi-

[a]This work was funded in part by NIH Grants HL 40424, HL 42299, HL 37669, and HL 24935.

bronectin, and laminin.[20–22] The integrins represent transmembrane receptors that have been proposed to integrate information from the extracellular matrix to the internal cytoplasm of the individual cells.[23,24]

One of the primary events in the development of the heart that occurs after septation is morphological formation of the ventricular chambers and the growth of the myocytes by hypertrophy and limited hyperplasia.[7] These events are profoundly influenced by both physical and chemical factors.[25] The mechanical influences such as tension and muscular contraction are dealt with elsewhere in this volume. The focus of this report is the chemical effects of the ECM on postseptational development, with particular emphasis on the collagen network and its receptor.

MATERIALS AND METHODS

Animals

Time-pregnant rats were obtained from Sprague-Dawley and sacrificed on specific days. Following anesthesia, fetuses were removed and decapitated. The hearts were dissected directly into 2% paraformaldehyde in Sorenson's phosphate buffer and processed for light or electron microscopy as previously described.[14,26]

Immunofluorescence Microscopy

Following fixation, the hearts were quenched with 0.1 M glycine and processed for double immunofluorescence or immunoperoxidase staining using antibodies against interstitial collagen types I and III and the receptors for B_1 integrin specific for interstitial collagens.[22] The antibodies for integrins were made from rat cardiac muscle following the procedures described by Gullberg *et al.*[22]

RESULTS AND DISCUSSION

Staining with antisera against interstitial collagens types I and III and fibronectin demonstrated the presence of very little collagen in association with the myocardium. Both types of antisera, however, showed the presence of these collagens in the forming valvular regions. Differences in the presence of either type I or type III could not be detected. Similar patterns in the myocardium were also seen with antisera against fibronectin.[8] Scanning electron microscopy of the developing hearts revealed little development of the connective tissue network. The surface of the myocytes appears relatively smooth; however, some regions show the formation of Z bands (FIG. 1). The bundles of collagen present at this time are usually associated with fibroblasts (FIG. 1).

The antibodies against the collagen receptor clearly stained regions where collagenous connective tissue would eventually be present, such as in the regions of valve formation and trabeculation (FIGURES 2, 3, and 4). The cardiac cushions, cardiac skeleton, trabeculae, and pericardium all showed the presence of the collagen receptor. Regions near the cardiac cushions showed invaginations of stain into the myocardium, indicating the strong correlation between the cushions and the connective tissue in the presumptive valve-forming region (FIG. 3). The trabeculae exhibited positive staining in 13-day fetal hearts (FIG. 4). As the ventricular chamber underwent changes in shape, the pattern of staining was always associated with regions where collagen deposition would be expected to be increased.

In later stages of development (neonatal), the connective tissue rapidly develops with the increased pressure observed after birth.[26] Previous studies indicate that the

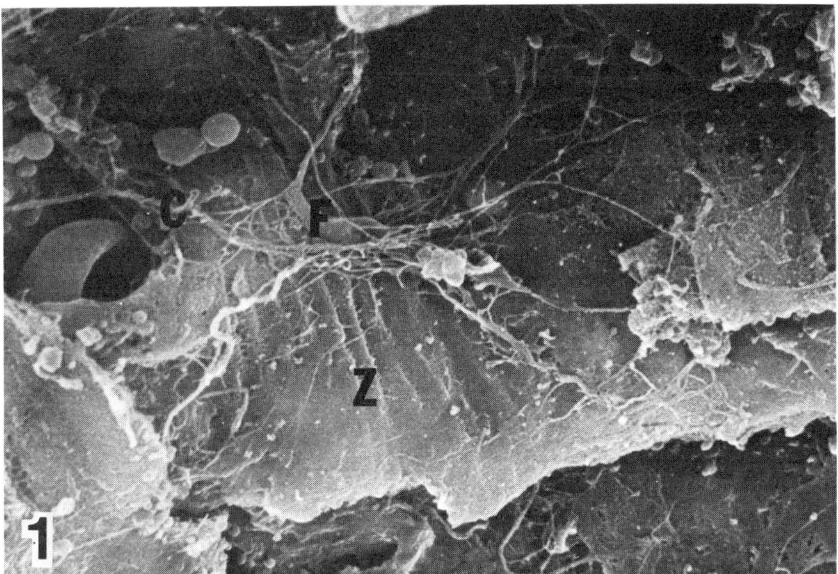

FIGURE 1. Scanning electron micrograph of developing myocytes showing collagen (C) associated with fibroblasts (F) on the surface of the myocytes. Note that the Z bands (Z) of the myocytes are incompletely developed.

connective tissue forms in response to increased pressure from both development and disease.[6]

Studies now indicate that receptors are present before the expression of the specific ECM components. The factor(s) that are responsible for the upregulation of the receptors are unknown; however, current data suggest that growth factors such as PDGF and TGF-β are both capable of regulating the synthesis of integrins as well as ECM components.[27,28] Recent investigations have shown that at least TGF-β is present in high titers at times when the integrins are also being expressed. Further investigations are necessary to determine the role of the growth factors and their potential role in regulation of both components of the ECM and the specific ECM receptors. It will be significant to determine how these factors are associated with the differentiation of the myocytes, as the integrins have been proposed to be molecules

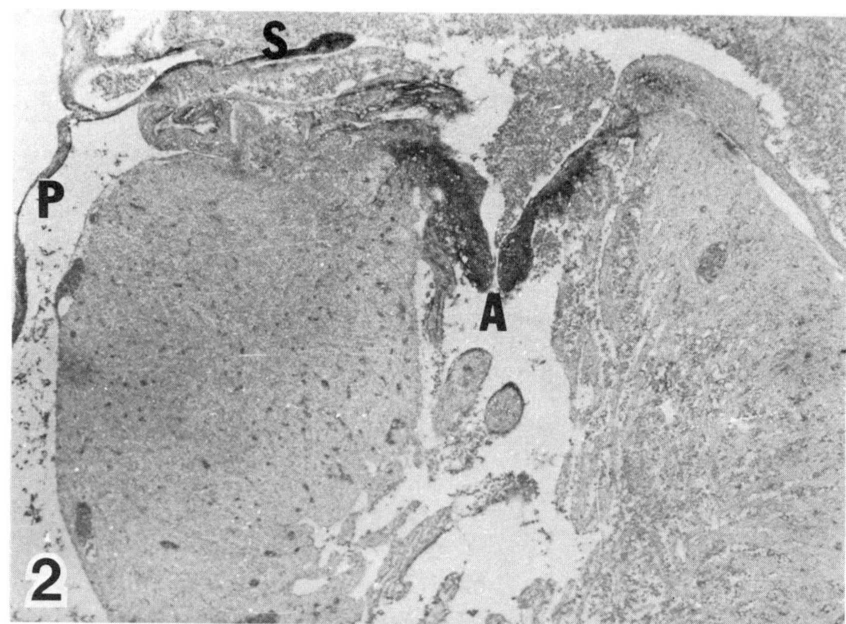

FIGURE 2. Immunohistochemical staining of a 19-day fetal rat heart with antibodies against the B_1 integrin, with specificity for collagen, showing the intense staining around the atrioventricular valves (A), pericardium (P), and projection of the pericardium between the atrium and ventricle to form the cardiac skeleton (S).

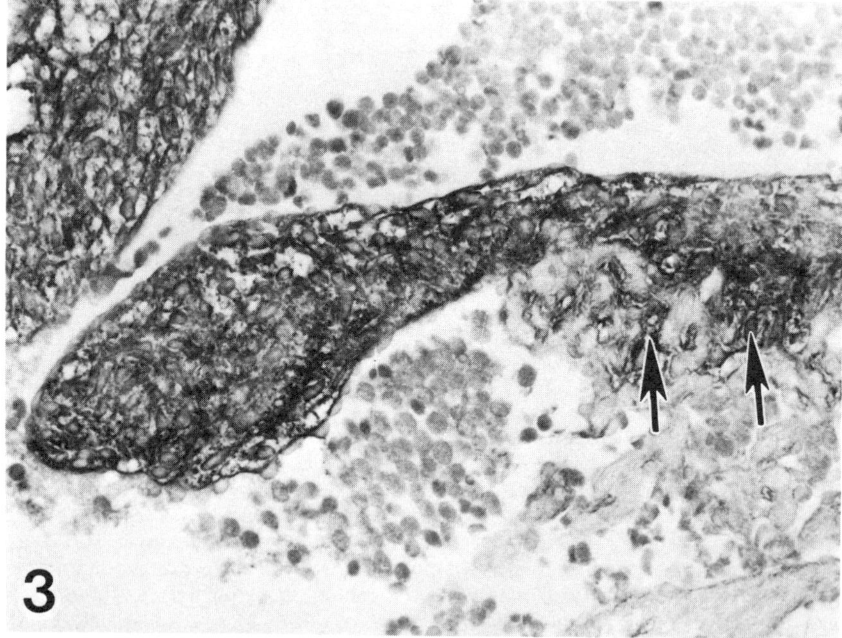

FIGURE 3. High magnification of immunohistochemical staining of 19-day fetal rat heart, showing the reaction product within the forming valve as well as in the myocardium (arrows).

that translate information from the ECM across the sarcolemma to the cytoskeleton.[24,29,30]

ACKNOWLEDGMENTS

The authors would like to thank Benny Davidson and Caleb Roberts for their technical assistance.

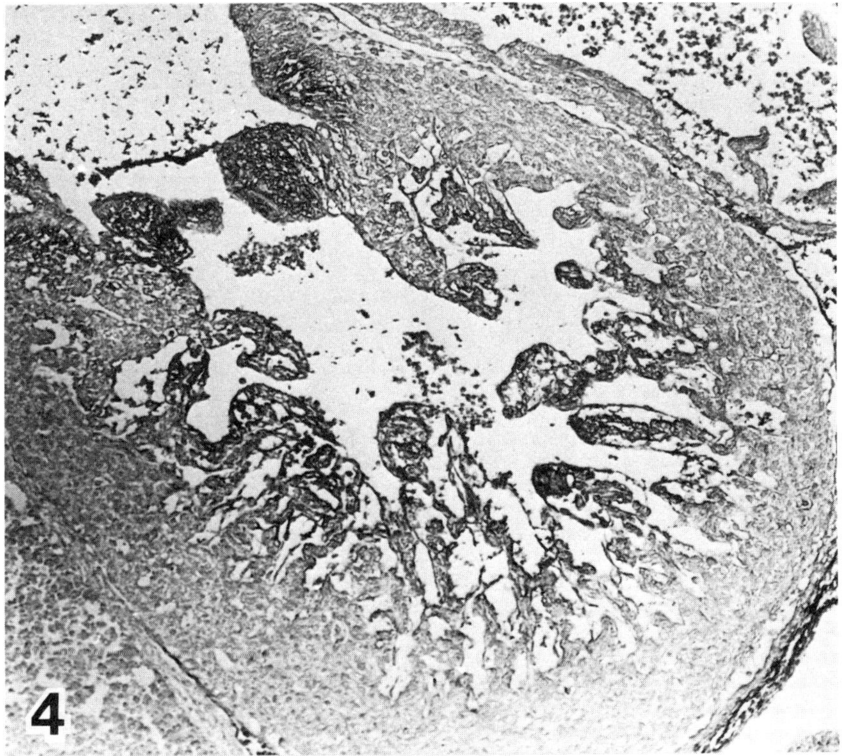

FIGURE 4. Immunohistochemical staining of 15-day fetal rat heart showing the intense reaction product associated with the trabeculae of the left ventricle as well as in the endocardial cushions and adjacent myocardium.

REFERENCES

1. EDELMAN, G. M. 1986. Annu. Rev. Cell Biol. **2:** 81–116.
2. BISSELL, M. J., H. G. HALL & G. PARRY. 1982. J. Theor. Biol. **99:** 31–68.
3. ECKBLOM, P., D. VESTWEBER & R. KEMLER. 1986. Annu. Rev. Cell Biol. **2:** 27–48.
4. RUNYAN, R. B., J. VERSALOVIC & B. D. SHUR. 1988. J. Cell Biol. **107:** 1863–1872.
5. KROTOSKE, D. M., C. DOMINGO & M. BRONNER-FRASER. J. Cell Biol. **103:** 1061–1071.

6. BORG, T. K. & L. TERRACIO. 1988. Issues in Biomedicine. T. Robinson, Ed. S. Karger AG. Basal.
7. TERRACIO, L. & T. K. BORG. 1988. Heart Failure **4:** 114-124.
8. BORG, T. K., R. GAY & L. D. JOHNSON. 1982. Collagen Relat. Res. **2:** 211-218.
9. BORG, T. K., M. XUEHUI, L. HILENSKI, N. VINSON & L. TERRACIO. 1989. *In* Congenital Heart Defects. A. Takao, Ed. Aseni Press. Tokyo, Japan.
10. BORG, T. K., T. SULLIVAN & J. IVY. 1982. Scanning Electron Microsc. **IV:** 1775-1784.
11. ROBINSON, T. F., S. M. FACTOR, J. M. CAPASSO, J. M. WHITTENBURG, O. O. BLUMENFELD & S. SEIFTER. 1987. Cell Tissue Res. **249:** 247-255.
12. SHEKHONIN, B. V., S. P. DOMOGATSKY, G. L. IDELSON & V. E. KOTELIANSKY. 1988. J. Mol. Cell. Cardiol. **20:** 501-508.
13. KITTEN, G. T., R. R. MARKWALD & D. L. BOLENDER. 1987. Anat. Rec. **217:** 379-390.
14. LUNDGREN, E., D. GULLBERG, K. RUBIN, T. K. BORG, M. J. TERRACIO & L. TERRACIO. 1988. J. Cell. Physiol. **136:** 43-53.
15. KRUG, E., C. H. MJAATVEDT & R. R. MARKWALD. 1987. Dev. Biol. **120:** 348-355.
16. FUNDERBURG, F. M. & R. R. MARKWALD. 1987. J. Cell Biol. **103:** 2475-2487.
17. WOODS, A., J. COUCHMAN & M. HOOK. 1985. J. Biol. Chem. **260:** 10872-10879.
18. BORG, T. K. & L. TERRACIO. 1988. *In* Biology of Isolated Adult Cardiac Myocytes. W. Clark, R. Decker & T. BORG, Eds. Elsevier. New York.
19. TERRACIO, L. & T. K. BORG. 1988. *In* Biology of Isolated Adult Cardiac Myocytes. W. Clark, R. Decker & T. Borg, Eds. Elsevier. New York.
20. RUOSLAHTI, E. & M. D. PIERSCHBACHER. 1987. Science **238:** 491-497.
21. HYNES, R. O. 1987. Cell **48:** 549-554.
22. GULLBERG, D., L. TERRACIO, T. K. BORG & K. RUBIN. 1989. J. Biol. Chem. **264:** 12686-12694.
23. TERRACIO, L., D. GULLBERG, K. RUBIN & T. K. BORG. 1989. Anat. Rec. **223:** 62-71.
24. HORWITZ, A., F. DUGGAN, C. BUCK, M. C. BERKERLE & K. BURRIDGE. 1986. Nature **320:** 531-533.
25. TERRACIO, L., B. MILLER & T. K. BORG. 1988. In Vitro **24:** 53-58.
26. BORG, T. K., L. D. JOHNSON & R. GAY. 1983. Dev. Biol. **97:** 417-423.
27. IGNOTZ, R. & J. MASSAGUE. 1986. J. Biol. Chem. **261:** 4337-4345.
28. THOMPSON, N. L., K. C. FLANDERS, J. M. SMITH, L. R. ELLINGSWORTH, A. B. ROBERTS & M. B. SPORN. 1989. J. Cell Biol. **108:** 661-669.
29. HILENSKI, L. L., L. TERRACIO, R. SAWYER & T. K. BORG. 1989. Scanning Microscopy **3:** 535-548.
30. TERRACIO, L., A. TINGSTRÖM, W. H. PETERS III & T. K. BORG. 1990. A potential role for mechanical stimulation in cardiac development. Ann. N.Y. Acad. Sci. This volume.

Voltage-Dependent Gating of Gap Junctional Conductance in Embryonic Chick Heart[a]

RICHARD D. VEENSTRA

Department of Pharmacology
State University of New York
Health Science Center
Syracuse, New York 13210

INTRODUCTION

Gap junctions are well-established very early in cardiac development, as evidenced by the presence of synchronous electrical activity in the chick heart by the 9-somite stage (30-35 h).[1] Besides the obvious function of electrical coupling associated with normal cardiac function, gap junction channels are of sufficient size (10-20 Å in diameter) to permit the intercellular diffusion of small molecules of up to 1000 daltons in size in mammalian cells.[2-4] Such molecules could include second messengers and morphogens that act as regulatory or inductive signals during embryonic development.[5,6] The evidence that gap junctions play a direct role in the cell-cell transfer of developmental signals remains largely correlative,[7,8] but this concept has gained support from recent experiments that demonstrate that disruption of junctional communication by injection of gap junction antibodies can produce pattern defects in developing tissues.[9,10] A key factor in the process is the regulation of junctional permeability that restricts the movement of the intracellular signal-carrying molecule. Several factors have been reported to affect short-term or long-term regulation of gap junction communication, including intracellular pH, intracellular Ca^{2+}, and a variety of protein kinases.[6] One regulatory mechanism that is often found to regulate gap junctional communication in developing embryonic tissues, but not in adult tissues, is transjunctional voltage (V_j). These observations are summarized in TABLE 1, including recent reports of V_j-dependent cardiac gap junctions in paired embryonic chick ventricular myocytes.[15,16] This process in 7-day embryonic heart shares many of the functional characteristics of voltage-dependent gap junctions as first described in amphibian blastomeres.[11,16] This report summarizes these observations by employing a quantitative (Boltzmann) model to derive parameters that express the relative voltage sensitivity of the system. Key assumptions about the model's gating kinetics were examined using macroscopic and single gap junction channel currents. Finally, these procedures were extended to include 4- and 14-day embryonic chick heart to determine whether changes in the V_j sensitivity occur during development.

[a] This work was supported by NIH Grant #HL-42220 and AHA Grant-in-Aid #880708.

TABLE 1. Transjunctional Voltage Dependence of Vertebrate Gap Junctions

Preparation	Voltage Gated (V_j)	Reference No.
Blastomeres		
amphibian	yes	11
Ambystoma	yes	11
Rana	yes	11
Xenopus	yes	11
fish	yes	12
squid	yes	13
Xenopus (connexin38)	yes	14
Embryonic heart		
7-day chick	yes	15, 16
Mammalian liver		
adult rat	no	17, 18
Mammalian heart		
adult rat	no	19, 20, 21
adult guinea pig	no	22, 23

METHODS

Ventricular tissue from 4-, 7-, or 14-day embryonic chick hearts was dissociated into its cellular components by modification of previously published procedures.[24,25] The resultant cell suspension contains 85-90% single cells plus several small clusters of two or more cells. Primary cultures containing $2 \times 10^{+5}$ cells/plate were prepared using solutions and methods as previously described.[26,27] Plates were washed with serum-free balanced saline solution after 22-28 h incubation *in vitro* immediately prior to experimentation and are termed 4-day, 7-day, or 14-day with reference to the age of the donor embryo.

All electrophysiological experiments were performed on paired myocytes at room temperature (20-22 °C) using standard whole-cell patch clamp procedures.[28] Macroscopic junctional current (I_j) and conductance (G_j) were measured directly using the double voltage-clamp technique with independent patch clamp amplifiers as previously described.[11,26,27] Initially, both cells (1 and 2) are voltage-clamped to the same membrane potential ($V_1 = V_2$) in order to determine the background holding currents ($I_1 = I_{m1}$ and $I_2 = I_{m2}$). Next, a transjunctional voltage (V_j) gradient is produced by depolarizing or hyperpolarizing V_1 while V_2 is held constant. Under these conditions, I_j is recorded as the change in I_2 (ΔI_2) during the V_j pulse ($V_j = V_2 - V_1$) and gives a direct measure of G_j when divided by V_j. Only ΔI_2 is taken as a measure of I_j, although I_j must be recorded as a current of opposite polarity and equal magnitude by the two voltage clamp circuits for V_1 and V_2 to be held constant ($\Delta I_1 = \Delta I_{m1} - I_j$; $\Delta I_2 = I_{m2} + I_j$).[11,26,27] Voltages and currents were stored on VCR tape with a Neuro-corder model DR-484 digitizer (Neuro Data Instruments, New York, NY) and transferred to an IBM PC/AT for final analysis.

RESULTS

To investigate the modulation of G_j by V_j in embryonic chick ventricular myocytes, V_1 was stepped from a holding potential of -40 mV ($= V_2$) for a duration of 1 s in

10 mV increments to produce V_j values ranging from -90 to $+90$ mV. To ensure that each V_j pulse was administered under identical conditions, a 5 s recovery interval ($V_1 = V_2 = -40$ mV; $V_j = 0$ mV) was included between tests pulses. Representative I_j traces generated by pulsing one 7-day embryonic chick ventricular cell pair to different V_j values are presented in FIGURE 1. It is evident from this example that I_j remains relatively constant for the entire duration of the pulse when $V_j \leq \pm 30$ mV.

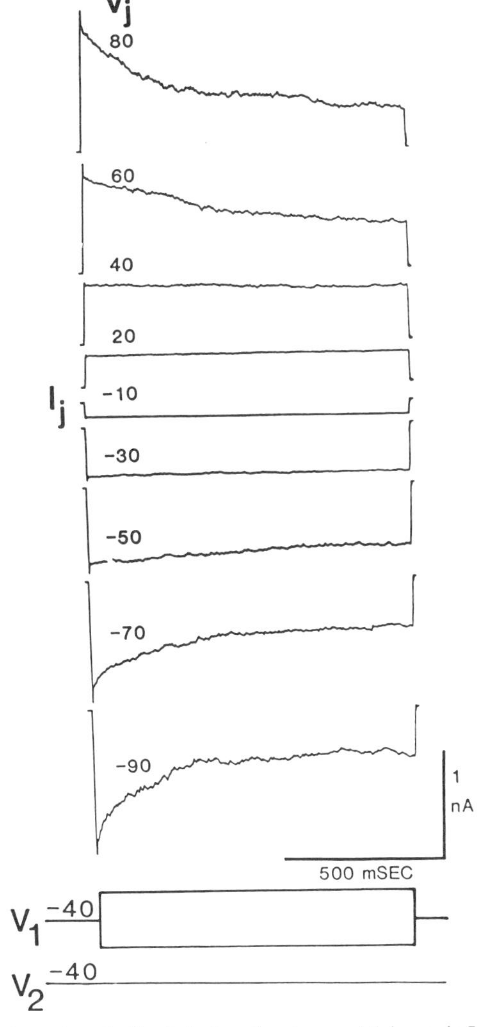

FIGURE 1. Voltage-dependent decline in I_j. Junctional current (change in I_2), during one second pulses to indicated V_j values, undergoes a time-dependent decay when V_j exceeds ± 30 mV. Instantaneous (onset of pulse) G_j values ranged from 10.8 to 12.5 nS, and steady-state (end of pulse) G_j values ranged from 3.6 to 11.8 nS for the currents shown. Low pass filter frequency = 200 Hz, and digital sample rate = 500 Hz. $V_1 = V_2 = -40$ mV, with V_1 stepped once every five seconds to new potentials ranging from -130 to $+50$ mV in 10 mV increments as indicated in the inset. Prep #7d815.

When $V_j > 30$ mV, however, I_j undergoes a time- and V_j-dependent decay towards new steady-state values. The instantaneous I_j, measured at the onset of the pulse, appears to rise linearly and decays more rapidly towards steady-state values as V_j increases.

The voltage-dependence of I_j is best illustrated by plotting the instantaneous and steady-state I_j values as a function of V_j, as shown in FIGURE 2. The instantaneous I_j-V_j relationship for the data shown in FIGURE 1 approximates a straight line with a slope of 11.9 nS over the entire voltage range. The steady-state I_j-V_j curve also has a linear slope of 11.5 nS within the range of ± 30 mV, but rectifies to a constant value above these voltages. The V_j-dependent rectification appears to be symmetrical about the origin, which suggests a bilateral voltage-gated mechanism.

Because instantaneous I_j (and G_j) remains linear with V_j, steady-state G_j (G_{ss}) was normalized to the initial G_j (G_{inst}) at the beginning of each pulse and plotted as a function of V_j. The results, taken from five different 7-day cell pairs, are summarized in FIGURE 3. V_j protocols were identical to that described for FIGURE 1, with the addition of reversing the order of the voltage protocol by stepping V_2 and holding V_1 constant at -40 mV ($V_j = V_1 - V_2$). The results were found to be similar whether V_1 or V_2 was stepped. Both trials are included in the final analysis of each experiment. Steady-state G_j decreases rapidly between V_j values of ± 40 to ± 80 mV, leveling off near 0.38 at ± 90 mV and approaching unity as V_j approaches 0 mV. This steady-state G_j-V_j curve has a similar shape to that reported for other voltage-dependent gap junctions, so the experimental data was fit using the same two-state (open-closed) model proposed by previous authors.[11] The solid line represents the best fit of the data, assuming a two-state Boltzmann distribution of the form

$$(G_{ss} - G_{min})/(G_{max} - G_{ss}) = \exp[-A(V_j - V_o)]$$

where V_o is the half-inactivation voltage for the voltage-sensitive conductance, and A is a constant expressing the strength of the interaction of the open channel with V_j.[11,29] The constant A is equivalent to nq/kT, where n is the equivalent number of electron charges (q) that act as the gating mechanism by sensing changes in V_j, and k and T

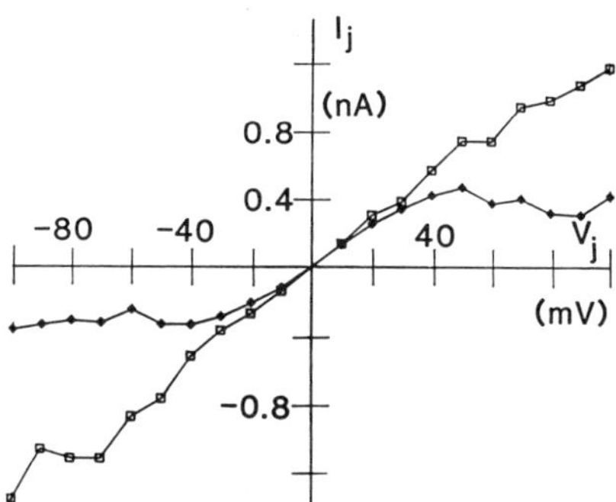

FIGURE 2. Instantaneous and steady-state I_j-V_j relationships of 7-day embryonic chick gap junctions. Instantaneous and steady-state I_j for the experiment shown in FIGURE 1 were plotted as a function of V_j. The instantaneous I_j-V_j relationship is linear with a slope 11.9 nS over the entire voltage range. The steady-state I_j-V_j relationship has a linear slope of 11.5 nS over the range of ± 30 mV, which approaches zero above $V_j = \pm 40$ mV. Key to symbols: $\square$ instantaneous I_j; $\diamond$ steady-state I_j.

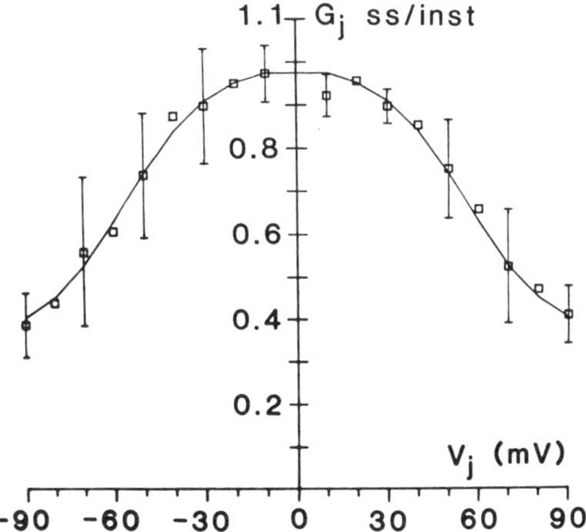

FIGURE 3. Voltage-dependent decline in steady-state G_j. Ratio of steady-state G_j/instantaneous G_j taken from five different 7-day cell pairs using the voltage protocol described in FIGURE 1. Each point represents the average ($\pm$SD) of five experiments. Error bars have been omitted from every other point for reasons of clarity. Steady-state G_j declines with increasing V_j in either direction. The solid line is a theoretical fit of the data assuming a two-state Boltzmann distribution (see text) with A = 0.70 and V_o = 56 mV. Prep #7d810, 7d812-15.

represent Boltzmann's constant and temperature in °K. For this graph, G_{max} = 1.0, G_{min} = 0.35, and G_{ss} are the experimentally derived steady-state G_j values. For the curve shown in FIGURE 4, n = 1.78 and V_o = 56 mV.

The model assumes the voltage-sensitive transition between the two states to be a first order, reversible process. As a test of this assumption, the time-dependent decay of G_j was examined. FIGURE 4 is a semilog plot of G_j for several V_j values based on the methods of Harris et al.[29] For each V_j, steady-state G_j was subtracted from time-dependent G_j and plotted as $\ln(G_j\text{-}G_{ss})$, with the y intercept given by $\ln(G_{inst})$ and the slope equal to $\ln(G_{inst}\text{-}G_{ss})$. These results are taken from a single 7-day cell pair. In all cases, the G_j-time relationship is linear, confirming a monoexponential decay process. The decay time constant is also observed to become faster with increasing V_j of either polarity, ranging from 133 ms at +90 mV to 1.136 s at −50 mV in this particular experiment.

The recovery of G_j upon returning to V_j = 0 mV was also examined to determine if this process followed a similar exponential time course. To address this question, a 20 mV, 100 ms prepulse was applied at different intervals following a 1 s inactivating V_j pulse to 80 mV. The purpose of the prepulse was to provide a measurement of G_j immediately prior to returning to an inactivating potential. At the end of the 20 mV prepulse, V_j was again stepped to 80 mV for 1 s, and instantaneous G_j measurements were obtained. Each experiment was normalized to the maximum G_j attained during the recovery phase, and the results of five experiments are summarized in FIGURE 5. In all five experiments, maximum G_j was achieved after a 5 s recovery interval, which did not increase further with longer recovery intervals of up to 10 seconds. G_j, observed at V_j = 20 (FIG. 5, top panel) or 80 mV (FIG. 5, middle panel), also follows an exponential time course with a rate constant of 1.1 second. This rate of recovery is five times slower than the decay rate constants presented in FIGURE 4 (225 ms at +80 mV). The instantaneous G_j at V_j = 80 mV varied by no more than 7% from

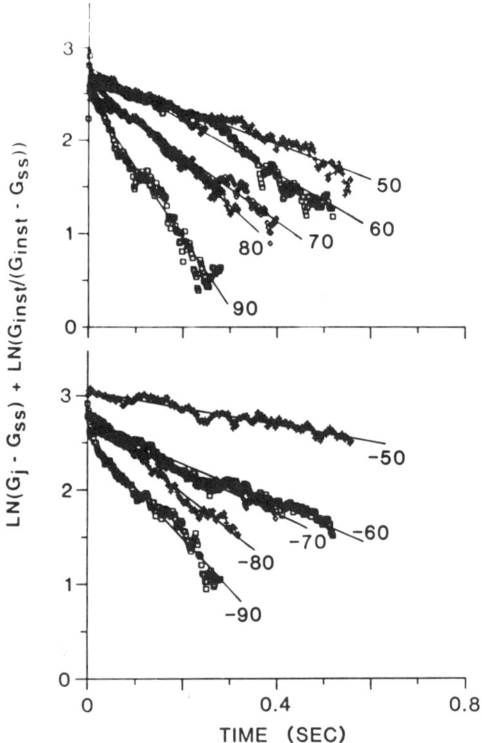

FIGURE 4. Time-dependent decay of G_j. A semilog plot of G_j versus time at several transjunctional potentials for the junctional currents illustrated in FIGURES 1 and 2. Each trace is best fit by a straight line indicative of a monoexponential function. The decay time constants become faster as V_j increases in either direction. Actual time constants are (in ms): -90, 186; -80, 256; -70, 432; -60, 467; -50, 1136; 90, 133; 80, 225; 70, 286; 60, 351; 50, 537. Based on methods of Harris *et al.*[29]

G_j values measured at $V_j = 20$ mV (FIG. 5, bottom panel), further indicating that G_j increases ohmically with the onset of large V_j values.

The above procedures were extended to cell pairs isolated from 4- and 14-day embryonic ventricular myocytes to determine if developmental differences in V_j-sensitivity were present. The same voltage protocol as that described in FIGURE 1 was used with one minor modification. The duration of the V_1 test pulse was lengthened from one to two seconds to provide a better measure of steady-state G_j in the ± 30 to ± 60 mV V_j range. The results are summarized in FIGURE 6. All three normalized steady-state G_j-V_j curves (4-day, 7-day, and 14-day embryonic heart) exhibit a V_j-dependent decline that approaches a minimum at ± 100 mV. There are subtle differences, however, in the shape of each curve, which are most pronounced in the lower range of potentials. Below V_j values of ± 50 mV, steady-state G_j becomes progressively higher with increasing developmental age, achieving differences of 30% between 4-day and 14-day heart (4-day $= 0.65 \pm 0.15$, 14-day $= 0.95 \pm 0.06$ at $V_j = \pm 30$ mV). The solid lines again represent the theoretical fit of the data assuming the same two-state Boltzmann distribution described above. A full comparison of the important parameters derived from the theoretical fit of the three G_j-V_j curves is presented in TABLE 2. The most striking feature is that the half-inactivation voltage, V_o, gradually shifts outward from 40 to 57 mV in 4-day and 14-day heart, respectively.

The model also assumes that the voltage-dependent changes in G_j are the result of gating of individual channels, although this was not possible to demonstrate in blastomere pairs. Single gap junction channel currents, however, can be observed in embryonic chick cell pairs under appropriate conditions ($G_j < 2$ nS).[26,27] In those experiments where single channel currents were observed during V_j pulses, the single

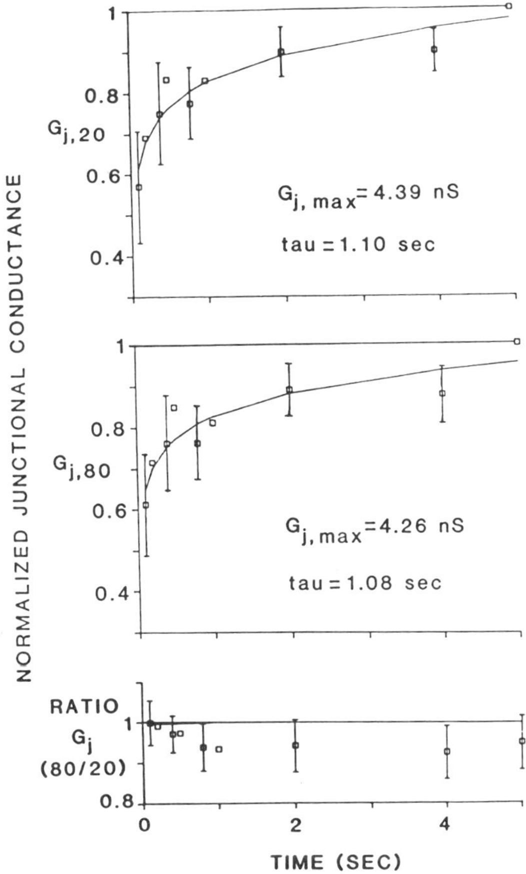

FIGURE 5. Time-dependent recovery of G_j. The time interval between 80 mV, 1 s V_j pulses ($V_1 = -80$ mV, $V_2 = 0$ mV), was varied between 0.1 to 5 s, and the recovery of G_j was examined by a 20 mV, 100 ms prepulse immediately preceding the next 80 mV pulse. G_j values at 20 mV (top panel) and instantaneous G_j at 80 mV (middle panel) are plotted as a function of the recovery interval. Each point represents the average ($\pm$ SD) of 5 experiments, and the solid line represents the exponential fit of the data. G_j increased exponentially with similar time constants for both curves, achieving a maximum at 5 s in all five experiments. Longer recovery intervals (8-10 s) did not produce any further increase in G_j. The ratio of instantaneous G_j, 80 mV/G_j, 20 mV (bottom panel) varied from 0.93 to 1.0. Prep #7d810, 7d812-15.

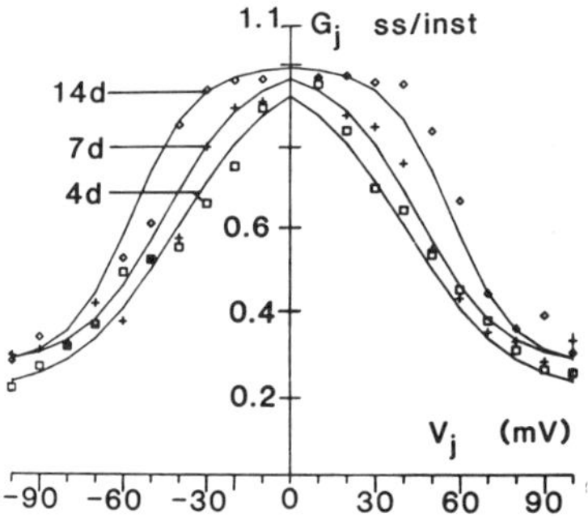

FIGURE 6. Normalized steady-state G_j-V_j relationship of 4-day, 7-day, and 14-day embryonic cardiac gap junctions. Normalized G_j-V_j curve for three developmental ages using the exact same procedures outlined in FIGURE 3 except for lengthening the V_j pulse duration from 1 to 2 seconds. Each symbol represents the average of 4 or more trials, and the line is the theoretical fit assuming the Boltzmann distribution described in the text. Pertinent experimental and theoretical parameters are summarized in TABLE 2. Key to symbols: □ 4-day; + 7-day; and ◇ 14-day.

gap junction channel current-voltage relationship was linear, with a slope of 145 pS (data not shown). These results are consistent with previous observations in embryonic chick heart and suggest that the channels themselves do not rectify.[27]

Repetitive V_j pulses to inactivating potentials exhibit channel behavior which, when averaged together, resemble the time-course of I_j decay observed in high conductance junctions. This point is illustrated in FIGURE 7, where the junctional current obtained by averaging five individual I_j traces from a 14-day cell pair with an instantaneous $G_j < 0.6$ nS is displayed. Each arrow marks the closure of an individual gap junction channel, and it is readily observed that two or more channel closures occur during each pulse to $V_j = +80$ mV. The single channel conductance of these events averaged 175 pS in this experiment. The decay of the average current follows an exponential time course with a time constant of 207 ms, nearly identical to the value observed in FIGURE 4 ($V_j = 80$ mV, $\tau = 225$ ms).

DISCUSSION

From the above findings in embryonic chick heart, it is obvious that I_j is time- and voltage-dependent. There are four possible mechanisms that could explain this

TABLE 2. Developmental Differences in V_j-Dependent Embryonic Chick Gap Junctions

		Experimental Values			Theoretical Parameters	
Age	N^a	G_{max}	G_{min}	A	V_o (mV)	n^b
4-day	8	1.0	0.20	0.055	41	1.39
7-day	4	1.0	0.27	0.068	45	1.72
14-day	4	1.0	0.27	0.088	57	2.22

[a] N = number of trials included in averaged data.
[b] n = number of equivalent electron charges.

time- and voltage-dependent decline in I_j: series resistance errors in clamping the junction (*i.e.* electrode rectification); local ion depletion/accumulation across the junctional membrane (*i.e.* junctional equilibrium potential alterations); reductions in single channel conductance (channel rectification); and reductions in the open-state probability of gap junction channels (all-or-none gating).

The first hypothesis was tested by applying the double whole-cell patch clamp

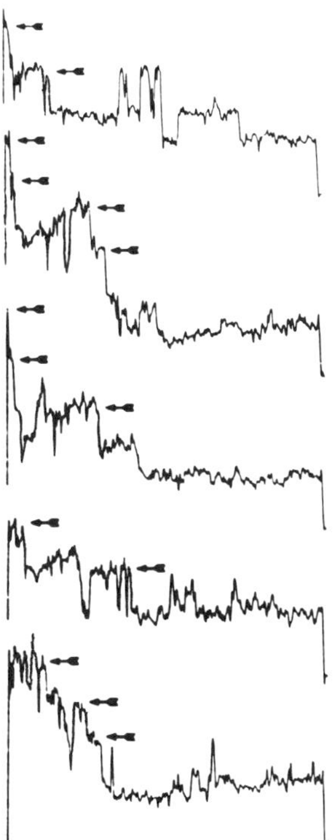

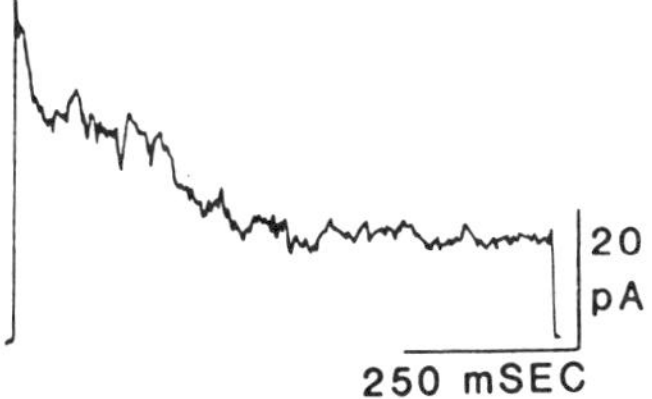

FIGURE 7. Time-dependent closure of single gap junction channels; a train of 80 mV, 750 ms V_j pulses applied in 0.5 s intervals to a 14-day cell pair with G_j < 0.6 nS. All five individual V_j pulses (top five traces) reveal the closure (arrows) of two or more gap junction channels (channel conductance = 170 pS) during the pulse. The bottom trace represents the ensemble average of the above five traces, and the decay phase of the average current can be fit by an exponential function with a time constant of 207 milliseconds. Prep #fd804.

technique to a single 7-day embryonic chick ventricular cell and measuring the electrode response to voltage pulses analogous to the protocol used to examine V_j-dependence. During repetitive 1 s, 80 mV voltage pulses between the two electrodes, currents of opposite polarity and equal amplitude were recorded (data not shown). The currents remained constant for the duration of each pulse and measured 6.15 nA in amplitude. This corresponds to a resistance of 13 MΩ, which is equivalent to the series resistance of the two electrodes. This observation confirms that electrode resistance does not increase during a large amplitude V_j pulse, even when the current flow is five- to sixtyfold higher than I_j recorded from a cell pair.

Double voltage clamp experiments on septal membranes of earthworm median giant axons reveal a time-dependent relaxation of I_j, which also becomes faster with increasing voltage.[30] This phenomenon was shown to be dependent on the local accumulation of an impermeant anion on one side of the junctional membrane and depletion on the other, resulting in changes in the equilibrium potentials for permeant ions across the junction. This time-dependent change in junctional equilibrium potential produces current-dependent current relaxations during the pulse, with time constants of 3-6 seconds. Upon returning to $V_j = 0$ mV, slow time-dependent tail currents are observed as the ions reequilibrate after the pulse. The V_j-dependent currents presented here have decay time constants ranging from 0.1 to 1 s, and tail currents were not observed when stepping back to $V_j = 0$ mV (FIG. 1). This result supports the conclusion that I_j relaxation in cardiac gap junctions does not result from current-dependent ion depletion/accumulation effects on the gap junction.

The two remaining plausible explanations for the V_j dependence of I_j involve two properties of the single gap junction channels, conductance changes and gating behavior. From single-channel current-voltage relationships in embryonic chick heart, it is apparent that the single channel conductance is V_j-independent.[16,27] When successive chick gap junction channel current records obtained in response to a train of 80 mV V_j pulses are signal averaged together, an exponential time course is produced with a decay time constant of 207 milliseconds. This is remarkably similar to the time course observed in high conductance junctions (FIGURES 1 and 4) and is consistent with previous observations in this preparation.[16] Thus, all experimental observations to date support the conclusion that I_j (and G_j) declines as a result of all-or-none gating of a population of V_j-sensitive gap junction channels. The basis of the residual V_j-insensitive I_j remains to be determined. One hypothesis is that there is a second population of gap junction channels with a open-state probability near 1.0 that may be closed only by exposure to known uncoupling agents, such as low pH or octanol.

There are numerous similarities between the voltage-dependent behavior of chick cardiac gap junctions and the gap junctions of amphibian blastomeres.[11] In all cases, the relaxation of I_j became more rapid with increasing V_j; the normalized G_j-V_j curves contain a voltage-insensitive component of G_j, and the voltage-sensitive component of the V_j-G_j curve can be adequately described by a two-state Boltzmann distribution. The amphibian blastomere gap junctions exhibit a stronger voltage dependence, with a calculated gating charge (n) of 6 electrons, half-maximal G_j at a transjunctional voltage (V_o) of 15 mV, and a voltage-insensitive G_j of only 5% of maximum. The steady-state G_j-V_j curves of embryonic chick heart gap junctions exhibit a more gradual slope (n = 1-2), larger half-inactivation voltage $(V_o = 40\text{-}57$ mV), and a larger voltage-insensitive G_j component (20-30% of maximum) than most other embryonic gap junctions.

There is a gradual increase in V_o with developmental age in the chick heart from 41 to 57 mV between the ages of 4 and 14 days, suggesting a loss of V_j sensitivity with development. Observations in neonatal rat and hamster cardiac gap junctions also reveal a voltage- and time-dependent decay in I_j, but only when $V_j \geq \pm 60$ mV.[31,32] The V_j dependence in neonatal rat apparently disappears as G_j of newly forming gap junctions increases,[31] an observation consistent with the lack of V_j dependence in adult mammalian myocardium.[19-23] Although it is tempting to conclude that cardiac gap junctions progressively lose their voltage sensitivity during the developmental process by a shift in V_o towards larger potentials, final proof awaits verification of a lack of V_j dependence in adult chicken or the presence of V_j-dependent gap junctions in fetal mammalian heart. Some of the discrepancies regarding the V_j dependence of cardiac gap junctions could be attributed to differences between chick and mammalian heart. The basis for the apparent disappearance of V_j dependence as G_j increases in newly forming gap junctions also requires further verification. Furthermore, information about the molecular basis of the age-dependent shift in V_o would be helpful in developing an understanding of the conformational changes involved in channel gating.

Definitive proof that V_j-dependent gap junctions play a role in developmental signaling awaits confirmation of two distinct events. First, evidence that electrical field potentials exist within the developing embryo that can account for intercellular permeability barriers must be demonstrated. In the early mammalian zygote, gap junctional communication is well-established in the 8 cell stage when the blastomeres flatten against one another in a process called compaction.[33,34] As a result of this compression, the outer blastomeres acquire, for the first time, a cell surface polarity in the form of an apical/basolateral polarization. This early polarization is followed by localization of mitochondria and Na^+,K^+-ATPase activity to the basolateral surface, which is believed to be causally related to formation of the blastocoele, trophectoderm, and inner cell mass.[34] In an interesting vibrating probe mapping study, Wiley and Nuccitelli[34] propose that an apical-basal transcellular current exists prior to compaction, which further promotes blastomere polarity. Is it also possible that these transcellular currents affect junctional permeability by a voltage-gated mechanism? Such a role has been proposed, but awaits further verification.[35] Second, identification of the morphogenic molecules and proof that they diffuse through gap junctions must also be demonstrated. To date, only two "morphogens" (one being free intracellular Ca^{2+} concentration) have been identified.[36] Obviously, there is still much to be discovered about the mechanisms of establishing morphogenic patterns. Nonetheless, there is mounting evidence (although largely circumstantial) to support the hypothesis that embryonic gap junctions serve a functional role in transmitting developmental signals and that junctional permeability can be modulated by intercellular potentials.

ACKNOWLEDGMENT

I am grateful to Mark Chilton for his technical assistance in tissue culture preparation and data analysis.

REFERENCES

1. FUJII, S., A. HIROTA & K. KAMINO. 1981. Optical indications of pace-maker potential and rhythm generation in early embryonic chick heart. J. Physiol. **312:** 253-263.
2. FLAGG-NEWTON, J., I. SIMPSON & W. R. LOEWENSTEIN. 1979. Permeability of the cell-to-cell membrane channels in mammalian cell junction. Science **205:** 404-407.
3. SCHWARZMANN, G., H. WIEGANDT, B. ROSE, A. ZIMMERMAN, D. BEN-HAIM & W. R. LOEWENSTEIN. 1981. Diameter of the cell-to-cell junctional membrane channels as probed with neutral molecules. Science **213:** 551-553.
4. IMANAGA, I., M. KAMEYAMA & H. IRISAWA. 1987. Cell-to-cell diffusion of fluorescent dyes in paired ventricular cells. Am. J. Physiol. **252:** (Heart Circ. Physiol. 21): H223-H232.

5. CAVENEY, S. 1985. The role of gap junctions in development. Ann. Rev. Physiol. **47:** 319-335.
6. LOEWENSTEIN, W. R. 1987. The cell-to-cell channel of gap junctions. Cell **48:** 725-726.
7. GREEN, C. R. 1988. Evidence mounts for the role of gap junctions during development. Bioessays **8**(1): 7-10.
8. WARNER, A. 1988. The gap junction. J. Cell. Science **89:** 1-7.
9. WARNER, A. E., S. C. GUTHRIE & N. B. GILULA. 1984. Antibodies to gap junctions selectively disrupt junctional communication in the early amphibian embryo. Nature **311:** 127-131.
10. FRASER, S. E., C. R. GREEN, H. R. BODE & N. B. GILULA. 1987. Selective disruption of gap junctional communication interferes with a patterning process in Hydra. Science **237:** 49-55.
11. SPRAY, D. C., A. L. HARRIS & M. V. L. BENNETT. 1981. Equilibrium properties of a voltage-dependent junctional conductance. J. Gen. Physiol. **77:** 77-93.
12. WHITE, R. L., D. C. SPRAY, A. C. CARVALHO & M. V. L. BENNETT. 1982. Voltage-dependent gap junctional conductance between fish embryonic cells. Soc. Neurosci. Abstr. **8:** 944 (Abstr.).
13. SPRAY, D. C., R. L. WHITE, A. C. CAMPOS DE CARVALHO, A. L. HARRIS & M. V. L. BENNETT. 1984. Gating of gap junction channels. Biophys. J. **45:** 219-230.
14. EBIHARA, L., E. C. BEYER, K. I. SWENSON, D. L. PAUL & D. A. GOODENOUGH. 1989. Cloning and expression of a Xenopus embryonic gap junction protein. Science **243:** 1194-1195.
15. CHEN, Y.-H., R. L. PENROD & R. L. DeHAAN. 1988. Conductance of gap junctions in embryonic heart cells is voltage dependent. Abstr. Int. Congress Cell Biol. **4:** 234 (Abstr.).
16. VEENSTRA, R. D. 1989. Voltage-dependent gating of embryonic cardiac gap junction channels. Biophys. J. **55:** 152a (Abstr.).
17. SPRAY, D. C., R. D. GINSBERG, E. A. MORALES, Z. GATMAITAN & I. M. ARIAS. 1986. Electrophysiological properties of gap junctions between dissociated pairs of rat hepatocytes. J. Cell Biol. **103:** 135-144.
18. REVERDIN, E. C. & R. WEINGART. 1988. Electrical properties of the gap junctional membrane studied in rat liver cell pairs. Am. J. Physiol. **254**(Cell Physiol. 23): C226-C234.
19. METZGER, P. & R. WEINGART. 1985. Electric current flow in cell pairs isolated from adult rat hearts. J. Physiol. **366:** 177-195.
20. WHITE, R. L., D. C. SPRAY, A. C. CAMPOS DE CARVALHO, B. A. WITTENBERG & M. V. L. BENNETT. 1985. Some electrical and pharmacological properties of gap junctions between adult ventricular myocytes. Am. J. Physiol. **249**(Cell Physiol. 18): C447-C455.
21. WEINGART, R. 1986. Electrical properties of the nexal membrane studied in rat ventricular cell pairs. J. Physiol. **370:** 267-284.
22. KAMEYAMA, M. 1983. Electrical coupling between ventricular paired cells isolated from guinea-pig heart. J. Physiol. **336:** 345-357.
23. NOMA, A. & N. TSUBOI. 1987. Dependence of junctional conductance on proton, calcium and magnesium ions in cardiac paired cells of guinea-pig. J. Physiol. **382:** 193-211.
24. DeHAAN, R. L. 1970. The potassium-sensitivity of isolated embryonic heart cells increases with development. Dev. Biol. **23:** 226-240.
25. VEENSTRA, R. D. & R. L. DeHAAN. 1986a. Electrotonic interactions between aggregates of chick embryo cardiac pacemaker cells. Am. J. Physiol. **250** (Heart Circ. Physiol. 19): H453-H463.
26. VEENSTRA, R. D. & R. L. DeHAAN. 1986b. Measurement of single gap junction channel currents from cardiac gap junctions. Science **233:** 972-974.
27. VEENSTRA, R. D. & R. L. DeHAAN. 1988. Cardiac gap junction channel activity in embryonic chick ventricle cells. Am. J. Physiol. **254**(Heart Circ. Physiol. 23): H170-H180.
28. HAMILL, O. P., A. MARTY, E. NEHER, B. SAKMANN & F. J. SIGWORTH. 1981. Improved patch-clamp techniques for high-resolution current recording from cells and cell-free membrane patches. Pfluegers Arch. **391:** 85-100.
29. HARRIS, A. L., D. C. SPRAY & M. V. L. BENNETT. 1981. Kinetics of a voltage-dependent junctional conductance. J. Gen. Physiol. **77:** 95-117.

30. BRINK, P. R., R. T. MATHIAS, S. W. JASLOVE & G. J. BALDO. 1988. Steady-state current flow through gap junctions. Effects on intracellular ion concentration and fluid movement. Biophys. J. **53:** 795-807.

31. ROOK, M. B., H. J. JONGSMA & A. C. G. VAN GINNEKEN. 1988. Properties of single gap junctional channels between isolated neonatal rat heart cells. Am. J. Physiol. **255**(Heart Circ. Physiol. 24): H770-H782.

32. VEENSTRA, R. D. 1990. Comparative physiology of cardiac gap junction channels. *In* Biophysics of Gap Junction Channels. C. Peracchia, Ed. CRC Press. Boca Raton, FL. In press.

33. LEE, S., N. B. GILULA & A. E. WARNER. 1987. Gap junctional communication and compaction during preimplantation stages of mouse development. Cell **51:** 851-860.

34. WILEY, L. M. & R. NUCCITELLI. 1986. Detection of transcellular currents and effect of an imposed electric field on mouse blastomeres. *In* Progress in Clinical and Biological Research. R. Nuccitelli, Ed. Vol. 210, Ionic Currents in Development: 197-204. Alan R. Liss, Inc. New York.

35. HARRIS, A. L., D. C. SPRAY & M. V. L. BENNETT. 1983. Control of intercellular communication by voltage dependence of gap junctional conductance. J. Neuroscience 3(1): 79-100.

36. NUCCITELLI, R. 1986. Introduction. *In* Progress in Clinical and Biological Research. R. Nuccitelli, Ed. Vol. 210, Ionic Currents in Development: xv-xxiii. Alan R. Liss, Inc. New York.

Elastogenic Cells in the Developing Cardiovascular System

Smooth Muscle, Nonmuscle, and Cardiac Neural Crest

THOMAS H. ROSENQUIST AND ARTHUR C. BEALL

The Heart Development Group
Department of Anatomy
Medical College of Georgia
Augusta, Georgia 30912-2000

INTRODUCTION

Elastogenesis is initiated in the cardiovascular system of the avian embryo at the interface between the myocardial cuff of the truncus arteriosus and the truncal ectomesenchyme at an early stage of development, and then the elastogenic phenotype is deployed in an orderly downstream sequence.[1] The ectomesenchyme, which propagates elastogenesis, is derived from neural crest[1] that migrates from an area we now may refer to as the "cardiac" neural crest (CNC).[2] Cells of the CNC develop into the elastic mediae of the great vessels[3] and into the truncal septum[4] whose cells express soluble tropoelastin for the entire duration of their function, that is, incubation days 5-8.[1]

The presence of an elastic matrix has obvious implications for the length-tension relationships of the behavior of the embryonic outflow vessels. These relationships, however, are a result of the interaction of both passive (elastic matrix) and active (smooth muscle contractile) factors.[5,6] Thus elastogenesis and the smooth muscle phenotype are closely related in structure and function; indeed elastogenesis is generally recognized as a basic quality of vascular smooth muscle.[7,8] Therefore we hypothesized that the smooth muscle phenotype would be expressed in the same temporal and geographic sequence as the elastogenic phenotype in the outflow vessels, among the same cells of CNC origin. We were encouraged by the studies of Clark,[9] which showed that the time of deployment of the elastic matrix, incubation days 3-5.5, was also a time of dramatic change in the hemodynamics of the developing chicken cardiovascular system. Furthermore the truncal septum is composed of elastogenic smooth muscle cells.[10]

The results of the present study, however, show that the phenotype "elastogenic" (positive binding of antitropoelastin[1]) and the phenotype "smooth muscle" (positive binding of antismooth muscle alpha-actin[10]) are not mutually inclusive in time or space in the outflow tract, and the presence of smooth muscle in the outflow vessels is not contingent upon the arrival of cells from the CNC.

MATERIAL AND METHODS

Fertile Arbor Acre chicken eggs (Central Soya of Athens, GA) were incubated at 38° C and a relative humidity of 97%. Embryos were collected after each of the following incubation intervals: 2 days(2d), 3d, 4.5d, 6d, 8d, 9d, 10d, 12d, 14d, and 19d.

Another set of fertile Arbor Acre chicken eggs from the same source was incubated simultaneously with a set of Japanese quail eggs from the breeding colony of the Heart Development Group of the Medical College of Georgia. After 24-36 h in 100% humidity, quail [donor] and chicken [host] eggs were prepared for microsurgery[11] at Hamburger-Hamilton[12] stage 9. The chicken neural fold over somites 1-3 was excised bilaterally and then was replaced by the homotypic quail neural fold. After the tissue was transplanted, the eggs were sealed and replaced in the incubator. Quail-chicken chimeric embryos were collected after total incubation periods of 4.5d, 6d, 7d, and 8d. In these embryos the cells derived from cardiac neural crest could be identified by the unique configuration of the nucleolus in the quail cell nucleus.[13] Tissue from some of these chimeric embryos has been used in a previous study reported by this laboratory.[1]

Embryos of 2d-10d and the heart-lung-great vessel aggregates of older embryos were placed in a nonaldehyde fixative (methacarn[14]) at 4° C for 12-24 hours. Then they were processed through alcohols and xylenes at 4° C into low melting point "paraplasts" at 57° C. We have found the best preservation of both anatomic detail and epitopes for immunohistochemistry with this procedure.[1] Sections of 10 micrometers were cut and mounted serially on glass slides.

Sections were rehydrated and incubated at 37° C in phosphate-buffered saline, pH 7.4, with 0.5% bovine serum albumin (PBS/BSA). Then they were incubated with 20 microliters/section of the diluted primary antibodies detailed below for 1 h at 37° C, rinsed with PBS, and incubated with 20 microliters/section of the appropriate secondary antibody, labeled in all cases with rhodamine. (For best contrast of the secondary antibody against the brilliant blue-green autofluorescence of some embryonic proteins, fluorescein should be avoided during immunofluorescence studies of embryonic tissues[1]). Each slide carried four or more sections. One section on each slide received neither the primary nor the secondary antibody, one section received only the secondary antibody, and the two or more remaining sections received both the primary and the secondary antibody. Details of the primary antibodies are given below; the ratios that are given are for our empirically optimum working dilutions of the antibodies in PBS/BSA.

Monoclonal antismooth muscle alpha-actin clone 1A4,[15] ascites 1:200, (Sigma) was localized with the secondary antibody, rhodamine-labeled rabbit antimouse IgG 1:10 (ICN Immunobiochemicals). Polyclonal rabbit antisoluble tropoelastin primary antibody (gift of Dr. Judith Foster) 1:10 was localized with the secondary antibody, rhodamine-labeled goat antirabbit IgG 1:10 (Sigma). Finally all sections were rinsed well with PBS/BSA, and coverslips were mounted over the sections with Elvanol, (DuPont). Sections were observed and photographed in a Zeiss Standard WL or a Zeiss Axioskop microscope under green epifluorescence: exciter filter BP 510-560, dichromatic beam splitter FT 580, and barrier filter DP 590. Photographs were taken on Kodak Tri-X film.

RESULTS

Smooth Muscle Alpha-Actin (SMAA)

Anti-SMAA was bound to myocardial cells along the entire length of the primitive tubular ventricle in the 2d embryonic heart (FIG. 1A). The area of myocardium that expressed SMAA was reduced to the distal part of the myocardial cuff of the truncus arteriosus by 3d (FIG. 1B) and was reduced further, by 4.5d, to a ring of cells at the most distal extremity of the myocardial cuff (FIG. 1C).

The layer of mesenchymal cells nearest the endothelium in the dorsal aorta, 2d-6d, expressed SMAA (FIGURES 1 and 4A). By about 4.5d aortic arch arteries III, IV, and VI also expressed SMAA along their entire length, from the dorsal aorta to the heart where the arterial SMAA was contiguous with that of the truncal septum; all of the branches of the dorsal aorta and the aortic arch arteries expressed SMAA

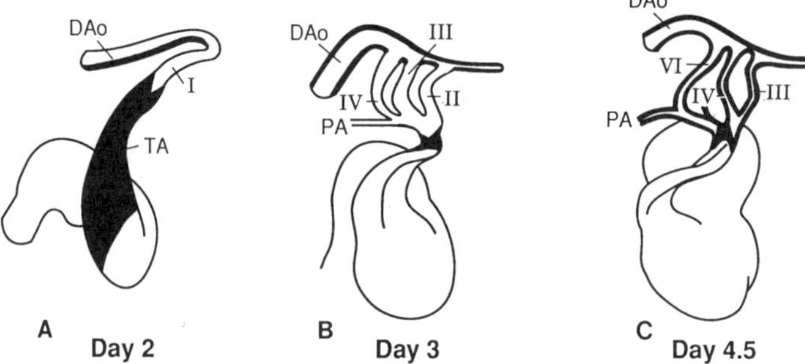

FIGURE 1. Diagrammatic representation of the primary distribution of smooth muscle alpha-actin (SMAA) in the primal vessels, incubation days 2-4.5, is shown in dense black. DAo = dorsal aorta; TA = truncus arteriosus; PA = pulmonary artery; I, II, III, IV, and VI = aortic arch arteries.

(FIGURES 1C and 4B). In the arch arteries as in the dorsal aorta and all other vessels, SMAA was expressed in a narrow band of cells adjacent to the endothelium (FIG. 4B).

The localization of neural crest-derived cells in the aortic arch arteries of the 4.5d and 6d chimeric embryos indicated that the periendothelial cells binding SMAA were nonectomesenchymal cells of chicken origin (FIG. 5). The cardiac neural crest cells in transit through the aortic arches were identified by their distinctive quail nuclei; no cell so identified expressed SMAA. On the other hand the cells expressing SMAA in the aortic arch arteries were indistinguishable from those expressing SMAA in the dorsal aorta, where there were no neural crest cells.[3] These data indicate that the smooth muscle cells in the primal arteries are not of neural crest origin.

The same pattern of expression of SMAA continued at 6d, when the dorsal aorta, the aortic arch arteries from the dorsal aorta to the heart, and all of the branches of the large arteries showed periendothelial SMAA (FIGURES 2A and 6A). At 8d the periendothelial binding of anti-SMAA was retracted downstream relative to the heart, so that the proximal part of arch arteries IV and VI was negative, and a fairly long stretch of the outflow was without smooth muscle (FIGURES 2B and 6B).

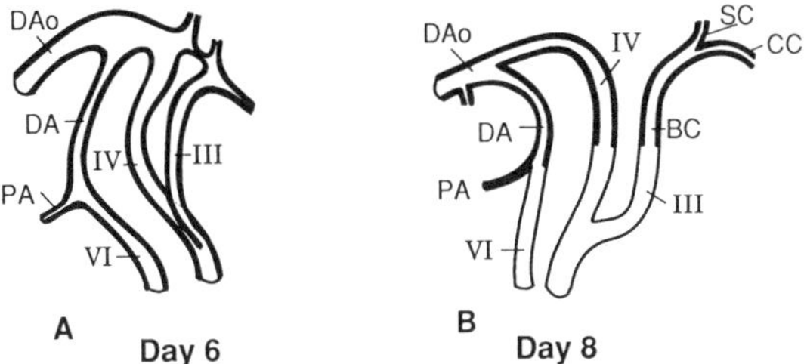

FIGURE 2. Distribution of SMAA during septation. By day 8 it is absent from the proximal great vessels. DAo = dorsal aorta; PA = pulmonary artery; DA = ductus arteriosus; BC = brachiocephalic; CC = common carotid; SC = subclavian; III, IV, and VI = aortic arch arteries.

By 10d the periendothelial SMAA was also retracted relative to the heart in the arteries of arch III, which did not express the protein until they branched into the subclavian and carotid arteries. The distribution of SMAA was otherwise as before, except now the coronary arteries were well-developed and showed intense binding of anti-SMAA from their origins, whereas the aorta from which they arose was SMAA-negative (FIGURES 3A,7A).

By 12d a second focus of SMAA was obvious: cells of the great vessel mediae other than the periendothelial layer began to express SMAA. This second phase of the expression of SMAA was observed first in the cells nearest the heart and then at progressively more distal or downstream sites (FIG. 3B), and was obvious first in the medial cells nearer the adventitia and later in the cells nearer the lumen (FIG. 7A): in these two respects the deployment of the second phase of SMAA expression was similar to the deployment of the elastic matrix. In vessels branching from the aortic arch arteries (*e.g.,* the intrapulmonary arteries or the subclavian artery), the periendothelial form persisted throughout the time course of this study, apparently expanding by addition of new cell layers in the larger vessels (FIG. 7B).

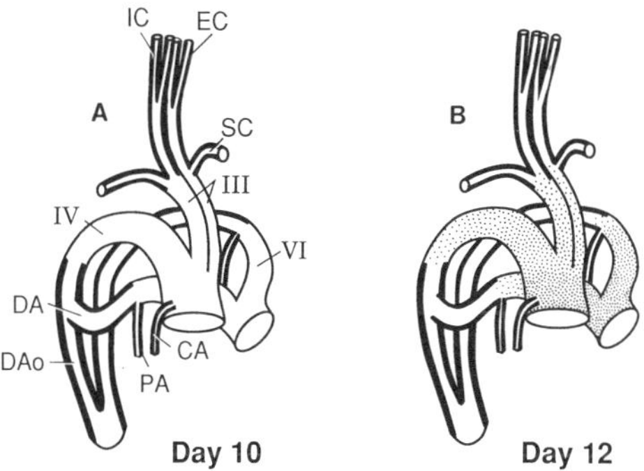

FIGURE 3. At day 10 (**A**) primary SMAA (dense black) is absent from all of the proximal aortic arch arteries. By day 12 (**B**) the secondary expression of the protein (stippling) has extended from the heart downstream along the great vessels. IC = internal carotid; EC = external carotid; CA = carotid artery. For other abbreviations, see legends of FIGURES 1 and 2.

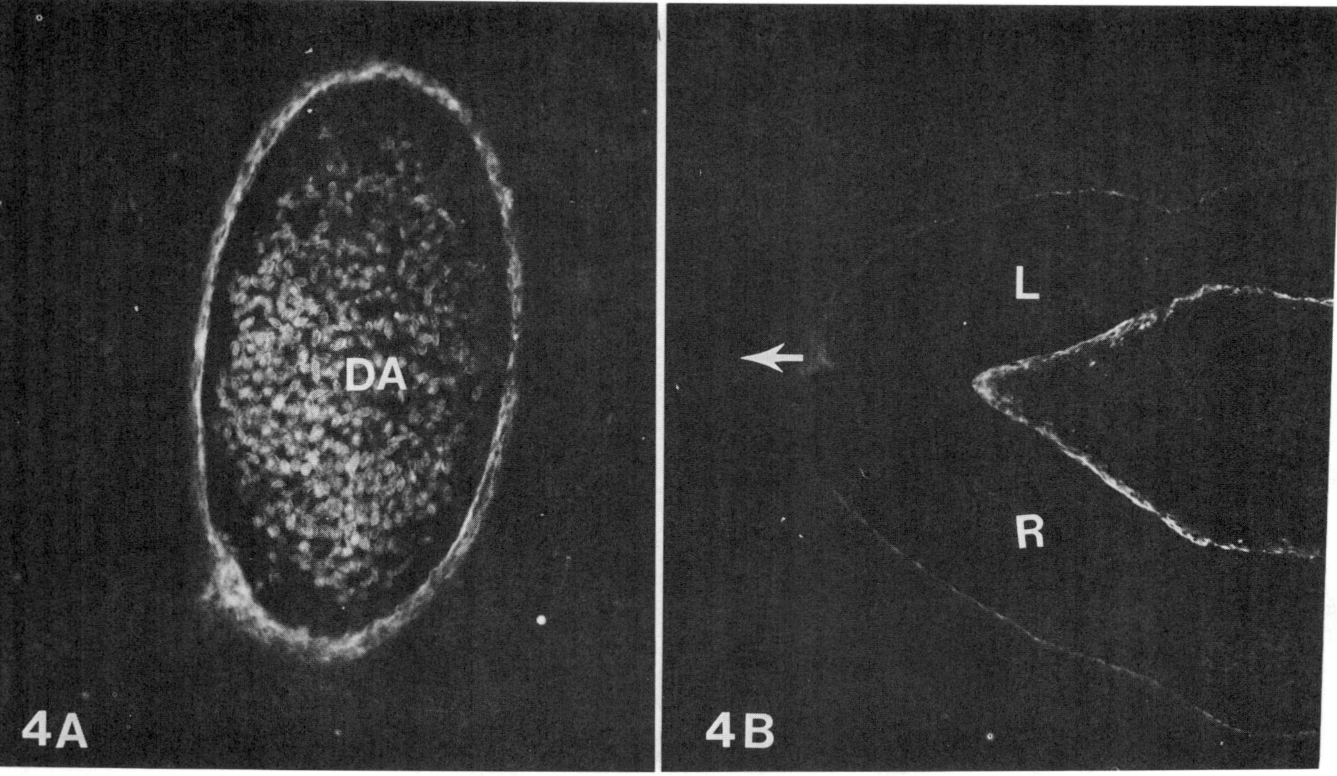

FIGURE 4. Immunofluorescence of anti-SMAA. **A:** In the dorsal aorta (DA) there is a layer, 1-2 cells thick, of SMAA-positive cells immediately adjacent to the endothelium; day 2–day 6 (shown). Luminal blood cells show bright autofluorescence; $\times$ 1000. **B:** Left and right aortic arch III of a 4-day chicken embryo; more SMAA typically is expressed in the ventral wall of the vessel than in the dorsal wall in the earliest stages of its appearance. Arrow points dorsad; $\times$ 400.

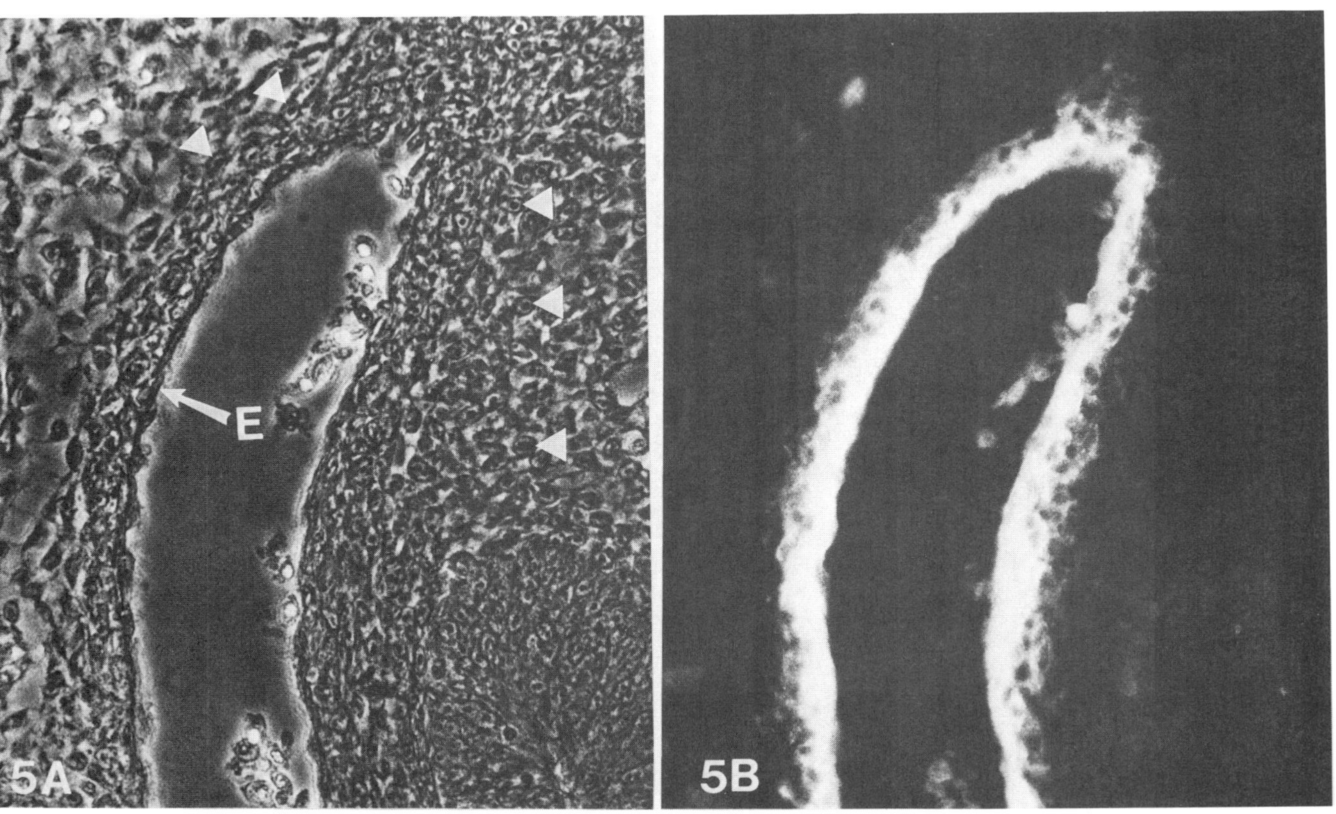

FIGURE 5. Aortic arch IV from a 4-day chimeric embryo; immunofluorescence of anti-SMAA; $\times$ 1700. **A:** Phase contrast; the endothelium (E) is evident and helps to locate the sites of SMAA positivity that are shown in **B.** The quail nuclei of the migrating neural crest cells can be seen clearly by their unique "bull's-eye" nucleus (arrowheads). **B:** Same section as **A;** epiillumination; comparing **A** with **B** it may be seen that cells of quail origin do not express SMAA.

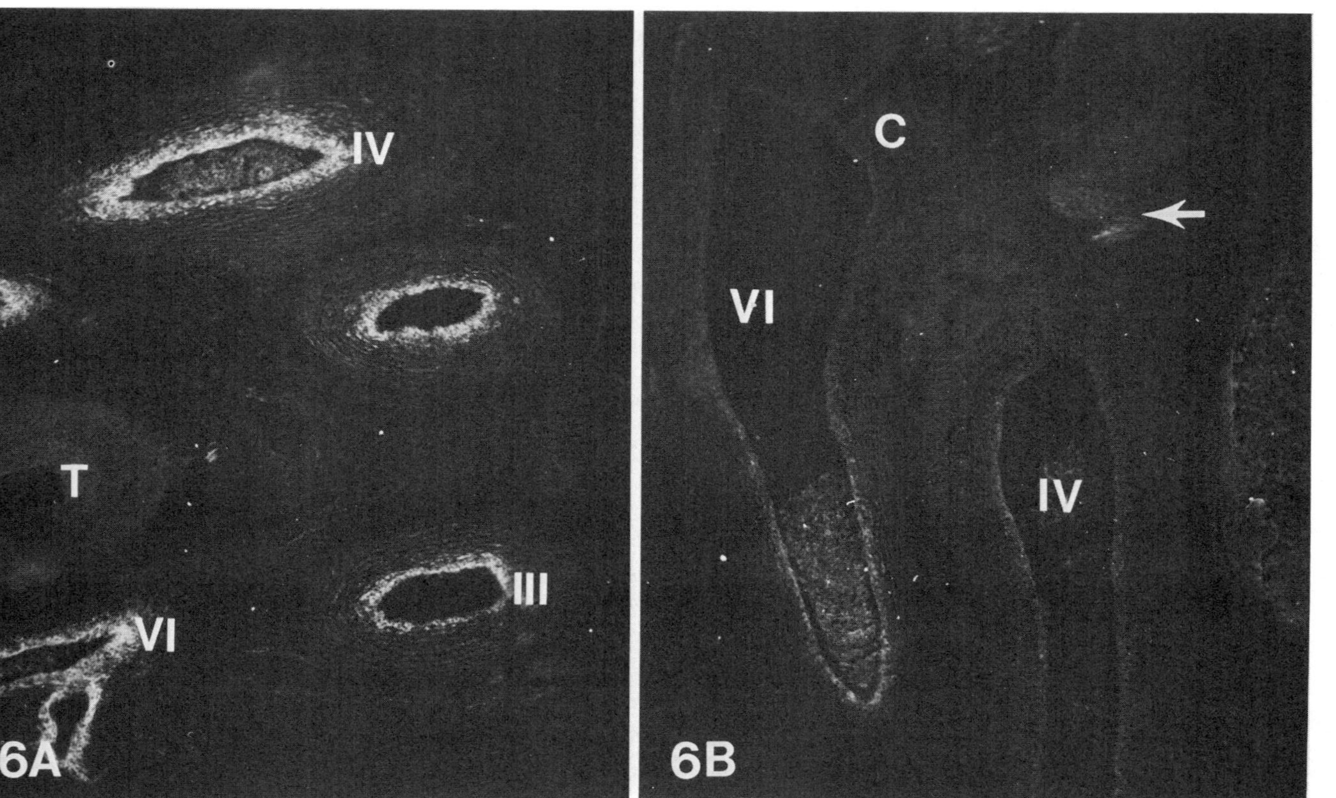

FIGURE 6. Immunofluorescence of anti-SMAA, both under epiillumination, 9-day chicken embryo; $\times$ 400. **A:** Downstream from the heart and dorsad as far as the thorax (T), SMAA is located only nearest the lumen in arches III, IV, and VI; the mediae are well-laminated. At lower left, arch VI gives rise to the pulmonary artery proper, whose entire wall expresses SMAA. **B:** The great vessels nearest the valve cusps (C) are without SMAA, whereas the pulmonary trunk (VI) retains a slight reaction for SMAA downstream. The myocardial cuff (arrow) at the base of the aorta (IV) also has a slight reaction for SMAA.

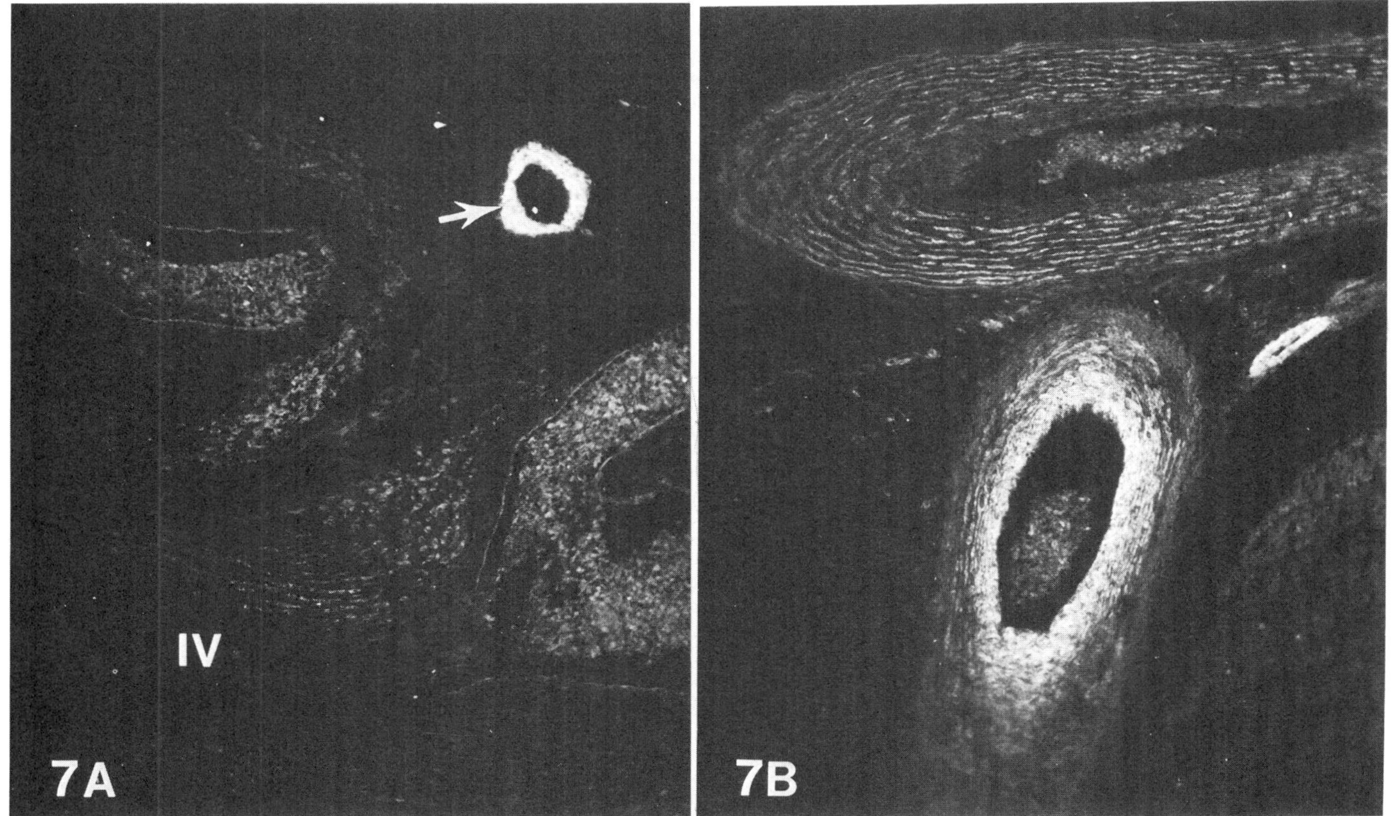

FIGURE 7. Immunofluorescence of anti-SMAA, both under epiillumination; × 400. A: In the proximal aorta (IV) of a 12-day chicken embryo, SMAA-positive cells are obvious in the outer laminae of the media. Directly above the aorta, the outer laminae of the pulmonary trunk shows the same reaction site. A coronary artery (arrow) is highly reactive. B: In the 14-day chicken embryo, aortic arch artery III (top) has SMAA throughout the media but not near the lumen, whereas its branch, the subclavian artery (below), has dense periendothelial SMAA as well as laminar SMAA. A small muscular artery is at the right.

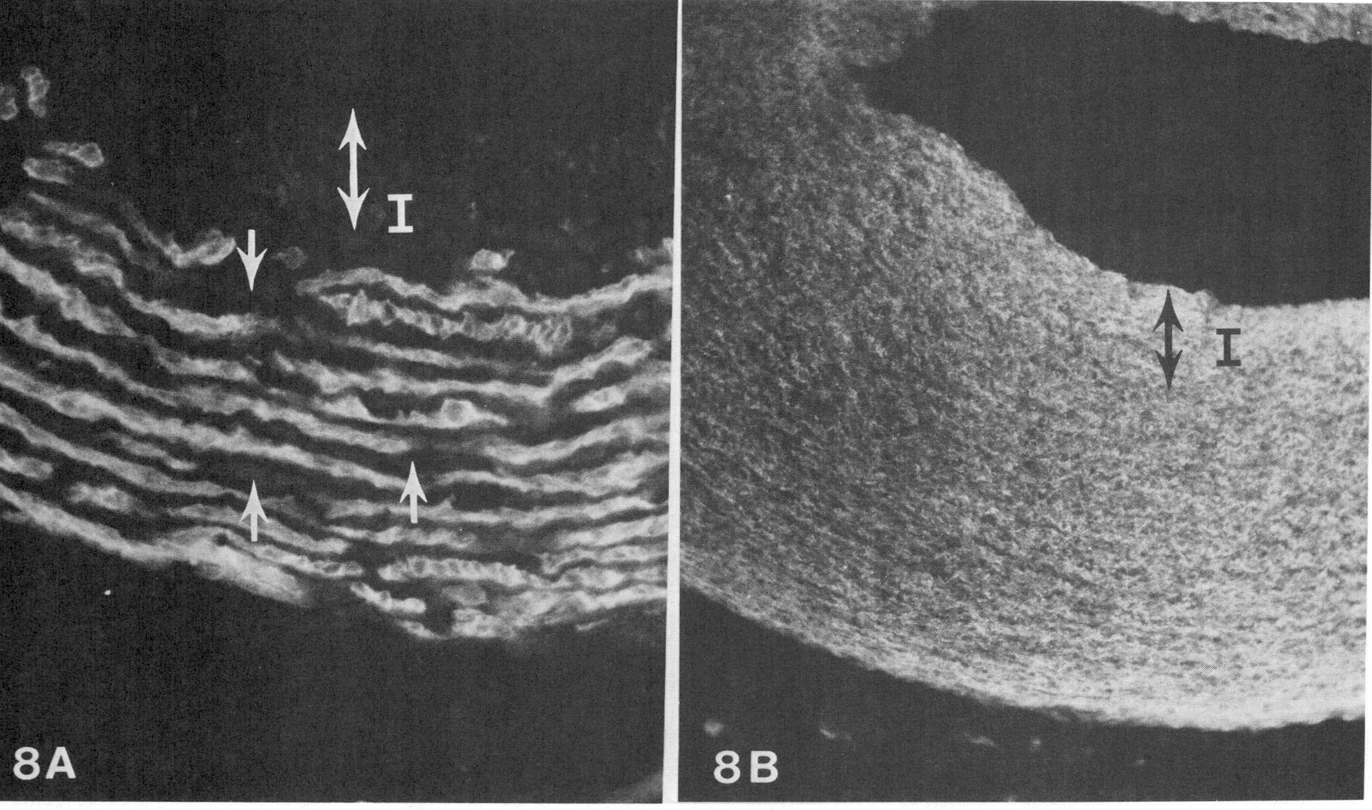

FIGURE 8. Immunofluorescence of 14-day chicken embryo aorta, both under epiillumination; $\times$ 1700. **A:** SMAA-positive cells in laminae in the media are contiguous with occasional SMAA-negative cells (arrows); the intima (I) is SMAA-negative. **B:** All of the cells and all of the intercellular spaces of the media and the intima are STE-positive.

At about 12d the cells in the walls of the great vessels were arranged in distinct laminae of mostly SMAA-positive cells, separated by an elastic matrix; between 12d and 14d a second population of cells arose that was SMAA-negative (FIG. 8A), but which remained elastogenic (FIG. 8B). These cells appeared first in the laminae of smooth muscle cells and were contiguous with them as shown at 14d (FIG. 8A). Later, SMAA-negative (nonmuscle) cells separated from the contiguous smooth muscle cells; they were then found among the elastic laminae as reported previously.[16,17]

Thus there appears to be two distinct formats for deployment of SMAA: an early or primal phase during which a periendothelial, nonectomesenchymal, nonelastogenic layer of cells expresses SMAA throughout the arterial tree; and a second, much later phase during which SMAA is expressed centrifugally from the heart by the ectomesenchymal cells that have appropriated the mediae of the great vessels, and that have obtained a well-ordered elastic lamination in advance of their expression of SMAA (see below).

Soluble Tropoelastin (STE)

None of the cells expressing SMAA in the primal arteries ever expressed STE; thereafter the binding of the antibody against STE was identical with what has been described previously.[1] Expression of STE was initiated in the ectomesenchymal cells at their interface with the myocardial cuff of the truncus arteriosus at day 3; then STE was deployed downstream. By 6d aortic arch arteries III, IV, and VI were STE-positive as far dorsal as the esophagus, and by 8d the entire length of the aortic arch arteries and the dorsal aorta were expressing STE (FIG. 9). Well-laminated vessels were apparent after about 8d. The results of the downstream deployment of STE are summarized in FIGURE 10.

DISCUSSION

The data presented here may be interpreted as follows: The primal arteries of arches III, IV, and VI and the dorsal aorta all contain smooth muscle cells that are not elastogenic, and which are not of neural crest origin. In the vessels that never receive a contribution from the cardiac neural crest (CNC), for example, the intrapulmonary arteries or the subclavian arteries,[3] the definitive mediae of the vessels appear to undergo uninterrupted development by addition of more layers of mesenchymal smooth muscle.

In the vessels that receive CNC on the other hand, the developmental history is more complex. The CNC cells populate the aortic arches by incubation day 3, but they express neither STE nor SMAA upon their arrival. Instead they remain quiescent (at least with respect to these proteins) until the vanguard CNC cells arrive at the myocardial cuff of the truncus arteriosus; then they stop migrating and differentiate into an elastogenic phenotype. Thereafter the cells behind the vanguard also differentiate in an orderly downstream progression that is perfectly symmetrical among the aortic arch arteries until all of them are elastogenic, that is, about incubation day 5.5. As the definitive elastic laminae become formed the primal smooth muscle cells disappear downstream from the heart, about as far along the great vessels as their first branch point. The fate of these cells is not known from these data; they may be replaced as the structure and function of the vessels is assumed by CNC, or they may become transformed into some other phenotype.

Smooth muscle derived from the CNC cells appears much later, after incubation day 10, and appears first nearer the heart. Most of the cells of the mediae of the great vessels become smooth muscle. Then another cell type appears among the smooth muscle cells that is a nonmuscle elastogenic cell; it appears to be derived from smooth muscle cells.

It is of some interest that the cardiac neural crest cells expressed neither SMAA nor STE while they were in transit, and when they began to express STE or SMAA it was at the terminus of their migration: it may mean that these cells have no special function in the aortic arch arteries per se in the preseptation embryo.

The expression by a cell of SMAA is necessary and sufficient for its designation as smooth muscle.[15,18,19] Because SMAA has been found only in cells that have the capacity to contract[15] it may be assumed that the very youngest arteries in the chicken embryo (2 incubation days) have that capacity, according to the results of this study. Therefore they must have a role in the control of blood flow. There are no nerves present for them to respond to, but there may be some soluble vasoactive factors present, and the primal smooth muscle may have some primitive receptors for

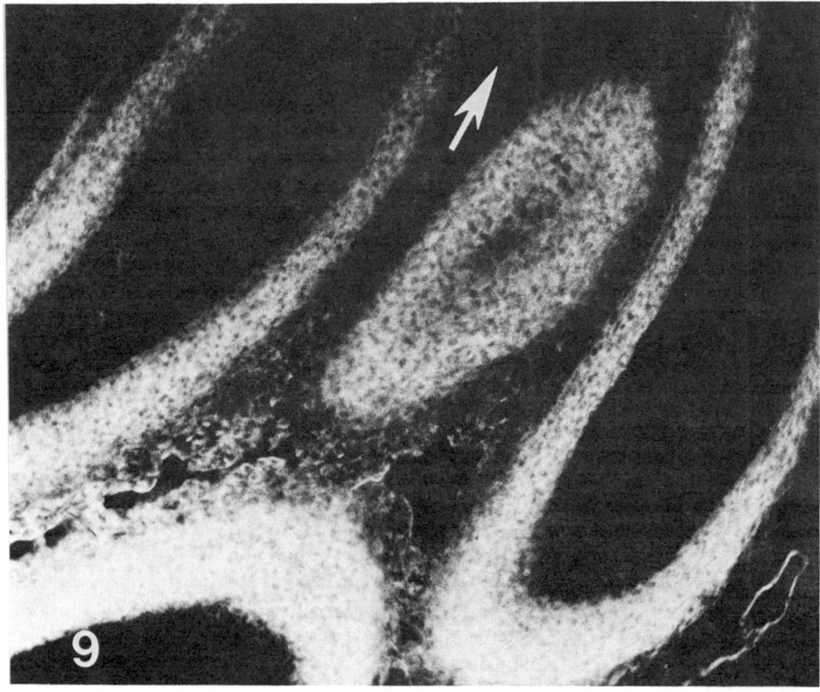

FIGURE 9. Immunofluorescence of anti-STE in the 8-day chicken embryo. All of the aortic arch arteries are empirically equal in binding intensity at any given dorsoventral level; the intensity is reduced dorsad (arrow) or downstream from the heart.

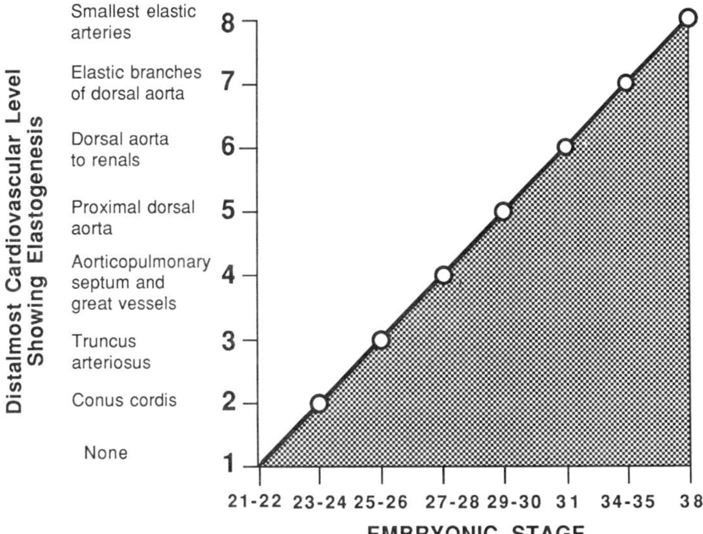

FIGURE 10. Summary of the sequence of deployment of STE downstream from the heart; Hamburger-Hamilton stages 21-38 or incubation days 3-12. (Rosenquist *et al.*[1] With permission of Alan R. Liss, Inc.)

them.[9,20,21] There is no elastin in these vessels, but they may still have the capacity to behave elastically: in vessels as small as these, and at the high pulse rates of the embryo[22] the hyaluronate-rich matrix in the surrounding mesenchyme will be elastic rather than viscous.[23] Therefore the length-tension relationships may be dependent upon both the passive and the active behavior of the vessels, even in the primal arteries.

The potential for active change of the length-tension relationships in these primal arteries, their descent from cells other than CNC, and the apparent nonfunctioning state of the preseptation CNC cells may all help explain the ability of young embryos to maintain normal hemodynamics,[24] including peak systolic dorsal aorta pressure[25] even when the general morphology of the aortic arch arteries is altered as a result of ablation of the CNC.[26] In the scenario presented by the data of this study, the primal arteries may actively accommodate for any induced alterations of vessel size, and their ability to do so is independent of the neural crest. Indeed these data indicate that neural crest-derived smooth muscle cells are not present at all until about two days after the completion of septation, and consequently their presence or absence could not relate to the putative active accomodation of the earliest arteries.

The presence of SMAA in the primitive ventricle is consistent with (1) earlier work that reported that expression of SMAA marked the beginning of differentiation of the cardiac myocyte,[27] and (2) the peristaltic contractions of the primitive ventricle that are obvious in any specimen of chicken embryonic heart after 2 or 3 days of incubation.

These findings have demonstrated the geographic and temporal relationships of two proteins that are significant contributors to cardiovascular function; these data may serve, therefore, to help interpret studies of the physiology of the embryonic cardiovascular system, especially related to the role of the cardiac neural crest.

REFERENCES

1. ROSENQUIST, T. H., J. R. MCCOY, K. L. WALDO & M. L. KIRBY. 1988. Origin and propagation of elastogenesis in the developing cardiovascular system. Anat. Rec. **221:** 860-871.
2. KIRBY, M. L., K. L. TURNAGE & B. M. HAYS. 1985. Characterization of conotruncal anomalies following ablation of "cardiac" neural crest. Anat. Rec. **213:** 87-93.
3. LELIEVRE, C. S. & N. M. LEDOUARAIN. 1975. Mesenchymal derivatives of the neural crest: analysis of chimeric quail and chick embryos. J. Embryol. Exp. Morphol. **34:** 125-154.
4. KIRBY, M. L., T. F. GALE & D. E. STEWART. 1983. Neural crest cells contribute to normal aorticopulmonary septation. Science **220:** 1059-1061.
5. DOBRIN, P. B. 1978. Mechanical properties of arteries. Physiol. Rev. **58:** 397-460.
6. MURPHY, R. A. 1984. Assessment of vascular smooth-muscle mechanisms using isolated segments of the vessel wall. Ann. Biomed. Engineer. **12:** 451-462.
7. KELLY, D. E., R. L. WOOD & A. C. ENDERS. 1984. Bailey's Textbook of Microscopic Anatomy. **8:** 253-261. Williams and Wilkins. Baltimore.
8. SIMIONESCU, N. & M. SIMIONESCU. 1988. The cardiovascular system. *In* Cell and Tissue Biology. L. Weiss, Ed. **10:** 353-400. Urban & Schwartzenberg. Baltimore.
9. CLARK, E. B. 1984. Hemodynamic control of the chick embryo cardiovascular system. *In* Congenital Heart Disease. Causes and Processes. J. J. Nora & A. Takao, Eds.: **26:** 377-385. Futura Publishing. Mt. Kisco, NY.
10. BEALL, A. C. & T. H. ROSENQUIST. 1990. Smooth muscle cells of neural crest origin form the aorticopulmonary septum in the avian embryo. Anat. Rec. In press.
11. NARAYANAN, C. H. 1970. Apparatus and current techniques in the preparation of the avian embryos for microsurgery and for observing embryonic behavior. Bioscience **20:** 868-871.
12. HAMBURGER, V. & H. HAMILTON. 1951. A series of normal stages in the development of the chick embryo. J. Morphol. **88:** 49-92.
13. LEDOUARAIN, N. M. 1982. The Neural Crest. Cambridge University Press. Cambridge, U.K.
14. PUCHTLER, H., F. S. WALDROP, S. N. MELOAN, M. TERRY & H. CONNER. 1970. Methacarn (methanol-Carnoy) fixation. Histochemie **21:** 97-116.
15. SKALLI, O., P. ROPRAZ, A. TRECZIAK, G. BENZONANA, D. GILLESSEN & G. GABBIANI. 1986. A monoclonal antibody against alpha-smooth muscle actin: a new probe for smooth muscle differentiation. J. Cell Biol. **103:** 2787-2796.
16. HUGHES, A. F. W. 1943. The histogenesis of the arteries of the chick embryo. J. Anat. **77:** 266-287.
17. JAFFEE, O. C. 1967. The development of the arterial outflow tract in the chick embryo. Anat. Rec. **158:** 35-42.
18. SKALLI, O., J. VANDERCKHOVE & J. GABBIANI. 1987. Actinisoform pattern as a marker of normal or pathological smooth-muscle and fibroblastic tissues. Differentiation **33:** 232-238.
19. GABBIANI, G., E. SCHMID, S. WINTER, C. CHAPONNIER, C. DE CHASTONAY, J. VANDERCKHOVE, K. WEBER & W. W. FRANKE. 1981. Vascular smooth muscle cells differ from other smooth muscle cells: predominance of vementin filaments and a specific alpha-type actin. Proc. Natl. Acad. Sci. USA **78:** 298-302.
20. IGNARRO, L. J. & F. E. SHIDEMAN. 1968. Appearance and concentrations of catecholamines and their biosynthesis in the embryonic and developing chick. Exp. Ther. **159:** 38-48.
21. ROTH, J., D. LEROITH, J. SHILOACH *et al.* 1982. The evolutionary origins of hormones, neurotransmitters and other extracellular chemical messengers. N. Engl. J. Med. **306:** 523-527.
22. CLARK, E. B. & N. HU. 1982. Developmental hemodynamic changes in the chick embryo from stages 18-27. Circ. Res. **51:** 810-815
23. BALASZ, E. A. & D. A. GIBBS. 1970. The rheological properties and biological function of hyaluronic acid. *In* Chemistry and Molecular Biology of the Intercellular Matrix. E. A. Balazs, Ed.: Vol. III: 1241-1253. Academic Press. New York.

24. JACKSON, W. F., H. GAULDIN, H. TOMITA & L. LEATHERBURY. 1990. Neural crest ablation does not alter ventricular pressure or estimated cardiac output despite altered morphology. Ann. N.Y. Acad. Sci. This volume.
25. LEATHERBURY, L., D. S. BRADEN, H. TOMITA, H. E. GAULDIN & W. F. JACKSON. 1990. Hemodynamic changes: Wall stresses and pressure gradients in neural crest–ablated chick embryos. Ann. N.Y. Acad. Sci. This volume.
26. BOCKMAN, D. E., M. E. REDMOND, K. W. WALDO, H. DAVIS & M. L. KIRBY. 1987. Effect of neural crest ablation on development of the heart and arch arteries in the chick. Am. J. Anat. **180:** 332-341.
27. RUZICKA, D. L. & R. J. SCHWARTZ. 1988. Sequential activation of alpha-actin genes during avian cardiogenesis: vascular smooth muscle alpha-actin marks the onset of cardiomyocyte differentiation. J. Cell Biol. **107:** 2575-2586.

Role of Sympathetic Innervation in Cardiac Development *in Oculo*[a]

DIANE C. TUCKER AND CLARA H. GAUTIER

School of Social and Behavioral Sciences
Department of Psychology
University of Alabama at Birmingham
Birmingham, Alabama 35294

Although cardiac production of growth factors is known to support survival of cardiac sympathetic innervation, the possibility that sympathetic innervation may influence cardiac development is less thoroughly explored. Sympathetic innervation could affect heart development directly, through altering contractile activity or through interacting with hormonal stimulation. Experiments in both intact animals and using model systems are necessary to elucidate sympathetic influences on cardiac development.

SYMPATHETIC CONTROL OF CARDIAC DEVELOPMENT *IN OCULO*

Experiments in intact animals suggest that the effect of sympathetic innervation on cardiac growth depends on the developmental stage of the heart. Kirby and colleagues produced sympathetically aneural chick hearts by removal of the neural crest giving rise to sympathetic neurons and found that both the morphology and size of the heart was normal.[1] During the perinatal period when the heart is growing primarily by cell division,[2] a single injection of the β-adrenergic receptor agonist, isoproterenol, inhibited ongoing cell division.[3] Conversely, chemical sympathectomy extended the period of cardiac cell proliferation.[4] In mature hearts where growth occurs by cellular hypertrophy,[2] chronic treatment with isoproterenol produces cardiac hypertrophy.[5] Chronic propranolol treatment inhibited growth in postmitotic juvenile rabbit hearts and increased the intrinsic beating rate as measured from isolated, perfused hearts.[6] Together these data suggest that adrenergic stimulation inhibits cardiac cell division, but promotes cellular hypertrophy. In intact animals, however, direct effects of sympathetic stimulation cannot be separated from hemodynamic consequences or from the potentiation of hormonal influences on heart development.

[a] This work was supported by NIH HL39048, NIH HL42258, and March of Dimes 5-651. D. C. Tucker is an Established Investigator of the American Heart Association.

SYMPATHETIC INFLUENCES ON CARDIAC MYOCYTES *IN VITRO*

Sympathetic control of cardiac growth and function has been examined in cultures of isolated myocytes and in transplanted hearts. Simpson and colleagues demonstrated that norepinephrine stimulation produced growth of nondividing myocytes from neonatal hearts[7,8] that was mediated by α_1-adrenergic receptor stimulation. More recent studies indicate that α-adrenergic receptor stimulation activates the phosphatidyl inositol system, stimulates protein kinase C, and increases expression of the *c-myc* oncogene mRNA.[8,9] Beating in these isolated ventricular myocytes was observed after simultaneous α_1- and β-adrenergic stimulation.[8] Co-culture with sympathetic neurons transforms the chronotropic response of ventricular myocytes from tachycardia to bradycardia, presumably through induction of a pertussis toxin-sensitive guanine nucleotide-binding protein (N_i).[10] Because disruption of the relationships among cell types may alter the response of myocytes to sympathetic stimulation, experiments in which the developing heart is transplanted into a controlled milieu complement cell culture experiments.

DEVELOPMENT OF EMBRYONIC HEART IN THE ANTERIOR EYE CHAMBER

We have used the anterior eye chamber of an adult rat to examine the effects of sympathetic innervation on mammalian cardiac development. When grafted into the anterior eye chamber, embryonic atrial, ventricular, or whole heart grafts become vascularized from the iris plexus and continue to beat and grow for several months. Our initial studies[11] have confirmed the reports of others[12,13] that the grafted heart becomes functionally innervated by sympathetic and parasympathetic nerves *in oculo*. In addition, we have demonstrated that embryonic heart differentiates into adult-like myocardium *in oculo*[14] and that the spontaneous beating is pacemaker-driven.[15]

Morphologic Development of Heart Grafts in Oculo

Morphologic studies indicate that embryonic heart tissue continues to differentiate *in oculo*.[14] Electron microscopic examination of embryonic heart at the time of implantation *in oculo* showed bundles of myofibrils that were loosely organized and often oriented at sharp angles to each other (FIG. 1A). Compared to mature myocardium, myofibrils and mitochondria were sparse, and intercalated discs were incompletely developed. Tritiated thymidine studies showed that myocyte cell division continued through the second week *in oculo*, a postgestational age equivalent to a 5-day postnatal heart; after 10 weeks *in oculo*, however, no evidence of dividing myocytes was found.[14] By 5 weeks *in oculo*, myocytes had assumed an elongated shape, and myofibrils were plentiful and mature in appearance, with clear M-lines and Z-lines. The distribution

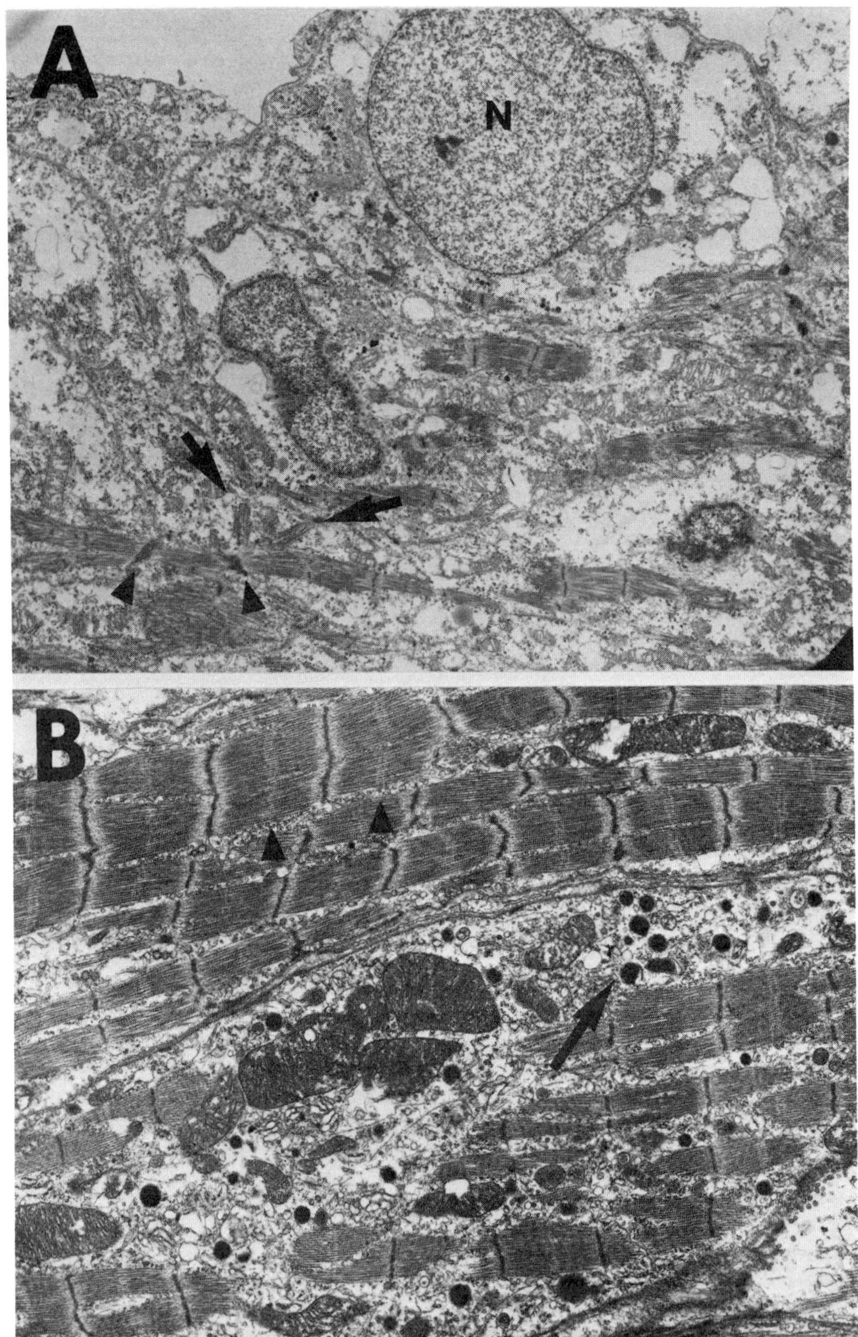

FIGURE 1. See legend on opposite page.

of mitochondria and myofibrils was characteristic of adult myocardium and showed clear differentiation from the embryonic state at implantation. The appearance of mature myocardium *in oculo* is illustrated by the 3.5-month-old atrial graft shown in FIGURE 1B; atrial granules were prominent, and both M-lines and Z-bands were evident in the large bundles of well-organized myofibrils.

Myocardium maturing *in oculo* differed in several ways from heart growing *in situ*. Myocytes maturing *in oculo* remained smaller than postnatal myocytes and, perhaps as a consequence of the small cell size, did not develop a T-tubular system.[14] Polarization of myofibrils within myocytes *in oculo* was less consistent, and alignment of cells within the tissue showed greater variability than in myocardium maturing *in situ* (FIG. 2). We hypothesize that the force generated during pumping of the intact heart organizes the parallel alignment of myofibrils and myocytes. Without the organizing force of a physiologic workload, some of the disorganization of myofibrils and myocytes in embryonic heart is retained *in oculo*. Terracio's experiments with cultured myocytes indicate that myocytes align perpendicular to the line of stretch[16,17] and are consistent with our observations. By most criteria, however, myocytes do differentiate from embryonic to adult morphology *in oculo*, suggesting that the *in oculo* model system can be used to examine neural and hormonal controls of cardiac growth and differentiation.

Pacemaker Development in Oculo

When grafted *in oculo*, embryonic heart beats spontaneously. In collaboration with W. T. Woods Jr., we investigated whether the beating of grafts was driven by a distinct pacemaker or resembled the beating syncytium observed when ventricular myocytes are dissociated and maintained *in vitro*. We identified a site of earliest activation in grafts that was consistently located at the junction between the iris and the graft.[15] Action potentials recorded from this region showed the phase IV depolarization characteristic of the sinoatrial pacemaker. Because similar pacemakers were observed in grafted tissues that lacked their own pacemaker (*i.e.*, ventricular and atrial appendage grafts), we hypothesized that a new pacemaker may develop when embryonic heart is grafted onto the surface of the iris. Studies are currently underway to determine the fate of the original pacemaker and to determine whether grafting *in oculo* induces formation of a new pacemaker in embryonic heart. Because the spontaneous beating of *in oculo* grafts is initiated by a pacemaker that resembles the sinoatrial pacemaker, we have used the *in oculo* model to examine neural and hormonal influences on the intrinsic pacemaker rate established during development.

Innervation of Hearts Grafted in Oculo

Grafts into the anterior eye chamber become innervated by collaterals of the sympathetic, parasympathetic, and sensory nerves to the iris. When innervated, grafts

---

◄—FIGURE 1. Panel **A** is an electron micrograph of ventricular myocardium from 13 day rat embryo. Myofibrils are sparse and poorly organized and aligned (arrows). Intercellular junctions (arrowheads) are immature. Magnification, × 4960. Panel **B** is an electron micrograph of atrial embryonic myocardium cultured *in oculo* for 2.5 months. Myofibrils are well-developed with M-lines (arrowheads) and Z-bands. Atrial granules are prominent (arrow). Magnification, × 5420.

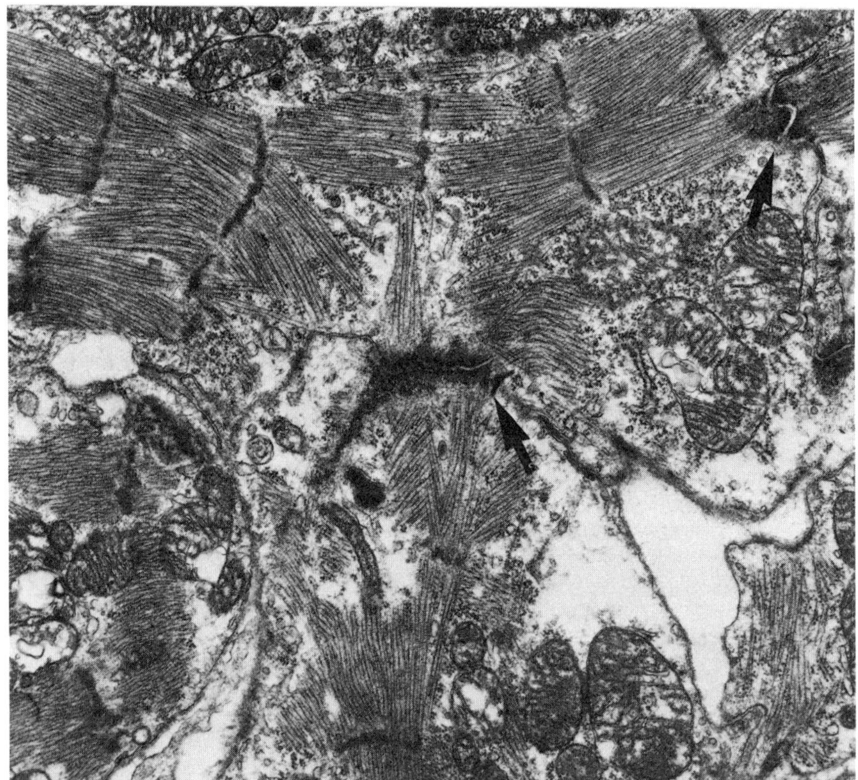

FIGURE 2. Electron micrograph of ventricular myocardium from a 12 day rat embryo *in oculo* for 2 weeks. The alignment of myofibrils has retained the disorganization characteristic of embryonic heart. Intercalated discs (arrows) have begun to assume a mature appearance. Magnification, × 14,275.

change beating rate with changes in ambient light.[11–13] Glyoxylic acid-induced fluorescence studies revealed sympathetic fibers in heart tissue within one week after grafting. FIGURE 3 shows the development of bradycardic responses to light stimulation during the first two weeks after grafting. After 8 weeks *in oculo* we observed a dense network of catecholamine-containing fibers in grafted hearts with substantial norepinephrine content in the grafts (2.6 ng/mg).

Sympathetic innervation of grafts can be prevented by surgical denervation of the eye chamber prior to grafting of heart tissue. Permanent denervation of the eye chamber is accomplished by removal of the ipsilateral superior cervical ganglion (SCG); this does not alter sympathetic innervation of the contralateral eye chamber.[11,18,19] Bjorklund[18] and Kessler[19] reported that sympathetic denervation of the anterior eye chamber resulted in induction of tyrosine hydroxylase-like and neuropeptide Y-like immunoreactivity in cholinergic neurons; Kessler[19,20] reported that iris sympathectomy resulted in increased levels of substance P in sensory nerves. In our experiments, embryonic hearts are grafted into the sympathetically denervated and intact eye chambers of adult host rats. In both conditions, grafts are perfused by the host circulation; therefore, differences between grafts are likely to result from differences in the neural environment of the innervated and denervated eye chambers.

Culture of Heart in Sympathetically Denervated Eye Chambers

To test the hypothesis that growth and pacemaker rate of embryonic rat heart is altered by neural stimuli, atria from E-12 rat embryos were grafted into sympathetically denervated and intact eye chambers of 34 adult host rats.[11] Growth and beating rate were monitored for 8 weeks. Growth was estimated by measuring the surface dimension of grafts using a micrometer in a surgical microscope. Beating rate was estimated from the time required for 20 contractions.

Catecholamine content assayed from a sample of grafts confirmed that sympathetic denervations were permanent and that grafts into intact eye chambers were innervated by norepinephrine-containing fibers.[11] Atria grafted into sympathetically denervated eye chambers grew significantly less than grafts into intact eye chambers (see FIG. 4).[11] Beating rate of grafts was recorded from permanently implanted extraocular electrodes after 2.5 months *in oculo*. A combined β-adrenergic and muscarinic receptor blockade was used to estimate intrinsic beating rate of grafts. As shown in FIGURE 5, a faster intrinsic beating rate was recorded from grafts in sympathetically denervated eye chambers, suggesting that the neural environment may modulate the intrinsic rate established by the pacemaker during development.

Cografting of an Additional Source of Sympathetic Neurons

We hypothesized that an additional source of sympathetic innervation would potentiate the growth and increase the intrinsic beating rate of sympathetically innervated grafts. C. H. Gautier and I tested this hypothesis by grafting an SCG from

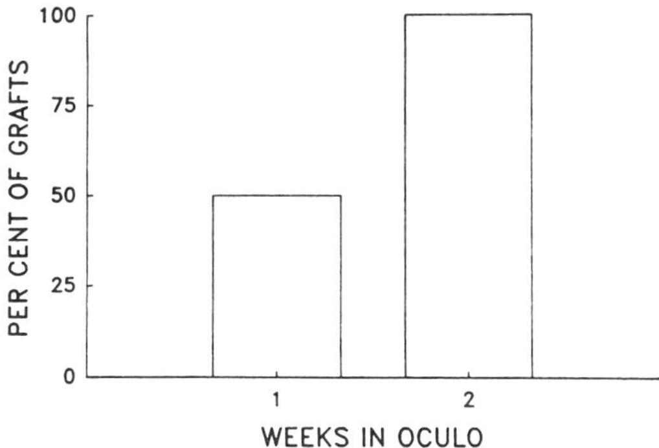

FIGURE 3. Development of bradycardic response to light stimulation in 8 whole embryonic hearts grafted *in oculo*. Hosts were dark-adapted for 20 minutes. Bradycardic responses to light stimulation were observed in 50% of grafts that had been *in oculo* for 1 week and in 100% of grafts *in oculo* for 2 weeks.

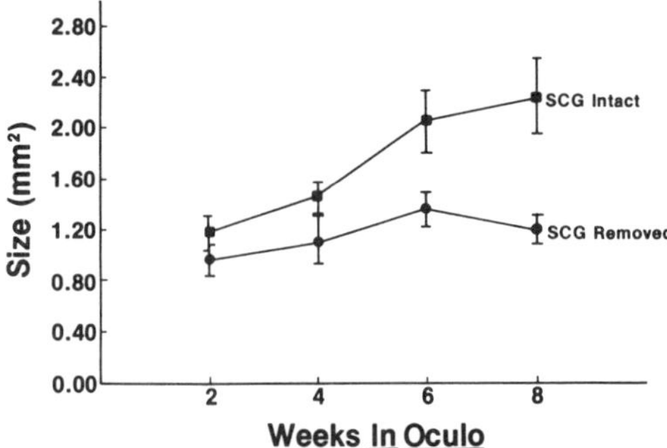

FIGURE 4. Growth of atrial grafts into sympathetically innervated and denervated eye chambers was estimated by measuring the long axis of the graft and the width perpendicular to the long axis. By 6 weeks *in oculo* grafts in sympathetically innervated eye chambers were larger than grafts in denervated eye chambers. Data are mean $\pm$ SEM. (D. C. Tucker & R. Gist.[11] With permission from *Circulation Research.*)

a neonatal rat and an embryonic whole heart into the anterior eye chamber. All grafts were made into intact eye chambers. In each host, one eye chamber contained a grafted SCG and a 12 day gestation rat heart; the other eye chamber contained only an embryonic heart graft. Immunohistochemistry for tyrosine hydroxylase performed in the laboratory of B. J. Davis confirmed that cografted neurons survived and innervated the graft (FIG. 6). Graft surface dimension and beating rate were measured immediately after implantation (week 0) and after 4 and 8 weeks *in oculo.* Cografting of an SCG with embryonic hearts did not alter growth *in oculo* ($p > .10$; see FIG. 7).

Beating rate was measured from grafts while hosts were tranquilized with diazepam. Profile analysis indicated that by 8 weeks beating rate was slower in grafts co-cultured with an SCG than in control grafts ($F(2,18) = 4.97, p < .02$; FIG. 8). To determine the source of the slower beating rate in grafts co-cultured with an SCG, extraocular electrodes were implanted and rates were recorded while hosts were unanesthetized.

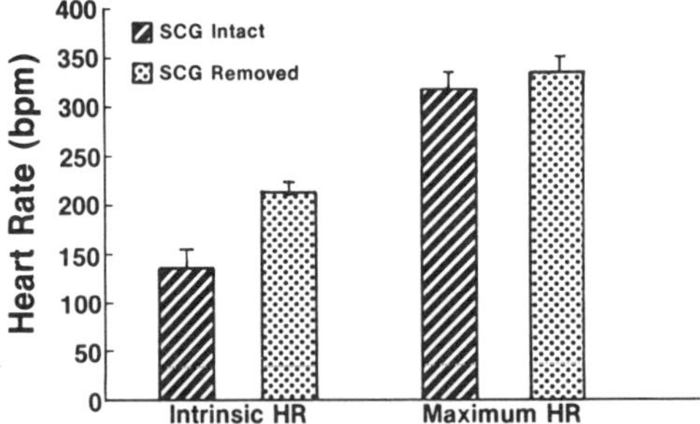

FIGURE 5. Intrinsic and maximal *in oculo* heart rate. Intrinsic heart rate was estimated from sympathetically innervated and noninnervated grafts after combined treatment of the host with the β_1-adrenergic antagonist, atenolol (1 mg/kg, s.c.), and the muscarinic antagonist, methylatropine (10 μg/kg, s.c.). Maximal heart rate was estimated by treatment of hosts with the β-adrenergic agonist, isoproterenol (1 μg/kg, s.c.). Intrinsic heart rate was lower in sympathetically innervated grafts than in noninnervated grafts; maximal heart rates did not differ. (D. C. Tucker & R. Gist.[11] With permission from *Circulation Research.*)

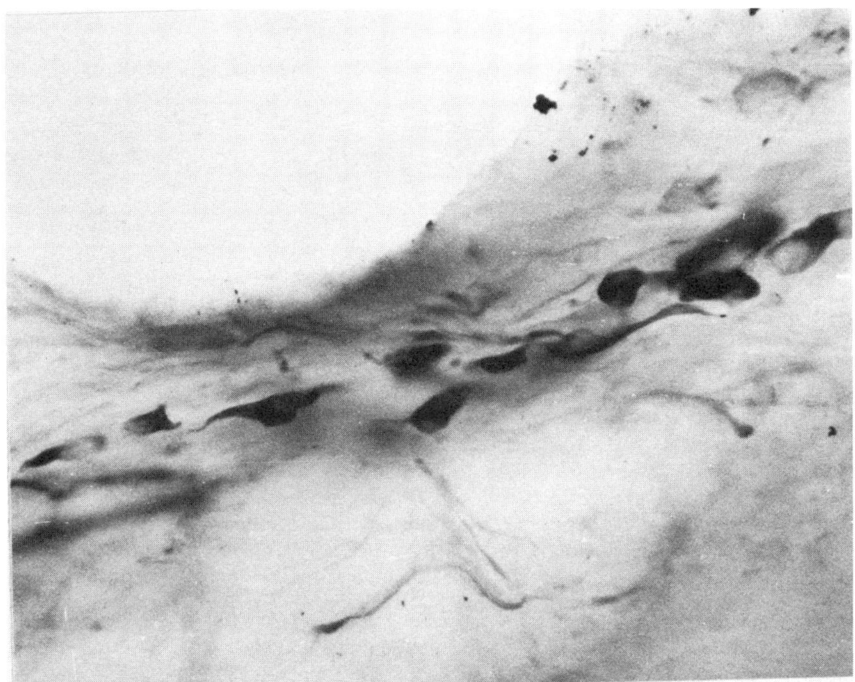

FIGURE 6. Photomicrograph illustrating tyrosine hydroxylase immunoreactive neurons on the surface of an embryonic heart graft indicates that neurons from the superior cervical ganglion grafted with the embryonic heart survived the 10 week culture period *in oculo.*

Baseline rates were recorded with host rats in a darkened chamber, resulting in low parasympathetic and high sympathetic tone to the eye chamber. As in the measurement at 8 weeks *in oculo,* rates were slower in hearts co-cultured with a neonatal SCG ($F(1,11) = 11.93; p < .01$; FIG. 9). When the muscarinic receptor blocker, atropine methyl nitrate (0.1 mg/kg, s.c., Sigma, St. Louis), was administered to the host rat, the difference in beating rate disappeared, suggesting increased parasympathetic control of beating rate in co-cultured grafts. The β-adrenergic receptor blocker, atenolol (1 mg/kg, s.c., ICI Americas, Wilmington, DE), was administered after responses to methylatropine were recorded to produce a combined β-adrenergic and muscarinic

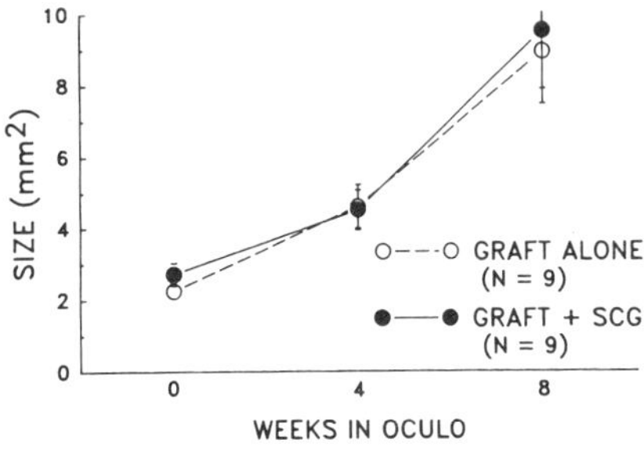

FIGURE 7. Co-culture of superior cervical ganglion (SCG) and heart: effects on growth. Growth of embryonic heart grafts was estimated by measuring surface dimensions of grafts as in FIGURE 4. Hearts grafted with an SCG showed no greater growth than hearts grafted alone.

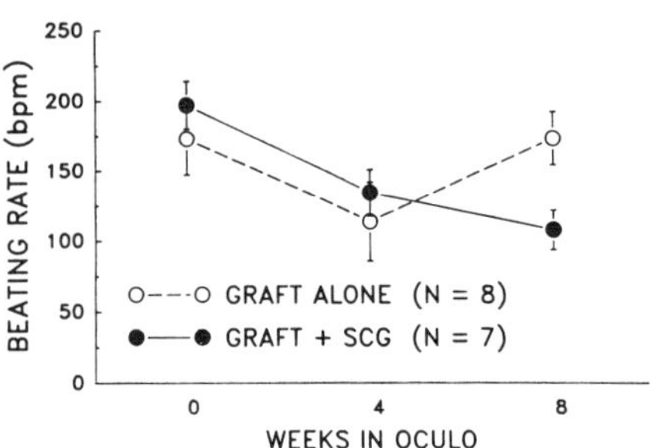

FIGURE 8. Co-culture of SCG and heart: effects on beating rate. Beating rate of grafts was determined by the time required for 20 sequential contractions while hosts were tranquilized with diazepam. Beating rate was slower in hearts co-cultured with an SCG at 8 weeks *in oculo*.

blockade from which intrinsic beating rate could be estimated. Neither the intrinsic beating rate or the bradycardic response to atenolol treatment differed between co-cultured and control grafts ($p > .10$; FIG. 9).

These data suggest that exposure to an additional source of sympathetic neurons is not sufficient to increase growth of embryonic heart cultured *in oculo*. Baseline beating rate was, however, slower in grafts maturing with a cografted SCG, due to a relative increase in parasympathetic inhibitory control. One likely interpretation is that the cografted sympathetic neurons compete with endogenous sympathetic neurons for trophic factors produced by the heart grafts,[20–23] resulting in reduced functional sympathetic control of beating rate. Inasmuch as cografted sympathetic neurons receive no preganglionic stimulation, they are unlikely to provide functional sympathetic control of beating rate.

Summary

Embryonic heart cultured *in oculo* differentiates into adult-like heart tissue, increases in size, and maintains spontaneous activity driven by a defined pacemaker. The growth and beating rate of embryonic heart maturing *in oculo* are modulated by its neural milieu. Culture in a sympathetically denervated eye chamber compromised

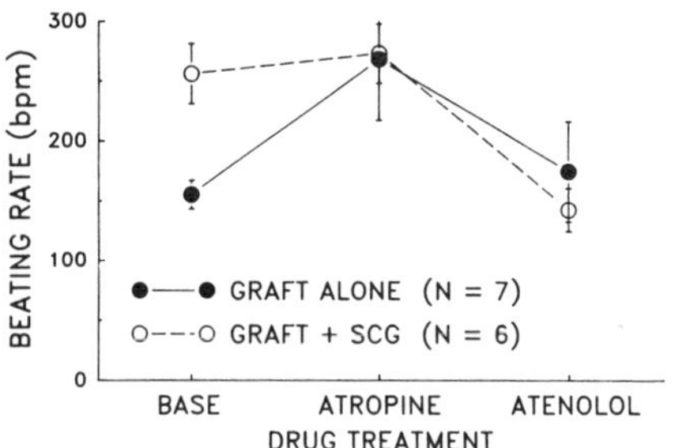

FIGURE 9. Co-culture of SCG and heart: autonomic controls of beating rate. The autonomic controls of beating rate and intrinsic beating rate of grafts were measured from chronically implanted electrodes. The baseline beating rate was slower in grafts co-cultured with an SCG. Treatment of the host with methylatropine (10 μg/kg, s.c.) to block parasympathetic control eliminated the beating rate difference. Intrinsic rate, estimated after combined β-adrenergic and muscarinic receptor blockade, did not differ between conditions.

growth and increased intrinsic beating rate. Exposure to an additional source of sympathetic neurons increased parasympathetic control of heart rate but did not alter growth or intrinsic beating rate. Because eye chamber sympathectomy alters neurotransmitter expression in parasympathetic and sensory neurons, it is possible that the growth inhibition observed in heart grafts is not a direct consequence of preventing sympathetic innervation. This possibility is being tested in additional experiments.

ACKNOWLEDGMENTS

The authors wish to thank Dr. S. P. Bishop and Dr. P. G. Anderson for providing the electron micrographs and Dr. B. J. Davis for performing the tyrosine hydroxylase immunohistochemistry.

REFERENCES

1. KIRBY, M. & D. STEWART. 1984. Adrenergic innervation of the developing chick heart: Neural crest ablations to produce sympathetically aneural hearts. Am. J. Anat. **171:** 295-305.
2. CLUBB, F. J. JR. & S. P. BISHOP. 1984. Formation of binucleated myocardial cells in the neonatal rat: An index for growth hypertrophy. Lab. Invest. **50:** 571-577.
3. CLAYCOMB, W. C. 1976. Biochemical aspects of cardiac muscle differentiation. J. Biol. Chem. **251:** 6082-6089.
4. KUGLER, J. D., P. C. GILLETTE, S. P. GRAHAM, A. GARSON JR., M. A. GOLDSTEIN & H. K. THOMPSON JR. 1980. Effect of chemical sympathectomy on myocardial cell division in the newborn rat. Pediatr. Res. **14:** 881-884.
5. TSE, J., J. R. POWELL, C. A. BASTE, R. E. PRIEST & J. F. KUO. 1979. Isoproterenol-induced cardiac hypertrophy: Modifications in characteristics of beta-adrenergic receptor, adenylate cyclase, and ventricular contraction. Endocrinology **105:** 246-255.
6. NAYLER, W. G., A. SLADE, E. M. VAUGHAN WILLIAMS & C. E. YEPEZ. 1980. Effect of prolonged beta-adrenoceptor blockage on heart weight and ultrastructure in young rabbits. Br. J. Pharm. **68:** 201-213.
7. SIMPSON, P. & S. SAVION. 1982. Differentiation of rat myocytes in single cell cultures with and without proliferating of nonmyocardial cells. Circ. Res. **50:** 101-116.
8. SIMPSON, P. 1985. Stimulation of hypertrophy of cultured neonatal rat heart cells through an α_1-adrenergic receptor and induction of beating through an α_1- and β_1-adrenergic receptor interaction. Circ. Res. **56:** 884-894.
9. STARKSEN, N. F., P. C. SIMPSON, N. BISHOPRIC, S. R. COUGHLIN, W. M. F. LEE, J. A. ESCOBEDO & L. T. WILLIAMS. 1986. Cardiac myocyte hypertrophy is associated with c-myc protooncogene expression. Proc. Natl. Acad. Sci. USA **83:** 8348-8350.
10. STEINBERG, S. F., E. D. DRUGGE, J. P. BILEZIKIAN & R. B. ROBINSON. 1985. Acquisition by innervated cardiac myocytes of a pertussis toxin-specific regulatory protein linked to the α_1-receptor. Science **230:** 186-188.
11. TUCKER, D. C. & R. GIST. 1986. Sympathetic innervation alters growth and intrinsic heart rate of fetal rat atria maturing *in oculo.* Circ. Res. **59:** 534-544.
12. OLSON, L. O. & A. SEIGER. 1976. Beating intraocular hearts: Light-controlled rate by autonomic innervation from host iris. J. Neurobiol. **7:** 193-203.
13. TAYLOR, D., A. SEIGER, R. FREEDMAN, L. OLSON & B. HOFFER. 1978. Electrophysiological analysis of reinnervation of transplants in the anterior chamber of the eye by the autonomic ground plexus of the iris. Proc. Natl. Acad. Sci. USA **75:** 1009-1012.

14. BISHOP, S. P., P. G. ANDERSON & D. C. TUCKER. 1990. Morphologic development of the rat heart growing *in oculo* in the absence of hemodynamic work load. Circ. Res. **66**.
15. TUCKER, D., C. SNIDER & W. T. WOODS JR. 1988. Pacemaker development in embryonic rat heart cultured *in oculo*. Pediatr. Res. **23**: 637-642.
16. TERRACIO, L., A. TINGSTRÖM, W. H. PETERS III & T. K. BORG. 1990. A potential role for mechanical stimulation in cardiac development. Ann. N.Y. Acad. Sci. This volume.
17. TERRACIO, L., B. MILLER & T. K. BORG. 1988. Effects of cyclic mechanical stimulation of the cellular components of the heart: *in vitro*. In Vitro. **24**: 53-58.
18. BJORKLUND, H., T. HOKFELT, M. GOLDSTEIN, L. TERENIUS & L. OLSON. 1985. Appearance of the noradrenergic markers tyrosine hydroxylase and neuropeptide Y in cholinergic nerves of the iris following sympathectomy. J. Neurosci. **5**: 1633-1643.
19. KESSLER, J. A., W. O. BELL & I. B. BLACK. 1983. Interactions between the sympathetic and sensory innervation of the iris. J. Neurosci. **3**: 1301-1307.
20. KESSLER, J. A. 1985. Parasympathetic, sympathetic, and sensory interactions in the iris: Nerve growth factor regulates cholinergic ciliary ganglion innervation *in vivo*. J. Neurosci. **5**: 2719-2725.
21. KORSCHING, S. & H. THOENEN. 1983. Nerve growth factor in sympathetic ganglia and corresponding target organs of the rat: Correlation with density of sympathetic innervation. Proc. Natl. Acad. Sci. USA **80**: 3513-3516.
22. SHELTON, D. L. & L. F. REICHARDT. 1984. Expression of the β-nerve growth factor gene correlates with the density of sympathetic innervation in effector organs. Proc. Natl. Acad. Sci. USA **81**: 7951-7955.
23. HEUMANN, R., S. KORSCHING, J. SCOTT & H. THOENEN. 1984. Relationship between levels of nerve growth factor (NGF) and its messenger RNA in sympathetic ganglia and peripheral target tissues. EMBO J. **3**: 3183-3189.

Development of Cholinergic Neuroeffector Transmission in the Avian Heart

Implications for Regulatory Mechanisms[a]

ACHILLES J. PAPPANO

Department of Pharmacology
University of Connecticut Health Center
Farmington, Connecticut 06032

INTRODUCTION

The embryonic heart is a most suitable model for experimental evaluation of the development of autonomic neuroeffector junctions. There have been many studies of the morphological and functional development of postganglionic cholinergic nerves that carry signals for the parasympathetic (vagus) nervous system. The salient ontogenetic features of cholinergic neuroeffector transmission will be reviewed, and selected problems that have emerged in connection with the onset or regulation of neuroeffector transmission will be discussed. There are two postulates that will be presented and developed. First, muscarinic agonists can stimulate the aneural embryonic chick heart, and this phenomenon can be manifested later in development and in adult animals, that is, it is not a phenomenon peculiar to the aneural embryonic heart. Second, a single transmitter, acting on pharmacologically indistinguishable receptors, can initiate opposite or antagonistic effects characterized by "fade" of the dominant response.[1]

CHOLINERGIC NEUROEFFECTOR TRANSMISSION

Cholinergic transmission to the sinoatrial (SA) node of the embryonic chick heart was detected on the twelfth embryonic (12E) day and was registered as an inhibition of the primary cardiac pacemaker.[2] Excitation of intracardiac vagal nerves reduced the rate of diastolic depolarization and hyperpolarized the membrane by acting on atropine-sensitive muscarinic receptors (mAChR). Functional vagal innervation of

[a] The author's work is supported by Grant HL-13339 from the USPHS.

the embryonic chick ventricle was first detected on 13E and was registered as inhibition of the positive inotropic effect of exogenously applied isoproterenol.[3] Cardioinhibition by vagal stimulation occurred at a time when the sensitivity of the SA node to muscarinic agonist[4] and the number of mAChR in both atrium and ventricle had increased.[3,5] These findings regarding functional innervation are consistent with reports concerning the ontogenetic expression of the cholinergic phenotype, including the appearance of high affinity choline uptake (maximum at 10E to 12E),[6] morphologically mature cardiac parasympathetic ganglia (11E),[7] and choline acetyltransferase activity (13E)[8] in the embryonic chick heart. Additionally, they are in accordance with descriptions of the anatomical innervation of the embryonic chick heart by the vagus nerve whose rudimentary atrial and bulbar plexuses are first detected at the end of the first week *in ovo.*[9] There is no evidence yet available to exclude the possibility that vagal fibers seen in 4E to 5E embryonic chick hearts are sensory in nature.[10,11]

There is an important feature of muscarinic drug action that remains to be solved in connection with the onset of cholinergic neuroeffector transmission. The electrical signal associated with SA node pacemaker inhibition by muscarinic agonists changes well before vagal innervation. When acetylcholine (ACh) or carbamylcholine (CCh) inhibited pacemaking in the SA node of 4E chicks, the membrane depolarized.[12] As shown in FIGURE 1, CCh depolarized the SA node membrane with Na^+ in the bathing medium and hyperpolarized in the absence of Na^+. This membrane potential change is opposite the hyperpolarization characteristic of the adult SA node pacemaker and seen two days later in the same tissue of the embryonic chick. The mechanism for the depolarization was attributed to an increased membrane conductance to Na^+ through tetrodotoxin (TTX)-insensitive channels.[12] The eventual ontogenetic appear-

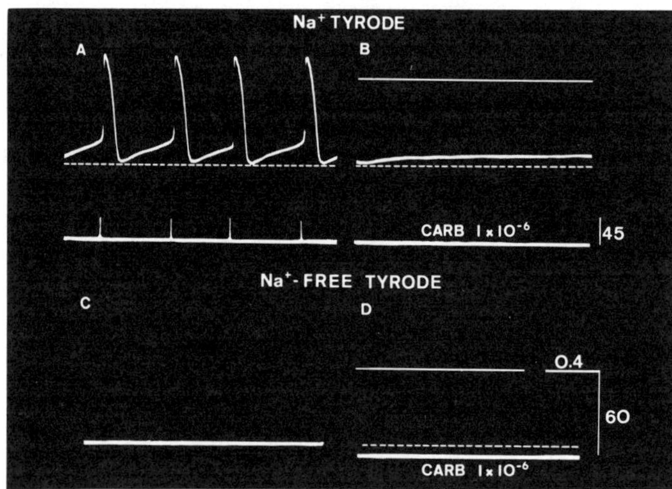

FIGURE 1. CCh (10^{-6}M) depolarizes SA node cell membrane when pacemaking is transiently inhibited. In the presence of Tyrode's solution with 149 mM Na^+, SA node pacemaker activity (A) is inhibited by CCh (B), and the membrane is depolarized. C: Removal of external Na^+ (replaced by Tris $^+$) caused pacemaking to cease. In D, addition of CCh hyperpolarized the membrane. The presence of a mAChR-regulated Na channel permitted depolarization, and mAChR-regulated K channel activation could be detected only when external Na was removed. (A. J. Pappano.[12] With permission from the *Journal of Pharmacology and Experimental Therapeutics.*)

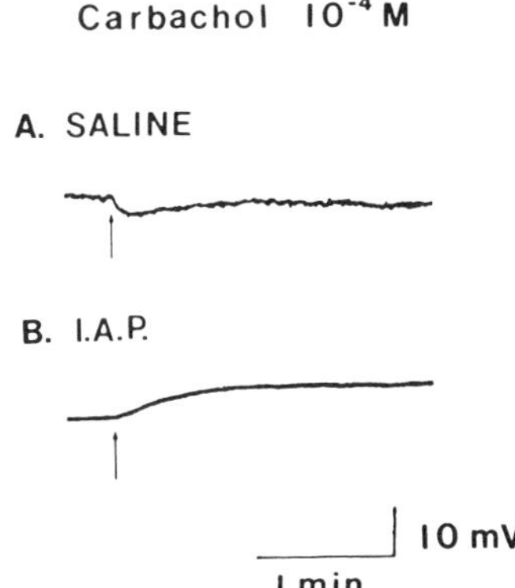

FIGURE 2. Effect of islet-activating protein (IAP) on atrial membrane response to CCh (10^{-4}M). A: Control recording from an atrial cell of a hatched chick pretreated with saline. CCh evokes a hyperpolarization that fades with time. B: Recording from atrial cell of a chick that received IAP two days earlier. CCh elicits membrane depolarization whose time course parallels the fade of the hyperpolarization seen in A. (Tajima *et al.*[14] With permission from *Circulation Research.*)

ance of muscarinic agonist-induced hyperpolarization due to increased K^+ conductance paralleled the increased membrane conductance to this ion.[11]

A more complete understanding of the significance of muscarinic agonist-induced depolarization was not available until recently. In the presence of pertussis toxin, the hyperpolarization of SA node and atrial cells (FIG. 2A) caused by ACh and CCh in hatched chicks was blocked, presumably by inactivation of the transducer proteins (Gi/Go) that link mAChR with K^+ channel activation and with adenylate cyclase inhibition.[13–15] The fact that ACh and CCh depolarized the membrane (FIG. 2B) and elicited a positive inotropic action by way of the mAChR was attributed to an unmasking of these phenomena by pertussis toxin.[15] Of particular interest was the observation that the depolarization depended upon extracellular Na^+ and was resistant to TTX. As in embryonic chick SA node, the actions of muscarinic agonists in atria from hatched chicks treated with pertussis toxin were independent of catecholamines and the adrenergic nervous system.[15] Actually, in SA node cells from hatched chicks treated with pertussis toxin, CCh consistently depolarized the membrane and in many preparations accelerated pacemaking activity.[16] Atropine selectively antagonized the depolarization and acceleration of the SA node caused by ACh.

In guinea pig ventricular muscle, choline esters increased intracellular Na^+ activity and exerted a positive inotropic effect by an action on mAChR.[17,18] Moreover, the stimulant actions of choline esters were independent of endogenous catecholamines.[17] In light of the observations by Korth and Kühlkamp and our own, we developed a single ventricular myocyte model (guinea pig) to evaluate the mechanism for the stimulant action of muscarinic agonists with the voltage clamp technique.

In the presence of either Ba^{2+} (0.2 mM) or Cs^+ (20 mM), CCh and ACh depolarized single ventricular myocytes and evoked an inward current when the membrane was clamped at the resting potential of -75 mV.[19] The current generated by CCh was observed in the presence of TTX to block voltage-dependent Na^+ entry, Cd^{2+} to block voltage-dependent Ca^{2+} entry, Cs^+ (Ba^{2+} and tetraethylammonium) to block i_{K1}, and ouabain to block the Na pump. Nevertheless, the CCh-induced current depended upon the transmembrane Na^+ gradient (FIG. 3) and the reversal potential, for the action of CCh shifted by 61 mV per tenfold change of external Na^+.[19] These findings confirm and extend those of Korth and Kühlkamp and verify their assumption concerning the mechanism for muscarinic agonist-induced increments of intracellular Na^+ activity. Additionally, our results are consistent with the hypothesis that Na^+ entry is the first step in a series of reactions that culminate in a positive inotropic effect.[19]

It must be noted that activation of phospholipase C[15,18] or of phospholipase D[19] have been considered in order to provide intracellular messengers for the "stimulant" actions of certain muscarinic agonists on various cardiac tissues. There is as yet,

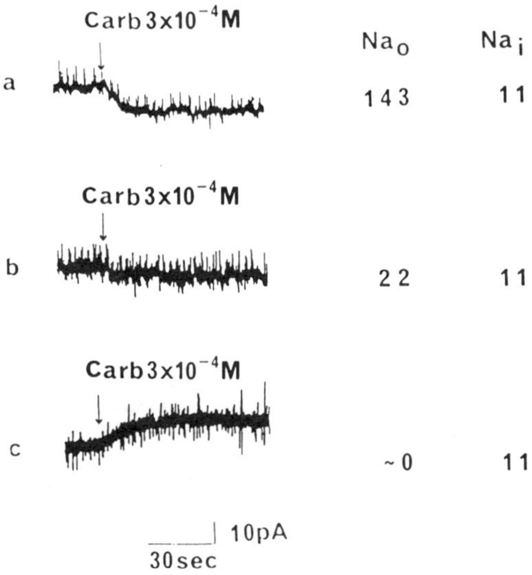

FIGURE 3. Effect of transmembrane Na^+ gradient on direction of CCh-induced membrane current in isolated guinea pig ventricular myocytes. The bathing solution contained (mM): $MgCl_2$, 2.3; HEPES, 10; glucose, 5.5; $BaCl_2$, 2.0; $CdCl_2$, 0.1; TTX, 0.01; and isotonic replacement of N-methyl-D-glucamine$^+$ for Na^+ in b and c. The pipette solution contained (mM); Cs aspartate, 66; CsCl, 20; $MgCl_2$, 5.5; Na_2 creatine phosphate, 5; NaH_2PO_4, 1; TEA-Cl, 20; EGTA, 5; HEPES, 5; and K_2ATP, 10. The holding potential was -40 mV, and each record was taken from a separate cell. The right-hand columns indicate the extracellular ($[Na^+]_o$) and intracellular ($[Na^+]_i$) concentrations of Na. When the Na gradient is inward (a,b), the CCh-induced current is inward in direct proportion to the size of the gradient. When the Na gradient is outward (c), the current induced by CCh is also outward. (Unpublished experiment of K. Matsumoto and A. Pappano).

however, no conclusive evidence for or against the participation of inositol trisphosphate (IP_3) or of diacylglyceral (DAG) as intracellular mediators.

There are many examples of paradoxical stimulation of the heart either by vagal stimuli or by exogenously applied muscarinic agonists.[20] In rabbit Purkinje fibers[1] and in SA node,[21] there is a "rebound" decrease in K conductance and increase of spontaneous impulse frequency, respectively, upon removing ACh or CCh from the bathing solution. Furthermore, it has been suggested that endogenously released or exogenously applied ACh can increase Na^+ conductance in SA node cells from rabbit,[22] cat,[23] and dog.[24] Paradoxical stimulation of the SA node by the vagus and postvagal tachycardia are atropine-sensitive phenomena that have been attributed to the increased Na conductance.[23,24] When the results from adult and embryonic hearts are compared, it may be suggested that the Na-dependent depolarization and stimulation by ACh or CCh in the aneural embryonic heart can be manifested later in life under various conditions. While particularly evident when either the transducer proteins, Gi/Go, are inactivated or the muscarinic-regulated K channel is blocked, there is reason to suspect that fade of the negative responses and rebound from them are expressions of muscarinic stimulation of Na entry in adult hearts.

SUMMARY

A brief outline of the ontogenesis of cholinergic neuroeffector transmission in the embryonic chick heart is given. It is important to define the development of neuroeffector transmission to evaluate the possible effects on postjunctional membrane properties. The membrane response of the aneural chick heart undergoes a qualitative change to muscarinic agonist at a time well before cholinergic innervation. This suppressed response can be revealed later in life, even in adults, when provision is made to exclude Gi/Go and or K channel activity.

ACKNOWLEDGMENT

Thanks are due to Dr. Kazuo Matsumoto (Saitama Medical School) for providing unpublished records shown in FIGURE 3.

REFERENCES

1. CARMELIET, E. & K. MUBAGWA. 1986. Desensitization of the acetylcholine-induced increase of potassium conductance in rabbit cardiac Purkinje fibres. J. Physiol. (London) **371:** 239-255.
2. PAPPANO, A. J. & K. LÖFFELHOLZ. 1974. Ontogenesis of adrenergic and cholinergic neuroeffector transmission in chick embryo heart. J. Pharmacol. Exp. Ther. **191:** 468-478.
3. SULLIVAN, J. K., S. SOROTA, C. ZOTTER & A. J. PAPPANO. 1985. Is muscarinic receptor number in avian ventricle regulated by vagal innervation? *In* Cardiac Morphogenesis. V. J. Ferrans, G. Rosenquist & C. Weinstein, Eds.: 253-266. Elsevier Science Publishing Co., Inc. New York.
4. LÖFFELHOLZ, K. & A. J. PAPPANO. 1974. Increased sensitivity of sinoatrial pacemaker to acetylcholine and to catecholamines at the onset of autonomic neuroeffector transmission in chick embryo heart. J. Pharmacol. Exp. Ther. **191:** 479-486.
5. KIRBY, M. L. & R. S. ARONSTAM. 1983. Atropine-induced alterations of normal development of muscarinic receptors in the embryonic chick heart. J. Mol. Cell. Cardiol. **15:** 685-696.

6. KIRBY, M. L. & D. E. STEWART. 1983. Neural crest origin of cardiac ganglion cells in the chick embryo: Indentification and extirpation. Dev. Biol. **97:** 433-443.

7. KIRBY, M. L., T. A. WEIDMAN & J. W. McKENZIE. 1980. An ultrastructural study of the cardiac ganglia in the bulbar plexus of the developing chick heart. Dev. Neurosci. **3:** 174-184.

8. ROSKOSKI, R. JR., R. I. McDONALD, L. M. ROSKOSKI, W. J. MARVIN & K. HERMSMEYER. 1977. Choline acetyltransferase activity in heart: Evidence for neuronal and not myocardial origin. Am. J. Physiol. **233:** H642-H646.

9. ROMANOFF, A. L. 1960. The Avian Embryo: Structural and Functional Development. The MacMillan Company. New York.

10. HIGGINS, D. 1983. The ontogeny of the response of the avian embryo heart to autonomic neurotransmitters and to neurotransmitter-like drugs. Pharm. Ther. **20:** 53-77.

11. PAPPANO, A. J. 1977. Ontogenetic development of autonomic neuroeffector transmission and transmitter reactivity in embryonic and fetal hearts. Pharmacol. Rev. **29:** 3-33.

12. PAPPANO, A. J. 1972. Sodium-dependent depolarization of non-innervated embryonic chick heart by acetylcholine. J. Pharmacol. Exp. Ther. **180:** 340-350.

13. SOROTA, S., Y. TSUJI, T. TAJIMA & A. J. PAPPANO. 1985. Pertussis toxin treatment blocks hyperpolarization by muscarinic agonists in chick atrium. Circ. Res. **57:** 748-758.

14. TAJIMA, T., Y. TSUJI, S. SOROTA & A. J. PAPPANO. 1987. Positive vs negative inotropic effects of carbachol in avian atrial muscle: Role of N_i-like protein. Circ. Res. **61**(Suppl. I): I-105-I-111.

15. TAJIMA, T., Y. TSUJI, J. H. BROWN & A. J. PAPPANO. 1987. Pertussis toxin-insensitive phosphoinositide hydrolysis, membrane depolarization, and positive inotropic effect of carbachol in chick atria. Circ. Res. **61:** 436-445.

16. AGNARSSON, U., T. TAJIMA & A. J. PAPPANO. 1988. Carbachol depolarizes and accelerates pacemaker activity in the sinoatrial node of chicks treated with pertussis toxin. J. Pharmacol. Exp. Ther. **247:** 150-155.

17. KORTH, M. & V. KÜHLKAMP. 1985. Muscarinic receptor-mediated increase of intracellular Na^+-ion activity and force of contraction. Pfluegers Arch. **403:** 266-272.

18. KORTH, M. & V. KÜHLKAMP. 1987. Muscarinic receptors mediate negative and positive inotropic effects in mammalian ventricular myocardium: Differentiation by agonists. Br. J. Pharmacol. **90:** 81-90.

19. MATSUMOTO, K. & A. J. PAPPANO. 1989. Sodium-dependent membrane current induced by carbachol in single guinea-pig ventricular myocytes. J. Physiol. (London) **415:** 487-502.

20. LÖFFELHOLZ, K. & A. J. PAPPANO. 1985. The parasympathetic neuroeffector junction of the heart. Pharmacol. Rev. **37:** 1-24.

21. BOYETT, M. R. & A. ROBERTS. 1987. The fade of the response to acetylcholine at the rabbit isolated sino-atrial node. J. Physiol. (London) **393:** 171-194.

22. TODA, N. & T. C. WEST. 1967. Interactions of K, Na and vagal stimulation in the S-A node of the rabbit. Am. J. Physiol. **212:** 416-423.

23. BURKE, G. H. & F. R. CALARESU. 1972. An experimental analysis of the tachycardia that follows vagal stimulation. J. Physiol. (London) **226:** 491-510.

24. CHIBA, S., M. N. LEVY & H. ZIESKE. 1975. Chronotropic response to acetylcholine injected into the sinus node artery of the isolated atrium of the dog. Cardiovasc. Res. **9:** 127-133.

Developmental Changes in Alpha Adrenergic Modulation of Ventricular Pacemaker Function[a]

MICHAEL R. ROSEN[b] AND RICHARD B. ROBINSON

*Departments of Pharmacology and Pediatrics and
Division of Developmental Pharmacology
Columbia University College of Physicians and Surgeons
New York, New York 10032*

INTRODUCTION

This report will summarize research we and our associates have performed on the alpha-adrenergic modulation of cardiac rhythm. Our specific interest is in the developmental changes that occur in this control mechanism. We shall demonstrate that alpha-adrenergic receptor stimulation not only serves an important modulatory function with respect to cardiac rhythm, but that receptor-effector coupling and its physiologic expression change developmentally.

METHODS

Studies are performed on cardiac myocytes in monolayer cell culture alone or in co-culture with sympathetic neurons. We also study isolated cardiac tissues and intact animals. To prepare the cell cultures, the ventricles of 1-2-day-old Wistar rats are minced and disaggregated into single cells by a previously described trypsin treatment.[1] The cells are suspended at a concentration of 500,000/mL and preplated for 45 minutes to remove nonmuscle cells. For the biochemistry experiments, the nonattached cells are then plated directly into petri dishes coated with protamine sulfate or fibronectin, whereas for the pharmacology experiments they are plated onto coated glass cover slips within the dishes. Single neurons are prepared from the paravertebral sympathetic ganglia of 3-4-day-old Wistar rats using a trypsin disaggregation.[1] The neurons are plated several hours before the muscle, using a ratio of 1:4 between neuronal and myocardial cells at the time of plating. All cells are grown in minimal

[a] These studies were supported by USPHS-NHLBI Grant HL-28958. Dr. Robinson is an Established Investigator of the New York Heart Association.

[b] Address for correspondence: Michael R. Rosen, M.D., Department of Pharmacology, Columbia University, College of Physicians and Surgeons, 630 West 168th Street, P&S 7-517, New York, NY 10032.

essential medium with antibiotic and 10% horse serum, as well as 20 ng/mL nerve growth factor (NGF). The medium is changed after 24 hours and again three days later. Cultures are generally studied 5 days after plating.

Isolated tissue studies are performed using Purkinje fiber bundles excised from the hearts of neonatal and adult dogs. Dogs are anesthetized with pentobarbital sodium, 30 mg/kg, i.v. or i.p. (neonates, only), and their hearts are removed through a thoracotomy. Purkinje fiber bundles are excised from the right and left ventricles and mounted in a tissue chamber perfused with modified Tyrode's solution maintained at approximately 37° C and gassed with 95% O_2 and 5% CO_2. Tissues are impaled with 3 M KCl-filled glass microelectrodes, and the transmembrane potentials and automatic rhythms are recorded. The calibration of the equipment and details of the method have been described previously.[2,3]

Intact Animal Studies

Neonatal rats are divided into three groups at birth and injected subcutaneously with either NGF, a saline placebo, or NGF antibody daily through day 9 of life. On days 1 and 10 of life we record the ECG. Animals are sacrificed on days 10-11, their hearts are removed, and the ventricular septa are dissected free and mounted in a tissue bath perfused with Tyrode's solution, as above. Bipolar silver wires, insulated to the tips with Teflon, are used to record surface electrograms, which are displayed continuously on a strip chart recorder.[4,5]

RESULTS

Neonatal rat myocytes plated in tissue culture before day 2 of life respond to alpha-adrenergic stimulation with an increase in automatic rate.[1] This increase in automaticity is blocked by prazosin, but not by propranolol, atropine, or adenosine deaminase. Hence, in ventricular myocytes, obtained from a young animal whose heart has minimal or no sympathetic innervation, the effect of alpha-adrenergic innervation is to increase impulse initiation. Moreover, this positive chronotropic action can be attributed to an alpha-adrenergic rather than a beta-adrenergic, muscarinic, or purinergic mechanism.

By contrast, when myocytes from animals of the same age are co-cultured with sympathetic neurons, the response to alpha-adrenergic stimulation in two-thirds of the co-cultures is a decrease in automaticity (FIG. 1). This decrease is also attenuated by prazosin and unmodified by propranolol, atropine, or adenosine deaminase.[1] That the co-cultures are, in fact, innervated has been demonstrated in three types of experiments: ultrastructural studies that showed areas of close apposition between muscle and nerve cells; physiologic studies in which tyramine, which induces neural catecholamine release, increased automaticity in nerve-muscle co-cultures, but not in pure myocyte cultures; and nerve stimulation by way of electrodes.[6]

Subsequent studies have established the necessity of close nerve-muscle contact if there is to be maturation of alpha-adrenergic responsiveness from excitation to inhibition of automaticity. This has been done by placing pure myocyte cultures on cover slips adjacent to nerve-muscle co-cultures in the same petri dish.[7] Catecholamines released from nerves by tyramine readily increase the automaticity of the myocytes on both cover slips, indicating that substances released by nerves can diffuse through the bulk environment. The pure myocyte cultures persist, however, in a positive chronotropic response to alpha agonist, suggesting that whatever substance provides the neural signal for maturation to the myocyte, it is not distributed into the bulk phase (or is unavailable in sufficient quantity to induce maturation). Additional studies have indicated that the "signal" that induces maturation of the alpha response is not norepinephrine or acetylcholine. We are continuing to seek the identification of this signal.

There is a small decrease in the number of α_1-adrenergic receptors in membranes

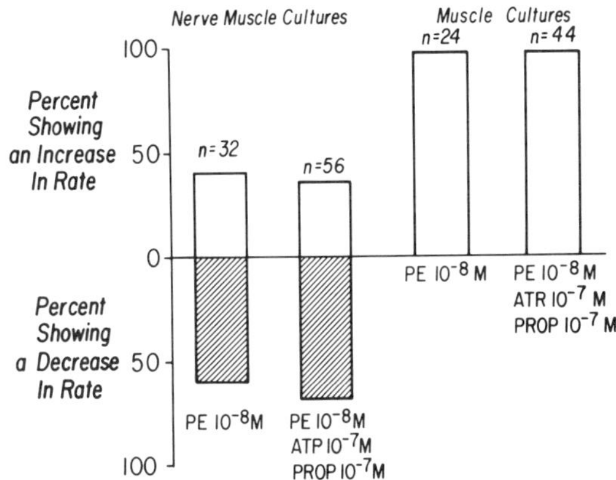

FIGURE 1. Chronotropic response of cardiac myocytes, cultured alone or co-cultured with sympathetic neurons to phenylephrine (PE), 1×10^{-8}M. Sixty percent of the nerve-muscle co-cultures exhibited a negative chronotropic response to phenylephrine, 1×10^{-8}M. This decrease in rate persisted in 63% of the nerve-muscle cultures in the presence of atropine (ATR) (1×10^{-7}M) and propranolol (PROP) (1×10^{-7}M). All of the noninnervated myocyte cultures exhibited increases in rate that persisted in the presence of atropine and propranolol. (E. D. Drugge *et al.*[1] With permission from *Circulation Research.*)

from adult rat ventricle, compared to the neonate, but no change in affinity.[8] Given that the alpha receptor, itself, does not change importantly in number or affinity for agonist in the time required for maturation of the alpha response, we have looked elsewhere for a cause for maturation. The next level of receptor-effector coupling considered has been the GTP regulatory proteins. We have been particularly interested in the 41 kDa family of pertussis toxin substrates, as one of the group, G_i, has been shown to modulate cardiac function through its role in muscarinic receptor-effector coupling.[9] As shown in FIGURE 2A, in noninnervated myocytes in tissue culture, the 41 kDa family of pertussis toxin substrates is present in only a limited amount. The protein seen here presumably includes G_i, as noninnervated myocytes from other mammalian species demonstrate a normal response to cholinergic agonists.[10] In the innervated cultures (FIG. 2B), however, the amount of 41 kDa pertussis toxin substrate is markedly increased, and this increase coincides with the change from alpha-adrenergic excitation to inhibition of automaticity. The cause and effect relationship of the

41 kDa substrate to alpha-adrenergic inhibition of automaticity is such that when nerve-muscle cocultures are incubated with pertussis toxin to an extent that the substrate is fully ADP-ribosylated and functionally inactivated, the alpha response reverts to excitation of automaticity despite the persistence of sympathetic innervation (FIG. 2B).[11] Hence, this series of experiments demonstrates that for isolated cell systems

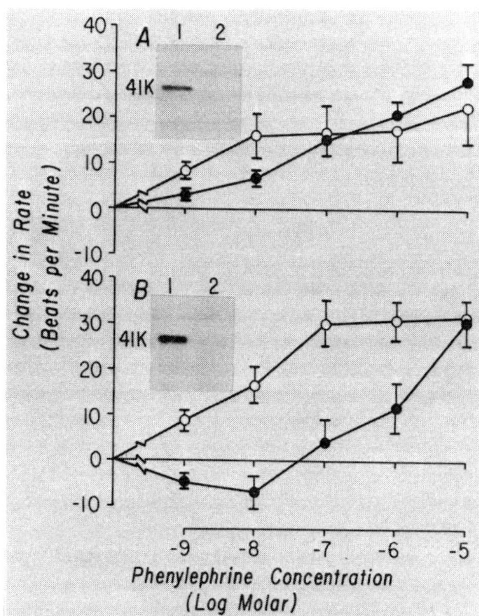

FIGURE 2. The effect of pertussis toxin on the chronotropic response of noninnervated and innervated cardiac myocytes in culture. Noninnervated myocytes (A, filled symbols, n = 10) respond to phenylephrine with an exclusive increase in rate of beating, whereas for innervated myocytes the average response to phenylephrine (1-10 nM) is a reduction in beating rate (B, filled symbols, n = 10). When the cultures are assessed for the amount of pertussis toxin substrate by the ADP-ribosylation reaction, the co-cultures are enriched (compare lane 1 of insets B and A). Other myocyte cultures (A, unfilled symbols, n = 10) and nerve-muscle co-cultures (B, unfilled symbols, n = 18) were exposed to pertussis toxin (0.5 μg/mL) for 16-24 hours before testing with phenylephrine. The noninnervated cultures show no change in their positive chronotropic response to phenylephrine; nerve-muscle co-cultures, however, now show an exclusive increase in beating rate. The in vitro ADP-ribosylation assay shows complete endogenous ADP-ribosylation after in vivo incubation with pertussis toxin in both situations (lane 2 of both insets). (J. P. Bilezikian et al.[21] With permission from Molecular and Cellular Biochemistry.)

a clear relationship of sympathetic innervation to development of 41 kDa regulatory proteins and maturation of alpha responsiveness occurs.

Isolated Tissue Studies

Although the abovementioned studies establish the essential role of the 41 kDa pertussis toxin substrate in the modulation of alpha-adrenergic responsiveness, they do not provide information on the function of the system *in situ*, or on the mechanism whereby the substrate permits alpha agonists to reduce automaticity. These studies have been performed in isolated neonatal and adult canine Purkinje fibers and rat ventricle and in disaggregated adult canine Purkinje myocytes.

In isolated neonatal rat ventricular septa and neonatal canine Purkinje fibers, alpha-adrenergic stimulation tends to increase automaticity.[1,12] In the adults of both species the tendency is for automaticity to decrease. A difference between the species' responses is seen in the fact that 100% of adult rat ventricles and only 60-75% of canine Purkinje fibers show a decrease in automaticity in response to phenylephrine (the remainder of canine fibers show an increase). The same relationship of sympathetic neural development to maturation of alpha-adrenergic responsiveness described above for cells in culture appears to hold for the isolated tissues.[3] Moreover, a temporal relationship has been shown for the development of sympathetic innervation and of the 41 kDa pertussis toxin substrate. That is, with development from fetal through neonatal dog there are parallel increases in sympathetic innervation and in the presence of the 41 kDa pertussis toxin substrate.[13,14] There also are developmental changes in myocardial alpha receptors, which decrease in number in the canine heart from the fetus through the adult.[15] As in rat heart, however, these changes do not occur within the same time frame as that in alpha responsiveness. Moreover, in rat ventricles there is a dramatic difference in the nature of the guanine nucleotide regulatory protein coupled to the neonatal and adult myocardial α_1 receptor. In both cases, agonist binding is affected by guanine nucleotides, suggesting an interaction of a G protein with the receptor, but in the neonate this interaction is totally unaffected by pertussis toxin. In the adult, the ability of guanine nucleotides to affect agonist binding is reduced but not eliminated by pertussis toxin. Thus, the neonatal cardiac α_1-adrenergic receptor is linked to a G protein that is not a substrate for pertussis toxin, whereas the adult receptor is linked to both pertussis toxin sensitive and insensitive G proteins.[8]

There is also evidence in adult fibers for a temporal relationship between the presence of the regulatory protein and the inhibition of automaticity by α_1-adrenergic stimulation. For example, in adult Purkinje fibers with intact sympathetic innervation, ADP ribosylation of the 41 kDa substrate by pertussis toxin results in a loss of alpha-adrenergic inhibition of automaticity.[2] In this setting, automaticity increases. Other data obtained from canine experiments suggest that once the nerve has signaled the development of the 41 kDa protein, it is no longer necessary for the protein's maintenance. Specifically, treatment of adult dogs with 6-hydroxydopamine for two weeks results in loss of functional sympathetic terminals (reflected in low tissue norepinephrine content and absent tyramine response), yet the levels of 41 kDa substrate remain unchanged, and the response to alpha agonist remains inhibitory of automaticity.[2]

Given that the 41 kDa substrate is a central factor in the maturation of the alpha response, it, nonetheless, does not explain why there is a decrease or an increase in automaticity. To consider the mechanism, we have turned our attention from the modulator (*i.e.,* the 41 kDa pertussis toxin substrate) to the subcellular processes it might modulate. Of particular interest are the pacemaker current, itself, and the metabolic pumps that might modify pacemaker activity. Experiments in other laboratories[16,17] have suggested that alpha-adrenergic stimulation does not affect the pacemaker current. By contrast, studies of disaggregated adult canine Purkinje myocytes have shown that an outward current is increased.[18] This current persists in the presence of barium, is blocked by dihydroouabain, and has been identified as the Na-K pump current. Moreover, the ability of alpha agonists to stimulate the current is lost following treatment with pertussis toxin. Other evidence that alpha agonists stimulate Na-K pump current comes from experiments using ion sensitive electrodes.[19] Alpha agonist (phenylephrine, 2×10^{-8} M) has been shown to decrease intracellular sodium activity from 9.9 ± 1.5 mM to 6.1 ± 1.3 mM ($p < .05$), consonant with reducing automaticity of adult canine Purkinje fibers. That this action on aNa_i is not secondary to changes occurring in automatic beating rate has been shown in two ways: first, by determining the change in aNa_i (0.2 mM), induced by altering the drive rate of Purkinje fibers to encompass the range of spontaneous rates seen in the automatic fibers (10-30 b/min); second, by demonstrating that in two-thirds of fibers driven at a constant rate, alpha agonists persist in decreasing aNa. These effects of alpha agonist on aNa_i are blocked by prazosin but not propranolol.

Hence, primary stimulation of the Na-K pump appears to be the mechanism whereby alpha agonists decrease automaticity in adult fibers. In addition, alpha agonists decrease an outward K current, which appears to be iK_1, an action that would tend to increase automatic rate.[18] This action, too, is dependent on the 41 kDa pertussis toxin substrate. Inasmuch as the actions of alpha agonists on Na-K pumping and on outward current have opposing effects on automaticity, it is likely that the ultimate magnitude of rate change results from whatever balance is achieved between the two.

The mechanism(s) responsible for the pertussis toxin insensitive excitation of automaticity in neonatal fibers has not yet been determined. This may reflect an iK_1-dependence that is unrelated to the 41 kDa substrate. It could be derived from stimulation of pacemaker current, or inhibition of Na-K pump function, or an entirely different pathway. This question remains to be answered.

Studies in the Intact Animal

We have been studying the relationship of sympathetic innervation to alpha-adrenergic responsiveness in the intact animal, as a means to comprehending the physiologic implications of the system. In the adult dog with normal sympathetic innervation, but complete heart block (induced by formalin injection of the His bundle), epinephrine infusion decreases ventricular automaticity, an effect blocked by phentolamine, but not propranolol.[20] Hence, alpha stimulation does modulate automaticity in the intact adult ventricle.

We also have investigated the role of nerve growth in the neonatal rat. Littermate rat pups are injected with NGF, the antiserum to nerve growth factor, or placebo on days 1-10 of life.[4,5] Evidence that NGF accelerates and the antiserum inhibits sympathetic growth is obtained by measuring tissue norepinephrine levels, by observing the response of isolated ventricle to tyramine, and by staining the ventricles using tyrosine hydroxylase. With all three procedures it is apparent that nerve growth is accelerated in the NGF-treated animals and is interfered with in the antiserum-treated animals. In addition, the 41 kDa pertussis toxin substrate appears elevated in the NGF-treated animals and decreased in the antiserum-treated animals. Finally, ECG recordings reveal an abnormally long Q-T interval in the antiserum-treated animals. (By contrast, the Q-T intervals of placebo and NGF-treated animals are comparable.) Work is currently proceeding to evaluate the mechanism for this long Q-T interval, as well as its possible role in arrhythmogenesis.

CONCLUSIONS

We have demonstrated that with development of the heart there is a change in alpha-adrenergic responsiveness of the ventricular conducting system from excitation to inhibition of automaticity. Moreover, we have shown that the critical factors in this pattern are the development of the sympathetic nervous system and of a GTP regulatory protein that is a pertussis toxin substrate. We have shown, as well, that the substrate appears to link the receptor to the Na-K pump, thereby effecting the decrease in automaticity.

We have considered, also, some of the questions that remain in our understanding of this regulatory system. We are confident that continued investigation of this pathway not only will provide further insights into alpha-adrenergic modulation and its changes with development, but will be useful in understanding the regulation of other cardiac-humoral interactions.

REFERENCES

1. DRUGGE, E. D., M. R. ROSEN & R. B. ROBINSON. 1985. Neuronal regulation of the development of the alpha adrenergic chronotropic response in the rat heart. Circ. Res. **57:** 415-423.
2. ROSEN, M. R., S. F. STEINBERG, Y-K. CHOW, J. P. BILEZIKIAN & P. DANILO JR. 1988. The role of a pertussis toxin sensitive protein in the modulation of canine Purkinje fiber automaticity. Circ. Res. **62:** 315-323.
3. REDER, R., P. DANILO JR. & M. R. ROSEN. 1984. Developmental changes in alpha adrenergic effects on canine Purkinje fiber automaticity. Dev. Pharm. Ther. **7:** 94-108.
4. MALFATTO, G., T. ROSEN, L. SUN, S. STEINBERG, P. DANILO JR. & M. R. ROSEN. 1988. Sympathetic innervation in neonatal rats induces a GTP regulatory protein that modulates alpha adrenergic effects on ventricular automaticity. Pediatr. Res. **23:**(Suppl.I): 1401.
5. MALFATTO, G., S. F. STEINBERG, T. S. ROSEN, L. S. SUN & M. R. ROSEN. 1988. Long Q-T interval and abnormal alpha adrenergic receptor-effector coupling. Circulation **78:** II-557.
6. ROBINSON, R. B. 1985. Models of cardiac development: transplants, organ culture, cell dispersion and cell culture. *In* The Developing Heart. M. Legato, Ed.: 69-94. Kluwer-Nijhoff. Boston.
7. DRUGGE, E. D. & R. ROBINSON. 1987. Trophic influence of sympathetic neurons on the cardiac alpha adrenergic response requires close nerve-muscle association. Dev. Pharm. Ther. **10:** 47-59.
8. HAN, H. M., S. F. STEINBERG, R. B. ROBINSON & J. P. BILEZIKIAN. 1988. Developmental changes in coupling of alpha$_1$ adrenergic receptors to GTP binding regulatory proteins in the rat heart. FASEB J. **2:** A620.
9. PFAFFINGER, P. J., J. M. MARTIN, D. D. HUNTER, N. M. NATHANSON & B. HILLE. 1985. GTP-binding proteins couple cardiac muscarinic receptors to a K channel. Nature **317:** 536-538.
10. LANE, M. A., A. SASTRE, M. LAW & M. M. SALPETER. 1977. Cholinergic and adrenergic receptors on mouse cardiocytes *in vitro.* Dev. Biol. **57:** 254-269.
11. STEINBERG, S. F., E. D. DRUGGE, J. P. BILEZIKIAN & R. B. ROBINSON. 1985. Acquisition by innervated cardiac myocytes of a pertussis toxin-specific regulatory protein linked to the alpha$_1$ receptor. Science **230:** 186-188.
12. ROSEN, M. R., A. J. HORDOF, J. ILVENTO & P. DANILO JR. 1977. Effects of adrenergic amines on electrophysiologic properties and automaticity of neonatal and adult canine cardiac Purkinje fibers. Circ. Res. **40:** 390-400.
13. DANILO JR., P. 1985. Electrophysiology of the fetal and neonatal heart. *In* The Developing Heart. M. Legato, Ed.: 21-38. Martinus Nijhoff. Boston.
14. ROSEN, M. R., P. DANILO JR., R. B. ROBINSON, A. SHAH & S. F. STEINBERG. 1988. Sympathetic neural and α-adrenergic modulation of arrhythmias. *In* The Sudden Infant Death Syndrome P. J. Schwartz, D. P. Southall & M. Valdes-Dapena. Ed.: **533:** 200-209. Annals of the New York Academy of Sciences. New York.
15. BUCHTHAL, S. D., J. P. BILEZIKIAN & P. DANILO JR. 1987. Alpha$_1$-adrenergic receptors in the adult, neonatal and fetal heart. Dev. Pharm. Ther. **10:** 90-99.

16. HAUSWIRTH, O., H. D. WEHNER & R. ZOSKOVEN. 1976. Alpha adrenergic receptors and pacemaker current in cardiac Purkinje fibers. Nature **263:** 155-157.
17. TSIEN, R. W. 1974. Effects of epinephrine on the pacemaker potassium current of cardiac Purkinje fibers. J. Gen. Physiol. **64:** 293-319.
18. SHAH, A., I. S. COHEN & M. ROSEN. 1988. Stimulation of cardial alpha$_1$ receptors increases Na/K pump activity via a pertussis toxin sensitive pathway. Biophys. J. **54:** 219-225.
19. ZAZA, A., R. P. KLINE & M. R. ROSEN. 1987. Effects of alpha-adrenergic stimulation on intracellular Na activity. Circulation **76:** IV-62.
20. HORDOF, A. J., E. ROSE, P. DANILO JR. & M. R. ROSEN. 1982. Alpha and beta adrenergic effects of epinephrine on ventricular pacemakers in dogs. Am. J. Physiol. **242:** H677-H682.
21. BILEZIKIAN, J. P., S. F. STEINBERG, E. M. HORN, R. B. ROBINSON & M. R. ROSEN. 1988. G protein-adrenergic interactions in the heart. Mol. Cell. Biochem. **82:** 5-11.

The Development of Physiologic Responsiveness to Muscarinic Stimulation in Embryonic Chick Heart

Relationship to Increased Levels of Pertussis Toxin Substrates

JOEY V. BARNETT, STEVEN M. SHAMAH, AND
JONAS B. GALPER

Department of Medicine
Cardiovascular Division
Brigham and Women's Hospital
and
Harvard Medical School
Boston, Massachusetts 02115

INTRODUCTION

The ability of embryonic chick heart to respond to muscarinic and beta-adrenergic stimulation does not develop coordinately. Prior to days 4–5 *in ovo,* both beta-adrenergic receptors, as demonstrated by the binding of the beta-adrenergic antagonist (-)-[^{3}H]dihydroalprenolol,[1] and muscarinic receptors, as measured by the binding of the muscarinic antagonist [^{3}H]QNB,[2] are present on the cell membrane of the developing embryonic chick heart cell. However, although the beta-adrenergic agonist-mediated increase in beating rate and adenylate cyclase activity[1,3] is demonstrable in hearts prior to day 4–5 *in ovo,* muscarinic agonists exert relatively little effect on beating rate at this stage of development.[2,4] These data suggest that at this stage, which corresponds to the time of ingrowth of the vagus nerve, muscarinic receptors are not coupled to a physiologic response in the heart. Hence, the embryonic chick heart offers a good model for the study of factors that couple muscarinic receptors to a physiologic response.

At present, five forms of the muscarinic receptor have been described.[5] Some of these have been associated with particular muscarinic responses in a given tissue type. Whether isoform shifts of muscarinic receptors are involved in the appearance of new physiologic responses to muscarinic stimulation during embryonic development of the heart has not been determined. The guanine nucleotide regulatory proteins that couple muscarinic receptors to a physiologic response now include a family of at least four proteins, α_o, α_{i-1}, α_{i-2}, and α_{i-3},[6] which are substrates for ADP-ribosylation by pertussis toxin and α_p, which is coupled to hormonal stimulation of phospholipase C activation and is not a pertussis toxin substrate.[7] Because muscarinic receptors are present in embryonic chick heart cells 3.5 days *in ovo*,[2] the absence of a physiologic response in these cells to muscarinic stimulation might be due to the absence of a specific isoform of the muscarinic receptor required to couple agonist binding to a given effector molecule, the absence of the appropriate guanine nucleotide binding protein to couple the muscarinic receptor to a physiologic response, or the absence of an appropriate effector to mediate a specific physiologic response. In experiments presented here, we will determine whether developmental changes in levels of guanine nucleotide regulatory proteins may be associated with the embryonic development of the muscarinic cholinergic response in the chick heart. The relationship between changes in levels of G proteins and the coupling of muscarinic receptors to inhibition of adenylate cyclase activity will be determined.

MATERIAL AND METHODS

Heart cell cultures were prepared by a modification of the method of DeHaan.[8] Embryonic age was determined by the method of Hamberger and Hamilton.[9] Embryos were removed from embryonated Leghorn chicken eggs at the indicated embryonic age; hearts were removed, atria and ventricle separated, and the tissue incubated with 0.025% (w/v) trypsin in Ca^{2+}/Mg^{2+}-free Hanks' balanced salt solution at 37 °C for 8 minutes. The trypsin solution was removed and diluted into medium M199 containing 50% heat-inactivated horse serum at room temperature. After successive trypsinizations, suspensions of trypsinized cells were sedimented at 1000 rpm and resuspended in growth medium containing 6% fetal calf serum at a density of 1.6×10^5 cells/cm^2 in 100 mm petri dishes (Falcon, Oxnard, CA), and incubated at 37 °C in a humidified atmosphere of 5% CO_2, 95% air. Unless otherwise indicated, cells were used from experiments on culture day three.

Preparation of Tissue for Adenylate Cyclase Assay and ADP-Ribosylation

Hearts of chick embryos of the indicated gestational age were suspended in TMSD buffer (50 mM Tris-HCl, 1 mM EDTA, 0.2 M sucrose, and 0.6 mM dithiothreitol, and 75 mM NaCl), Dounce homogenized, and filtered through gauze at 4 °C. The filtrate was adjusted to approximately 0.5 mg protein/cc, and 50 μL samples were assayed in each tube. The addition of a mixture of protease inhibitors, 16 μg/mL lima bean trypsin inhibitor, 9 μg/mL leupeptin, 0.18 mg/mL 1,10 phenanthroline, 1.4 mM EGTA, and the surface active antibiotic alamethicin (14 μg/mL) markedly improved reproducibility.

Adenylate Cyclase Activity

Adenylate cyclase activity was determined as described by Neer.[10] The reaction mixture was 0.4 mM [^{3}H]ATP (specific activity 50-80 μC_i/mM), 12 mM $MgCl_2$, 10 mM phosphocreatine, 0.84 U creatine phosphokinase, 1.0 mM cAMP, 1 mM dithiothreitol, 75 mM NaCl, 100 μM GTP, 50 mM Tris HCl, 1 mM EDTA, 0.2 M sucrose, and protease inhibitors at the concentrations indicated. 1-Isoproterenol, carbamylcholine, and atropine were added in the order and the concentrations indicated in the text. Following incubation for 10 min at 37 °C, a diluting solution containing unlabeled cAMP, ATP, and [^{14}C]cAMP was added; the reaction mixture was boiled for 2 min and loaded onto Dowex AG50wX2 (Biorad, Inc.) columns; the cAMP peak was collected. Further separation of remaining adenine and guanine nucleotides was accomplished by Ba(OH)$_2$ and ZnSO$_4$ precipitation. Following Ba(OH)$_2$ and ZnSO$_4$ precipitation, recovery of [^{3}H]cAMP was determined by measurement of the ratio of [^{3}H] to [^{14}C] in an aliquot of the supernatant in a Beckman liquid scintillation counter. Recoveries of [^{3}H]cAMP were usually 40 percent.

ADP Ribosylation with Pertussis Toxin

ADP ribosylation was carried out for the times indicated at 37 °C. The assay mixture contained 10 μM NAD$^+$, 0.3-0.5 μCi [^{32}P]NAD, 2.5 mM ATP, 2 mM GTP, 10 mM isoniazid, 10 mM thymidine, 10 mM MgCl$_2$, 25 ng pertussis toxin, 10 mM phosphocreatine, 84 U creatine phosphokinase in a total volume of 25 microliters. Tissue homogenized in TMSD buffer was added to the reaction mixture at 50-100 μg/assay. The protease inhibitors, soybean trypsin inhibitor, lima bean trypsin inhibitor, and leupeptin were present at the concentrations described previously from the time of initial homogenization of the tissue. The reaction was stopped by the addition of 2% SDS in Laemmli sample buffer[11] followed by boiling for one minute. Analysis of peptides following ADP-ribosylation was performed on 9% acrylamide gels prepared according to Laemmli.[11] Dried gels were exposed to Kodak XAR film with or without enhancing screens for 1-2 days at -70 °C.

Immunoblotting

Antibodies were prepared and characterized as described previously.[12] Immunoblotting was carried out by a modification of the method of Towbin *et al.*[13] Specific antibody against bovine α_o was a gift of E. J. Neer.

RESULTS

Developmental Changes in Muscarinic Inhibition of Isoproterenol-Stimulated Adenylate Cyclase Activity

We previously determined that the level of isoproterenol stimulation of adenylate cyclase activity did not change during embryonic development of the chick heart between days 2.5 *in ovo* and 3 days posthatching. In order to determine whether muscarinic cholinergic inhibition of isoproterenol-stimulated adenylate cyclase activity increased with embryonic age, we compared the ability of various concentrations of carbamylcholine to inhibit isoproterenol-stimulated adenylate cyclase activity in homogenates of hearts from embryos 2.5, 3.5, and 10 days *in ovo* and three days posthatching. Isoproterenol (10^{-4} M) stimulated adenylate cyclase activity by 2260 pM/mg/10 min at each embryonic age studied. Data summarized in FIGURE 1 indicate that at day 2.5 *in ovo* carbamylcholine inhibited isoproterenol-stimulated adenylate cyclase activity by only 80 ± 16 (n = 7, SE) pmol/10 min/mg protein or 3.5 percent. Thus, inhibition increased at day 3.5 *in ovo* to 220 ± 12 (n = 7) pmol/10 min/mg or 10% of the isoproterenol-stimulated level. At day 10 *in ovo* carbamylcholine inhibited isoproterenol-stimulated adenylate cyclase activity 320 ± 30 (n = 8) pmol/10 min/mg or 29% of the isoproterenol-stimulated level, and at 3 days posthatching, inhibition increased to 1040 ± 28 pmol/10 min/mg (n = 5) or 46% of the isoproterenol-stimulated level. The total increase in the extent of inhibition during development was 13-fold. Furthermore, the sensitivity to carbamylcholine increased with embryonic age (FIG. 1) from an EC_{50} of 16.5 ± 5 μM in hearts 2.5 days *in ovo* to 0.6 ± 0.1 μM in homogenates of hearts 3 days posthatching. This represents a 26-fold increase in sensitivity of adenylate cyclase activity to inhibition by carbamylcholine during development.

Developmental Changes in Guanine Nucleotide-Binding Proteins Demonstrated by ADP-Ribosylation of Chick Heart Homogenates by Pertussis Toxin

Data summarized in FIGURE 1 indicates that between days 2.5 and 10 *in ovo* there is a significant increase in the ability of muscarinic agonists to inhibit isoproterenol-stimulated adenylate cyclase activity. Inasmuch as we have previously demonstrated that between days 2.5 and 10 *in ovo* muscarinic receptor number, as measured by the binding of [^{3}H]QNB, did not change,[2] one explanation for enhanced coupling of muscarinic receptors to adenylate cyclase inhibition is that between days 2.5 and 10 *in ovo* levels of guanine nucleotide regulatory proteins, which couple muscarinic receptors to inhibition of adenylate cyclase activity, increase.

In order to study developmental changes in levels of α_o and α_i, crude membrane preparations of embryonic chick hearts at various embryonic ages were preincubated with pertussis toxin in the presence of [^{32}P]NAD$^+$. Following polyacrylamide gel electrophoresis and autoradiography two specifically labeled bands appeared, one at 41 kDa and one at 39 kDa at each embryonic age (FIG. 2a). Densitometry scanning of the autoradiographs demonstrated that the intensity of the 39 kDa band increased 1.7-fold from days 2.5 to 3.5 *in ovo*, 1.5-fold from 3.5 to 10 *in ovo*, and was unchanged from day 10 until hatching. The 41 kDa band increased 1.5-fold from 2.5 to 3.5 days *in ovo* and was unchanged from days 3.5 to 10 *in ovo* (FIG. 2b).

Immunoblotting of the α_{39} Subunits of G_o at Various Embryonic Ages

Because measurement of levels of α_o and α_i by ADP-ribosylation with pertussis toxin may not accurately reflect the levels of these proteins because of difficulties due to inaccessibility of NAD or pertussis toxin to the substrate, studies with specific antibodies to α_{39} were carried out. These studies used proteins solubilized in 1% SDS-mercaptoethanol followed by polyacrylamide gel electrophoresis and electrotransfered to nitrocellulose followed by immunoblotting and autoradiography. Such studies are not complicated by the tertiary structure of the G protein or its association with

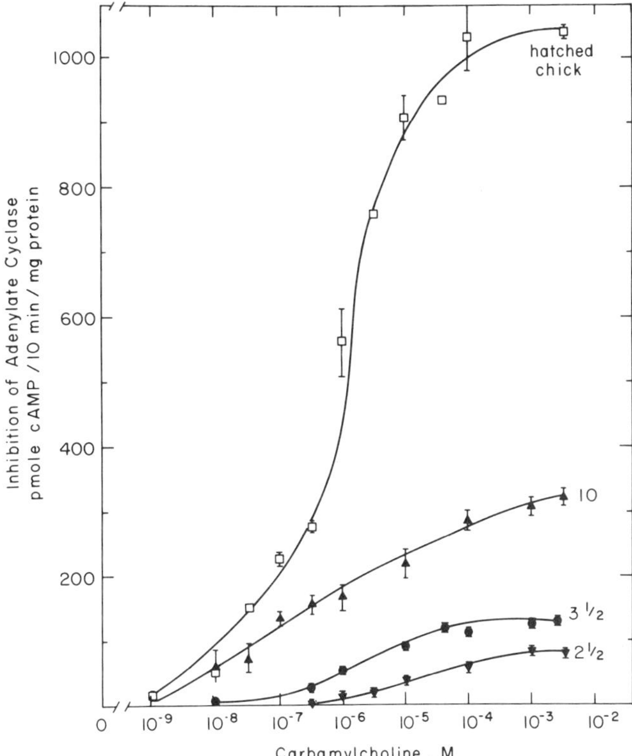

FIGURE 1. Effect of various concentrations of carbamylcholine on the inhibition of isoproterenol-stimulated adenylate cyclase activity at various developmental stages of embryonic chick heart. Assays of adenylate cyclase activity were carried out on homogenates of chick hearts from embryos at the ages indicated in the presence of 100 μM GTP, 80 mM Na$^+$, 10 μM isoproterenol, and the indicated concentrations of carbamylcholine. Data were plotted as inhibition of isoproterenol-stimulated adenylate cyclase activity (control isoproterenol-stimulated adenylate cyclase activity minus isoproterenol-stimulated adenylate cyclase activity in the presence of carbamylcholine). The data were the mean of n independent experiments; n = 3, 3, 5, and 3 for 2.5 days *in ovo*, 3.5 days *in ovo*, 10 days *in ovo*, and hatched chick, respectively. The levels of inhibition of adenylate cyclase by carbamylcholine were significantly different between any two ages by Student's *t* test. Those values for hatched chick without error bars represent single determinations. ▼, 2.5 days *in ovo*; ■, 3.5 days *in ovo*; ▲, 10 days *in ovo*; □, 3 days posthatched chick. (B. T. Liang *et al.*[19] With permission from the *Journal of Biological Chemistry.*)

membrane proteins or phospholipids. Studies of developmental changes in α_{39} levels measured by immunoblotting with anti-α_{39} demonstrated that α_{39} increased 2-fold between days 2.5 and 3.5 *in ovo*, increased 2-fold further between days 3.5 and 10 *in ovo*, but was unchanged between day 10 *in ovo* and 3 days posthatching. Hence the

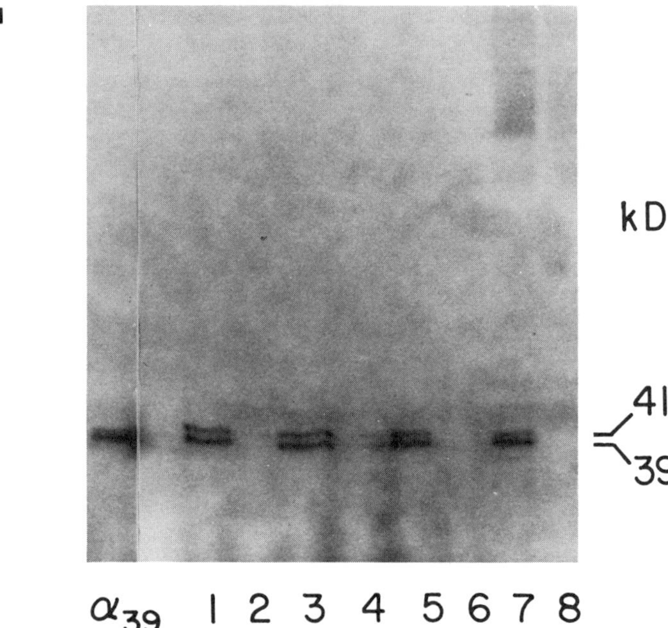

FIGURE 2a. Autoradiograph of embryonic chick heart proteins ADP-ribosylated with pertussis toxin in the presence of [^{32}P]NAD$^+$. Homogenates were prepared and incubated for 30 min at 37 °C with pertussis toxin and [^{32}P]NAD$^+$, solubilized, and subjected to polyacrylamide gel electrophoresis and autoradiography as described under MATERIAL AND METHODS. Each lane contains 100 μg of protein as determined by the method of Lowry.[14] Molecular weights were determined by plotting the distance migrated in millimeters for standard proteins stained with Coomassie blue versus the logarithm of their molecular weights. (B. T. Liang *et al.*[19] With permission from the *Journal of Biological Chemistry.*)

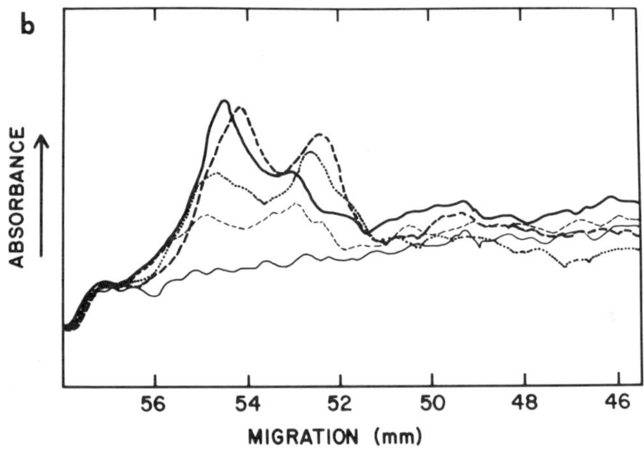

FIGURE 2b. Densitometry tracings of autoradiographs of α_{39} kDa and α_{41} kDa from **a.** Autoradiographs were scanned on an LKB laser densitometer and the base line for scans at each embryonic age superimposed. Data are typical of scans of 10 different determinations. ____, control base line; ----, 2.5 days *in ovo;* . . . . 3.5 days *in ovo;* ----, 10 days *in ovo;* ____, 3 days posthatched. (B. T. Liang *et al.*[19] With permission from the *Journal of Biological Chemistry.*)

development of increased responsiveness to muscarinic stimulation was associated with an increase in the levels of α_{39} and α_{41} (FIG. 3).

Developmental Changes in the Number of Muscarinic Receptors

In order to determine whether the increase in muscarinic inhibition of adenylate cyclase activity seen during embryonic development reflected changes in the number

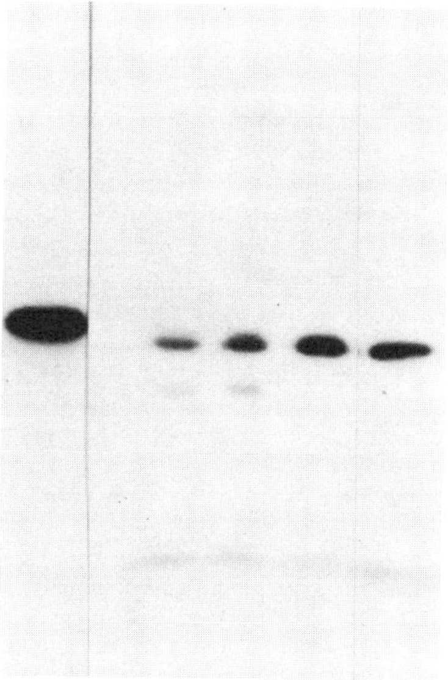

FIGURE 3. Immunoblot assay of α_{39}. Proteins were prepared and solubilized; polyacrylamide gel electrophoresis and immunoblotting were carried out as described under MATERIAL AND METHODS. Equal amounts of protein (100 µg) were loaded onto each lane. Lane 1: immunoblot of purified α_{39} from bovine brain; lane 2: immunoblot of samples from hearts 2.5 days *in ovo;* lane 3: 3.5 days *in ovo;* lane 4: 10 days *in ovo;* lane 5: 3 days posthatched. Data are typical of 10 experiments. (B. T. Liang *et al.*[19] With permission from the *Journal of Biological Chemistry.*)

of muscarinic receptors, we studied levels of muscarinic receptors as a function of embryonic age. Although we have previously demonstrated that muscarinic receptor number as measured by the binding of [³H]QNB was unchanged between days 2.5 and 18 *in ovo*,[2] studies of receptor number in embryos older than 18 days *in ovo* have not been carried out. Muscarinic receptor number was constantly at 212 fmol/mg protein between days 2.5 and 10 *in ovo*. Unlike our previous findings, however, receptor number increased 2.6-fold between day 10 and 3 days posthatching, from 200 ± 10 (n = 5) fmol/mg protein at day 10 *in ovo* to 270 ± 15 (n = 3) fmol/mg protein at day 14 *in ovo* to 520 ± 30 (n = 3) fmol/mg protein on the third day after hatching.

Correlations between Changes in the Ability of Muscarinic Agonist to Inhibit Adenylate Cyclase Activity and Changes in Levels of α_o and α_i

In order to determine whether a relationship existed between developmental changes in the number of muscarinic receptors, levels of α_{39} and α_{41}, and the appearance

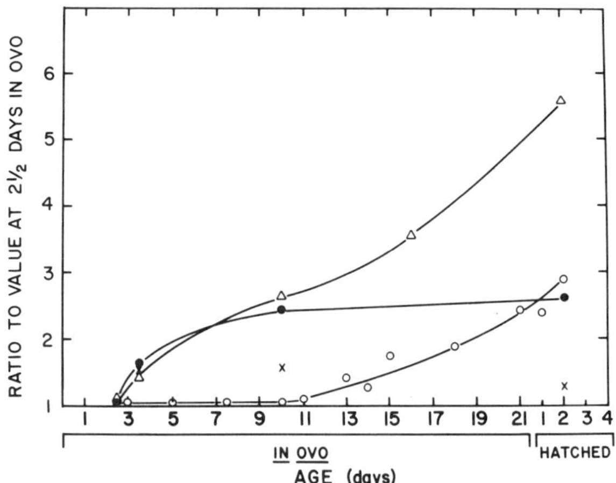

FIGURE 4. Comparisons between changes in muscarinic inhibition of adenylate cyclase, muscarinic receptor number, and α_{39} and α_{41} at each embryonic age were normalized by setting the value for each parameter at 2.5 days *in ovo* at one and determining the ratio of values at each embryonic age to the value at 2.5 days *in ovo*. The ratios for carbamylcholine inhibition of adenylate cyclase were determined from the data in FIGURE 1. The ratio for inhibition of adenylate cyclase activity in hearts 16 days *in ovo* represents the ratio of the mean of three separate determinations carried out in triplicate. Ratios for receptor number were determined by dividing the number of [³H]QNB-binding sites at each age by 200 fmol/mg of protein, the value at 2.5 days *in ovo*. Ratios for α_{39} and α_{41} were determined by dividing the relative area under the curve in FIGURE 2b for α_{41} at each embryonic age by the value for α_{41} at 2.5 days *in ovo* and the value for α_{39} at each embryonic age by the value for α_{39} at 2.5 days *in ovo*. △, inhibition of cyclase; ○, [³H]QNB-binding sites; ●, α_{39}; X, α_{41}. (B. T. Liang *et al.*[19] With permission from the *Journal of Biological Chemistry*.)

of increased sensitivity of adenylate cyclase to inhibition by muscarinic agonists, measurements of each of these parameters were normalized to their value at 2.5 days *in ovo* (FIG. 4). This allowed data for each measurement to be expressed as the extent of increase since day 2.5 *in ovo*. Hence, the inhibition of adenylate cyclase increased 2.7-fold between day 2.5 and day 10 *in ovo* while muscarinic number was constant. During the same time period, however, α_{39} increased 2.4-fold with a time course that closely paralleled the increase in muscarinic inhibition of adenylate cyclase activity. Between day 10 *in ovo* and 3 days posthatching, inhibition of adenylate cyclase increased 2.2-fold, and muscarinic receptor number increased 2.6-fold with a time course that closely paralleled the increase in inhibition of adenylate cyclase activity. During that time period the level of α_{39} remained constant. These data suggest that early in embryonic development, muscarinic inhibition of adenylate cyclase activity increases in parallel with the levels of α_{39}, whereas between day 10 *in ovo* and 3 days posthatching, inhibition of adenylate cyclase activity increases in parallel with receptor number. One explanation of these data is that early in embryonic development muscarinic receptors are present but uncoupled from inhibition of adenylate cyclase because levels of α_{39} in the cell are limiting. Subsequently, α_{39} increases to levels sufficient to couple existing receptors to a physiologic response, and the number of muscarinic receptors appears to limit the physiologic response.

DISCUSSION

The data presented here suggest that at a time during embryonic development when levels of α_o and α_i are increasing, muscarinic coupling to pertussis toxin-sensitive physiologic responses is also increasing. Muscarinic inhibition of isoproterenol-stimulated adenylate cyclase activity and the negative chronotropic response to muscarinic stimulation increase between these ages. The parallel increase in levels of these physiological responses with changes in levels of α_o and α_i supports the hypothesis that levels of guanine nucleotide regulatory proteins may be critical in regulating the level of coupling of receptors to a physiologic response in the cell.

The pertussis toxin-sensitive muscarinic responses are characterized by either complete lack of expression or a markedly decreased expression prior to ingrowth of the vagus nerve. This class of responses increases between days 2.5 and 12 *in ovo*. The pertussis-sensitive muscarinic responses are those most closely linked to the more classical negative inotropic and negative chronotropic response to muscarinic stimulation.

There is a striking parallel between developmental increases in the levels of α_o and α_i and the appearance of these pertussis toxin-sensitive muscarinic responses, a negative chronotropic response mediated by way of a pertussis toxin-sensitive activation of a K^+ conductance,[15,16] inhibition of adenylate cyclase activity, and stimulation of inositol phosphate production. One interpretation of these findings is that during embryonic development of the chick heart, levels of α_o and α_i are limiting, and their increased expression during development generates sufficiently high levels of the G-protein to permit coupling between muscarinic receptors and the effector systems involved. The presence of multiple isoforms of muscarinic receptor, however, suggest that alterations in the specificity of the G-protein that couples the muscarinic receptor to a given physiologic response may also reflect isoform switches in muscarinic receptors and phospholipase C during embryonic development. Five isoforms of the muscarinic receptor have been demonstrated and their interactions with at least three pertussis toxin substrates have been suggested.[17,18]

SUMMARY

Studies of the development of parasympathetic responsiveness in embryonic chick hearts have demonstrated that between days 2.5 and 10 *in ovo* the ability of muscarinic agonists to inhibit adenylate cyclase activity increases 10-fold in parallel with a 2.7-fold increase in the level of α_i and α_o. Thus, muscarinic inhibition of adenylate cyclase increases in parallel with an increase in α_o and α_i. These data suggest that changes in levels of guanine nucleotide regulatory proteins control, at least in part, the appearance of a parasympathetic response in the heart during embryonic development of the chick.

ACKNOWLEDGMENTS

The authors wish to thank Ms. Gretchen Hehn for able technical assistance and Ms. Barbara Zillman for typing the manuscript.

REFERENCES

1. ALEXANDER, R. W., J. B. GALPER, E. J. NEER & T. W. SMITH. 1982. Biochem. J. **204:** 825-830.
2. GALPER, J. B., W. KLEIN & W. A. CATTERALL. 1977. J. Biol. Chem. **252:** 8692-8699.
3. CULVER, N. G. & D. A. FISHMAN. 1977. Am. J. Physiol. **232:** R116-R123.
4. PAPPANO, A. & C. SKOWRONECK. 1974. J. Pharmacol. Exp. Ther. **191:** 109-118.
5. PERALTA, E. G., A. ASHKENAZI, J. WINSLOW, J. RAMACHANDRAN & D. J. CAPON. 1988. Nature **334:** 434-437.
6. JONES, D. T. & R. R. REED. 1987. J. Biol. Chem. **262:** 14241-14249.
7. COCKCROFT, S. & B. D. GOMPERTS. 1985. Nature **314:** 534-536.
8. DEHAAN, R. L. 1967. Dev. Biol. **16:** 216-249.
9. HAMBURGER, U. & H. L. HAMILTON. 1945. J. Morphol. **88:** 49-92.
10. NEER, E. J. 1978. J. Biol. Chem. **253:** 1498-1502.
11. LAEMMLI, U. K. 1980. Nature **227:** 680-685.
12. HUFF, R. M., J. M. AXTON & E. J. NEER. 1985. J. Biol. Chem. **260:** 10864-10871.
13. TOWBIN, H., T. STAEHELIN & J. GORDON. 1985. Proc. Natl. Acad. Sci. USA **76:** 4350-4353.
14. LOWRY, O. H., N. J. ROSEBROUGH, A. L. FARR & R. J. RANDALL. 1951. J. Biol. Chem. **193:** 265-275.
15. PFAFFINGER, P., J. MARTIN, D. HUNTER, N. NATHANSON & B. HILLE. 1985. Nature **317:** 536-538.
16. LOGOTHETIS, D. E., Y. KURACHI, J. B. GALPER, E. J. NEER & D. E. CLAPHAM. 1987. Nature **325:** 321-326.
17. KATAN, M., R. W. KRIZT, N. TOTTY, R. PHILIP, E. MEDUUM, R. A. ALDAPE, J. L. KNOPF & P. J. PARKER. 1988. Cell **54:** 171-177.
18. HAGA, K., H. UICHIYAMA, T. HAGA, A. ICHIYAMA, K. KANGAWA & H. MATSUO. 1989. Mol. Pharmacol. **35:** 286-294.
19. LIANG, B. T., M. R. HELLMICH, E. J. NEER & J. B. GALPER. 1988. J. Biol. Chem. **261:** 9011-9021.

Regulation of Receptor Function by Protein Phosphorylation

M. MARLENE HOSEY,[a] MADAN M. KWATRA,[b]
JUDITH PTASIENSKI,[a] AND
RICARDO M. RICHARDSON [a]

Department of Biological Chemistry and Structure
University of Health Sciences
The Chicago Medical School
North Chicago, Illinois 60064

INTRODUCTION

Recent studies have implicated protein phosphorylation as a widespread mechanism in the regulation of receptor function.[1-3] Many different types of receptors, including certain neurotransmitter and sensory receptors that couple to GTP binding proteins (G-proteins), certain neurotransmitter receptors that form ion channels, several growth factor receptors, some receptors that contain guanylate cyclase activity, and some of the steroid receptors, undergo phosphorylation at serine, threonine, or tyrosine residues. The mechanisms involved in receptor phosphorylation appear to be diverse and are not completely understood. In some instances, receptors that signal the formation of second messengers are regulated by protein kinases that are activated by the second messengers. For example, cAMP-dependent protein kinase and protein kinase C have been implicated in the regulation of β- and α_1-adrenergic receptors.[4-8] In other cases, receptors are known to autophosphorylate. The receptors for insulin and many growth factors autophosphorylate at tyrosine residues upon receptor activation.[3] In yet other instances, receptors are regulated by soluble receptor-"specific" protein kinases. For example, the light receptor rhodopsin is phosphorylated by a specific rhodopsin kinase,[9,10] whereas certain adrenergic and muscarinic cholinergic receptors are substrates for another relatively specific receptor kinase.[11-14,46] The consequences of receptor phosphorylation that have been described to date include desensitization, internalization, and activation. In the class of neurotransmitter receptors, it has been demonstrated that phosphorylation of β_1-, β_2-, and α_1-adrenergic, as well as nicotinic and muscarinic cholinergic receptors, occurs in intact cells, and appears to be involved in receptor desensitization, that is, the diminished responsiveness of the receptors to a given stimuli.[15-19]

This work will concentrate on muscarinic cholinergic receptors (mAChR), which

[a] Current address: Department of Pharmacology, Northwestern University Medical School, 303 E. Chicago Avenue, Chicago, IL 60611.

[b] Current address: Department of Pathology, Duke University Medical Center, Durham, NC 27710.

are activated by the neurotransmitter acetylcholine. Signal transduction through mAChR results in the modulation of a variety of effector systems, including attenuation of adenylyl cyclase,[20,21] hydrolysis of polyphosphoinositides,[22,23] activation of potassium channels,[24–26] and increased accumulation of cGMP.[27] Muscarinic receptors undergo densitization, that is, under certain conditions they exhibit diminished responsiveness.[28–31] The molecular basis of this process is not completely understood; however, recent evidence (see below) has suggested that the function of different mAChR subtypes may be regulated by the phosphorylation of the receptors.[31–37]

ARE CHANGES IN PROPERTIES OF CARDIAC MUSCARINIC RECEPTORS DURING DEVELOPMENT DUE TO PHOSPHORYLATION?

Receptor phosphorylation processes could conceivably participate in the regulation of receptors during cardiac development. It is well-established that the number and affinity of mAChR vary during development. Cardiac mAChR are present before innervation occurs.[38] The number of mAChR is relatively stable in the embryonic chick heart throughout development,[38–41] but increases 2-2.5-fold at birth.[40,41] In addition, the affinity of the mAChR for agonists, but not antagonists, varies during chick heart development; agonists bind with considerably higher affinity to the receptors in embryonic hearts than they do to receptors in newborn chick hearts.[40,41] If phosphorylation is important in regulating muscarinic receptor affinity and internalization, these developmental differences in receptor properties could, at least in part, reflect differences in the regulation of the receptors by phosphorylation.

MUSCARINIC RECEPTORS ARE PHOSPHORYLATED IN INTACT CARDIAC CELLS

Our laboratory has sought to understand if and how mAChR are regulated by phosphorylation. Because these receptors are present in very low amounts in cells, it is necessary to use methodology that allows for the study of the phosphorylation of the receptors. To do so, the intracellular ATP stores of chick ventricular slices are prelabeled by incubation of the tissue in ^{32}P-containing Tyrode's solution, and the receptors are purified by affinity chromatography under conditions to prevent dephosphorylation and proteolysis.[18] Receptor phosphorylation can be analyzed by gel electrophoresis and autoradiography of the purified receptors. Using such a strategy, it is possible to demonstrate that the mAChR are indeed phosphoproteins in chick cardiac cells.[18] The exciting finding[18,37] is that treatment of cardiac tissue with agonists markedly stimulates receptor phosphorylation (FIG. 1). All full muscarinic agonists tested stimulate receptor phosphorylation to the extent of 3-6 mol phosphate/mol of receptor. Phosphorylation cannot be induced by antagonists, but antagonists prevent the ability of agonists to induce mAChR phosphorylation.[18,37] The phosphoamino acids formed are serine and threonine.[37] These results were the first to demonstrate that mAChR undergo phosphorylation in intact cells and that this process is regulated by receptor activation.

MUSCARINIC RECEPTOR PHOSPHORYLATION CORRELATES WITH DESENSITIZATION

The functional consequence of mAChR phosphorylation appears to be related to receptor desensitization.[37] Early indirect studies by Burgoyne first suggested that phosphorylation of mAChR might lead to changes in receptor affinity.[32–34] In chick heart, conditions that induce receptor phosphorylation result in decreased affinity for muscarinic agonists (FIG. 2). Antagonist binding is unaffected.[37] The time courses for agonists to induce receptor phosphorylation and the decrease in receptor affinity are similar (FIG. 3). A functional consequence of the phosphorylation-induced decrease in affinity for agonists is also expressed as a decreased sensitivity of agonist-treated tissue to the negative inotropic effects of mAChR agonists.[37] These results provided the first direct, albeit initial, evidence suggesting a correlation between muscarinic receptor phosphorylation and desensitization. Whether or not similar mechanisms may play a role in the regulation of mAChR affinity during cardiac development is not known. We found that mAChR phosphorylation occurs in embryonic as well as newborn chick hearts;[18] however, a systematic characterization of this process has not yet been performed.

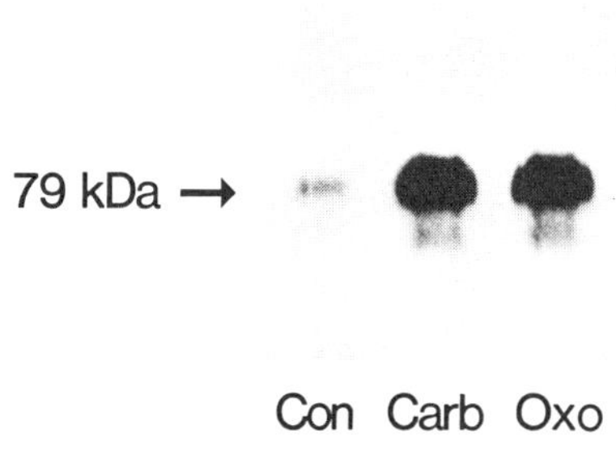

FIGURE 1. Autoradiogram depicting effects of agonists on the phosphorylation of chick heart muscarinic receptors *in situ*. Chick ventricular slices were incubated in oxygenated ^{32}P-containing Tyrode's solution at 37° C and then exposed to no drug (Con), 1 mM carbachol (Carb), or 0.1 mM oxotremorine (Oxo) for 15 min. Subsequently the mAChR were purified[18,37] by affinity chromatography and electrophoresed onto SDS gels. Shown is an autoradiogram of the resulting gel. The mAChR protein is indicated by the arrow at 79 kDa. (Kwatra *et al.*[37] With permission from the *Journal of Biological Chemistry*.)

MECHANISM OF MUSCARINIC RECEPTOR PHOSPHORYLATION

The mechanism(s) that are responsible for phosphorylation of mAChR are not known with certainty. *In situ* phosphorylation studies designed to identify the protein kinase(s) responsible for the phosphorylation of cardiac mAChR suggested that the kinase involved is not one of the well-characterized protein kinases that are regulated by second messengers, such as cyclic nucleotides, Ca^{2+}, or diacylglycerols.[37] Stimulation of cardiac slices with cyclic nucleotide analogues, activators of protein kinase C, calcium ionophores, and/or calmodulin antagonists does not modify mAChR phosphorylation in control or carbachol-treated slices.[37] Furthermore, activation of adenosine receptors, which use similar signaling pathways in cardiac cells, also does not modulate mAChR phosphorylation.[37] The results of these *in situ* phosphorylation studies suggest that either the phosphorylation of the chick heart muscarinic receptors requires agonist occupancy of the receptors, and/or is mediated by a receptor-specific protein kinase.

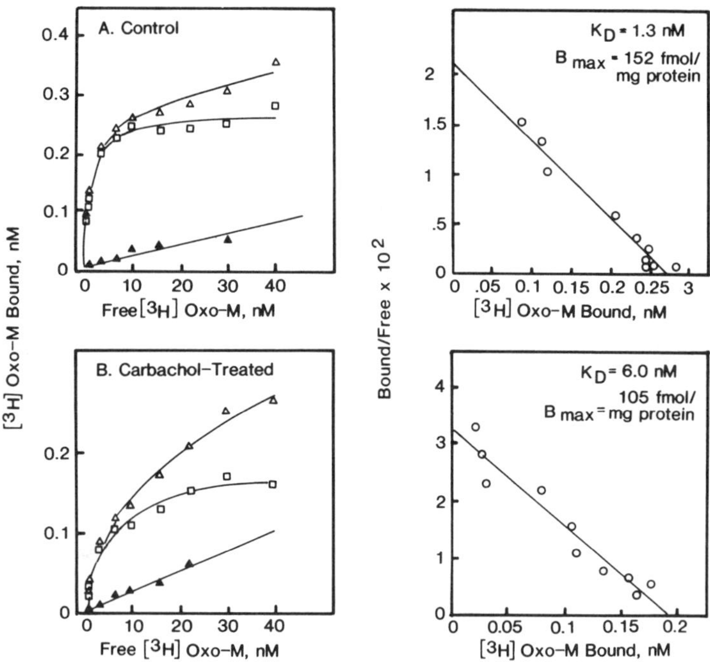

FIGURE 2. Saturation isotherms and Scatchard plots for [³H]oxotremorine-M binding to membranes prepared from control preparations and from preparations in which mAChR phosphorylation was induced by carbachol treatment. Chick ventricular slices were incubated in physiological media and exposed to either no drug (A) or to 1 mM carbachol for 30 min (B). Membranes were isolated under conditions to prevent dephosphorylation and assayed for [³H]oxotremorine binding at 20° C for 20 min.[37] The mean K_d in control preparations was 2.5 ± 0.3 nM, whereas the K_d in carbachol-treated preparations was 7.1 ± 0.4 nM (n = 5; $p <$ 0.001). No statistical differences in the B_{max} were found. (Kwatra *et al.*[37] With permission from the *Journal of Biological Chemistry.*)

The phosphorylation of cardiac muscarinic receptors by agonist-induced events has parallels to the agonist-dependent phosphorylation of adrenergic receptors. Recent studies concerning adrenergic receptors have implicated the participation of a novel protein kinase that only recognizes as substrate the agonist occupied forms of certain adrenergic receptors.[11–13] This enzyme, referred to as the β-adrenergic receptor kinase (β-AR kinase), does not appear to be regulated by any known second messengers, and effectively phosphorylates the agonist-occupied forms of the β_2- and the α_2-adrenergic receptors.[11–13] This process appears to be important in the homologous desensitization of β-adrenergic receptors.[11] In addition, indirect evidence has suggested that the enzyme β-AR kinase may be of general importance in regulating the phosphorylation of receptors coupled to adenylyl cyclase.[42,43] Cardiac mAChR, like β- and α_2-adrenergic receptors, couple to regulation of adenylyl cyclase.[20,21] In addition, recent molecular cloning studies have indicated that muscarinic receptors have structural homologies to adrenergic receptors.[44–46] In view of these similarities, it seems possible that the agonist-mediated phosphorylation of muscarinic receptors might occur through mechanisms similar to those implicated for adrenergic receptors. To test this possibility, we determined whether purified chick cardiac muscarinic receptors could serve as substrates for β-AR kinase *in vitro*. Using purified and reconstituted mAChR from chick heart, we succeeded in demonstrating that chick heart mAChR are excellent substrates for the β-AR kinase *in vitro*.[47] Phosphorylation is observed only when the receptors are occupied with agonist (FIG. 4); empty receptors and antagonist-occupied receptors are poor substrates for the enzyme.[47] The extent of phosphorylation catalyzed by β-AR kinase *in vitro* is 3-5 mol phosphate/mol receptor, and phosphorylation occurs on serine and threonine residues. Thus, many of the characteristics of the phosphorylation of mAChR by β-AR kinase *in vitro* are similar to what has been observed for agonist-induced phosphorylation of the receptors *in situ*. It is therefore tempting to suggest that β-AR kinase, or a similar enzyme, is responsible for the agonist-induced phosphorylation and desensitization of mAChR in intact cardiac cells.

Multiple mechanisms involving phosphorylation may be responsible for the regulation of muscarinic receptors. Such is the case for adrenergic receptors, which, in addition to β-AR kinase, are believed to also be regulated by cAMP-dependent protein kinase and protein kinase C.[4–8] Muscarinic receptors are known to activate phos-

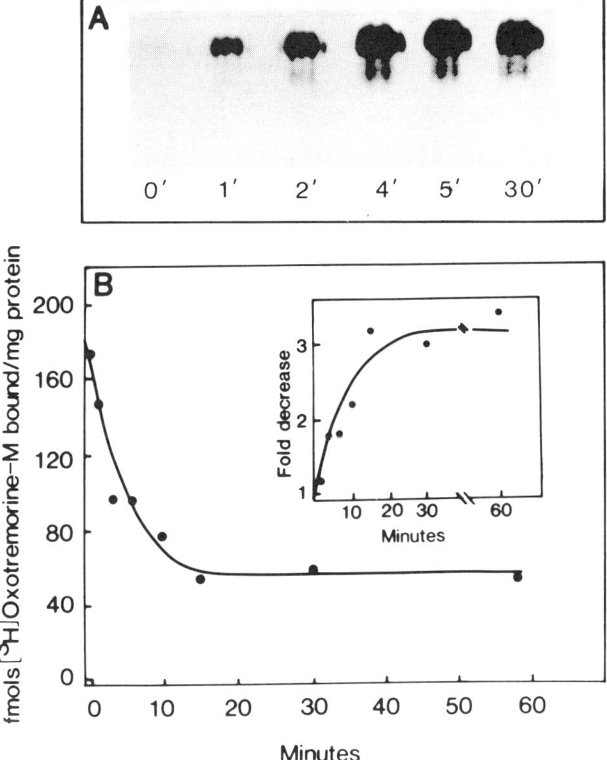

FIGURE 3. Time courses of carbachol-induced phosphorylation of muscarinic receptors and decrease in high-affinity agonist binding. Chick heart slices were exposed to 1 mM carbachol for the times indicated and examined subsequently for mAChR phosphorylation (panel A) or [³H]oxotremorine binding (panel B).

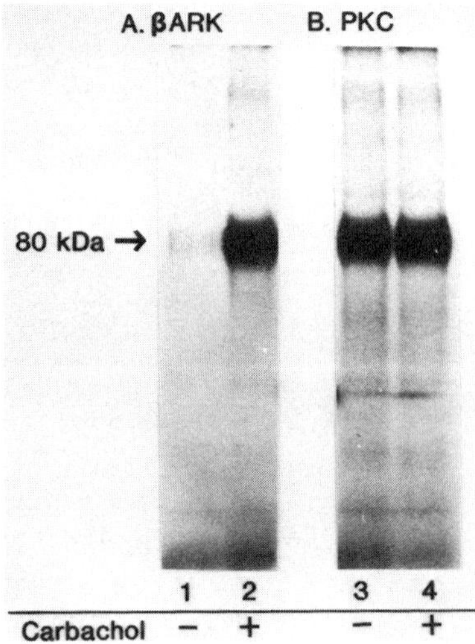

FIGURE 4. Phosphorylation of chick heart muscarinic receptors by the β-adrenergic receptor kinase and protein kinase C. Purified mAChR were reconstituted into liposomes made from chick heart lipids and incubated in the presence of [γ-^{32}P]ATP/Mg and purified preparations of either the β-adrenergic receptor kinase (A) or protein kinase C (B), in the presence or absence of 1 mM carbachol, as indicated. Incubations were at 37° C for 45 min and were terminated with SDS sample buffer. Samples were electrophoresed onto SDS gels. Shown is an autoradiogram of the resulting gel. Quantitation of the ^{32}P by scintillation counting indicated that the extent of phosphorylation by both kinases was approximately 3.5 mol phosphate/mol receptor.

phoinositide hydrolysis in cardiac cells,[22,23] which should lead to activation of protein kinase C. Activation of protein kinase C has been suggested to play a role in the down regulation of mAChR in neuroblastoma cells.[29,36] Thus, it was of interest to determine whether cardiac mAChR serve as substrates for protein kinase C. In recent *in vitro* studies we found the purified chick heart mAChR to be an excellent substrate for protein kinase C. The extent of phosphorylation of mAChR with protein kinase C *in vitro* is similar to that observed with β-AR kinase (FIG. 4). In marked contrast to the results obtained with β-AR kinase, however, phosphorylation catalzyed by protein kinase C is independent of agonist occupancy of the receptor (FIG. 4). The rate of phosphorylation of mAChR by protein kinase C is also much more rapid than that observed with β-AR kinase. The functional significance of the protein kinase C-catalyzed phosphorylation of mAChR remains to be determined.

PHOSPHORYLATION OF MUSCARINIC RECEPTOR SUBTYPES

An important question is whether phosphorylation is of general importance in the regulation of the function of mAChR subtypes. At least five subtypes of mAChR have been identified by molecular cloning of cDNAs.[45,46,49–51] In order to test the possibility that each of the mAChR subtypes are regulated by phosphorylation, it is necessary to determine whether each receptor subtype undergoes agonist-mediated phosphorylation in intact cells and, if so, if such phosphorylation has functional consequences. The subtype of mAChR in chick heart that is phosphorylated remains to be determined. Although most cardiac mAChR appear to be M2 receptors, it was suggested earlier that the chick heart mAChR may be an M1 subtype.[23] Therefore, as a first approach to defining which subtypes of mAChR are regulated by agonist-induced phosphorylation, we asked whether the porcine atrial mAChR, which are the prototypical M2 receptors,[45,46] undergo agonist-induced phosphorylation in intact tissue. As was observed in chick heart, porcine heart mAChR are phosphoproteins in intact cells, and agonists induce a marked increase in phosphorylation.[48] Many of the properties of the phosphorylation of the porcine and chick cardiac mAChR are similar. The pharmacological properties of the two receptors, however, are different (FIG. 5). In addition, peptide mapping of the purified receptors indicated that the two proteins possess structural differences.[48] Therefore it appears that the porcine and chick heart mAChR are distinct proteins. Nevertheless, the results of the phosphorylation studies show that the two mAChR undergo agonist-induced phosphorylation in intact cardiac cells, and that the characteristics of the phosphorylation processes are similar. It is as yet uncertain whether the pathways of receptor phosphorylation in chick and porcine cardiac tissue are the same or different, as only the chick system has been extensively analyzed. Further studies are planned to characterize the phosphorylation of each mAChR subtype, including the identification of the phosphorylation sites in each receptor, the identification of the protein kinase(s) responsible for the phosphorylation, and the functional significance of the phosphorylation reactions.

The studies performed to date strongly support the concept that mAChR are regulated by protein phosphorylation. It is likely that many more types of receptors will also be found to be regulated by protein phosphorylation. Once the processes underlying these events are more fully understood, they may contribute to our understanding of how receptor number and affinity is regulated in normal and abnormal cardiac development, as well as in aging and pathological conditions.

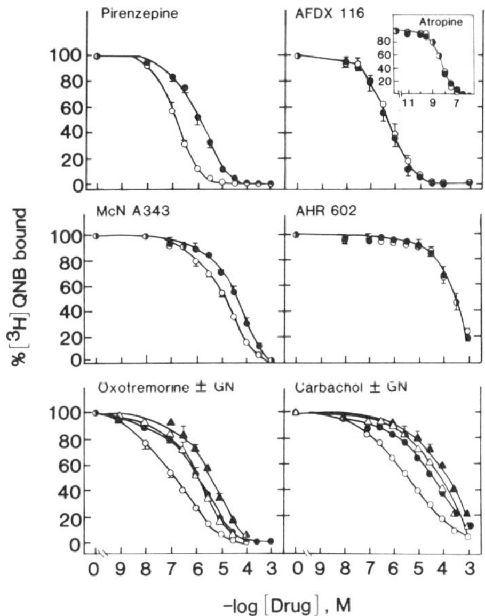

FIGURE 5. Competition of agonists and antagonists at muscarinic receptors in chick ventricular and porcine atrial membranes. Assays were performed using the antagonist [³H]quinuclidinyl benzilate (QNB) as the radioligand.[48] Data points shown are the mean of 3-5 experiments performed in duplicate. Hatch bars indicate the SEM. The effect of guanosine 5'-(β,γ-imido) triphosphate (GN) on the affinity of carbachol and oxotremorine for the chick (open triangles) and the porcine (closed triangles) was also determined. Open symbols, chick heart membranes; closed symbols, porcine atrial membranes. (Kwatra *et al.*[48] With permission from *Molecular Pharmacology.*)

REFERENCES

1. SIBLEY, D. R., J. L. BENOVIC, M. G. CARON & R. J. LEFKOWITZ. 1987. Cell **48:** 913-922.
2. HUGANIR, R. L. & P. GREENGARD. 1987. Trends Pharmacol. Sci. **8:** 472-477.
3. RAMACHANDRAN, J. & A. ULLRICH. 1987. Trends Pharmacol. Sci. **8:** 28-31.
4. BENOVIC, J. L., L. J. PIKE, R. A. CERIONE, C. STANISZEWSKI, T. YOSHIMASA, J. CODINA, M. G. CARON & R. J. LEFKOWITZ. 1985. J. Biol. Chem. **260:** 7094-7101.
5. LEEB-LUNDBERG, L. M. F., S. COTECCHIA, A. DEBLASI, M. G. CARON & R. J. LEFKOWITZ. 1987. J. Biol. Chem. **262:** 3098-3105.
6. SIBLEY, D. R., P. NAMBI, J. R. PETERS & R. J. LEFKOWITZ. 1984. Biochem. Biophys. Res. Commun. **121:** 973-979.
7. KELLEHER, D. J., J. E. PESSIN, A. E. RUOHO & G. L. JOHNSON. 1984. Proc. Natl. Acad. Sci. USA **81:** 4316-4320.
8. CLARK, R. B., M. W. KUNKEL, J. FRIEDMAN, T. J. GOKA & J. A. JOHNSON. 1988. Proc. Natl. Acad. Sci. USA **85:** 1442-1446.
9. PALCZEWSKI, K., J. H. McDOWELL & P. A. HARGRAVE. 1988. Biochemistry **27:** 2306-2313.
10. SHICHI, H. & R. L. SOMERS. 1978. J. Biol. Chem. **253:** 7040-7046.
11. BENOVIC, J. L., R. H. STRASSER, M. G. CARON & R. J. LEFKOWITZ. 1986. Proc. Natl. Acad. Sci. USA **83:** 2797-2801.
12. BENOVIC, J. L., F. MAYOR, C. STANISZEWSKI, R. J. LEFKOWITZ & M. G. CARON. 1987. J. Biol. Chem. **262:** 9026-9032.
13. BENOVIC, J. L., J. W. REGAN, M. HIROAKI, F. MAYOR, S. COTECCHIA, L. M. LEEB-LUNDBERG, M. G. CARON & R. J. LEFKOWITZ. 1987. J. Biol. Chem. **262:** 17251-17253.
14. BENOVIC, J. L., A. DEBLASI, W. C. STONE, M. G. CARON & R. J. LEFKOWITZ. 1989. Science **246:** 235-240.
15. STADEL, J. M., P. NAMBI, R. G. L. SHORR, D. F. SAWYER, M. G. CARON & R. J. LEFKOWITZ. 1983. Proc. Natl. Acad. Sci. USA **80:** 3173-3177.
16. STRASSER, R. H., D. R. SIBLEY & R. J. LEFKOWITZ. 1986. Biochemistry **25:** 1371-1377.
17. LEEB-LUNDBERG, L. M. F., S. COTECCHIA, J. W. LOMASNEY, J. F. DEBERNARDIS, R. J. LEFKOWITZ & M. G. CARON. 1985. Proc. Natl. Acad. Sci. USA **82:** 5651-5655.
18. KWATRA, M. M. & M. M. HOSEY. 1986. J. Biol. Chem. **261:** 12429-12432.
19. MILES, K., D. T. ANTHONY, L. L. RUBIN, P. GREENGARD & R. L. HUGANIR. 1987. Proc. Natl. Acad. Sci. USA **84:** 6591-6595.
20. MURAD, F., Y. M. CHI, T. W. RALL & E. W. SUTHERLAND. 1962. J. Biol. Chem. **237:** 1233-1238.
21. JACOBS, K. H., K. AKTORIES & G. SCHULTZ. 1979. Naunyn-Schmiedeberg's Arch. Pharmakol. **310:** 113-119.
22. BROWN, J. H. & S. L. BROWN. 1984. J. Biol. Chem. **259:** 3777-3781.
23. BROWN, J. H., D. GOLDSTEIN & S. B. MASTERS. 1985. Mol. Pharmacol. **27:** 525-531.
24. GILES, W. & S. J. NOBLE. 1976. J. Physiol. (Lond.) **261:** 103-123.
25. BREITWIESER, G. E. & G. SZABO. 1985. Nature **317:** 538-540.
26. PFAFFINGER, P. J., J. M. MARTIN, D. D. HUNTER, N. M. NATHANSON & B. HILLE. 1985. Nature **317:** 536-538.
27. GEORGE, W. J., J. B. POLSON, A. G. O'TOOLE & N. D. GOLDBERG. 1970. Proc. Natl. Acad. Sci. USA **66:** 398-403.
28. NATHANSON, N. M. 1987. Annu. Rev. Neurosci. **10:** 195-236.
29. EL-FAKAHANY, E. E., B. E. ALGER, W. S. LAI, T. A. PITLER, P. F. WORLEY & J. M. BARABAN. 1988. FASEB J. **2:** 2575-2583.
30. MCKINNEY, M. & E. RICHELSON. 1984. Annu. Rev. Pharmacol. Toxicol. **24:** 121-146.
31. BURGOYNE, R. D. 1986. Trends Biochem. Sci. **12:** 208-209.
32. BURGOYNE, R. D. 1980. FEBS Lett. **122:** 288-292.
33. BURGOYNE, R. D. 1981. FEBS Lett. **127:** 144-148.
34. BURGOYNE, R. D. 1983. J. Neurochem. **40:** 324-331.
35. HO, A. K. S. & J. H. WANG. 1985. Biochem. Biophys. Res. Commun. **133:** 1193-1200.
36. LILES, W. C., D. D. HUNTER, K. E. MEIER & N. M. NATHANSON. 1986. J. Biol. Chem. **261:** 5307-5313.

37. KWATRA, M. M., E. LEUNG, A. C. MAAN, K. K. MCMAHON, J. PTASIENSKI, R. D. GREEN & M. M. HOSEY. 1987. J. Biol. Chem. **262:** 16314-16321.
38. GALPER, J. B., W. KLEIN & W. A. CATTERALL. 1977. J. Biol. Chem. **252:** 8692-8699.
39. RENAUD, J. F., J. BARHANIN, D. CAVEY, M. FOSSET & M. LAZDUNSKI. 1980. Dev. Biol. **78:** 184-200.
40. HOSEY, M. M. & J. Z. FIELDS. 1981. J. Biol. Chem. **256:** 6395-6399.
41. HOSEY, M. M., K. K. MCMAHON, A. M. DANCKERS, C. M. O'CALLAHAN, J. WONG & R. D. GREEN. 1985. J. Pharmacol. Exp. Ther. **232:** 795-801.
42. STRASSER, R. H., J. L. BENOVIC, M. G. CARON & R. J. LEFKOWITZ. 1986. Proc. Natl. Acad. Sci. USA **83:** 6362-6366.
43. MAYOR, F., J. L. BENOVIC, M. G. CARON & R. J. LEFKOWITZ. 1987. J. Biol. Chem. **262:** 6468-6471.
44. KUBO, T., K. FUKUDA, A. MIKAMI, A. MAEDA, H. TAKAHASHI, M. MISHINA, T. HAGA, K. HAGA, A. ICHIYAMA, K. KANGAWA, M. KOJIMA, H. MATSUO, T. HIROSE & S. NUMA. 1986. Nature **323:** 411-416.
45. KUBO, T., A. MAEDA, K. SUGIMOTO, I. AKIBA, A. MIKAMI, H. TAKAHASHI, T. HAGA, K. HAGA, A. ICHIYAMA, K. KANGAWA, H. MATSUO, T. HIROSE & S. NUMA. 1986. FEBS Lett. **209:** 367-372.
46. PERALTA, E. G., J. W. WINSLOW, G. L. PETERSON, D. H. SMITH, A. ASHKENAZI, J. RAMACHANDRAN, M. I. SCHIMERLIK & D. J. CAPON. 1987. Science **236:** 600-605.
47. KWATRA, M. M., J. L. BENOVIC, M. G. CARON, R. J. LEFKOWITZ & M. M. HOSEY. 1989. Biochemistry **28:** 4543-4547.
48. KWATRA, M. M., J. PTASIENSKI & M. M. HOSEY. 1989. Mol. Pharmacol. **35:** 553-558.
49. BONNER, T. I., N. J. BUCKLEY, A. C. YOUNG & M. R. BRANN. 1987. Science **237:** 527-532.
50. PERALTA, E. G., A. ASHKENAZI, J. W. WINSLOW, D. H. SMITH, J. RAMACHANDRAN & D. J. CAPON. 1987. EMBO J. **6:** 3923-3929.
51. BONNER, T. I., A. C. YOUNG, M. R. BRANN & N. J. BUCKLEY. 1988. Neuron **1:** 403-410.

Development of Gap Junctions

ROBERT L. DeHAAN AND YAN-HUA CHEN

Department of Anatomy and Cell Biology
Emory University
Health Science Center
Atlanta, Georgia 30322

THE ROLE OF GAP JUNCTIONS IN EMBRYONIC DEVELOPMENT

Gap junctions allow communication among cells of most multicellular organisms, permitting the flow of ions and small molecules from cell to cell.[1,2] Ample evidence indicates that the intercellular communication mediated by these junctions is important during development.[3-5] This evidence is of three kinds, showing that junctional conductance among cells of embryos changes with time in developmentally significant ways, that spatially organized patterns of decoupling create junctionally coupled compartments that correspond to regions of specific developmental fate, and that experimental perturbation of junctional communication can cause developmental defects. We will first consider the data that underlies each of these ideas and then discuss how these results relate to development of the heart.

Degree of Cell Coupling Changes with Development

Junctional communication between embryonic cells was first described in the Squid embryo by Potter *et al.*[6] These workers noted that gap junctional communication was ubiquitous among the blastomeres without regard to developmental fate and speculated that this pathway might provide a channel for the exchange of information needed to direct development. Since then, some degree of gap junctional communication—measured by the transfer of dyes or marker molecules, or by electrical resistance across junctions—has been observed in a wide variety of embryos, both vertebrate and invertebrate. In many cases, the degree of coupling changes systematically during development. For example, insect larvae grow progressively through a series of molt/ intermolt cycles. During each cycle, the cells of the larval epidermis experience a short burst of mitotic activity and a longer period of synthetic activity. Caveny and co-workers have shown that cell communication by way of gap junction channels rises and falls in phase with these cycles.[7] Intercellular resistance is lowest when the cells are secreting new cuticle and highest when the cuticle is complete, shortly before mitotic activity begins. Application of L-glutamate (0.5 mM) to epidermal cells cultured *in vitro* caused a dramatic decrease in intercellular resistance, mimicking the natural fall in resistance that follows mitosis.[7]

In the developing vertebrate heart systematic changes in cell coupling are manifested in a dramatic increase in propagation velocity of action potentials (TABLE 1). Adult cardiac tissue has gap junctions that connect the cardiac myocytes into an electrical syncytium.[8] Conduction velocities ranging from 400 to 2000 mm/s in different parts of the heart ensure that the action potential (AP) propagates throughout the organ in a fraction of a second, that is, at a rate that is optimal for the hemodynamic pumping of blood through the organ. In the embryo, as soon as differentiation has proceeded far enough that cardiac myocytes are able to generate electrical activity, the cells are connected by low-resistance junctions that support AP propagation, but at a much lower rate. Using a multiple-site optical recording system and a voltage-sensitive dye, Komuro *et al.*[9] recorded the early spontaneous APs from 25 locations simultaneously in the early chick heart. In the 28-30 h embryo, when the heart tube is about 0.5 mm long and consists of about 3000 cells, the linear caudorostral con-

TABLE 1. Developmental Increase in Propagation Velocity of the Chicken Cardiac Action Potential

Stage	Tissue	Velocity (mm/s)	Reference No.
28-hour	Ventrical	1	10
2-day	Ventrical	17	12
3-day	Ventrical	45	12
4-day	Ventrical	93	12
13-day	Atrium	400-500	11a
Adult	Atrium	500-800	12a
Adult	Ventrical	500-900	12b

duction velocity was about 1 mm/second. Thus, it took about 0.5 s for the excitation wave to propagate throughout the heart, nearly the same as in the adult. Mechanical contractions begin at 36 h, and by 2 days the excitation wave that sweeps anteriorward from the left caudal pacemaker region produces a rhythmic peristaltic contraction that initiates the circulation of the blood. At about 3 days, as the atria form and become functional, a prominent atrioventricular (AV) delay appears that results from slow propagation through the AV canal. This reduced rate of propagation through the AV canal remains a feature of the heart during the rest of its development. Measuring by either fresh weight or total cell number, the heart increases by more than 1000-fold in size during embryogenesis,[10] although the time required for the spread of excitation remains relatively constant. Propagation matches the increasing size of the early heart because the conduction velocity increases apace in the ventricle. For example, action potential propagation through the chick ventricle increases from 17 mm/s to 93 mm/s between 2 days and 4 days of development.[12] That is, between 30 h and 4 days, conduction velocity in the ventricle increases roughly 100 times, matching almost exactly the growth in cell number.[11] It is presumed that enhanced junctional coupling and a resultant decrease in resistance to intercellular ion flow contributes to this increasing conduction velocity. The rate of action potential propagation through the heart, however, is determined by at least three parameters in addition to intercellular resistance: the dimensions of the individual cells, the resistance in the intercellular clefts, and the shape of the action potential upstroke. All of these parameters change with development in the embryonic heart. Therefore, the contribution that junctional resistance makes to the increase in conduction velocity remains to be determined.

Junctionally Coupled Compartments Have Specific Fates

Tissue-wide changes in junctional coupling with time, like those in the insect epidermis and avian heart, are presumed to play an important development role, but that role is not understood. By contrast, spatially organized changes in intercellular junctional resistance within a tissue could, in principle, define local domains or compartments that might result in different developmental pathways being taken. Alternatively, graded levels of junctional conductance from cell to cell within a tissue could allow the formation of gradients of developmentally significant "determinants" that could define the spatial organization of a part of the body plan. A "model" gradient of charged marker molecules has been established in an *in vitro* cell system that could be altered iontophoretically.[11] Recent findings in both insect and mouse embryonic systems are consistent with such mechanisms. For example, injection of dye into cells of the Drosophila wing imaginal disk revealed that the epithelium is segregated into multiple communication compartments.[13,14] Within each compartment, dye diffusion is rapid, but each compartment is separated from its neighbors by a narrow band of cells at the border (two to three cells wide) that exhibit only a very low level of coupling. Of greatest potential importance is the fact that the location of these restriction boundaries appears to coincide with lineage compartment borders mapped with lineage analysis.[14,15] Inasmuch as it is known that lineage compartments are determined by the expression of insect pattern-determining genes,[16] these results suggest that junctional communication might play an important role in the organizing pattern. Confirmatory evidence of this hypothesis was obtained from dye-injection experiments in the wing disk epithelium of the engrailed mutant of Drosophila, showing that the dye-diffusion compartments matched the mutant lineage compartments.[15,17]

Similar dye injection studies in pre- and postimplantation mouse embryos revealed that coupling is initiated at the late 8-cell stages, as the time differentiation first begins.[18,19] Initially, the entire embryo is coupled, but shortly after implantation, as the inner cell mass and trophoblast differentiate, they establish separate communication compartments that separate from each other. Upon further differentiation, the inner cell mass cells become further segregated into a number of additional communication compartments. For example, in the 7.5-day primitive streak-stage mouse embryo, coupling within each germ layer is extensive, but dye-diffusion between germ layers and between the inner cell mass and the extraembryonic layers becomes restricted. Later, within the germ layers, especially the epiblast layer, cells become segregated into box-like diffusion compartments[15] that may be related to developmental fate.

The appearance of restrictions in dye coupling between groups of embryonic cells raises the question of whether the changes in coupling are the cause or effect of cell determination. In the molluscan embryo, Lymnaea, it is known precisely from cell lineage studies when different sets of larval cells are determined.[20] Recent evidence indicates that in this system, larval cells become uncoupled from the rest of the embryo concomitant with or after their developmental fate is determined, but not before. By uncoupling, the larva is subdivided into a number of communication compartments with different prospective fates, separated by communication-incompetent larval cells. These communication compartments are congruent with mosaic developmental compartments established by early ooplasmic segregation,[21] but further development within the compartments is characterized by regulative mechanisms. That is, after deletion of a cell or group of cells within a compartment destined to form a specific embryonic component, the loss is compensated by the remaining cells of the compartment that are equipotential, suggesting that junctional communication is required for maintenance of differentiative instructions.[22]

An interesting tissue-culture model in which such junction-restricted diffusion compartments can form is the cellular reaggregate of chick or mouse cells. After dissociation of embryonic tissues, maintenance of the cells in suspension on a gyratory shaker allows them to reaggregate. Indirect evidence that cells can quickly reestablish gap junctional communication was derived first from the observation that such aggregates, composed of embryonic chick heart cells, took on a coordinated rhythmic beat within a few hours after reassociation.[23] The high degree of cell coupling among cells within an aggregate has since been measured directly,[24,25] and the process of coupling between newly apposed clusters of chick heart cells[26] and newly paired rat neonatal heart cells[27] has been analyzed.

Even when two or more different types of cells reassociate, the aggregate initially forms a single communication compartment, in which each cell preserves its histotypical identity. Such heterotypic cell aggregates, however, progressively sort into homotypic groups of cells and form multiple compartments. Junctional communication within each group is maintained, but it is reduced or lost between the cells at the boundaries of each intra-aggregate cluster.[28] The relationship between cell sorting and cell coupling is one that needs further investigation.

Agents That Affect Cell Coupling Perturb Development

The conductance or permeability of gap junction channels is influenced by a wide variety of agents,[29] including cytoplasmic pH and pCa (the negative log of calcium concentration);[30–34] second messengers, such as intracellular nucleotides,[35,36] and calmodulin,[37] as well as other effectors of kinase-dependent phosphorylation, such as growth factors;[38,39] and the products of growth-regulating genes.[40,41] In addition, antibodies against gap junction protein[42,43] and several lipophilic substances, including some alkanols, anesthetics, and fatty acids,[44–48] have profound effects on junctional coupling. These agents all appear to work by altering the open-state probability or open time of gap junction channels. In several tissue systems, it has been demonstrated that application of agents that reduce junctional coupling disturbs normal developmental pathways.

In the embryo of the South African clawed toad, *Xenopus laevis,* the blastomeres are also well-coupled. Between the 8-cell and 32-cell stage, lucifer yellow infected into a blastomere readily diffuses to surrounding blastomeres. To test whether antibodies to the major 27 kDa gap junction protein of liver (now termed Connexin32)[49] would block cell-cell communication in Xenopus, the antibodies were injected into the right dorsal blastomere of embryos at the 8-cell stage.[42] This blastomere is normally destined to give rise to the head ectoderm and mesoderm on the embryo's right side. Injections of buffer, preimmune sera, and a neutral antibody raised against matrix glycoprotein were used as controls. After two further rounds of cell division, lucifer yellow was injected into a blastomere neighboring one of those carrying the antibody or control substance. After injection of any of the control reagents, dye transfer into the previously injected cell occurred in 70-80% of the experiments, whereas in embryos previously injected with antibody the incidence of dye diffusion fell to 18 percent. The embryos that failed to transfer dye also showed complete block of electrical coupling in the antibody-containing region. These junctional antibody-loaded cells continued cleaving in harmony with their uninjected neighbors. But these embryos generated a high proportion of tadpoles with defects that were related to the developmental fate of the injected blastomere. Sixty-three percent of the antibody-injected tadpoles had varying degrees of right/left head asymmetry, and in severe cases, the tadpoles failed to form eyes or trigeminal ganglia on the right side. Thus, blocking cell communication had serious consequences for embryonic development.[50]

In the fresh water coelenterate, hydra, detailed developmental studies have been possible because of the animal's relatively simple body plan, consisting of a head and a foot at opposite ends of a cylindrical epithelial body column. The cells of the body column are well-coupled by gap junctions, as demonstrated with dye diffusion and electrical measurements.[51] Head regeneration after microsurgery in hydra is controlled by separate gradients of two developmental morphogens, a head activation factor and a head inhibition factor.[51,52] When hydra were loaded with the same anti-Connexin32 used by Warner et al., by briefly permeabilizing the epithelium with dimethyl sulfoxide, dye diffusion from cell to cell was blocked. In this condition, grafting experiments demonstrated that the gradient of head inhibition factor was also disrupted,[51,52] again suggesting the importance of junctional communication for normal development.

GAP JUNCTIONS IN THE EMBRYONIC HEART

As noted above, in embryonic[26,33] and adult[8] heart tissue, gap junctions connect the cells of the cardiac fibers and mediate action potential propagation. A major difference in the function of those gap junctions, however, has been reported. Adult heart gap junctions are not voltage-sensitive. Their conductance has proven consistently to be unaffected by either membrane potential of the cells or transjunctional potential.[34,53,54] In early experiments from this laboratory,[33] designed to test the voltage dependence of junctional conductance, we varied the voltage across the junction between a pair of embryonic chick heart cells in small (5 mV) incremental steps. The results we obtained indicated that junctional conductance in these embryonic heart cells was independent of potential, as in the adult heart.[33,55] In more recent studies,[29] however, we have applied larger transjunctional voltage steps (10, 20, 30. . . . .80 mV) in sequence, returning to 0 voltage difference between each step, and have found that the current that crossed the junction was not linear with the step potential difference. With steps larger than ± 20 mV, current across the junction was large initially, and then it inactivated from the initial peak to a voltage-dependent steady-state level in a manner comparable to the behavior of gap junctions in amphibian or Fundulus blastomeres.[56] With independent voltage-clamp circuits applied to each member of a pair (FIG. 1A), V_1 was held constant whereas V_2 was stepped to more positive or negative levels to establish the transjunctional potential (V_j, defined as $V_1 - V_2$), as shown (FIG. 1B). At each step in V_j greater than about ± 20 mV, the current across

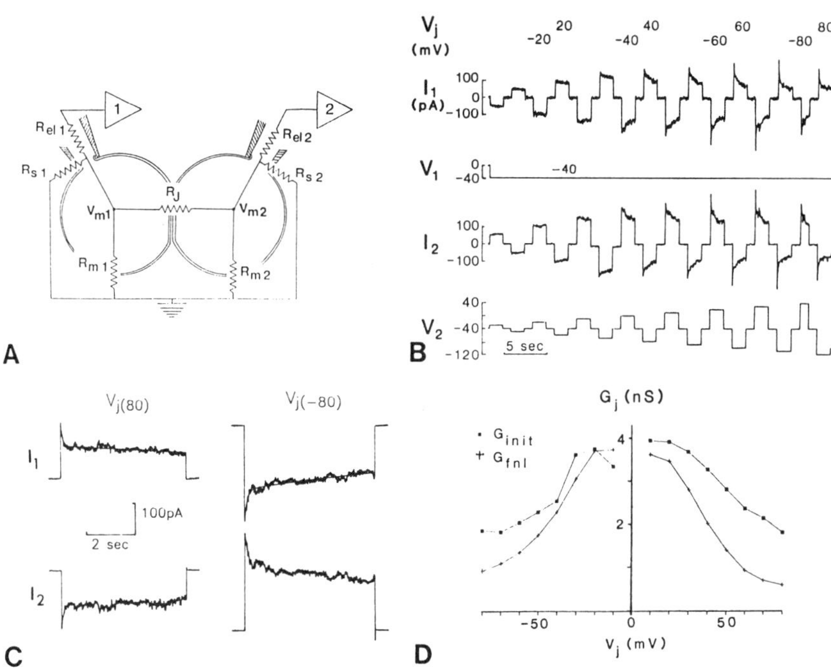

FIGURE 1. Dependence of junctional current (I_j) and conductance (G_j) on the potential (V_j) applied across the junction between a pair of coupled embryonic chick ventricle cells. **A:** Schematic diagram of the two-electrode patch clamp. Gigaseals were obtained on each member of a pair of cells, and the membrane patches were ruptured to achieve the whole-cell clamp configuration. The labeled components are access resistance (R_{el1}, R_{el2}); seal resistance (R_{s1}, R_{s2}); nonjunctional membrane resistances (R_{m1}, R_{m2}); junctional resistance (R_j); and membrane potential (V_{m1}, V_{m2}). Typical values for the named resistances were R_{el}, 5-15 MΩ; R_s, 5-50 GΩ; R_m, 2-5 GΩ; R_j, 0.05-5 GΩ. It was usually convenient to express the intercellular coupling pathway in units of junctional conductance ($G_j = 1/R = 0.2$-20 nS). Cells were bathed in balanced salt solution (BSS) containing (in mM) NaCl, 142; KCl, 2.5; MgSO$_4$, 0.8; NaH$_2$PO$_4$, 0.9; CaCl$_2$, 1.8; dextrose, 5.5; Hepes, 10 (pH 7.4). Tetrodotoxin (300 nM) was added to block sodium currents. **B:** I_1 ($=I_j$) and I_2 ($= -Ij+I_m$) in response to the voltage sequence shown in V_2. V_1 ($= V_H$) is held constant at -40 mV, whereas V_2 is stepped through a series of 1.6 s pulses at $+10$, $+20...+$ 80 mV from V_H, with each voltage step separated from the next by 1 s at V_H. This produces a series of steps in V_j at increments of $\pm$ 10 mV. Positive steps of V_2 cause negative pulses of V_j and inward (downward) steps in I_1, indicating that the direction of the current is into cell 1 across the junction. Steps in V_2 and V_H to more negative membrane potentials produce outward junctional current (seen as upward-going steps in I_1). **C:** I_1 and I_2 in response to 5 s pulses of $V_{j(80)}$ ($V_1 = 0$ mV; V_2 stepped to -80 mV from a 5 s period at $V_2 = 0$ mV; left) and $V_{j(-80)}$ ($V_1 = -80$ mV; V_2 stepped to 0 mV; right). In both polarities I_j is fit with a biexponential curve. For $V_{j(80)}$, $\tau_1 = 63.4$ ms, $\tau_2 = 156$ s; for $V_{j(-80)}$, $\tau_1 = 101.9$ ms, $\tau_2 = 9.7$ seconds. **D:** The G_j-V_j relation shows an asymmetric decline of junctional conductance as V_j is increased, both at the beginning (G_{init}) and end (G_{fnl}) of each 1.6 s pulse. The electrodes were filled with IPS#57, which contained (in mM) K-glut, 120; NaCl, 15; KH$_2$PO$_4$, 1; MgCl$_2$, 4; CaCl$_2$, 4.7; EGTA, 5; Hepes, 10 (pH 7.1); ATPNa$_2$, 3; Creatine-PO$_3$Na$_2$, 3; and cAMP, 0.033. Free Ca^{2+} was calculated to be 4×10^{-6} M. (Panels A, B, D, pair 101387; panel C, pair 111287B).

the junction (I_1) was largest initially and then decayed with what appears to be more than one time constant. The rapidly decaying spike is particularly pronounced at V_j = ± 50 mV and greater. The responses to ± 80 mV steps in V_j could be fit with biexponential kinetics (FIG. 1C), with a fast time constant on the order of 100 ms and a slow one of many seconds. Interestingly, with the inter-pulse period at 0 mV held at only one second, the current response to a positive V_j step was smaller than that to a negative pulse and had a much longer slow time constant. For example, the conductance at the end of the 1.6 s pulses to 80 mV (as in FIG. 1B) was 27.6 $\pm$ 5.0% of the peak value, whereas with -80 mV it was 38.8 $\pm$ 7.2% (mean $\pm$ SEM, N = 5). At the end of a 5 s pulse to ± 80 mV, the difference between positive and negative values was even greater (FIG. 1C). That is, current met a lower conductance flowing across the junction from cell one to cell two (FIG. 1D) and decayed away more slowly than in the opposite direction. When the interpulse period of 0 mV across the junction was also extended to 5 s, however, this apparent rectification disappeared.

Are these findings relevant to the adult mammalian heart? Even when substantial voltage differences were applied between pairs of adult ventricular myocytes under voltage clamp control, junctional conductance was unaffected.[34,53,54] The electrical properties of embryonic ventricle cells, however, bear a closer resemblance to those of adult pacemaker cells than to adult ventricular myocytes.[57] In both the adult sinoatrial (SA)[58] and AV[59] nodes, and in the ventricle compromised by ischemia[60] or drugs,[61] appreciable propagation delays and voltage gradients may appear across the cell junctions with each beat. In such circumstances, where electrical interactions are dominated by junctional conductance,[62,63] voltage-dependent junctions would have profound effects. This possibility requires further exploration.

Differences in the voltage sensitivity of embryonic and adult gap junctions raises an interesting question. Do the gradual changes in cell communication with development, described above, reflect quantitative changes in the regulation of the gap junction channels, or are embryonic and adult gap junctions qualitatively different? Suggestive evidence for such a qualitative difference comes from experiments in which Xenopus oocytes are caused to express adult rat liver junctional channels. Oocytes injected with cDNA prepared from adult rat liver formed coupling junctions when pressed together in pairs.[64] The properties of these newly expressed liver junctions, however, differed from those that normally couple Xenopus blastomeres. Conductance of the endogenous Xenopus embryonic channels was sensitive to junctional voltage, was only weakly affected by increases in intracellular calcium, but was sharply reduced by cytoplasmic acidification. By contrast, the cDNA-directed channels had properties like those of adult liver. They were voltage-insensitive, closed by small increases in calcium, and relatively unaffected by cytoplasmic acidification. Injection of oocytes with cDNA prepared from Xenopus oocyte RNA caused the expression of voltage-sensitive, embryonic junctional protein, which differed only slightly from the endogenous blastomeric gap junctions.[65] As we learn more about the molecular nature of the complex family of Connexin genes,[49] questions about developmental differences may be clarified.

REFERENCES

1. SPRAY, D. C., R. L. WHITE, V. VERSELIS & M. V. L. BENNETT. 1985. General and comparative physiology of gap junction channels. *In* Gap Junctions. M. V. L. Bennett & D. C. Spray, Eds.: 139-153. Cold Spring Harbor Laboratory. New York.

2. NEYTON, J. & A. TRAUTMANN. 1986. Physiological modulation of gap junction permeability. J. Exp. Biol. **124:** 93-114.

3. PITTS, J. D. 1972. Direct interaction between animal cells. *In* Cell Interactions. L. G. Silvestri, Ed.: 277-285. North Holland. Amsterdam.

4. WOLPERT, L. 1978. Gap junctions: channels for communication in development. *In* Intercellular Junctions and Synapses. J. Feldman, N. B. Gilula & J. Pitts, Eds.: 83-94. Chapman and Hall. London.

5. NAGAJSKI, D. J., S. C. GUTHRIE, C. C. FORD & A. E. WARNER. 1989. The correlation between patterns of dye transfer through gap junctions and future developmental fate in Xenopus: the consequences of u.v. irradiation and lithium treatment. Development **105:** 747-752.

6. POTTER, D. D., E. J. FURSHPAN & E. S. LENNOX. 1966. Connection between cells of the developing squid as revealed by electrophysiological methods. Proc. Natl. Acad. Sci. USA **55:** 328-336.

7. CAVENY, S. 1988. Developmental physiology of insect gap junctions. *In* Gap Junctions. E. L. Hertzberg & R. G. Johnson, Eds.: 495-504. Alan R. Liss. New York.

8. PAGE, E. & C. K. MANJUNATH. 1986. Communicating junctions between cardiac cells. *In* The Heart and Cardiovascular System. H. A. Fozzard *et al.,* Eds.: 573-600. Raven Press. New York.

9. KOMURA, H., A. HIROTA, T. YADA, T. SAKAI, S. FUJII & K. KAMINO. 1985. Effects of calcium on electrical propagation in early embryonic precontractile heart as revealed by multiple-site optical recordings of action potentials. J. Gen. Physiol. **85:** 365-382.

10. DEHAAN, R. L. 1988. Embryonic origin of the heartbeat. *In* The Heart. J. W. Hurst *et al.,* Eds.: 72-76. 7th ed. McGraw-Hill. New York.

11. COOPER, M. S., J. P. MILLER & S. E. FRASER. 1989. Electrophoretic repatterning of charged cytoplasmic molecules within tissues coupled by gap junctions by externally applied electric fields. Dev. Biol. **132:** 179-188.

11a. LIEBERMAN, M. & A. PAES DE CARVALHO. 1965. The spread of excitation in the embryonic chick heart. J. Gen. Physiol.**49:** 365-379.

12. ARGUELLO, C., J. ALANIS, O. PANTOJA & B. VALENZUELA. 1986. Electrophysiological and ultrastructural study of the atrioventricular canal during the development of the chick embryo. J. Mol. Cell. Cardiol. **18:** 499-510.

12a. STURKIE, P. D. 1986. Heart: contraction, conduction and electrocardiography. *In* Avian Physiology. P. D. Sturkie, Ed.: 67-190. Springer. New York.

12b. LEWIS, T. 1915. The spread of excitatory process in the vertebrate heart. V. The bird's heart. Philos. Trans. R. Soc. Lond. A/B **207:** 298.

13. WEIR, M. P. & C. W. LO. 1982. Gap junctional communication compartments in Drosophila wing disk. Proc. Natl. Acad. Sci. USA **79:** 3232-3235.

14. WEIR, M. P. & C. W. LO. 1984. Gap junctional communication compartments in Drosophila wing imaginal disk. Dev. Biol. **102:** 130-146.

15. LO, C. W. 1988. Communication compartments in insect and mammalian development. *In* Gap Junctions. E. L. Hertzberg & R. G. Johnson, Eds.: 505-514. Alan R. Liss. New York.

16. LAWRENCE, P. A. 1981. The cellular basis of segmentation in insects. Cell **26:** 3-10.

17. WEIR, M. P. & C. W. LO. 1985. An anterior/posterior communication compartment border in engrailed wing disks: possible implications for Drosophila pattern formation. Dev. Biol. **110:** 84-90.

18. LO, C. W. & N. B. GILULA. 1979. Gap junctional communication in the preimplantation mouse embryo. Cell **18:** 399-409.

19. LO, C. W. & N. B. GILULA. 1979. Gap junctional communication in the postimplantation mouse embryo. Cell **18:** 411-422.

20. VERDONK, N. H. & J. A. M. VAN DEN BIGGELAAR. 1983. Early development and the formation of germ layers. *In* The Mollusca, Vol. 3, Development. N. H. Verdonk, J. A. M. Van den Biggelaar & A. S. Tompa, Eds.: 91-122. Academic Press. New York.

21. SERRAS, F. & J. A. M. VAN DEN BIGGELAAR. 1987. Is a mosaic embryo also a mosaic of communication compartments? Dev. Biol. **120:** 132-138.

22. VAN DEN BIGGELAAR, J. A. M. & F. SERRAS. 1988. Determinative decisions and dye-

coupling changes in molluscan embryo. *In* Gap Junctions. E. L. Hertzberg & R. G. Johnson, Ed.: 483-493. Alan R. Liss. New York.

23. DeHaan, R. L. & H. G. Sachs. 1972. Cell coupling in developing systems: the heart-cell paradigm. Curr. Top. Dev. Biol. **7:** 193-228.

24. DeHaan, R. L. & H. A. Fozzard. 1975. Membrane response to current pulses in spheroidal aggregates of embryonic heart cells. J. Gen. Physiol. **65:** 207-222.

25. Clay, J. R., L. J. DeFelice & R. L. DeHaan. 1979. Parameters of current noise derived from voltage noise and impedance in chick embryonic heart cell aggregates. Biophys. J. **28:** 169-184.

26. DeHaan, R. L., E. H. Williams, D.L. Ypey & D. E. Clapham. 1981. Intercellular coupling of embryonic heart cells. *In* Perspectives in Cardiovascular Research, vol. 5. Mechanisms of Cardiac Morphogenesis and Teratogenesis. T. Pexieder, Ed.: 299-316. Raven Press. New York.

27. Rook, M. B., H. J. Jongsma & A. C. G. van Ginnekin. 1988. Properties of single gap junction channels between isolated neonatal rat heart cells. Am. J. Physiol. Heart: **255:** H770-H782.

28. Pitts, J. D. & E. Kam. 1985. Communication compartments in mixed cell cultures. Exp. Cell Res. **156:** 439-449.

29. DeHaan, R. L., Y. H. Chen & R. L. Penrod. 1989. Voltage dependence of junctional conductance in the embryonic heart. *In* Molecular and Cellular Mechanisms of Antiarrhythmic Agents. L. Hondeghem, Ed.: 19-43. Futura Publishing Co. Mount Kisco, NY.

30. Spray, D. C., A. Campos de Carvalho & M. V. L. Bennett. 1986. Sensitivity of gap junctional conductance to H ions in amphibian embryonic cells is independent of voltage sensitivity. Proc. Natl. Acad. Sci. USA **83:** 3533-3536.

31. Spray, D. C., J. C. Saez, J. M. Burt, T. Watanabe, L. M. Reid, E. L. Hertzberg & M. V. L. Bennett. 1988. Gap junctional conductance: multiple sites of regulation. *In* Gap Junctions. E. L. Hertzberg & R. G. Johnson, Eds.: 227-244. Alan R. Liss. New York.

32. Burt, J. M. & D. C. Spray. 1988. Single channel events and gating behavior of the cardiac gap junction channel. Proc. Natl. Acad. Sci. USA **85:** 3431-3434.

33. Veenstra, R. D. & R. L. DeHaan. 1988. Cardiac gap junction channel activity in embryonic chick ventricle cells. Am. J. Physiol.:Heart H170-H180.

34. Noma, A. & N. Tsuboi. 1987. Dependence of junctional conductance on proton, calcium and magnesium ions in cardiac paired cells of guinea-pig. J. Physiol. **382:** 192-211.

35. Saez, J. C., D. C. Spray, A. C. Nairn, E. L. Hertzberg, P. Greengard & M. V. L. Bennett. 1986. cAMP increases junctional conductance and stimulates phosphorylation of the 27-kDa principal gap junction polypeptide. Proc. Natl. Acad. Sci. USA **83:** 2473-2477.

36. DeMello, W. C. & P. van Loon. 1987. Influence of cyclic nucleotides on junctional permeability in atrial muscle. J. Mol. Cell. Cardiol. **19:** 83-94.

37. Peracchia, C. 1988. The calmodulin hypothesis for gap junction regulation six years later. *In* Gap Junctions. E. L. Hetrzberg & R. G. Johnson, Eds.: 267-284. Alan R. Liss. New York.

38. Maldonado, P. E., B. Rose & W. R. Loewenstein. 1988. Growth factors modulate junctional cell-to-cell communication. J. Membr. Biol. **106:** 203-210.

39. Mehta, P. P., J. S. Bertram & W. R. Loewenstein. 1989. The action of retinoids on cellular growth correlates with their actions on gap junctional communication. J. Cell Biol. **108:** 1053-1065.

40. Azarnia, R., S. Reddy, T. E. Kmiecik, D. Shalloway & W. R. Loewenstein. 1988. The cellular src gene: regulation of communication and growth. *In* Gap Junctions. E. L. Hertzberg & R. G. Johnson, Eds.: 423-434. Alan R. Liss. New York.

41. Bargiello, T. A., L. Saez *et al.* 1987. The drosophila clock gene *per* affects intercellular junctional communication. Nature **328:** 686-688.

42. Warner, A. E., S. C. Guthrie & N. B. Gilula. 1984. Antibodies to gap junctional protein selectively disrupt communication in the early amphibian embryo. Nature **311:** 127-131.

43. Young, J. D-E., Z. A. Cohn & N. B. Gilula. 1987. Functional assembly of gap junctional

conductance in lipid bilayers: demonstration that the major 27 kd protein forms the junctional channel. Cell **48:** 733-743.

44. WOJTCZAK, J. A. 1985. Electrical uncoupling induced by general anesthetics: a calcium-independent process? *In* Gap Junctions. M. V. L. Bennett & D. C. Spray, Eds.: 13-22. Cold Spring Harbor Laboratory. New York.

45. WHITE, R. L., D. C. SPRAY, A. CAMPOS DE CARVALHO, B. A. WITTENBERG & M. V. L. BENNETT. 1985. Some electrical properties of gap junctions between adult ventricular myocytes. Am. J. Physiol:Cell **249:** C447-C455.

46. BURT, J. 1989. Uncoupling of cardiac cells by doxyl stearic acids: specificity and mechanism of action. Am. J. Physiol:Cell **256:** C913-C924.

47. GIAUME, C., C. RANDRIAMAMPITA & A. TRAUTMANN. 1989. Arachidonic acid closes gap junction channels in rat lacrimal glands. Pfluegers Arch. **413:** 273-279.

48. SPRAY, D. C., J. NERBONNE, A. CAMPOS DE CARVALHO, A. L. HARRIS & M. V. L. BENNETT. 1984. Substituted benzyl acetates: a new class of compounds that reduce gap junctional conductance by cytoplasmic acidification. J. Cell Biol. **99:** 174-179.

49. BEYER, E. C., D. L. PAUL & D. A. GOODENOUGH. 1987. Connexin43: a protein from rat heart homologous to a gap junction protein from liver. J. Cell Biol. **105:** 2621-2629.

50. WARNER, A. E. 1985. Antibodies to gap junction protein: probes for studying cell interactions during development. *In* Gap Junctions. M. V. L. Bennett & D. C. Spray, Eds.: 275-288. Cold Spring Harbor Laboratory. New York.

51. FRASER, S. E., C. R. GREEN, H. R. BODE & N. B. GILULA. 1987. Selective disruption of gap junctional communication interferes with a patterning process in hydra. Science **237:** 49-55.

52. FRASER, S. E., C. R. GREEN, H. R. BODE, P. M. BODE & N. B. GILULA. 1988. A perturbation analysis of the role of gap junctional communication in developmental patterning. *In* Gap Junctions E. L. Hertzberg & R. G. Johnson, Eds.: 515-526. Alan R. Liss. New York.

53. KAMEYAMA, M. 1983. Electrical coupling between ventricular paired cells isolated from guinea pig heart. J. Physiol. **336:** 345-357.

54. WEINGART, R. & P. MAURER. 1988. Action potential transfer in cell pairs isolated from adult rat and guinea pig ventricles. Circ. Res. **63:** 72-80.

55. VEENSTRA, R. D. & R. L. DeHAAN. 1988. Cardiac gap junction channel activity in embryonic chick ventricle cells. Am. J. Physiol.:Heart **254:** H170-H180.

56. HARRIS, A. L., D. C. SPRAY & M. V. L. BENNETT. 1981. Kinetic properties of a voltage-dependent junctional conductance. J. Gen. Physiol. **77:** 95-117.

57. DeHAAN, R. L. 1980. Differentiation of excitable membranes. Curr. Top. Dev. Biol. **16:** 117-164.

58. JALIFE, J. 1984. Mutual entrainment and electrical coupling as mechanisms for synchronous firing of rabbit sino-atrial pace-maker cells. J. Physiol. **356:** 221-243.

59. PAES DE CARVALHO, A., B. F. HOFFMAN & M. P. CARVALHO. 1969. Two components of the cardiac action potential. I. Voltage time course and the effects of acetylcholine on atrial and nodal cells of the rabbit heart. J. Gen. Physiol. **54:** 607-635.

60. KLEBER, A. G., C. B. RIEGGER & M. J. JANSE. 1987. Electrical uncoupling and increase of extracellular resistance after induction of ischemia in isolated, arterially perfused rabbit papillary muscle. Circ. Res. **61:** 271-279.

61. COLE, W. C., J. B. PICONE & N. SPERELAKIS. 1988. Gap junction uncoupling and discontinuous propagation in the heart. A comparison of experimental data with computer simulations. Biophys. J. **53:** 809-818.

62. JOYNER, R. W. & F. J. L. VAN CAPELLE. 1986. Propagation through electrically coupled cells. How a small SA node drives a large atrium. Biophys. J. **50:** 1157-1164.

63. VEENSTRA, R. D. & R. L. DeHAAN. 1986. Electrotonic interactions between aggregates of chick embryo cardiac pacemaker cells. Am. J. Physiol: Heart **250:** H453-H463.

64. DAHL, G., T. MILLER, D. PAUL, R. VOELLMY & R. WERNER. 1987. Expression of functional cell-cell channels from cloned rat liver gap junction complementary DNA. Science **236:** 1291-1293.

65. EBIHARA, L., E. C. BEYER, K. I. SWENSON, D. L. PAUL & D. A. GOODENOUGH. 1989. Cloning and expression of a Xenopus embryonic gap junction protein. Science **243:** 1194-1195.

Potassium Channels and the Repolarization of Cardiac Cells[a]

L. J. DeFELICE, W. N. GOOLSBY, AND
M. MAZZANTI

Anatomy and Cell Biology
Emory University School of Medicine
Atlanta, Georgia 30322

INTRODUCTION

Though all currents are involved in each phase of the action potential, K currents in particular help repolarize heart cells, allowing them to beat again. Naming potassium as the repolarizing ion, however, is convention rather than a strict definition of its role. Though all currents interact in the free-running membrane, it is permissible to consider the contribution of each to the overall potential. The balance of the inward and outward currents causes some cells to beat spontaneously, as in the SA node, and requires others to be stimulated, as in the ventricle. Knowing the magnitude of a particular current at every moment allows a precise statement of how that current helps shape the action potential. This article shows how to calculate the contribution of each action current to the action potential, and it demonstrates how to measure the action currents directly.

How does a particular class of channels contribute to the action potential? The traditional answer depends on a model of the voltage-dependent, time-variant conductance of the ion. The model of the current is usually derived from step-protocol, voltage-clamp experiments.[1-4] Driving a particular model with an action potential is one way to deduce the action current associated with an individual current. This paradigm, which Hodgkin and Huxley[5] introduced around 1950 to study K and Na currents in squid axons, is the principal means of studying neurons, heart cells, and other excitable tissues. The patch-clamp technique Neher and Sakmann[6] introduced in 1976 allows single-electrode, whole-cell voltage-clamp of individual cells.[7] The protocols used in the patch-clamp technique most often retain the basic Hodgkin-Huxley approach.

One way to look at the established method of finding action currents is to recognize that with traditional instruments it is impossible to measure current (voltage clamp) and voltage (current clamp) at the same time and place. Current meters and volt meters are too dissimilar to connect to the same membrane. Thus, we do not generally measure action potentials and action currents at the same time, and we are as a rule forced to go through the modeling procedure to answer the original question. Bren-

[a] This work was supported by the National Institutes of Health HL-27385.

necke and Lindemann[8] found a way to measure the current and voltage at nearly the same time by using a fast switching technique. Although this method is applied frequently to avoid using two electrodes in voltage-clamp experiments, it has not been exploited to measure the action currents.

Thus virtually all reconstructions of cardiac action potentials derive from step-protocol, voltage-clamp experiments, which are most often performed on multicellular preparations measuring macroscopic currents (Purkinje fibers;[9] adult ventricle;[10] SA node;[11] Purkinje fibers incorporating pumps and concentration changes;[12] and embryonic chick atrium[13]). Few models derive from single-cell experiments or single-channel data.[14,15] To describe the currents, most researchers will use variations of the basic Hodgkin-Huxley formulas, the principal differences being in the equation parameters. The HH formulas have physical meaning easily translatable to the single-channel domain.[7,16] Some modelers use empirical formulas to describe ion currents, for example, the i_x current,[13] which are useful for calculations but are difficult to interpret.

We have developed a new method for finding the action currents. In this article we apply the method to the delayed-rectifier current, I_K, to show how it contributes to the action potential and repolarization. The new method relies on single-channel data; therefore the separation of currents is less of a problem than it is using macroscopic data. Furthermore, the reconstruction of the action current and its contribution to the action potential[7,16,36,37] relies on data obtained during beating[17-21] and conditions that traditional methods are unable to reproduce.

The new technique depends on isolating a small area of membrane on a beating heart cell using a conventional patch-clamp electrode.[17] We measure the current through the patch membrane and monitor the voltage from the rest of the cell. We thus obtain current while measuring the voltage; however, the data are from different places, which is just the reverse of the Brennecke-Lindemann[22] situation. The assumption, therefore, is that the channel in the patch is representative of its kind outside the patch. The extension to many channels of one kind, or many channels of more than one kind, is straightforward. Though we discuss automaticity in heart cells, the method would apply to any other cell, spontaneously active or externally driven.

THEORY

Suppose the potential across a cell membrane is the same everywhere, a situation that is approximated in small, spontaneously beating, isolated heart cells. In such a cell the current flows normal to the membrane, and the following condition holds:

$$C(dV/dt) + \sum_i I_i(t) = 0$$

where the sum is over all ionic currents. For the sake of argument, let us assume that only Na and K currents flow through the membrane, and let I represent the macroscopic variable. In this case the above equation becomes:

$$dV = -I_K \, dt/C - I_{Na} \, dt/C$$

If there were more than two currents, other terms would then add to the right hand side of the equation. Let the macroscopic currents be written:

$$I[V(t)] = N \text{ times } i[V(t)] \text{ times } p[V(t),t]$$

where N is the total number of channels of a certain kind, and i is the microscopic variable. This formula expresses the prevailing view of channels, namely, (1) on the time scale of our experiments, N is a constant, (2) the open-channel current, i, depends on the membrane voltage, and i varies with time only if V does, and (3) the open-channel probability, p, however, has an explicit dependence on time as well as on voltage. In a voltage-clamp experiment, V is a constant, and the equation reduces to:

$$I(t) = Nip(t)$$

which is valid at a particular voltage. In a free-running membrane, V changes each time a channel opens or closes, which alters the current, which changes the voltage, and so on.

For our purposes we lump this diverse interaction, mediated through voltage in a free-running membrane, into the average over many action currents thus:

$$\langle i(t) \rangle = i[V(t)] \text{ times } p[V(t),t]$$

and therefore write in succinct form:

$$I(t) = N\langle i(t) \rangle$$

where $\langle i(t) \rangle$ is average action current through a particular kind of channel. The average thus includes variations that occur in the open-channel current and the open-channel probability, and the equation is valid for any recurring process. Assume $\langle i_K(t) \rangle$ and $\langle i_{Na}(t) \rangle$ are obtained by averaging over action potentials, then integrating dV from 0 to t results in an expression for the action potential in terms of the underlying currents:

$$V(t) = V(0) - N_K \int_o^t \langle i_K(u) \rangle \, du/C - N_{Na} \int_o^t \langle i_{Na}(u) \rangle \, du/C$$

where u is a dummy variable and $V(0)$ is a constant of integration, which we set to zero. We rewrite this expression as:

$$V(t) = V_K(t) + V_{Na}(t)$$

V_K is the part of the action potential due to K, V_{Na} is the part due to Na, and so on for other channels if they are present.

Thus we arrive at a relationship between the potential due to the K current and the K current itself:

$$V_K(t) = - N_K \int_o^t \langle i_K(u) \rangle \, du/C$$

In our experiments, we measure the delayed-rectifier current, $\langle i_K(t) \rangle$, and calculate V_K from the above equation. In principle the same procedure could be carried out with separate patches containing the inward-rectifier I_{K1} channels. Although we were able to record delayed-rectifier channels when the patch electrode contained bath solution (a required condition for the above equations to be valid), it proved impossible to measure inward-rectifier channels unless the electrode contained high K, because the conductance of the channels is too low in normal bath solution. For this reason we applied the above analysis to I_K channels but not I_{K1} channels. At present we are able to discuss the contribution of $V_{K1}(t)$ to the action potential only by extrapolating from experiments with 60 mM K in the cell-attached pipette.

METHODS

Embryonic ventricle cells were prepared by enzymatic digestion of 7-day chick embryo hearts, following the procedure of DeHaan.[23] After 12 to 24 hours in tissue culture medium, and immediately before the experiment, we washed the cells with bath solution at room temperature. The composition of the bath in all experiments was (in mM) 130 Na, 1.3 K, 1.5 Ca, 0.5 Mg, 1 SO_4, 133.5 Cl, 5 dextrose, and 10 HEPES, pH 7.35. The whole-cell electrode contained an intracellular-like solution consisting of 140 K, 0.1 Ca, 2 Mg, 122.1 Cl, 1.1 EGTA, and 10 HEPES, pH 7.4. The cell-attached electrode contained bath solution in the delayed-rectifier experiments in FIGURE 1 but a high K solution in the inward-rectifier experiments in FIGURE 2, with K replacing Na to bring the pipette to 60 mM K.

The patch electrodes were made from borosilicate glass (Corning 7052) using a programmable puller (Sachs-Flaming, PC-84, Sutter Instrument). After coating with Sylgard (Technical Products, Inc.) and fire polishing the tip to 1-3 mm diameter, the electrodes had resistances of 4-10 megohms. The cell-attached patch electrode for current and whole-cell electrode for voltage electrodes were usually 5 to 10 μm apart. Breaking the patch in the current electrode and switching to current clamp initially showed the same voltage as the whole-cell electrode; thus the membranes of the single cells we used in these experiments were at the same voltage.

List EPC5 and EPC7 amplifiers were used to measure the voltage and the current from the two electrodes, which we then recorded and stored on a Panasonic VCR. We analyzed the data off-line on a Nicolet 4094 oscilloscope and an IBM-AT, using software developed in our laboratory. To compare the data with theoretical models, as we do in FIGURE 1, we simulated the K action currents from ensembles of K channels obeying a specific kinetic scheme. This procedure required a program that simulates free-running membranes. The program, MACROCHAN,[24] is available on request.

RESULTS

The characteristics of I_K and I_{K1}, and the criteria we use to distinguish them in the free-running and voltage-clamped cells, are reviewed in Mazzanti & DeFelice.[21]

The Delayed Rectifier

The data in FIGURE 1 are from a spontaneously beating 7-day chick ventricle cell in bath solution. The action potential reproduced in the FIGURE is representative of the series of action potentials from this cell. Individual delayed-rectifier openings occurred during each beat (not shown), and the trace below the action potential in FIGURE 1a is the average delayed-rectifier current over 40 beats. We compare the experimental average in FIGURE 1a with the theoretical average in FIGURE 1b, calculated from a model of the delayed-rectifier current driven with this same action potential. The model we used is from Shrier and Clay[13] (their I_{x2} current). It is based

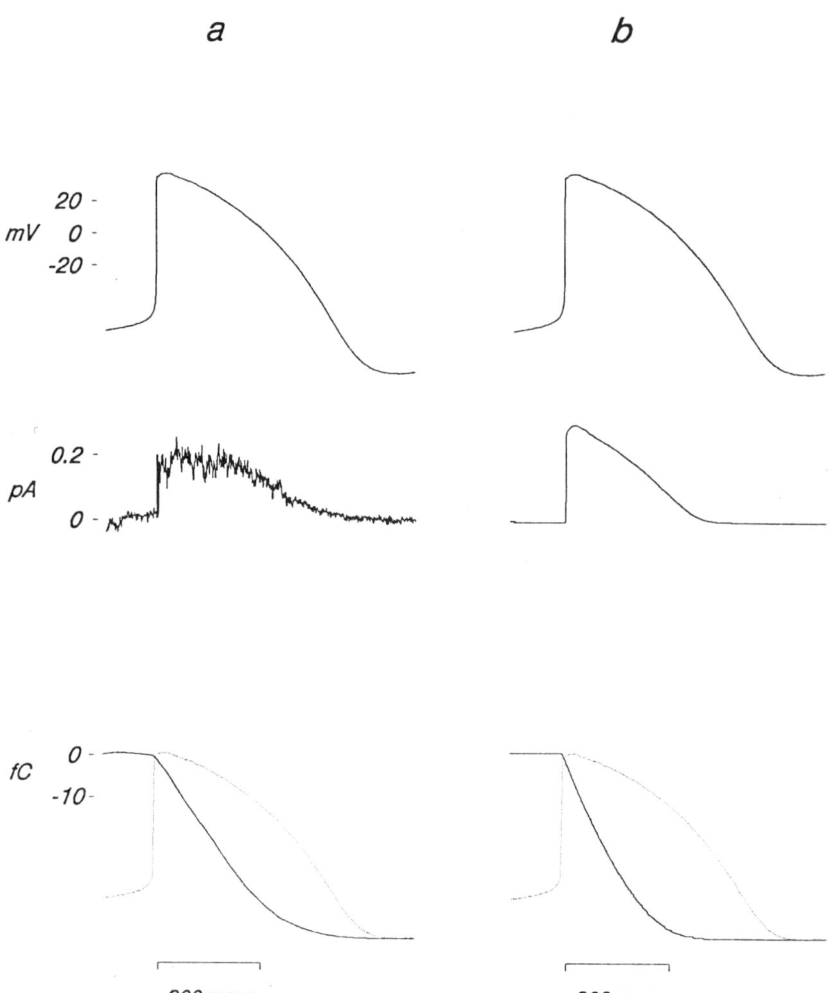

FIGURE 1. The delayed-rectifier. **a:** The top trace is an action potential recorded from a single, spontaneously beating, 7-day chick ventricle cell isolated in tissue culture. The noisy trace just below is an ensemble average of over 40 beats of the current through a single delayed-rectifier channel, $\langle i(t) \rangle$, isolated in a cell-attached patch on the same cell. The capacitive current and leak current were removed by averaging blank traces and subtracting. Below the current trace we replot the action potential (stippled) and superimpose it on the inverted time integral of the delayed-rectifier current, $-\int \langle i(u) \rangle dt$, integrated from 0 to t. The calculation results in the accumulated delayed-rectifier charge, given in units of 10^{-15} coulombs. **b:** The top trace is the same measured action potential, which we now use to drive the Shrier-Clay[15] model for the delayed-rectifier current. The middle trace plots the theoretical action current during the action potential (arbitrary units), which should be compared to the measured current on the same row in panel **a.** Similarly, compare the theoretical inverted time integral of the current at the bottom of panel **b** with the experimental integral in panel **a.**

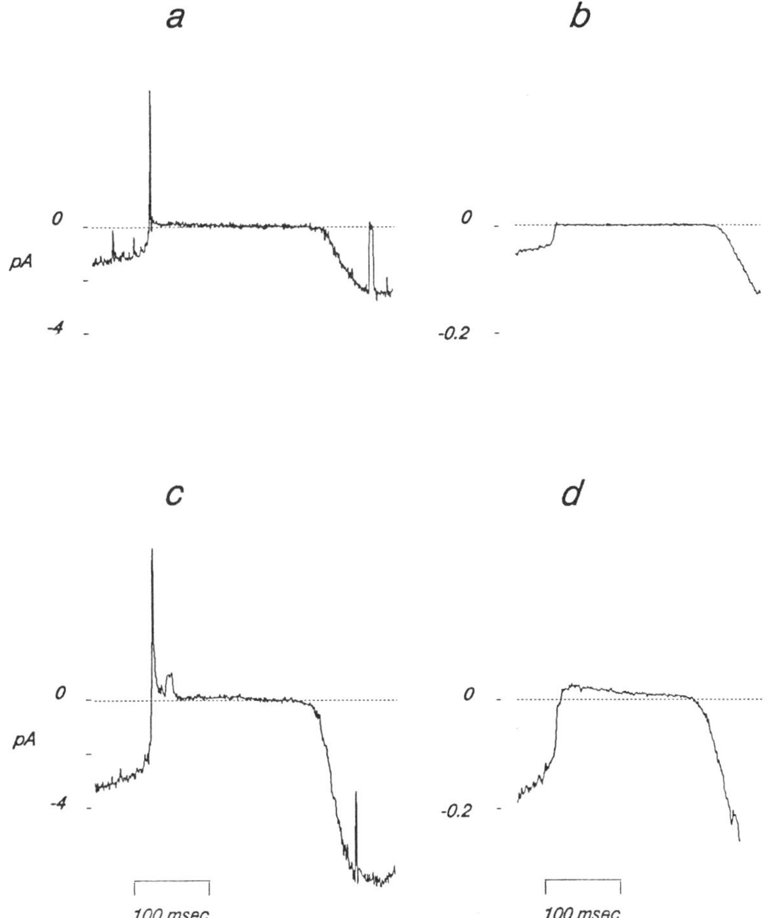

FIGURE 2. The inward rectifier. **a:** An individual action current from a patch containing one inward-rectifier channel. The bath solution is the same as in FIGURE 1, but the pipette solution on the cell-attached patch is the 60 mM K solution (see METHODS). **b:** The ensemble average of 40 action currents like the one in **a. c:** An individual action current from a patch containing at least three inward-rectifier channels. Otherwise, the conditions are as in **a. d:** The ensemble average of 40 action currents like the one in **c.**

on a two-microelectrode, step-protocol voltage clamp study of the repolarization currents in embryonic chick atrial heart cell aggregates. We took the model literally except for the reversal potential, which we set equal to our experimental value of -75 mV. In spite of the differences in preparation and technique, there is qualitative agreement between the data and the model. Note that virtually no delay exists in the onset of I_K following the upstroke. The principal reason for the rapid onset of the delayed-rectifier current at the upstroke is that delayed-rectifier channels in late diastolic depolarization have already moved toward the open state and are ready to conduct.[21]

The bottom row in FIGURE 1 redraws the action potential superimposed on the integrals of the experimental and the theoretical action currents. The integrals have been inverted, according to theory, and are arbitrarily scaled to the height of the action potential.

The Inward Rectifier

The experiments in FIGURE 2 follow the same protocol as the experiments in FIGURE 1 with one important exception: the cell-attached patch pipette now contains 60 mM K. The reason we used the 60 K solution is that the inward-rectifier channel has an extremely low conductance in normal external K and is virtually undetectable (see DISCUSSION). FIGURES 2a and b are from the same patch on a beating cell (action potential not shown). The sharp upward current corresponds to the rapid upstroke of the action potential, which in this case was not subtracted. FIGURE 2a is a sample action current, and FIGURE 2b is the average of 40 traces like the one on the left. In this particular patch, there was only one inward-rectifier channel in the patch, as judged by the lack of multiple openings in the inward direction in over 100 beats. Under these conditions, the inward-rectifier conducted current only in the diastolic phase of the action potential, not during the plateau in which the average current is zero.

The patch in FIGURES 2c and d contained at least three inward-rectifier channels. In patches with three or more inward-rectifier channels in the patch, and with high K in the pipette (greater than 40 mM), it is always possible to observe an average outward current during the plateau. We have argued previously[21] that this outward current is through the same inward-rectifier channels evident in the inward direction: it has the expected reversal potential and conductance, and the outward and inward components increase proportionally as the number of channels in the patch increase.

Because we do not know how inward-rectifier channels behave with normal K in the pipette, we can only guess at their kinetics from experiments like the one in FIGURE 2. For this reason, we did not integrate the I_{K1} current. In normal K we would expect I_{K1} to be smaller (inward and outward) than it is in high K (FIG. 2d), and the reversal potential would occur in the diastolic phase.

DISCUSSION

The problem we addressed in this chapter is how delayed-rectifier channels and inward-rectifier channels contribute to the repolarization of the cardiac action potential. To answer this question, we studied the behavior of these two kinds of channels in a free-running, unclamped membrane.

The Delayed Rectifier

For I_K we were able to show how the physiological current repolarizes the membrane during an action potential. Notwithstanding the presence of other channels, the shape of the inverted integral (Fig. 1a, bottom trace) describes the exclusive contribution of the delayed-rectifier channels. These experiments do not, however, tell us the magnitude of that contribution, which can only come from knowing the number of delayed-rectifier channels in the particular cell that gave rise to this action potential. Only the total number of potentially available delayed-rectifier channels, N_K, is needed to give the scale, not a model of its kinetics. The details of the channel kinetics and the channel conductance are contained in the averages we measure.

In the reconstruction in Figure 1, we used data from the 60 pS conductance state of the delayed rectifier.[21,25] Evidence mounts for multiple conductance states in the delayed rectifier.[26] At least three open states exist in our preparation in normal external K, 15 pS, 30 pS, and 60 pS, but all have the same kinetics as the 60 pS state. Our calculations are therefore unaffected by this complication except with regard to the magnitude of the total delayed-rectifier current. The 15 and 60 pS states of the delayed rectifier also appear in heart,[26–27] the node of Ranvier,[28] and the squid giant axon.[29]

Properly scaled, Figure 1a shows the contribution of the delayed rectifier to the action potential. Delayed-rectifier repolarization begins immediately after the upstroke and brings the potential down continuously throughout the plateau. From previous measurements, the density of delayed-rectifier channels is the order of 10 channels per cell.[21,25,28] Assuming a cell area of 500 μm^2 gives a nominal density of N = .02/μm^2. For a membrane capacitance of 1 $\mu F/cm^2$, the scaling factor is $N/C = 2/pF$.

From Figure 1a (bottom), the average total charge that moves through one delayed-rectifier channel during an action potential is 43.5 fC (270,000 K ions). The nominal density of 10 channels/cell implies a voltage change of:

$$\Delta V_K = -2/pF \times \Delta 43.5 \, fC = -87 \, mV$$

Under the above assumptions, this voltage would be the repolarization due to the delayed-rectifier channels, assuming a total of 10 were potentially available. The slope of the line through the linear part of the curve is:

delayed-rectifer charging rate $= -.175 \, fC/ms$

which gives a nominal value of:

delayed-rectifier repolarization rate $= -0.35 \, V/s$

The exact rate would depend on the actual number of channels in the cell. The total repolarization that occurs during this charge movement is 125 mV. If we assumed the entire amount is due to delayed-rectifier channels, 14 of them would have to be present in this particular cell. Other channels besides the delayed rectifier and the inward rectifier also contribute, however; thus the exact contribution of a particular channel type depends on independent knowledge of the channel number.

Though there is qualitative agreement between theory and experiment for the delayed rectifier, the theoretical current in Figure 1b gives a much faster repolarization rate of -0.59 V/second. Besides the uncertainties mentioned above, disparities could reflect the preparations or the conditions. The Shrier-Clay[15] model describes experiments on aggregates of atrial cells and might not apply to isolated ventricle cells. Another possibility is that step-protocol, voltage-clamp experiments do not reproduce conditions in beating heart cells, for example, variations in the concentration of internal ions. The delayed rectifier does not appear to depend on internal Ca;[32] however, other factors such as the K reversal potential may be different in beating cells.[21]

The Inward Rectifier

We were unable to measure the physiological action current for I_{K1} because the conductance of inward-rectifier channels in normal K is too small (less than 3 pS in 1.5 mM K).[21] We may only extrapolate from experiments in high external K.

The peak of the outward current in a patch containing at least three inward-rectifier channels in 60 mM K is roughly 0.03 pA (FIG. 2d), or about 0.01 pA/channel. This value includes the average conductance and kinetics of the channel during a beat. With extrapolation we might expect the peak in 1.5 mM K to be 1.5/60 = .025 times smaller, or 0.0025 pA/channel. This value is roughly 100th the size of the outward current through a delayed-rectifier channel (FIG. 1a). The ratio of inward-rectifier to delayed-rectifier channels, however, in this tissue is about $(2/\mu m^2)/(1/50\ \mu m^2) = 100$. From these calculations we might conclude that the net outward current through inward-rectifier channels makes an equivalent contribution to repolarization as the net outward current through delayed-rectifier channels.

This conclusion would be premature. First, we do not know how to extrapolate accurately, and the above proportionality is only a crude approximation. The inward-rectifier channel has multiple conductance states in high K,[31–33] but perhaps only one in normal K.[21] The normal reversal potential and driving forces in beating cells are unknown and may be different in beating and nonbeating cells. Second, even if we model these specific effects and incorporate them into our extrapolation procedure, we are unable to evaluate all the possibilities. For example, the large currents that flow inward in high K might wash out internal ions such as Mg and Ca, which we know influence I_{K1} rectification.[34,35] Until experiments are done at physiological concentrations, the actual contribution of the inward rectifier to excitability is speculative.

SUMMARY

What is the contribution of a particular potassium current to the repolarization of cardiac myocytes? The traditional answer to this question requires clamping the cells with step voltages, finding models that describe how individual currents depend on voltage and time, driving these models with action potentials to calculate the action currents, and evaluating the contribution of each pathway to repolarization from the action currents. Another method is to measure the action currents directly from beating cells. We isolated potassium channels in cell-attached patches and averaged the current over many beats. The average channel current, $\langle i(t) \rangle$, is a miniature version of the action current through corresponding channels in the membrane outside the patch. The time integral of this current, scaled by channel density, N, and membrane capacity, C, is the contribution of that particular pathway to the action potential:

$$V_i(t) = -N_i \int_o^t \langle i(u) \rangle\ du/C$$

Using this procedure,[36,37] we have found that the delayed rectifier, I_K, turns on virtually without delay following the upstroke of the action potential and gradually declines during the plateau and repolarization phases, having nearly the shape of the action potential itself. The inward rectifier, I_{K1}, may conduct little current during the plateau and is under the control of internal Ca. The traditional method of measuring action currents from step voltage-clamp records gives qualitatively similar results. Differences may arise because factors other than voltage modulate potassium currents in beating cells.

ACKNOWLEDGMENTS

We wish to thank John Pooler, John Clay, and Robert DeHaan for reading the manuscript and making suggestions for its improvement, and we acknowledge B. J. Duke-Cuti for preparing the tissue cultures and solutions used in these experiments.

REFERENCES

1. GILES, W. & E. R. SHIBATA. 1985. Voltage clamp of bullfrog cardiac pacemaker cells: A quantitative analysis of K currents. J. Physiol. **368:** 265-292.
2. HUME, J. R. & A. UEHARA. 1985. Ionic basis of the different action potential configurations of the guinea-pig. J. Physiol. **366:** 525-544.
3. SIMMONS, M. A., T. CREAZZO & H. C. HARTZELL. 1986. A time- and voltage-sensitive K current in single cells from frog atrium. J. Gen. Physiol. **88:** 739-755.
4. SHIBASAKI, T. 1987. Conductance and kinetics of delayed rectifier K channels in nodal cells of the rabbit heart. J. Physiol. **387:** 227-250.
5. HODGKIN, A. L. & A. F. HUXLEY. 1952. A qualitative description of membrane current and its application to conduction in nerve. J. Physiol. **117:** 440-544.
6. For a summary of the technique see B. Sakmann & E. Neher. 1983. Single-Channel Recording. Plenum Press. New York.
7. DeFELICE, L. J. & J. CLAY. 1983. Membrane channel and membrane potential from single-current kinetics. *In* Single-Channel Recording. B. Sakmann & E. Neher, Eds. Plenum Press. New York.
8. BRENNECKE, R. & B. LINDEMANN. 1974. Theory of a membrane voltage clamp with discontinuous feedback through a pulsed current clamp. Rev. Sci. Instrum. **45:** 184-188.
9. McALLISTER, R. E., D. NOBLE & R. W. TSIEN. 1975. Reconstruction of electrical activity of cardiac Purkinje fibres. J. Physiol. **251:** 1-59.
10. BEELER, G. W. & H. REUTER. 1977. Reconstruction of the action potential of ventricle myocardial fibers. J. Physiol. **268:** 177-210.
11. YANAGIHARA, K. A., A. NOMA & H. IRISAWA. 1980. Reconstruction of the SA node pacemaker potential based on voltage clamp experiments. Jpn. J. Physiol. **30:** 841-857.
12. DiFRANCESCO, D. & D. NOBLE. 1985. A model of cardiac electrical activity incorporating ionic pumps and concentration changes. Philos. Trans. R. Soc. Lond. Biol. Sci. B **307:** 353-398.
13. SHRIER, A. & J. R. CLAY. 1987. Repolarization currents in embryonic chick atrial heart cell aggregates. Biophys. J. **50:** 861-874.
13a. CLAY, J. R., C. E. HILL, D. ROITMAN & A. SHRIER. 1988. Repolarization current in embryonic chick atrial heart cells. J. Physiol. **403:** 525-537.
13b. CLAY, J. & A. SHRIER. 1981. Analysis of subthreshold pacemaker currents in chick embryonic heart cells. J. Physiol. **321:** 471-490.
14. CLAPHAM, D. E. 1988. A brief review of single channel measurements from isolated heart cells. *In* The Heart Cell in Culture. A. Pinson, Ed. CRC Press. Boca Raton, FL.
15. COHEN, I. S., N. B. DATYNER, G. A. GINTANT & R. P. KLINE. 1986. Time-dependent outward currents in the heart. *In* The Heart and Cardiovascular System. H. M. Fozzard, Ed. Raven Press. New York.

16. CLAY, J. R. & L. J. DEFELICE. 1983. Relationship between membrane excitability and single channel open-close kinetics. Biophys. J. **42:** 151-157.

17. FISCHMEISTER, R., L. J. DEFELICE, R. J. AYER JR., R. LEVI & R. L. DEHAAN. 1984. Channel currents in embryonic chick heart cells. Biophys. J. **46:** 267-272.

18. LEVI, R. & L. J. DEFELICE. 1986. Na-conducting channels in cardiac membranes in zero Ca. Biophys. J. **50:** 11-19.

19. MAZZANTI, M. & L. J. DEFELICE. 1987a. Regulation of the Na-conducting Ca channel during the cardiac action potential. Biophys. J. **51:** 115-121.

20. MAZZANTI, M. & L. J. DEFELICE. 1987b. Na channel kinetics during the spontaneous heart beat in chick ventricle cells. Biophys. J. **52:** 95-100.

21. MAZZANTI, M. & L. J. DEFELICE. 1988. K channel kinetics during the spontaneous heart beat in chick ventricle cells. Biophys. J. **54:** 1139-1148.

22. BRENNECKE, R. & B. LINDEMANN. 1974. Design of a fast voltage clamp for biological membranes using a discontinuous feedback. Rev. Sci. Instrum. **45:** 656-661.

23. DEHAAN, R. L. 1967. Regulation of spontaneous activity and growth of embryonic chick heart cells in tissue culture. Dev. Biol. **16:** 216-249. Also see FUJII, S., R. K. AYER & R. L. DEHAAN. 1988. Development of the fast Na current in early embryonic chick hearts. J. Membr. Biol. **101:** 209-223.

24. DEFELICE, L. J., W. GOOLSBY & D. HUANG. 1986. Membrane noise and excitability. *In* Noise in Physical Systems. A. D'Amico & P. Mazzetti, Eds. 35-45. Elsevier Science Publishers B. V. Amsterdam.

25. CLAPHAM, D. E. & L. J. DEFELICE. 1984. Voltage-activated K channels in embryonic chick heart. Biophys. J. **45:** 40-42.

26. BENNETT, P., L. MCKINNEY, R. KASS & T. BEGENISICH. 1985. Delayed rectification in the calf cardiac Purkinje fiber: evidence for multiple conductance states. Biophys. J. **48:** 553-567.

27. CLAPHAM, D. E. & D. E. LOGOTHETIS. 1988. Delayed-rectifier K current in embryonic chick heart ventricle. Am. J. Physiol. **254:** H192-H197.

28. CONTI, F., B. HILLE & W. NONNER. 1984. Non-stationary fluctuations of the K conductance of the node of Ranvier of the frog. J. Physiol. **353:** 199-230.

29. IIANO, I., C. A. WEBB & F. BENZANILLA. 1988. Potassium conductance of the squid giant axon. J. Gen. Physiol. **92:** 179-196.

30. KASS, R. S. 1984. Delayed rectification in the cardiac Purkinje fiber is not activated by intracellular Ca. Biophys. J. **45:** 837-839.

31. SAKMANN, B. & G. TRUBE. 1984a. Conductance properties of a single inwardly-rectifying K channel in ventricle guinea-pig. J. Physiol. **347:** 641-657.

32. SAKMANN, B. & G. TRUBE. 1984b. Voltage-dependent inactivation of inwardly-rectifying single-channel currents in the guinea-pig. J. Physiol. **347:** 659-683.

33. KELL, M. J. & L. J. DEFELICE. 1988. Surface charge in cardiac inward-rectifier channels measured from single-channel conductance. J. Membr. Biol. **102:** 1-10.

34. MATSUDA, H., A. SAIGUSA & H. IRISAWA. 1987. Ohmic conductance through the inwardly rectifying K channel and blocking by internal Mg. Nature **325:** 156-159.

35. MAZZANTI, M. & D. DIFRANCESCO. 1989. Intracellular Ca modulates K-inward rectification in cardiac myocytes. Pfluegers Arch. Eur. Physiol. **413:** 322-324.

36. DEFELICE, L. J. 1983. Reconstruction of the nerve action potential from single-channel fluctuations. Am. Phys. Soc. Bull. **28:** 358a.

37. DEFELICE, L. J. & R. LEVI. 1984. Reconstructing the cardiac action potential from single-channel kinetics. IUPAB 8th International Biophysics Congress. Bristol.

Regulation of Muscarinic Receptor and G-Protein Expression during Cardiac Development

NEIL M. NATHANSON

Department of Pharmacology, SJ-30
University of Washington
Seattle, Washington 98195

INTRODUCTION

Acetylcholine released from parasympathetic nerve terminals acts on muscarinic acetylcholine receptors (mAChR) on the cardiac cell surface to decrease both the rate (negative chronotropic effect) and force (negative inotropic effect) of contraction of the heart. Muscarinic receptors thus play a key role in the regulation of cardiac function. Muscarinic receptors mediate their physiological responses both by the alteration of intracellular second messengers and by the regulation of ion channel function with no involvement of second messengers. Both types of physiological responses are mediated by the action of one or more GTP-binding regulatory proteins (G-proteins), which couple mAChR both to enzymes such as an adenylate cyclase or phospholipase C and to ion channels such as an inwardly rectifying cardiac potassium channel (see Nathanson[1] for review). This chapter will summarize some recent studies from the laboratory on the regulation and development of the number and function of muscarinic receptors and G-proteins in the heart.

ONTOGENESIS OF CARDIAC mAChR RESPONSIVENESS DURING AVIAN DEVELOPMENT

Pappano and Skowronek[2] first showed in 1974 that atria isolated from chicks after three days of embryonic development exhibited a greatly diminished mAChR-mediated

[a] This research was supported by a Grant-in Aid from the American Heart Association and by the National Institutes of Health (HL30639). N. M. Nathanson is an Established Investigator of the American Heart Association.

negative chronotropic response compared to atria from later stages of development. Radioligand binding studies by Galper *et al.*[3] and Renaud *et al.*[4] subsequently showed that there were similar numbers of mAChR binding sites in hearts from 3-4-day-old embryos and in hearts from 5-6-day-old chick embryos (which had a much larger mAChR-mediated negative chronotropic response). In addition, these binding studies suggested that the affinity of the mAChR for agonists and antagonists was similar at various ages. Thus, the defect in the coupling of the mAChR to the negative chronotropic response did not seem to reside in the mAChR itself. Later binding studies by Halvorsen and Nathanson,[5] however, which compared the regulation of agonist binding to the mAChR by guanine nucleotides in membranes from 4 day embryonic chick atria to that in membranes from 5 day and 8 day embryonic atria, suggested that the interaction of the mAChR with the G-proteins was impaired. They found that the ability of guanine nucleotides to regulate agonist binding to the mAChR, an effect that results from the interaction of the receptor with its G-proteins, was greatly reduced at 4 days of development. Halvorsen and Nathanson[5] then used several biochemical assays to show that there were also functional differences in the G-proteins at this time. As further functional assays for the G-proteins, they determined dose-response curves for the regulation of agonist binding by guanine nucleotides and for guanine nucleotide-dependent inhibition of adenylate cyclase activity. Much higher concentrations of guanine nucleotides were required in both cases to produce effects at 4 days compared to 5 and 8 days of development. These results thus suggested that there were either decreased amounts of G-proteins or the presence of inactive forms of the G-proteins at early stages of development.

In order to examine the G-proteins directly, Halvorsen and Nathanson[5] labeled the G-protein alpha subunits using islet-activating protein (IAP) secreted by *Bordetella pertussis* and [^{32}P]NAD and determined their levels after separation by one- and two-dimensional gel electrophoresis and visualization by autoradiography. Two labeled polypeptides with molecular weights of 41-42,000 and 39,000 were observed after one-dimensional SDS gel electrophoresis. (Later studies using partial proteolysis showed that these two polypeptides yielded distinct peptide maps.[6] Immunological studies[7] indicated that the higher molecular weight species corresponded at least in part to $G_{i\alpha}$, and the lower molecular weight species corresponded both to $G_{o\alpha}$ and to a second form of $G_{i\alpha}$.) Each molecular weight species could be further resolved into two isoelectric forms by two-dimensional gel electrophoresis. At four days of development the acidic form of the 39,000 kilodalton polypeptide represented only a minor portion (16%) of the total IAP-labeled material. This isoform increased approximately 2.4-fold by embryonic day 5 and increased 3.4-fold by day 8, when it represented 55% of the total IAP-labeled material. These studies thus demonstrated that there were both physical and functional changes in the G-proteins in the chick heart during embryonic development, which occurred at the same time as the onset of the mAChR-mediated negative chronotropic response. This raised the possibility that these changes in the G-proteins could be responsible for the onset of mAChR responsiveness. Although it was known at that time that the G-proteins could couple the mAChR to inhibition of adenylate cyclase activity, there was also good evidence available indicating that cAMP or other diffusible second messengers were not involved in the mAChR-mediated negative chronotropic response (see Nathanson[1] for references). These results therefore suggested that, if the changes in G-proteins were related to the ontogenesis of responsiveness, a G-protein may directly couple the mAChR to activation of cardiac inwardly rectifying potassium channel, which is responsible for the negative chronotropic effect. Subsequent biochemical and electrophysiological experiments have demonstrated that G-proteins can indeed couple muscarinic receptors to potassium channels.[8-14]

TISSUE-SPECIFIC REGULATION OF MUSCARINIC RECEPTORS AND G-PROTEINS DURING CHICK CARDIAC DEVELOPMENT

Cardiac mAChR are coupled to different physiological responses in atria and ventricles (reviewed in Martin *et al.*[6]), and Kirby and Aronstam[15] reported that the level of mAChR may be regulated differentially in atria and ventricles during embryonic development. In order to examine the possibility of differential regulation of cholinergic signal transduction proteins in the atria and ventricles, Luetje *et al.*[7] determined the levels of G-protein subunits and mAChR during development of the embryonic chick heart. The levels of the G-protein polypeptides in atria and ventricles was determined using a quantitative immunoblot technique with monospecific affinity-purified antibodies specific for $G_{o\alpha}$, $G_{i\alpha}$, and G_β. The number of mAChR binding sites was determined using a radioligand filter binding assay with the muscarinic antagonist [^{3}H]quinuclidinyl benzilate. There were similar amounts of $G_{o\alpha}$, G_β, and mAChR in atria and ventricles at embryonic day 10, whereas the level of $G_{i\alpha}$ was 44% higher in atria than ventricles. Over the next five days, there were significant increases in the levels of $G_{o\alpha}$ (46% between day 10 and 15), G_β (80% between day 13 and 15), and mAChR (61% between day 10 and 12) and a 34% decrease in the level of $G_{i\alpha}$ in atria (between day 10 and 13). There were no changes in the levels of these polypeptides in the ventricles during this period of development.

To test if these changes in polypeptide levels were associated with alterations in functional responses mediated by the G-proteins, the inhibition of adenylate cyclase activity by both guanine nucleotides and muscarinic agonists in membrane homogenates from atria and ventricles was determined at various times in development. At embryonic day 10, adenylate cyclase activity was more sensitive to inhibition by muscarinic agonists in atria than in ventricles. This appeared to be correlated with the increased level of $G_{i\alpha}$ in atria. In addition, the atrial-specific increase in the level of G_β between day 13 and day 15 was associated with a loss of guanine nucleotide-mediated inhibition of basal adenylate cyclase activity in the atria. Thus, there are tissue-specific developmentally regulated changes in the levels of both muscarinic receptor and G-proteins in the chick heart that are associated with changes in the functional responses mediated by these polypeptides. Because these changes occur at the time of onset of functional cholinergic innervation of the chick heart, the expression of the mAChR and the G-proteins may be regulated in a tissue-specific fashion by the establishment of cholinergic innervation of the heart.

DEVELOPMENT OF G-PROTEINS IN MAMMALIAN HEART

Because of reports that suggested on the basis of IAP labeling that rat heart contained only $G_{i\alpha}$ and not $G_{o\alpha}$ and that the levels of $G_{i\alpha}$ were regulated in rat heart during development and by innervation,[16,17] we examined the levels of G-protein polypeptides and mRNA in neonatal and adult rat atria and ventricles by quantitative immunoblot, Northern blot, and quantitative RNA dot blot analyses.[18] The level of $G_{o\alpha}$ polypeptide was 5.2-fold higher in adult atria than in adult ventricles, and the level of $G_{o\alpha}$ mRNA was 3.4-fold higher. The amount of G_β polypeptide was 2.8-fold higher in adult atria than ventricles, although similar amounts of G_β mRNA were present in both tissues. There were developmental decreases in the level of $G_{i\alpha}$ polypeptide and mRNA in ventricles, in the level of G_β and $G_{o\alpha}$ mRNA in the ventricles, and in the levels of G_β and $G_{i\alpha}$-2 mRNA in the atria. There was also a developmental increase in the level of $G_{i\alpha}$-3 mRNA in the atria. Thus, there are tissue-specific and developmentally regulated differences in the expression of G-protein subunits in rat heart.

IMMUNOLOGICAL STUDIES OF THE CARDIAC mAChR

We have used preparations of mAChR,[19] purified from pig heart to homogeneity, to isolate nine monoclonal antibodies (mAbs) that specifically recognize the muscarinic receptor.[20] These antibodies were shown by enzyme-linked solid phase immunosorptive assays (ELISA) and by immunoblot analysis to have a high degree of specificity for the mAChR, as the antibodies recognized the purified porcine atrial mAChR, but did not react either with a control preparation of pig atrial glycoproteins from which the mAChR had been removed or with rod outer segment membranes (which contain large amounts of the structurally homologous protein rhodopsin). Some of these mAbs also cross-react with the mAChR solubilized from rat heart and can distinguish the mAChR in rat heart from those present in rat brain in immunoprecipitation experiments, suggesting that these antibodies are specific for the cardiac (M2) form of the receptor.

CONCLUSIONS

The levels of muscarinic receptors and G-proteins are regulated in both mammalian and avian hearts during development in a tissue-specific fashion. The availability of antibody and cDNA probes for these proteins should aid in the elucidation of the molecular mechanisms involved in the regulation of signal transduction proteins in the heart.

REFERENCES

1. NATHANSON, N. M. 1987. Annu. Rev. Neurosci. **10:** 195-236.
2. PAPPANO, A. J. & C. A. SKOWRONEK. 1974. J. Pharmacol. Exp. Ther. **191:** 109-118.
3. GALPER, J. B., W. L. KLEIN & W. A. CATTERALL. 1977. J. Biol. Chem. **252:** 8692-8699.
4. RENAUD, J. F., J. BARHANIN, D. CAVEY, G. FOSSET & M. LAZDUNSKI. 1980. Dev. Biol. **78:** 184-200.
5. HALVORSEN, S. W. & N. M. NATHANSON. 1984. Biochemistry **23:** 5813-5821.
6. MARTIN, J. M., E. M. SUBERS, S. W. HALVORSEN & N. M. NATHANSON. 1987. J. Pharmacol. Exp. Ther. **240:** 683-688.
7. LUETJE, C. W., P. GIERSCHIK, G. MILLIGAN, C. UNSON, A. SPIEGEL & N. M. NATHANSON. 1987. Biochemistry **26:** 4876-4884.
8. MARTIN, J. M., D. D. HUNTER & N. M. NATHANSON. 1985. Biochemistry **24:** 7521-7525.
9. ENDOH, M., M. MARUYAMA & T. IJIMA. 1985. Am. J. Physiol. **249:** H309-H320.
10. SOROTA, S., Y. TSUJI, T. TAJIMA & A. J. PAPPANO. 1985. Circ. Res. **57:** 748-58.

11. PFAFFINGER, P. J., J. M. MARTIN, D. D. HUNTER, N. M. NATHANSON & B. HILLE. 1985. Nature **317:** 536-538.
12. BREITWEISER, G. E. & G. SZABO. 1985. Nature **317:** 538-540.
13. CODINA, J., A. YATANI, D. GRENET, A. M. BROWN & L. BIRNBAUMER. 1987. Science **236:** 442-445.
14. LOGOTHETIS, D. E., Y. KURACHI, J. GALPER, E. J. NEER & D. E. CLAPHAM. 1987. Nature **325:** 321-326.
15. KIRBY, M. L. & R. S. ARONSTAM. 1983. J. Mol. Cell. Cardiol. **15:** 685-696.
16. STEINBERG, S. F., E. D. DRUGGE, J. P. BILZEEZIKIAN & R. B. ROBINSON. 1985. Science **230:** 186-188.
17. MURAKAMI, T. & H. YASUDA. 1986. Biochem. Biophys. Res. Commun. **138:** 1355-1361.
18. LUETJE, C. W., K. M. TIETJE, J. L. CHRISTIAN & N. M. NATHANSON. 1988. J. Biol. Chem. **263:** 13357-13365.
19. PETERSON, G. L., G. S. HERON, M. YAMAKI, D. S. FULLERTON & M. I. SCHIMERLIK. 1984. Proc. Natl. Acad. Sci. USA **81:** 4993-4997.
20. LUETJE, C. W., C. BRUMWELL, M. G. NORMAN, G. L. PETERSON, M. I. SCHIMERLIK & N. M. NATHANSON. 1987. Biochemistry **26:** 6892-6895.

Excitation-Contraction Coupling in Heart Cells

Roles of the Sodium-Calcium Exchange, the Calcium Current, and the Sarcoplasmic Reticulum[a]

W. J. LEDERER, J. R. BERLIN, N. M. COHEN,
R. W. HADLEY, D. M. BERS,[b] AND
M. B. CANNELL[c]

Department of Physiology
University of Maryland School of Medicine
Baltimore, Maryland 21201

[b]*Division of Biomedical Sciences*
University of California
Riverside, California 92521

[c]*Department of Pharmacology*
University of Miami School of Medicine
Miami, Florida 33101

INTRODUCTION

In heart muscle, electrical depolarization leads to a transient elevation of intracellular free calcium ($[Ca^{2+}]_i$) and contraction.[1] Many of the links between the electrical depolarization and the development of contraction in mammalian heart muscle have been studied. Nevertheless, important aspects of the process remain poorly defined. For example, the exact mechanism by which the depolarization of the heart cells leads to the calcium transient is still uncertain.

In this paper, we examine mechanisms important to excitation-contraction coupling in human, rat, and guinea-pig ventricular muscle. We compare properties of these mechanisms in neonatal and adult heart cells. We question how completely a simple model of calcium-induced calcium release (CICR)-linking depolarization to sarco-

[a]This work was supported by the NIH; fellowship support came from the Maryland Affiliate of the American Heart Association. Additional support for this work came from the University of Maryland Graduate School, Baltimore and the Medical Biotechnology Center of the Maryland Biotechnology Institute.

plasmic reticulum calcium release can explain all of our experimental data as well as the data of others. CICR postulates that calcium ions entering the heart can activate or "trigger" calcium release from the sarcoplasmic reticulum (SR) and thereby amplify the trigger signal.[2] The two principal sources of calcium that may provide the activating calcium for CICR are the sarcolemmal calcium channel and the Na/Ca exchanger. This signaling calcium can be considered to act with "high gain" if a small amount of calcium entering leads to a very large $[Ca^{2+}]_i$-transient. Conversely, the signaling calcium would act with "low gain" if the $[Ca^{2+}]_i$-transient were proportional to or largely due to the flux of signaling calcium itself. We suggest that neither a high- nor low-gain CICR mechanism can explain all of the data and conclude that a more sophisticated CICR mechanism is required. As an alternative or additional hypothesis, we suggest that a simple CICR mechanism combined with another process (such as voltage) may be the physiological mechanism of calcium release from the SR.[3]

METHODS

General

Adult rat and guinea pig ventricular myocytes were prepared by an enzymatic dissociation method,[3-5] and neonatal rat heart cells were maintained in short term primary culture.[6] The heart cells were voltage-clamped using a borosilicate patch-clamp pipette in whole-cell mode. Important conditions relevant to the experiment are given in the FIGURE legends.

Human Heart Cells

Human heart cells were obtained from the left ventricle of the recipient heart of patients undergoing cardiac transplantation for end-stage ischemic heart disease under conditions approved by the Human Volunteers Research Committee at the University of Maryland School of Medicine. The healthiest tissue was cut into 1 mm square pieces and dissociated enzymatically using a technique derived from that described by Escande *et al.*[7] using a physiological salt solution containing low calcium (.003 mM), 400 IU/mL of collagenase (Boehringer Mannheim, FRG), and 4 IU/mL protease type XIV (Sigma, St. Louis, MO). Continuous agitation was provided by bubbling with 100% O_2. After 40 minutes the supernatant was discarded and replaced by a similar solution containing collagenase only. After an additional 40 minutes, single cells were obtained and transferred to an enzyme-free salt solution containing 1-2 mM calcium.

Fluorescence Measurements of Intracellular Calcium

A. Fura-2

The cells were loaded with 30-75 μM of the potassium salt of fura-2 from the voltage-clamp pipette (see Cannell *et al.*[3] for details of pipette and superfusion solutions). The cells were illuminated sequentially with 340 and 380 nm light, and the fluorescence at 500 nm was recorded as photomultiplier tube current. After background subtraction, the ratio of fluorescence of 340 nm to 380 nm was obtained. The intracellular calcium was estimated using an *in vitro* calibration curve.

B. Indo-1

Low resistance patch-pipettes (0.4-1.5 MΩ) were filled with a solution containing (in mM) CsGlutamate 100, CsCl 20, PIPES 20, NaCl 10, K_2ATP 2.5, $MgCl_2$ 1, and Indo-1 (potassium salt) 0.05-0.07. pH was adjusted to 7.2. The superfusion solutions were similar to those used for the fura-2 experiments and contained (in mM) NaCl 145, KCl 4, $MgCl_2$ 1, $CaCl_2$ 2, glucose 10, and HEPES 10 with pH adjusted to 7.40 with NaOH. The apparatus used for the indo-1 experiments is shown diagrammatically in FIGURE 1. Cells were allowed to settle onto a glass coverslip that formed the bottom of a superfusion chamber.[8] The cells were voltage-clamped with a single patch-clamp pipette in a whole-cell voltage-clamp configuration and were transilluminated with red light to permit viewing with a video camera. Simultaneous measurement of calcium was achieved by illumination of the cells with 350 nm light provided by a xenon arc lamp and appropriate mirrors and filters. See also Peeters *et al.*[9] Photomultiplier tubes (PMT) were used to detect fluorescence at 400 and 500 nanometers.

RESULTS AND DISCUSSION

Sodium-Calcium Exchange and the ICa "Window" Current Effect $[Ca^{2+}]_i$

Human Heart Cells

FIGURE 2 shows records taken from a voltage-clamped ventricular muscle cell. This FIGURE shows voltage, current, $[Ca^{2+}]_i$, and cell shortening recorded simultaneously. $[Ca^{2+}]_i$ during rest is about 240 nM at a holding potential of -75 mV. Depolarization to -55 mV leads to an increase in $[Ca^{2+}]_i$ to about 290 nM. Thus resting $[Ca^{2+}]_i$ is sensitive to membrane potential. Peak $[Ca^{2+}]_i$ attained during a 60 mV depolarization from either holding potential is about 1 μM.[3,10,11]

In the steady state, the resting level of $[Ca^{2+}]_i$ reflects a balance between calcium entry and extrusion across the sarcolemma. Under steady-state conditions, intracellular calcium buffers or stores cannot affect the level of $[Ca^{2+}]_i$ set by the sarcolemma, because they cannot act as either an infinite store or source for calcium. The voltage dependence of the Na/Ca exchange will result in depolarization leading to a reduction in net calcium extrusion by the exchanger so that an increase in $[Ca^{2+}]_i$ will occur.[12–14] (This conclusion does not depend on the direction of the exchange process and may result from either a decrease in calcium efflux or an increase in calcium influx by way of the exchanger.) As $[Ca^{2+}]_i$ increases, however, the rate of net calcium extrusion by way of the exchanger will also increase until a new balance is achieved, albeit at a higher level of $[Ca^{2+}]_i$.[12,13] In comparison to this simple prediction of the effects of depolarization on the Na/Ca exchange, the effects mediated through calcium channels are more complex. The calcium influx by way of calcium channels is the product of

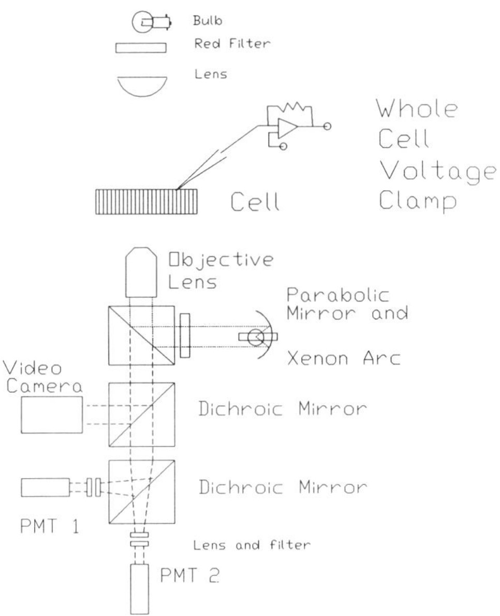

FIGURE 1. Schematic diagram of our fluorescence microscope. An inverted microscope designed to operate with epifluorescence illumination (Nikon Diaphot) has been modified to accept selected wavelengths of illuminating light produced by a xenon arc lamp fitted with appropriate filters. Light from the arc lamp at 350 nm is reflected by a dichroic mirror and focused onto a single cell using a 63 power, N.A. 1.25, Zeiss Neofluar objective. Red light is focused on the cell from above using our usual long-working distance condenser. All of the light from the cell (transmitted and fluorescent) is transmitted through the first dichroic mirror. The light is separated by the second dichroic mirror, with the red light reflected towards a video camera (Cohu CCD), whereas shorter wavelengths are transmitted towards a third dichroic mirror. This third mirror reflects light less than 450 nm towards a photomultiplier tube (PMT-1), whereas transmitted light is directed to PMT-2. Appropriate optics and filters are used to efficiently collect specific wavelengths of light. With this system, we use the calcium-sensitive indicator indo-1 (injected into the voltage-clamped heart muscle cell) to measure intracellular calcium, whereas the video camera is used to measure cell length, and the patch-clamp amplifier (Axon Instrument's Axopatch 1C) is used to measure membrane current. The data shown in FIG. 2 was collected with a system similar to the one shown, whereas data for FIGURES 3, 4, and 5 were collected using a slightly different arrangement and the calcium indicator fura-2 (see Cannell *et al.*[3]).

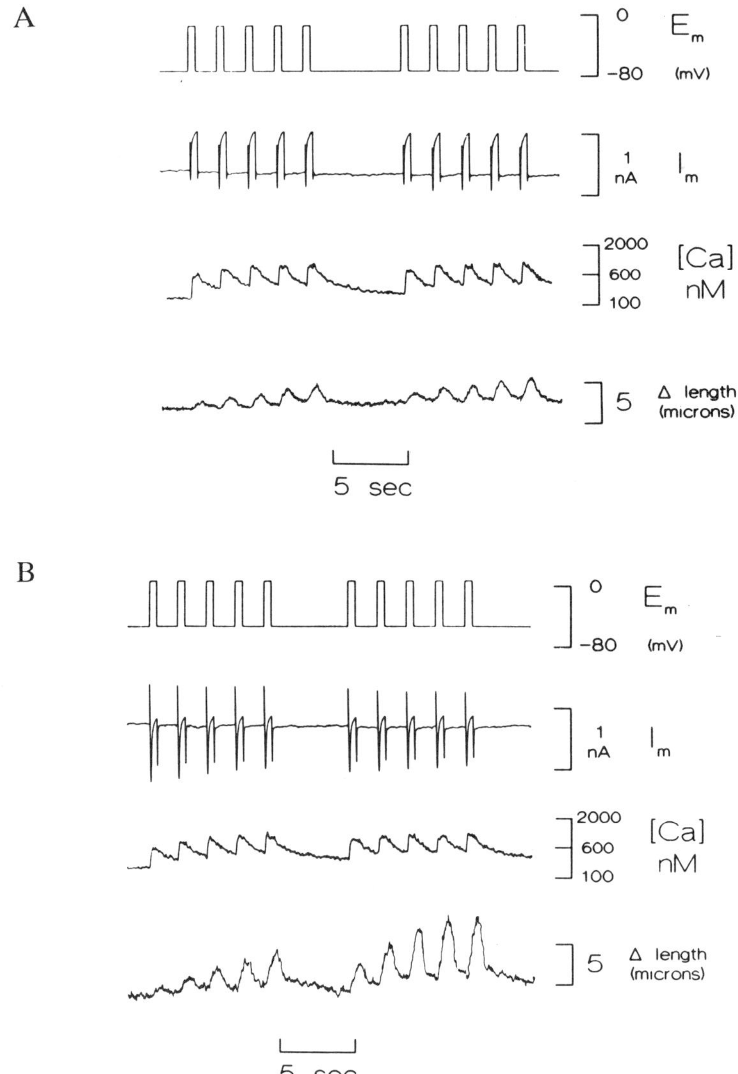

FIGURE 2. Effect of membrane potential and repetitive depolarizations on membrane current, intracellular calcium and cell length in adult human ventricular myoctyes. Indo-1 was loaded into the heart cells through the voltage-clamp pipette as described in the METHODS section. Cell length was measured using images obtained from a CCD video camera and length-measuring electronics. **A.** Human ventricular myocyte. Holding potential was -75 mV, and 500 ms depolarizations to -15 mV were applied. $[Ca^{2+}]_i$ at rest (before the depolarizing pulses were applied) is approximately 240 nM. The maximum systolic $[Ca^{2+}]_i$ in this experiment is just over 1 μM. **B.** Human ventricular myocyte. Holding potential was -55 mV, and depolarizations to $+5$ mV were applied. $[Ca^{2+}]_i$ at rest at -55 mV (before the depolarizing pulses were applied) was about 290 nM. Diastolic calcium, measured following a regularly applied voltage clamp depolarizing pulse, tended to exceed the resting $[Ca^{2+}]_i$ levels and depended on the voltage-clamp protocol as shown in both panels **A** and **B.**

the electrochemical gradient for calcium entry and the conductance of the channel. Were the conductance constant at all membrane potentials, depolarization would lead to a monotonic decrease in calcium influx through calcium channels. As the membrane depolarizes, however, the steady-state conductance increases until it is at a maximum at about 0 mV; it then decreases again. (The fact that the steady-state conductance is not zero over some range potentials leads to the so called "window current"[6]). At very negative and positive potentials (where the conductance may be approximately constant), changes in the electrochemical driving force should dominate the calcium influx. Once the membrane is depolarized to voltages where the window of conductance increases, the increase in conductance may more than offset the decrease in electrochemical gradient so that calcium influx increases. At even more positive potentials, influx will decrease again as both the decreasing electrochemical gradient and conductance decrease. Over the range of potentials examined, it seems likely that the changes in resting $[Ca^{2+}]_i$ will have resulted from changes in both Na/Ca exchange and calcium channel-mediated calcium fluxes.

A second important observation is that there is an increase in the magnitude of the contractions from beat to beat (or staircase) through each set of five depolarizations. This staircase could be due to an increase of resting $[Ca^{2+}]_i$, of SR Ca release, or of Ca influx (or some combination thereof). There is a progressive rise in the resting $[Ca^{2+}]_i$ as well as a decrease in diastolic cell length in each series (but especially apparent in FIG. 2B). It is also notable that the increase in the contractions is more dramatic than the increase in the amplitude of the $[Ca^{2+}]_i$ transients that are superimposed on this rising diastolic $[Ca^{2+}]_i$. Additionally, the peak I_{Ca} in FIGURE 2B decreases as the contractions increase. Thus, even though there may be progressive loading of the SR, it seems clear that the rising diastolic $[Ca^{2+}]_i$ plays a major role in this contraction staircase.

Can the Na/Ca Exchange Trigger Calcium Release from the Sarcoplasmic Reticulum?

Rat Ventricular Myocytes

In addition to any effects the Na/Ca exchange may have on resting calcium, it may influence calcium release from the SR. Although changes in resting calcium would be expected to influence the pool of calcium that can be released from the SR, it is also possible that calcium influx by way of the Na/Ca exchange may influence the mechanism of calcium release from the SR (see also FIG. 8).[15,16] In the CICR hypothesis, a calcium influx causes a local increase in $[Ca^{2+}]_i$ near calcium binding sites that regulate the calcium permeability of the SR. The increased occupancy of these binding sites then causes the SR calcium release channel to open, and calcium leaves the SR and enters the myoplasm. Although the calcium current is an obvious candidate for providing the calcium influx needed to trigger CICR, it is also possible that the Na/Ca exchange may play a role. To examine this possibility, we needed to abolish calcium influx by means of the calcium current while maintaining operation of the Na/Ca exchange. At very positive potentials calcium influx through calcium channels should decrease as the electrochemical gradient for calcium is reduced to zero. At such potentials, however, we would expect the calcium influx by way of the Na/Ca exchange to be stimulated,[17-20] so that it might be possible to activate the

CICR mechanism. As shown in FIGURE 3, depolarization to +100 mV did not result in a calcium transient (until the cell was repolarized; see below). Because depolarization to +10 mV evoked a typical calcium current and transient, there was no evidence that the failure to observe a response was due to either a failure of CICR or a lack of releasable calcium within the SR in these experiments. These data therefore suggest that calcium influx by way of the Na/Ca exchange cannot activate CICR under normal conditions. It must be noted, however, that this conclusion depends

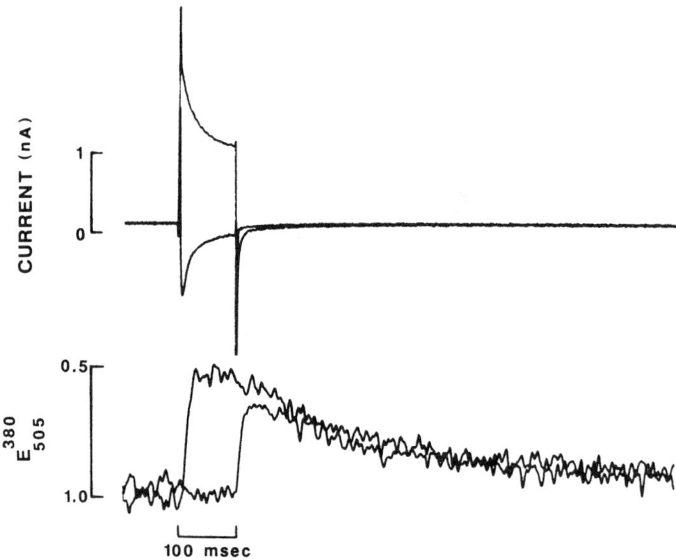

FIGURE 3. Effect of the sodium-calcium exchange on the activation of the calcium transient in adult rat ventricular myocytes. Membrane current is shown at the top, and fluorescence at 500 nm with illumination at 380 nm is shown at the bottom during and following depolarizations for 100 ms to +10 and +100 mV. Depolarizations to +100 mV produced no change in the fluorescence of voltage-clamped rat ventricular myocytes. Repolarization from +100, however, produced a repolarization calcium-transient. These results are compared to the effects of depolarizations to +10 mV. The absence of any fluorescence change on depolarizing to +100 mV is taken as evidence that virtually no calcium entry occurs under the conditions of these experiments where intracellular sodium concentration was 7.5 mM. (Cannell et al.[3] With permission from Science).

critically on the level of sodium within the cell. Inasmuch as the driving force for calcium influx by way of the exchanger is expected to have a cubic dependence on internal sodium, moderate increases in intracellular sodium may have large effects on calcium influx through the exchanger. Thus under conditions that increase intracellular sodium (and which were intentionally avoided in the experiment shown in FIG. 3), it may be possible to activate CICR by calcium influx on the exchanger.[15,16]

FIGURE 3 also shows that repolarization from +100 mV results in a calcium transient. This transient may be explained by the influx of calcium during the calcium "tail" current (that results from incomplete inactivation of the calcium current during the depolarization) activating CICR. It should be noted that the calcium tail current is brief (lasting only a few milliseconds), so that if the calcium transient arises from CICR, CICR must be both quickly activated and sensitive to calcium influx.

CICR Complexity: Voltage and Time Dependence of $[Ca^{2+}]_i$

FIGURE 4 shows an experiment in which the voltage dependence of the $[Ca^{2+}]_i$ transient and the calcium current were examined. Original records are shown in FIGURE 4A, whereas the results are summarized in FIGURE 4B. Examining the data between -60 and 0 mV, it is clear that the half maximum points of the calcium current and $[Ca^{2+}]_i$ transient occur at different potentials, with the half-maximal $[Ca^{2+}]_i$ transient occurring at a more negative potential than the half-maximal calcium current. In addition, there is a voltage range over which the $[Ca^{2+}]_i$ is almost maximal while the calcium current continues to increase. These results suggest that, if calcium release from the SR is activated by the calcium current, only a small calcium current is needed to initiate calcium release and that not all the calcium current is needed to achieve maximal release. At more positive potentials the amplitude of the calcium current decreases, a result that can be explained by the voltage approaching the reversal potential for the current. It is notable that the current amplitude has to decrease to about 60% of maximum before the $[Ca^{2+}]_i$ transient starts to decrease, a result that is consistent with the data that is seen during the ascending phase of the current-voltage relationship. These results can be explained if the CICR mechanism is very sensitive to the calcium influx occurring by way of the calcium current. Put another way, the CICR mechanism acts as a high gain system, where a small input (calcium current) results in a large response (calcium release from the SR). Thus once started, calcium release from the SR will tend to further activate CICR to ensure that calcium release continues to completion (which is also consistent with the observation that a brief tail current activates a $[Ca^{2+}]_i$ transient).

In contrast to this view, FIGURE 5 suggests that the SR calcium release never escapes control by the amplitude of the sarcolemmal calcium influx. This FIGURE shows, that as the duration of a depolarizing pulse is reduced, the amplitude of the $[Ca^{2+}]_i$ decreases. It is notable that, as soon as the cell is repolarized, the release of calcium appears to stop and the decline of the transient starts. Thus the amplitude of the $[Ca^{2+}]_i$ transient appears to be smoothly graded with the duration of the calcium current. This result is typical of a low gain system with no evidence of regeneration. It is notable that the tail currents do not activate calcium release in this experiment. These results do not appear easily explainable on the basis of a simple model of CICR, inasmuch as tail currents activate release from positive but not negative potentials and calcium release is not simply determined by the amplitude or duration of the calcium current. Thus if CICR is to regulate calcium release from the SR, it will have to be more complicated than the simple CICR hypothesis described earlier. Some of these results could be explained by a direct effect of voltage on calcium release, but this mechanism has trouble explaining the lack of release at positive potentials.

Because neither mechanism alone can explain all of our data, it is possible that calcium release from the SR is mediated by a combination of these mechanisms. In other words, calcium release from the SR may be mediated by a voltage and calcium current-dependent mechanism. (It should be noted that a more "complicated" CICR

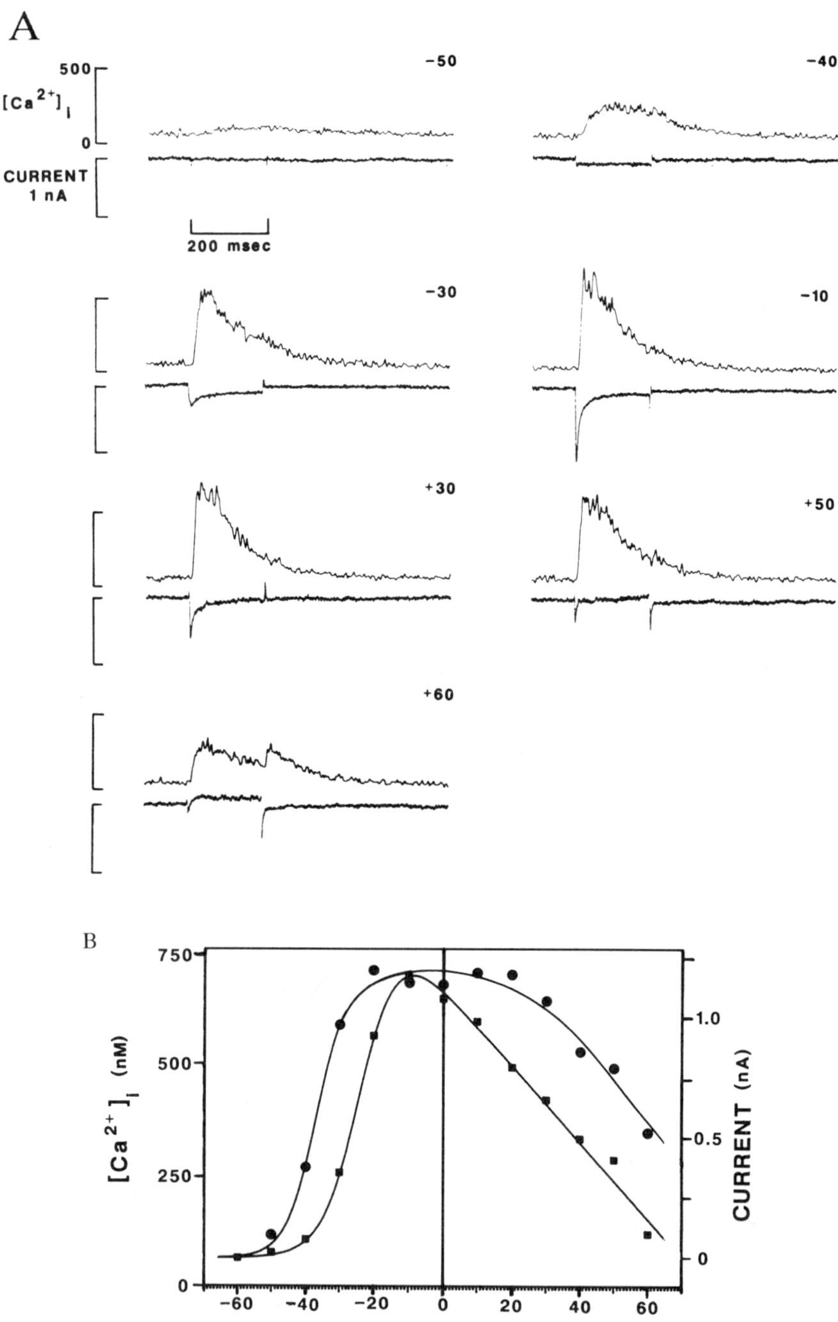

FIGURE 4. The voltage dependence of I_{Ca} and the $[Ca^{2+}]_i$ transient in adult rat ventricular myocytes. **A.** Original records showing the D600-sensitive current (I_{Ca}) and the $[Ca^{2+}]_i$-transients. **B.** Plot of the voltage dependence of I_{Ca} (filled squares) and of the $[Ca^{2+}]_i$ transient (filled circles). Twenty-five μM D600 was used to measure the D600-sensitive current. (Cannell *et al.*[3] With permission from *Science.*)

mechanism may be able to explain all of our data. The dual regulation system, however, is made more attractive by structural similarities between cardiac and skeletal muscle and our observation that the application of ryanodine can alter the voltage dependence of calcium-channel gating. This finding provides additional grounds for suggesting the converse effect: that calcium channel gating may also modify the properties of the SR release channel; see below.) The ryanodine result suggests that there may be "direct communication" between the sarcolemmal calcium channel and the ryanodine receptor/SR calcium-release channel.[21]

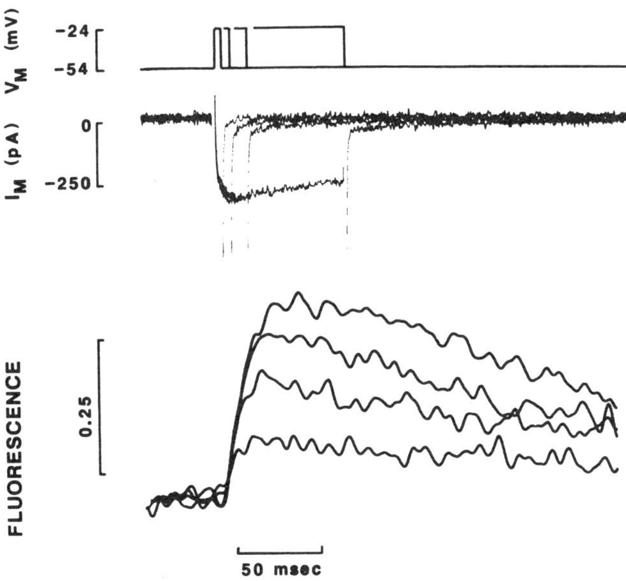

FIGURE 5. The duration-dependence of I_{Ca} and of the $[Ca^{2+}]_i$ transient in adult rat ventricular myocytes. The cell was depolarized from -54 mV to -24 mV for 100 ms for every 1.5 s. During every fourth depolarization, the duration varied. Records were obtained during 5, 10, 20, and 80 ms depolarizations. The voltage protocol is shown on top; the middle record shows membrane current, and the lower record shows changes in fluorescence measured at 500 nm during illumination with 380 nm light. (Cannell *et al.*[3] With permission from *Science.*)

Effect of Development on the Action of Ryanodine

Rat Ventricular Myocytes

We have studied the properties of I_{Ca} in neonatal and adult rat myocytes.[6,21] One particularly important difference between the two ages relates to I_{Ca} inactivation. FIGURE 6A shows the measured steady-state activation (d_∞) and inactivation (f_∞) parameters for I_{Ca} in neonatal ventricular myocytes. The overlap of d_∞ and f_∞ on the

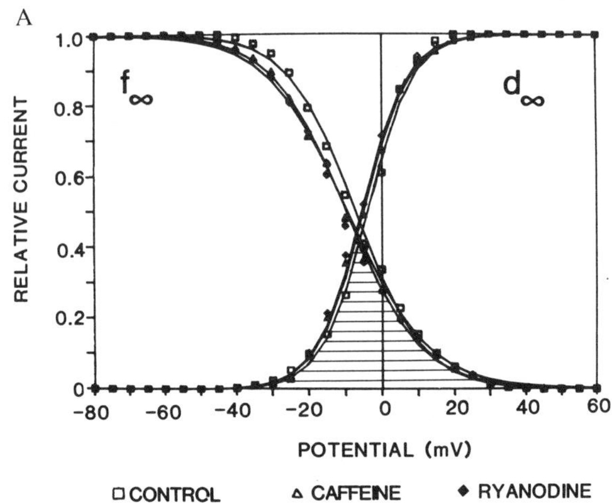

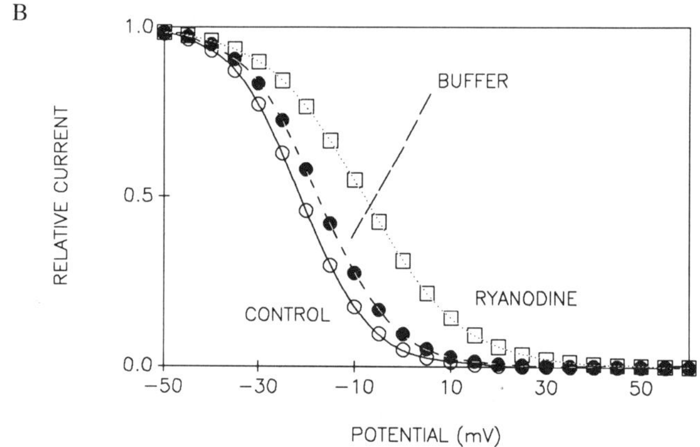

FIGURE 6. Action of ryanodine on the steady-state inactivation (f_∞) and activation (d_∞) variables of I_{Ca} in neonatal rat ventricular myocytes compared to that of adult rat ventricular myocytes. **A.** Neonatal cells. The application of ryanodine (10 μM) or caffeine (10 mM) produces no significant change in the d_∞ or f_∞ curves. **B.** Adult cells; steady-state inactivation. The effect of intracellular calcium buffering and ryanodine on f_∞. The open circles and solid line reflect the control values of f_∞; the open squares and the dotted line reflect the actions of ryanodine (10 μM) on f_∞ (in either the presence or absence of buffer). The "buffers" used include 10 mM or 20 mM EGTA and 10 mM BAPTA (all solutions were buffered to 100 nM $[Ca^{2+}]_i$). When buffer was dialyzed into the cell (in the absence of ryanodine), the f_∞ curve was shifted slightly to the right (filled circle with dashed line). When ryanodine was applied, there was a large shift of the f_∞ curve to the right. (Cohen & Lederer.[21] With permission from the *Journal of Physiology.*)

voltages axis represents the voltage range of the calcium "window" current.[6,21,22] It is clear that the overlap of the curves is significant and that neither ryanodine nor caffeine alters the curves. In adult ventricular myocytes, there is a large reduction in the magnitude of the overlap of the two curves and a shift to the left along the voltage axis of the window current. Although there is no effect of ryanodine on d_∞ (data not shown) in adult myocytes, there is a significant shift of f_∞ to the right along the voltage axis, which makes the voltage dependence of the f_∞ curve in adult cells appear like the voltage dependence of the f_∞ curve in neonatal cells (FIG. 6B). An important anatomical difference between these two cell types is the poorly developed sarcoplasmic reticulum of the neonatal myocytes.[21,23] Because I_{Ca} inactivation has been shown to be affected both by voltage and $[Ca^{2+}]_i$,[24–26] it is important to establish that the alteration of the f_∞ curve by ryanodine in adult myocytes is not simply due to the removal of the $[Ca^{2+}]_i$ transient. FIGURE 6B shows that buffering intracellular calcium shifted the f_∞ curve slightly to the right but that ryanodine was able to shift the f_∞ curve even further to the right (the effect of ryanodine on f_∞ was unchanged by the intracellular buffering). A direct communication between the sarcolemmal calcium channel and the SR calcium release channel is suggested. That ryanodine does not appear to significantly affect the sarcolemmal calcium channel directly is suggested, inasmuch as the application of ryanodine does not affect any parameter of the neonatal I_{Ca}. Additionally, the experiments with large concentrations of intracellular buffers suggest that the action of ryanodine on the adult heart cell is not mediated by $[Ca^{2+}]_i$ itself. We conclude therefore that ryanodine, by binding to its receptor on the calcium release channel of the SR, "indirectly" affects the sarcolemmal calcium channel through some "direct" link between the SR and sarcolemmal channels.[21] FIGURE 8 is a diagrammatic illustration of how we interpret this result, the results presented above, and the results of others. This model allows for both CICR and a voltage-dependent SR calcium release process to influence the release of calcium from the SR.

Charge Movement in Heart Cells

With either a CICR or a voltage-dependent mechanism for excitation-contraction coupling, the signal (sarcolemmal depolarization) must be transmitted to the target proteins. The signal is detected by voltage sensors that presumably are electrical dipoles or charges that are part of a membrane protein itself or are directly associated with it. Depolarization will apply a force on these signaling charges and lead to a conformational change in the membrane protein that could result in the opening of a channel or the transmission of the signal to another protein. Such hypothetical "intramembrane charges" will produce current when they move; these charges have been measured in nerve and skeletal muscle.[27–31] Recently we have measured these currents in single heart cells,[5] as have Bean and Rios,[32] Hanck *et al.*,[33] and Field *et al.*[34] FIGURE 7 shows typical records for ventricular cells from guinea pig (FIG. 7A) and from rat (FIG. 7B). We have been able to identify components correlated with the opening of both sodium channels and calcium channels. Although the sodium gating currents are approximately equal to those expected, given the estimated Na channel density, the calcium channel gating currents exceed the expected current by five- to ten-fold. At the present time, we can only speculate about the function of the excess charge movement. The estimate of calcium channel density or opening probability could be significantly erroneous. Latent calcium channels may give rise to such errors as could

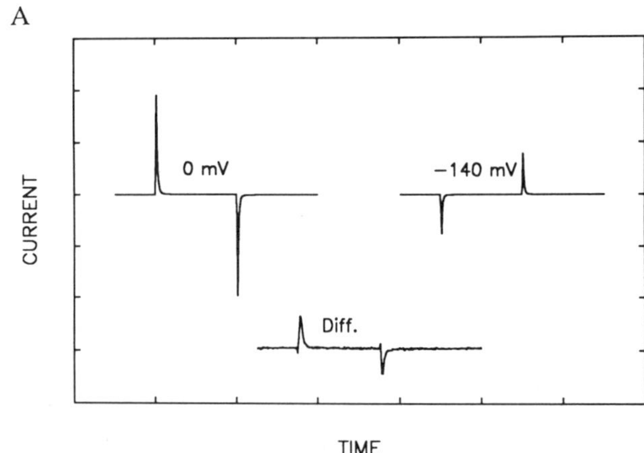

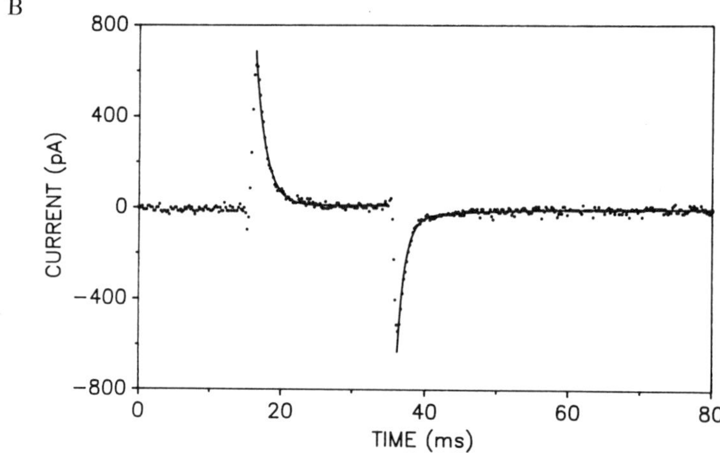

FIGURE 7. Intramembrane charge movement observed in guinea pig and rat ventricular myocytes. **A.** These records show capacitative currents obtained with a test depolarization from −100 mV to 0 mV (upper left), and a control hyperpolarization from −100 mV to −140 mV (upper right). The records were obtained from a guinea pig ventricular myocyte kept at room temperature (21° C). All ionic currents were blocked. The control is used to estimate the linear capacitance of the cell, and thus is scaled up and added to the test current. The difference current (bottom) represents charge movement during the test pulse. Additional experimental data suggest that the difference current reflects the intramembrane charge movement of sodium and calcium channels in these cells. The marks on the x-axis are at 20 ms intervals. The y-axis scale is 10 nA per division for the top traces and 1 nA per division for the difference current. **B.** Intramembrane charge movement is obtained in an adult rat ventricular myocyte. The dots are the data points obtained from charge movement measurements produced by a 20 ms voltage step from −100 to 0 mV. The lines are the least-square fits to the declining phases, the Q_{on} and Q_{off} transients. The Q_{on} transient is the charge movement elicited by the depolarization to 0 mV from the resting potential of −100 mV. The Q_{off} record is the charge movement elicited by the repolarization from 0 mV back to the resting potential of −100 mV. Q_{on} was fit with a single exponential with a time constant of 1.45 ms. Q_{off} was best fit with two exponentials that had time constants of 1.01 and 8.2 ms. (Hadley & Lederer.[5] With permission from the *Journal of Physiology.*)

"senile" and nonfunctional channels. One additional possibility is that a protein similar to the calcium channel is present in the membrane to act as a voltage sensor for the calcium release of the sarcoplasmic reticulum, but this protein does not conduct calcium ions.

Model for Excitation-Contraction Coupling in Heart Muscle

FIGURE 8 shows a diagram that may be adequate to explain the experimental data. It shows a sarcolemmal calcium channel that has two "binding" sites of calcium

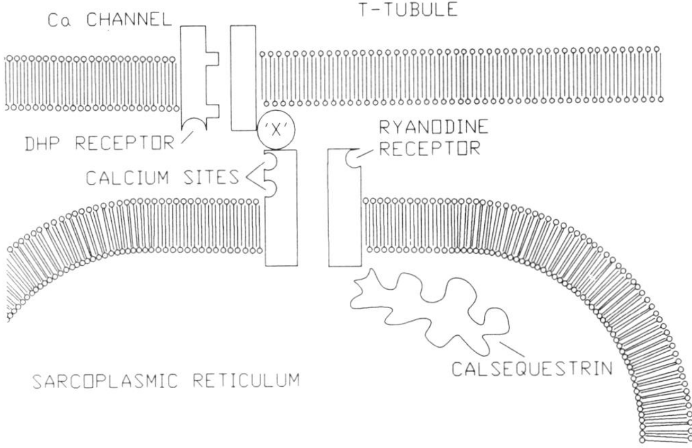

FIGURE 8. Schematic model of the interactions between sarcolemmal calcium channel, calcium-release channel from the sarcoplasmic reticulum, and other factors that regulate excitation-contraction coupling in heart muscle. A dihydropyridine (DHP) receptor is located on the sarcolemmal calcium channel. The pore of the calcium channel interacts with permeant ions to yield specific selectivity and conductance properties. The calcium-release channel in the sarcoplasmic reticulum is a very large protein, thought to contain four 450 kDa proteins. This calcium-release channel can bind calcium to activate the channel and can also bind to the channel to close the channel. The calcium-release channel also can bind ryanodine, which alters the behavior of the channel. The sarcoplasmic reticulum contains calcium-binding proteins such as calsequestrin. Any interactions between the sarcoplasmic-reticulum calcium release channel and the sarcolemmal calcium channel may depend on additional proteins (represented by the factor 'X'), but the nature of such links have not been elucidated.[21,37]

within the pore of the channel as has been suggested by recent experiments.[35,36] These binding sites may serve not only to regulate selectivity and permeation but (we speculate) also may affect inactivation of the channel and the communication of the channel with other proteins. A hypothesized linking protein, 'X,' may serve as a connection between the sarcolemmal calcium channel and at least some of the calcium-release channels in the sarcoplasmic reticulum. The calcium-release channel is the tetramer of 450 kDa subunits that contains the ryanodine receptor and calcium binding sites. Two calcium binding sites are illustrated in FIGURE 8, one of which is thought to regulate opening (activation) of the calcium release channel, whereas the other is thought to regulate closing (inactivation) of the calcium release channel.

SUMMARY

Experimental data do not support the idea that excitation-contraction coupling in heart muscle can be explained by a simple calcium-induced calcium release mechanism alone or a simple voltage-dependent calcium release mechanism alone. Our data on excitation-contraction coupling combined with the results of others suggest the need to either develop more complex and more sophisticated single-mechanism models, or to establish dual-control models.

ACKNOWLEDGMENTS

We are indebted to Dr. B. A. Reitz and Dr. W. A. Baumgartner of the Department of Surgery at the Johns Hopkins Hospital for their help in obtaining the human heart tissue.

REFERENCES

1. ALLEN, D. G. & J. R. BLINKS. 1978. Calcium transients in aequorin-injected frog cardiac muscle. Nature **273:** 509-513.
2. FABIATO, A. 1985. Simulated calcium current can both cause calcium loading and trigger calcium release from the sarcoplasmic reticulum of a skinned canine cardiac Purkinje cell. J. Gen. Physiol. **85:** 291-320.
3. CANNELL, M. B., J. R. BERLIN & W. J. LEDERER. 1987. Effect of membrane potential changes on the calcium transient in single rat cardiac muscle cells. Science **238:** 1419-1423.
4. MITRA, R. & M. MORAD. 1985. A uniform enzymatic method for dissociation of myocytes from hearts and stomachs of vertebrates. Am. J. Physiol. **249:** H1056-H1060.
5. HADLEY, R. W. & W. J. LEDERER. 1989. Intramembrane charge movement in guinea-pig and rat ventricular myocytes. J. Physiol. **415:** 601-624.
6. COHEN, N. M. & W. J. LEDERER. 1987. Calcium current in isolated neonatal rat ventricular myocytes. J. Physiol. **391:** 169-191.
7. ESCANDE, D., A. COULOMBE, J.-F. FAIVRE, E. DEROUBAIS & E. CORABOEUF. 1987. Two types of transient outward currents in adult human atrial cells. Am. J. Physiol. **252:** H142-H148.
8. CANNELL, M. B. & W. J. LEDERER. 1986. A novel experimental chamber for single-cell voltage-clamp and patch-clamp applications with low electrical noise and excellent temperature and flow control. Pfluegers Archiv. Eur. J. Physiol. **406:** 536-539.
9. PEETERS, G. A., V. HLADY, J. H. B. BRIDGE & W. H. BARRY. 1987. Simultaneous measurement of calcium transients and motion in cultured heart cells. Am. J. Physiol. **253:** H1400-H1408.
10. CANNELL, M. B., J. R. BERLIN & W. J. LEDERER. 1987. Intracellular calcium in cardiac myocytes: Calcium transients measured using fluorescence imaging. *In* Cell Calcium and

the Control of Membrane Transport. L. J. Mandel & D. C. Eaton, Eds.: 202-214. Rockefeller University Press. New York.

11. BERLIN, J. R., M. B. CANNELL & W. J. LEDERER. 1989. Cellular origins of the transient inward current, I_{TI}, in cardiac myocytes: role of fluctuations and waves of elevated intracellular calcium. Circ. Res. **65:** 115-126.

12. EISNER, D. A. & W. J. LEDERER. 1985. Na-Ca exchange: stoichiometry and electrogenicity. Am. J. Physiol. **248:** C189-C202.

13. EISNER, D. A. & W. J. LEDERER. 1989. The electrogenic sodium-calcium exchange. *In* Sodium-Calcium Exchange. T. J. A. Allen, D. Noble & H. Reuter, Eds.: 178-207. Oxford University Press. Oxford, England.

14. MULLINS, L. J. 1979. The generation of electric currents in cardiac fibers by Na/Ca exchange. Am. J. Physiol. **236:** C103-C110.

15. BERLIN, J. R., M. B. CANNELL & W. J. LEDERER. 1987. Regulation of twitch tension in sheep cardiac Purkinje fibers during calcium overload. Am. J. Physiol. **253:** H1540-H1547.

16. BERS, D. M., D. M. CHRISTENSEN & T. X. NGUYEN. 1988. Can Ca entry via Na-Ca exchange directly activate cardiac muscle contraction? J. Mol. Cell. Cardiol. **20:** 405-414.

17. KIMURA, J., A. NOMA & H. IRISAWA. 1986. Na-Ca exchange current in mammalian heart cells. Nature **319:** 596-597.

18. KIMURA, J., S. MIYAMAE & A. NOMA. 1987. Identification of sodium-calcium exchange current in single ventricular cells of guinea-pig. J. Physiol. **384:** 199-222.

19. EHARA, T., S. MATSUOKA & A. NOMA. 1989. Measurement of reversal potential of Na+-Ca++ exchange current in single guinea-pig ventricular cells. J. Physiol. **410:** 227-249.

20. BARCENAS-RUIZ, L., D. J. BUECKELMANN & W. G. WIER. 1987. Sodium-calcium exchange in heart: currents and changes in [Ca]i. Science **238:** 1720-1722.

21. COHEN, N. M. & W. J. LEDERER. 1988. Changes in the calcium current of rat heart ventricular myocytes during development. J. Physiol. **406:** 115-146.

22. ATTWELL, D., I. COHEN, D. EISNER, M. OHBA & C. OJEDA. 1979. The steady state TTX-sensitive ("Window") sodium current in cardiac Purkinje fibres. Pflugers Archiv. Eur. J. Physiol. **379:** 137-142.

23. HIRAKOW, R. & T. GOTOH. 1975. A quantitative ultrastructural study on the developing rat heart. *In* Developmental and Physiological Correlates of Cardiac Muscle. M. Lieberman & T. Sano. Eds.: 37-49. Raven Press. New York.

24. LEE, K. S., E. MARBAN & R. W. TSIEN. 1985. Inactivation of calcium channels in mammalian heart cells: Joint dependence on membrane potential and intracellular calcium. J. Physiol. **364:** 395-411.

25. HADLEY, R. W. & J. R. HUME. 1987. An intrinsic potential-dependent inactivation mechanism associated with calcium channels in guinea-pig myocytes. J. Physiol. **389:** 205-222.

26. KASS, R. S. & M. C. SANGUINETTI. 1984. Inactivation of calcium channel current in the calf cardiac Purkinje fiber: Evidence of voltage- and calcium-mediated mechanisms. J. Gen. Physiol. **84:** 705-726.

27. SCHNEIDER, M. F. & W. K. CHANDLER. 1973. Voltage-dependent charge movement in skeletal muscle: a possible step in excitation-contraction coupling. Nature **242:** 244-247.

28. HOROWICZ, P. & M. F. SCHNEIDER. 1981. Membrane charge moved at contraction thresholds in skeletal muscle fibres. J. Physiol. **314:** 595-633.

29. BEZANILLA, F. & C. M. ARMSTRONG. 1974. Gating currents of the sodium channels: Three ways to block them. Science **183:** 753-754.

30. GILLY, W. F. & C. S. HUI. 1980. Voltage-dependent charge movement in frog slow muscle fibres. J. Physiol. **301:** 175-190.

31. SCHEUER, T. & W. F. GILLY. 1986. Charge movement and depolarization-contraction coupling in arthropod vs. vertebrate skeletal muscle. Proc. Natl. Acad. Sci. USA **83:** 8799-8803.

32. BEAN, B. P. & E. RIOS. 1989. Non-linear charge movement in the membranes of mammalian cardiac ventricular cells. Components from Na and Ca channel gating. J. Gen. Physiol. **94:** 65-93.

33. HANCK, D. A., M. F. SHEETS & H. A. FOZZARD. 1988. Gating currents in single cardiac Purkinje cells. Biophys. J. **53:** 535a.

34. FIELD, A. C., C. HILL & G. D. LAMB. 1988. Asymmetric charge movement and calcium currents in ventricular myocytes of neonatal rat. J. Physiol. **406:** 277-297.
35. LANSMAN, J. B., P. HESS & R. W. TSIEN. 1986. Blockade of current through single calcium channels by Cd2+, Mg2+, Mg2+, and Ca2+: Voltage and concentration dependence of calcium entry into the pore. J. Gen. Physiol. **88:** 321-347.
36. HESS, P., J. B. LANSMAN & R. W. TSIEN. 1986. Calcium channel selectivity for divalent and monovalent cations: Voltage and concentration dependence of single channel current in ventricular heart cells. J. Gen. Physiol. **88:** 293-319.
37. LEDERER, W. J., M. B. CANNELL, N. M. COHEN & J. R. BERLIN. 1989. Excitation-contraction coupling in heart muscle. Mol. Cell. Biochem. **89:** 115-119.

Membrane Ion Channels in Cardiac Malformation and Disease

TONY L. CREAZZO, CANDACE ROSSIGNOL,
LESLIE HANCOCK, AND HARRIETT STADT

Department of Anatomy
Medical College of Georgia
Augusta, Georgia 30912

INTRODUCTION

Though nearly 1% of all live births are complicated by cardiovascular malformations,[1] nothing is known concerning the electrophysiology of cardiac myocytes in response to congenital heart defects. This is due largely to the lack of a reliable experimental model from which electrophysiological measurements can be made at the cellular level. Based on present knowledge of electrical activity in myocytes from hearts in various adult experimental models of heart disease, some differences as a result of congenital malformation would be expected. Cardiac malformation would be expected to increase the hemodynamic burden of the heart muscle. According to Braunwald[2] the mature heart basically depends on three mechanisms in order to compensate for an excessive hemodynamic burden and maintain cardiac output. These are (1) the Frank-Starling mechanism, (2) increased release of catecholamines by adrenergic nerves and the adrenal medulla, and (3) myocardial hypertrophy. Through the Frank-Starling mechanism the heart is intrinsically capable of varying its force of contraction on a beat-to-beat basis based on initial muscle (sarcomere) length. Catecholamines serve to increase muscle contractility and increase both Ca^{2+} and K^+ conductances[3,4] in the myocyte membrane, indirectly, through activation of beta-adrenergic receptors. If the excessive hemodynamic burden is prolonged the heart will respond with hypertrophy of the myocardium. Hypertrophy represents an intrinsic change in the cardiac myocyte characterized by accelerated protein synthesis[5] and, at least initially, increased contractility.[2] If the heart is not relieved of the excessive hemodynamic burden it will inevitably fail.[2]

Several changes in the electrical activity of myocytes have been associated with ventricular hypertrophy in a number of experimental models.[6] The most consistent observation is a prolongation of the action potential that may be accompanied by a more depolarized diastolic potential and less membrane depolarization during the plateau phase.[6,7] There are several underlying voltage and time-dependent Ca^{2+} and K^+ currents that may account for the prolonged action potential.[8] Unfortunately, there have been just two voltage clamp studies on myocytes from hearts with experimentally induced hypertrophy. Using the sucrose gap technique in cat papillary muscle, Ten Eik and colleagues[7] found both a reduction of the slow Ca^{2+} current and a reduction of time-dependent outward K^+ in hearts with right ventricular

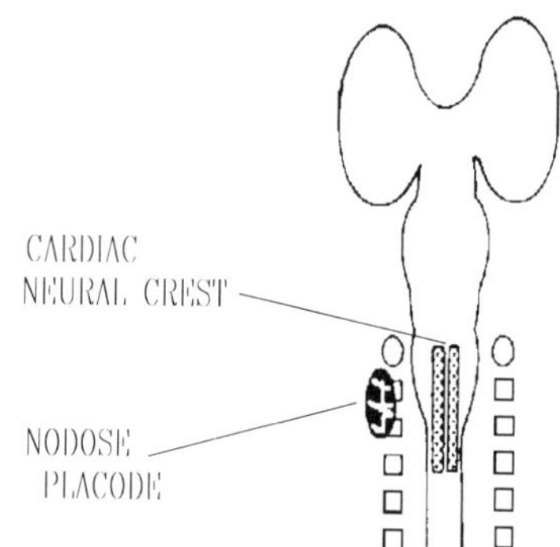

FIGURE 1. Diagram of the cephalic region of the stage 8 chick embryo, indicating the location of the cardiac neural crest and the nodose placodes. Bilateral ablation of these structures results in a heart with both PTA and an absence of parasympathetic innervation. Hearts were used in the studies described here only if diagnosed to have PTA by visual inspection.

hypertrophy. A more recent patch-clamp study by Kleiman and Houser,[9] also using the cat model, indicated a reduction of outward K^+ current and a slowing of Ca^{2+} current inactivation with no reduction of peak current. Though the data on Ca^{2+} current are contradictory these reports indicate that the prolongation of the action potential is due to a reduction of a time-dependent K^+ repolarization current, often referred to as the delayed rectifier or simply I_K. Presently, there are no voltage clamp studies addressing developmental changes in electrical activity associated with congenital cardiac malformations, despite the knowledge that malformations are often associated with myocardial hypertrophy.[1] We have sought to address this paucity of electrophysiological data by using an embryonic chick heart model developed and characterized by Kirby and colleagues (FIG. 1).[10,11]

PERSISTENT TRUNCUS ARTERIOSUS IN THE EMBRYONIC CHICK HEART

It is well-known that the postganglionic autonomic innervation to the heart is derived from specific subpopulations of migratory embryonic cells from the neural crest.[12–14] From the recent work of Kirby[10,11] it is now known that there are neural crest-derived ectomesenchymal cells that are essential for aorticopulmonary and conotruncal septation of the outflow region of the heart tube. These ectomesenchymal cells come from the same population of crest from which the parasympathetic intracardiac ganglion cells are derived. This region of "cardiac" neural crest extends from the midotic placode to the caudal region of somite 3. Ablation of the cardiac neural crest prior to migration results in failure of conotruncal and aorticopulmonary septation;[15] this is a congenital malformation known as persistent truncus arteriosus (PTA).[15,16] In this defect the output of both right and left ventricles exists through a common outflow tract. Interestingly, there is only a slight reduction in the number of intracardiac ganglion cells.[11] This occurs because migratory cells derived from the nodose placodes are able to "fill in" for the ablated cardiac neural crest.[11] The nodose placode cells, however, are unable to participate in septation of the outflow tract. Using a field stimulation technique we have recently determined that parasympathetic ganglion cells derived from the nodose placodes are functionally indistinguishable from those that are normally derived from the cardiac crest (Kirby, Creazzo, and Christiansen, submitted). Consequently, bilateral ablation of both the cardiac crest and the nodose placodes yields a heart that has PTA and an absence of parasympathetic innervation.[11] Preliminary evidence indicates that these hearts are hypertrophied (ratio of ventricle to whole embryo weight is increased 42%; Creazzo, unpublished).

CALCIUM CURRENT AND PTA

Calcium Current

Calcium current is voltage-activated by depolarizing the cell membrane to potentials positive to -50 mV[3,8] (examples in FIG. 2). It has been referred to as the slow inward current (I_{si} or I_{Ca}) to distinguish it from the voltage-activated inward sodium current that has much faster activation and inactivation kinetics. I_{Ca} is active during the plateau phase of the action potential and is essential for the initiation of the excitation-contraction coupling. Other functions may include the activation of various calcium-dependent enzymes,[17] such as protein kinase C.[17,18] More recent reports in-

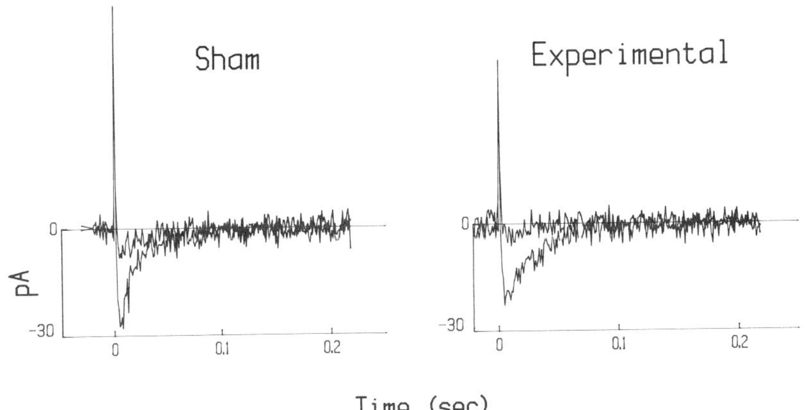

FIGURE 2. Examples of Ca^{2+} current traces in ventricular myocytes from sham and experimental (PTA) embryos in the presence and absence of 1 μM nifedipine. To produce these inward current transients the cells were depolarized from a holding potential of -80 mV to a test potential of 0 mV. The protocol was repeated in the same cells with nifedipine. The example traces were superimposed. In the presence of nifedipine (smaller traces), $I_{Ca.L}$ is blocked, and only $I_{Ca.T}$ is present. The composition of the extracellular solution was (in mM); $CaCl_2$ 1.8, CsCl 20, NaCl 110, $MgCl_2$ 1.8, Hepes (NaOH) 10, tetradotoxin 0.003, and glucose 0.5% (pH 7.3). The patch pipet solution contained (in mM); CsCl 120, $MgCl_2$ 4, EGTA 5, Hepes (CsOH) 10, Na_2ATP 3, Na_2GTP 0.4, and phosphocreatine 5 (pH 7.4). All experiments were conducted at room temperature (22-24°C).

dicate that I_{Ca} in the adult atrial myocardium is comprised of two conductances.[19] These are termed the low threshold or transient ($I_{Ca.T}$) and the long-lasting ($I_{Ca.L}$) calcium currents.[20] $I_{Ca.T}$, which shows both voltage-dependent activation and inactivation, is thought to play a role in pacemaking.[21] Peak activation occurs at about -30 to -20 mV, and its decay is rapid relative to $I_{Ca.L}$. $I_{Ca.T}$ antagonists include nickel, tetramethrin, and amiloride.[21,22] There are no known agonists. $I_{Ca.T}$ has been found to be either absent or an insignificant component of I_{Ca} in the ventricles of adult animals.[19] $I_{Ca.T}$, however, has recently been shown to be a much more significant component of I_{Ca} in the embryonic chick ventricle[23] (see FIG. 3 and discussion below).

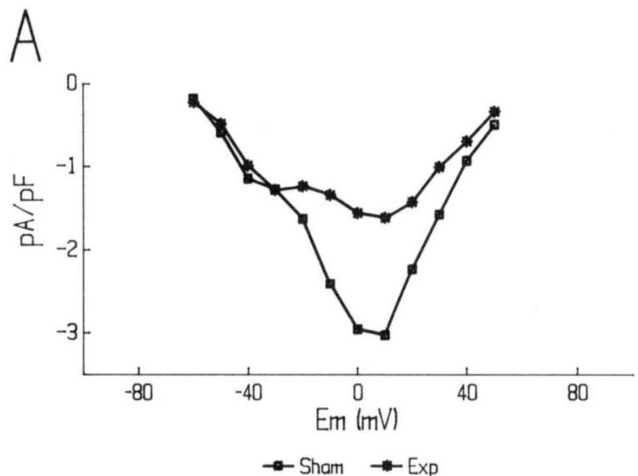

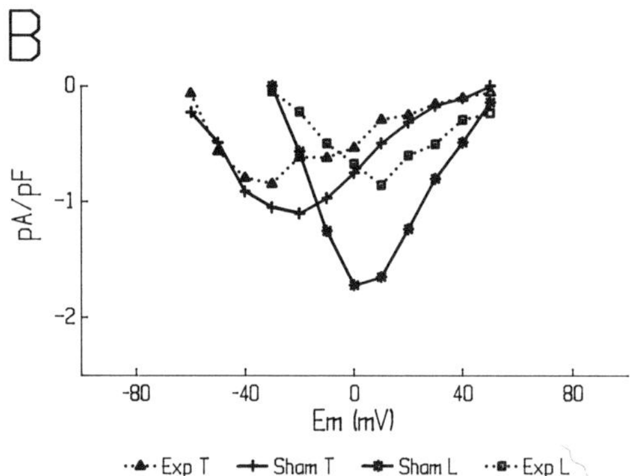

FIGURE 3. Current-voltage relationships (I-V) of peak Ca^{2+} current in ventricular myocytes from sham and experimental embryos. The results were normalized to cell capacitance. **A:** I-Vs of peak current from $E_{hold} = -80$ mV. Note the "shoulder" region at $E_{test} = -30$ mV and a second peak at $+10$ mV signifying the presence of both $I_{Ca.T}$ and $I_{Ca.L}$. The values at $E_{test} = -20, -10, 0, 10, 20$, and 30 mV are significantly different ($p < 0.05$, Student t test; sham: n $= 10$; exp: n $= 15$). **B:** $I_{Ca.T}$ and $I_{Ca.L}$ separated by nifedipine and voltage dependence, respectively. $I_{Ca.T}$ was visualized by blocking of $I_{Ca.L}$ with 1 μM nifedipine. The values were not statistically significant ($p > 0.1$; sham: n $= 6$; exp: n $= 6$). $I_{Ca.L}$ was visualized by inactivating $I_{Ca.T}$ (as well as a portion of $I_{Ca.L}$) with a 500 ms prepulse to -40 mV. The values at $E_{test} = -10, 0, 10$, and 20 mV were significant ($p < 0.05$; sham: n $= 6$; exp: n $= 6$).

Relatively more is known of $I_{Ca.L}$, which is found in both atrial and ventricular myocytes.[19,20] The L calcium channel is the receptor for the 1,4-dihydropyridines (DHP), and the gene coding for the DHP receptor/channel has been cloned.[24,25] $I_{Ca.L}$ has been called "long-lasting" because when barium ions are substituted for Ca^{2+} as the charge carrier, then the current inactivates very slowly.[19,20] Thus, the inactivation process, though not completely understood, appears to be largely Ca^{2+}-dependent.[26] Activation of $I_{Ca.L}$ begins at about -30 to -20 mV and peaks at $+10$ to $+20$ mV (see FIG. 3). Phosphorylation of the L channel by cyclic AMP-dependent protein kinase increases the probability that the channel will open, thereby increasing the magnitude of $I_{Ca.L}$.[3] Drugs such as the beta blockers will indirectly decrease $I_{Ca.L}$ by reducing intracellular cyclic AMP.[3] Calcium channel blockers such as nifedipine and verapamil act directly on the channel by way of specific receptors.[27] With the recent advent of the patch clamp and other molecular probes, knowledge of I_{Ca} has significantly increased, though there are still many unanswered questions. It should be noted that although $I_{Ca.T}$ and $I_{Ca.L}$ are distinguishable as "whole-cell" currents, there has not yet been an unequivocal separation of L and T currents at the single channel level. The difficulty has been that it is not possible to obtain accurate single channel measurements due to a very small conductance and rapid kinetics in normal physiological solutions.

Calcium Current in Hearts with PTA

Does PTA alter membrane conductance in the embryonic chick heart? To approach this question the whole-cell variation of the patch clamp technique[28,29] was employed to examine I_{Ca} in single ventricular myocytes in hearts from embryos with both PTA and an absence of parasympathetic innervation. Myocytes were obtained by an enzymatic dissociation procedure previously described by DeHaan.[23,30] Examples of inward Ca^{2+} current transients in the presence or absence of nifedipine are shown in FIGURE 2. Typically, I_{Ca} peaked within 10–20 ms, and decay was complete by 200 milliseconds. The DHP antagonist, nifedipine, decreased the current at positive potentials. A distinct shoulder region was apparent in the current-voltage relationships at about -30 mV, suggesting that I_{Ca} was composed of two conductances (FIG. 3A). These results were in accordance with a recent report that indicates that the embryonic chick ventricle contains both the DHP-sensitive $I_{Ca.L}$ and the low threshold DHP-insensitive $I_{Ca.T}$.[23] The current-voltage relationships for peak I_{Ca} indicated a twofold reduction of I_{Ca} at potentials positive to -30 mV in experimental hearts compared with shams. The results suggested a reduction in the peak amplitude of $I_{Ca.L}$, whereas $I_{Ca.T}$ appeared unaffected. These results were confirmed when $I_{Ca.T}$ and $I_{Ca.L}$ were examined separately (FIG. 3B). $I_{Ca.T}$ was viewed by blocking most of the $I_{Ca.L}$ with 1 μM nifedipine (FIGURES 2 and 3B). The results indicated that there was no difference in $I_{Ca.T}$ in myocytes from sham and experimental embryos. In order to visualize $I_{Ca.L}$ directly, a 500 ms prepulse to -40 mV was used to inactivate most or all of $I_{Ca.T}$. The current-voltage relationships in FIGURE 3B clearly demonstrate the reduction of $I_{Ca.L}$ in the ventricles from experimental hearts. In both sham and experimental ventricles the peak currents were somewhat smaller than would be expected from the I-V curves shown in FIGURE 3A because the prepulse to -40 mV also inactivated a portion of $I_{Ca.L}$.

The twofold reduction of $I_{Ca.L}$ in experimental ventricles could be explained by a comparable decrease in the number of L type Ca^{2+} channels present. To examine this possibility the number of DHP receptors was quantified using the high-affinity L channel antagonist, $(^+)[^3\mathrm{H}]\mathrm{PN200\text{-}110}$. Scatchard analysis of binding data indicated no difference in the number of DHP receptors in experimental ventricles (sham: [R] = 192 fmol/mg protein, K_d = 100 pM; experimental: [R] = 187 fmol/mg, K_d = 93 pM). These results suggest that $I_{Ca.L}$ in experimental ventricles was reduced by modulation of channel activity rather than channel number. The average total protein per ventricle was 1.1 mg for sham and 1.3 mg for the experimental (from 25 and 21 pooled ventricles, respectively). These data are a further indication that the hearts with PTA hypertrophied.

CONCLUSIONS

The results demonstrate a significant reduction of $I_{Ca.L}$ in hearts with PTA that was not due to a decrease in the number of calcium channels. These findings are similar to those reported by Ten Eik[7] in myocytes from hypertrophied myocardium. In order to evaluate the significance of these data several possibilities must be considered. The first consideration is that some or all of the decreased $I_{Ca.L}$ is due to the absence of parasympathetic innervation. This seems unlikely because parasympathetic innervation in the chick heart does not become functional until day 12[31] or at least one day later than the age at which the embryos used in this study were sacrificed. It remains a possibility that there is a neuronal "trophic factor" that is required for the development of $I_{Ca.L}$. In the skeletal-motor system, for example, it is well-known that efferent innervation plays an important developmental role in both distribution and gating of the nicotinic receptor-channel complex[32,33] that is not related to transmitter release. There is no compelling evidence, however, that neurotransmitters play a role of similar magnitude in heart development. In the future it will be possible to definitively determine whether parasympathetic innervation affects $I_{Ca.L}$ development because experimental hearts that have PTA along with functional innervation will be produced (Kirby, Creazzo, and Christiansen, submitted). Another consideration is that the stress of such a severe lesion causes a delay in the development of the mechanisms that regulate L channel activity. Though this possibility was not specifically addressed, the data indicate no development delay, at least in terms of ventricular weight and total protein. Further, a comparable increase in peak current density occurring during normal development through the ages of 7-15 days has not been observed (Creazzo, unpublished). Most likely, the reduction in $I_{Ca.L}$ is the result of the PTA.

What mechanism(s) could account for a decreased $I_{Ca.L}$ without a concomitant decrease in the number of L channels? It should not be surprising that cardiac stress might affect L channel function at the level of single myocytes. There are apparently multiple cellular mechanisms for regulating the activity of this channel. For example, there are enzymatic systems for phosphorylation and dephosphorylation of the channel protein.[34–37] Phosphorylation is thought to increase the open channel probability.[3] The presence of a specific DHP receptor site suggests regulation of the channel by an endogenous DHP-like molecule; at present there is some indirect evidence in support of this hypothesis.[38,39] Further, a recent report indicates that there is an endogenous peptide that acts to increase $I_{Ca.L}$ in cardiac myocytes by an apparently novel mechanism.[40] It will be important to determine the role that such mechanisms may play in cardiac malformation and other forms of excessive hemodynamic burden.

With regard to cardiac function, what is the significance of reduced $I_{Ca,L}$? $I_{Ca,L}$ appears to be an important factor in determining contractility[21] in the heart; therefore, a reduction in this current would be expected to reduce the force of contraction. Decreased $I_{Ca,L}$ would seem to be in conflict with the heart's apparent attempt to augment contractility through myocardial hypertrophy. In fact, both in humans and experimental models, the myocardium from stressed hearts generally exhibits decreased contractility even during early stages of compensatory hypertrophy.[2,6,7] Hence, the data discussed here suggest that decreased contractility in hypertrophied hearts is due to a reduction of $I_{Ca,L}$. Inasmuch as the chick embryos with PTA invariably die at day 12 or very shortly thereafter, it seems likely that the day 11 hearts used in this study are failing. Decreased $I_{Ca,L}$ may, therefore, be a contributing factor in heart failure. In addition, the data indicates that, at an early age, the embryonic heart is capable of responding much in the same way as the adult heart in the presence of an excessive hemodynamic burden. In summary, the embryonic chick heart with PTA represents a reliable model for the study of voltage-dependent membrane conductances during cardiac malformation and disease.

REFERENCES

1. FRIEDMAN, W. F. 1984. Congenital heart disease in infancy and childhood. *In* Heart Disease: A Textbook of Cardiovascular Medicine. E. Braunwald, Ed.: 941-1023. W. B. Saunders Company. Philadelphia, PA.
2. BRAUNWALD, E. 1984. Pathophysiology of Heart Failure. *In* Heart Disease: A Textbook of Cardiovascular Medicine. E. Braunwald, Ed.: 447-466. W. B. Saunders Company. Philadelphia, PA.
3. REUTER, H. 1983. Calcium channel modulation by neurotransmitters, enzymes and drugs. Nature **301:** 569-574.
4. BENNETT, P., L. MCKINNEY, T. BEGENISICH & R. S. KASS. 1986. Adrenergic modulation of the delayed rectifier potassium channel in calf cardiac Purkinje fibers. Biophys. J. **49:** 839-848.
5. RUSSO, L. A. & H. E. MORGAN. 1989. Control of protein synthesis and ribosome formation in rat heart. Diabetes Metab. Rev. **5:** 31-47.
6. COOPER, G., IV. 1987. Cardiocyte adaptation to chronically altered load. Annu. Rev. Physiol. **49:** 501-518.
7. TEN EICK, R. E., A. L. BASSETT & L. L. ROBERTSON. 1983. Possible electrophysiological basis for decreased contractility associated with myocardial hypertrophy in the cat: A voltage clamp approach. *In* Myocardial Hypertrophy and Failure. N. R. Alpert, Ed.: 245-259. Raven Press. New York.
8. NOBLE, D. 1984. The surprising heart: A review of recent progress in cardiac electrophysiology. J. Physiol. (London) **353:** 1-50.
9. KLEIMAN, R. B. & S. R. HOUSER. 1988. Calcium currents in normal and hypertrophied isolated feline ventricular myocytes. Am. J. Physiol. (Heart Circ. Physiol. **24**) **255:** H1434-H1442.
10. KIRBY, M. L., T. F. GALE & D. E. STEWART. 1983. Neural crest cells contribute to normal aorticopulmonary septation. Science **220:** 1059-1061.
11. KIRBY, M. L. 1988. Nodose placode contributes autonomic neurons to the heart in the absence of cardiac neural crest. J. Neurosci. **8:** 1090-1095.
12. NARAYANAN, C. H. & Y. NARAYANAN. 1980. Neural crest and placodal contributions in the development of the glosspharyngeal-vagal complex in the chick. Anat. Rec. **196:** 71-82.
13. LEDOUARIN, N. M. 1982. The Neural Crest. Cambridge U. P. London, England.
14. D'AMICO-MARTEL, A. & D. M. NODEN. 1983. Contributions of placodal and neural crest cells to avian cranial peripheral ganglia. Am. J. Anat. **166:** 445-468.

15. NISHIBATAKE, M., M. L. KIRBY & L. H. S. VAN MIEROP. 1987. Pathogenesis of persistent truncus arteriosus and dextroposed aorta in the chick embryo after neural crest ablation. Circulation **75:** 255-264.

16. MAIR, D. D., D. E. EDWARDS, V. FUSTER, J. B. SEWARD & G. K. DANIELSON. 1983. Truncus Arteriosus. *In* Heart Disease in Infants, Children, and Adolescents. F. H. Adams & G. C. Emmanouilides, Eds.: 400-410. Williams and Wilkins. Baltimore, MD.

17. ABDEL-LATIF, A. A. 1986. Calcium-mobilizing receptors, polyphosphoinositides, and the generation of second messengers. Pharmacol. Rev. **38:** 227-272.

18. WISE, B. C., B. L. RAYNOR & J. F. KUO. 1982. Phospholipid-sensitive Ca^{2+}-dependent protein kinase from heart: I. Purification and general properties. J. Biol. Chem. **257:** 8481-8488.

19. BEAN, B. P. 1985. Two kinds of calcium channels in canine atrial cells: Differences in kinetics, selectivity, and pharmacology. J. Physiol. (London) **86:** 1-30.

20. McCLESKEY, E. W., A. P. FOX, D. FELDMAN & R. W. TSIEN. 1986. Different types of calcium channels. J. Exp. Biol. **124:** 177-190.

21. HAGIWARA, N., H. IRISAWA & M. KAMEYAMA. 1988. Contribution of two types of calcium currents to the pacemaker potentials of rabbit sino-atrial node cells. J. Physiol. (London) **395:** 223-253.

22. TANG, C-M., F. PRESSER & M. MORAD. 1988. Amiloride selectively blocks the low threshold (T) calcium channel. Science **240:** 213-215.

23. KAWANO, S. & R. L. DeHAAN. 1989. The low-threshold current, I_T, is the major calcium-current in chick ventricular cells. Am. J. Physiol. **256:** H1505-H1508.

24. MAAN, A. C. & M. M. HOSEY. 1987. Analysis of the properties of binding of calcium-channel activators and inhibitors to dihydropyridine receptors in chick heart membranes. Circ. Res. **61:** 379-388.

25. TANABE, T., H. TAKESHIMA, A. MIKAMI, V. FLOCKERZI, H. TAKAHASHI, K. KANGAWA, M. KOJIMA, H. MATSUO, T. HIROSE & S. NUMA. 1987. Primary structure of the receptor for calcium channel blockers from skeletal muscle. Nature **328:** 313-318.

26. MENTRARD, D., G. VASSORT & R. FISCHMEISTER. 1984. Calcium-mediated inactivation of the calcium conductance in cesium-loaded frog heart cells. J. Gen. Physiol. **83:** 105-131.

27. HOSEY, M. M. & M. LAZDUNSKI. 1988. Calcium channels: Molecular pharmacology, structure and regulation. J. Membr. Biol. **104:** 81-105.

28. HAMILL, O. P., A. MARTY, E. NEHER, B. SAKMANN & F. J. SIGWORTH. 1981. Improved patch-clamp techniques for high-resolution current recording from cells and cell-free membrane patches. Pfluegers Arch. **391:** 85-100.

29. SIMMONS, M. A., T. L. CREAZZO & H. C. HARTZELL. 1986. A time-dependent and voltage-sensitive K^+ current in single cells from frog atrium. J. Gen. Physiol. **88:** 739-755.

30. NATHAN, R. D. & R. D. DeHAAN. 1979. Voltage clamp analysis of embryonic heart cell aggregates. J. Gen. Physiol. **73:** 175-198.

31. PAPPANO, A. J. & K. LÖFFELHOLZ. 1974. Ontogenesis of adrenergic and cholinergic neuroeffector transmission in chick embryo heart. J. Pharmacol. Exp. Ther. **191:** 468-478.

32. SAKMANN, B. & H. R. BRENNER. 1978. Change in synaptic channel gating during neuromuscular development. Nature **276:** 401-402.

33. CREAZZO, T. L. & G. S. SOHAL. 1983. Neural control of embryonic acetylcholine receptor and skeletal muscle. Cell Tissue Res. **228:** 1-12.

34. OSTERRIEDER, W., G. BRUM, J. HESCHELER, W. TRAUTWEIN, F. HOFMANN & V. FLOCKERZI. 1982. Injection of subunits of cyclic AMP-dependent protein kinase in to cardiac myocytes modulates Ca^{2+} current. Nature **298:** 576-578.

35. KAMEYAMA, M., F. HOFMANN & W. TRAUTWEIN. 1985. On the mechanism of beta-adrenergic regulation of the Ca channel in the guinea pig heart. Pfluegers Arch. **405:** 285-293.

36. KAMEYAMA, M., J. HESCHELER, G. MIESKES & W. TRAUTWEIN. 1986. The protein-specific phosphatase 1 antagonizes the beta-adrenergic increase of the cardiac Ca current. Pfluegers Arch. **407:** 461-463.

37. SPERELAKIS, N. 1988. Regulation of calcium slow channels of cardiac muscle by cyclic nucleotides and phosphorylation. J. Mol. Cell. Cardiol. (Supplement II) **20:** 75-105.

38. MANTIONE, C. R., M. E. GOLDMAN, B. MARTIN, G. T. BOLGER, H. W. M. LUEDDENS, S. M. PAUL & P. SKOLNICK. 1988. Purification and characterization of an endogenous protein modulator of radioligand binding to "peripheral-type" benzodiazepine receptors and dihydropyridine Ca^{2+}-channel antagonist binding sites. Biochem. Pharmacol. **37:** 339-347.
39. JANIS, R. A., A. V. SHRIKHANDE, D. E. JOHNSON, R. T. McCARTHY, A. D. HOWARD, R. GREGUSKI & A. SCRIABINE. 1988. Isolation and characterization of a fraction from brain that inhibits 1,4[^{3}H]dihydropyridine binding and L-type calcium channel current. FEBS Lett. **239:** 233-236.
40. CALLEWAERT, G., I. HANBAUER & M. MORAD. 1989. Modulation of calcium channels in cardiac and neuronal cells by an endogenous peptide. Science **243:** 663-666.

Myofibrillar Proteins in the Developing Heart[a]

RADOVAN ZAK, BLANCA CAMORETTI-MERCADO,
MADHU GUPTA, SMILJA JAKOVCIC,
NORIKO SHIMIZU, AND ALEXANDRE STEWART

*Departments of Medicine, Pharmacological and Physiological
Sciences, and Anatomy
University of Chicago
Chicago, Illinois 60637*

INTRODUCTION

The myogenesis of cross-striated muscles consists of three stages: determination of mesodermal stem cells to a myogenic lineage; differentiation of myogenic cells that initiates the expression of muscle-specific proteins; and modulation, when the muscle phenotype undergoes sequential changes as genes coding for some protein isoforms are induced, whereas others become repressed. Thus, as in other cells, the myogenic program includes progressive restriction of the developmental potential and specialization of function. Nevertheless, even in mature, fully functioning muscles, the phenotype is not static but is able to be modified depending on a multitude of epigenetic factors, such as the functional load and the hormonal and nutritional status of the animal. Therefore, muscle development is controlled by two sets of factors: intrinsic, that is, factors that govern the time-dependent pattern of muscle development occurring in the absence of contractile activity, such as cardiac morphogenesis, which takes place prior to the development of the circulatory system; and extrinsic, that is, factors that are related to muscle contractile activity and/or metabolic requirements. The existence of an intrinsic time-dependent program is illustrated in primary cultures where the basic events leading to myogenesis can be reproduced. The role of extrinsic factors is best documented by the phenotypic changes induced by the innervation of skeletal muscles by motoneurons of the heterologous discharge rate, or in the heart by altered hemodynamic load.[1] This remarkable ability to change the pattern of gene expression is referred to as phenotypic plasticity.

Myogenesis of the heart bears a resemblance to that known for skeletal muscle, but significant differences exist. In both skeletal and cardiac muscle the first stage of development consists of proliferation of stem cells, referred to as presumptive myoblasts, that possess no apparent identifiable characteristics to distinguish them from other types of proliferating cells. Later, these cells undergo various steps that convert

[a]This work was supported by U.S. Public Health Service Grants HL16637 and HL20592, and a Grant from the Muscular Dystrophy Association of America.

them to a muscle lineage. DNA hypomethylation is one of the events suggested to play a role in muscle lineage determination.[2] Recently, however, several myogenic factors, MyoD,[3] myogenin,[4] myd,[5] and myf-5[6] have been described as being required for skeletal muscle-specific expression. Whereas MyoD and myogenin are both expressed in skeletal muscle, they seem to be absent in cardiac muscle,[4] suggesting that different gene products are involved in the determination of the cardiac muscle cell lineage.

In the next stage, which can be considered as overt myogenesis, the committed myoblasts elongate and initiate synthesis of myofibrillar proteins that culminate in the appearance of cross-striations. In skeletal muscles these cells are referred to as myotubes, whereas in the heart they are referred to as developing myocytes.[7] In the heart, the differentiation of individual cells is not synchronized, and presumptive myoblasts and developing myocytes coexist initially. Eventually, however, more and more cells initiate the synthesis of cell-specific proteins, and all cells acquire myofibrils. With the accumulation of myofibrillar mass, the developing myocytes are gradually transformed to fully functioning adult myocytes. Myofibrillar acquisition by all cardiac cells contrasts with that in skeletal muscle, in which a sizable population of myogenic precursor cells (satellite cells) remains even in the adult muscle.[8] At present, myogenic cells have not been identified in the heart, although micrographs have shown that cells that bear a resemblance to satellite cells are observed to bind tightly to myocytes in adult rat ventricles.[9] Even at advanced stages of cytodifferentiation of cardiac cells, mitosis and cellular division still occur.[10] This duality of heart-specific protein expression and DNA synthesis is opposite from the situation in skeletal muscle, where only the myoblasts are able to proliferate during myogenesis. In skeletal myogenesis, once multinucleated myotube formation and synthesis of muscle-specific proteins begin, DNA synthesis in the incorporated myoblast nucleus is repressed. These multinucleated myotubes eventually become multinucleated "structural" syncytia, known as myofibers. Cardiac tissue, on the other hand, will form a "functional" syncytium because of tight, low-resistance junctions between the mostly binucleated myocytes.

FAMILY OF MYOFIBRILLAR PROTEINS

All myofibrillar proteins are known to exist as multiple isoforms.[1] In some cases this diversity is generated by different genes[11,12] and in others by alternative RNA splicing.[13,14] Although the functions for some isoforms are known in broad outlines, the relevance of each remains to be elucidated. Moreover, the molecular mechanisms that selectively activate these genes during differentiation and those that modulate the expression of different isoforms remain undefined.

The major known isoforms of myofibrillar proteins are listed in TABLE 1. The list is not complete. For example, additional distinct myosin heavy chains (HC) were described in fetal skeletal muscles, in extraocular muscles, in superfast and superslow muscles of the jaw, in the cardiac conduction system, and in the muscle spindle. In birds, the diversity might be even larger than in mammals because genomic clones for myosin HC that have been isolated indicate the presence of as many as thirty-one genes, possibly including pseudogenes.[15]

At this time, it is difficult to make generalizations concerning the biological meaning of muscle protein diversity. In some instances, such as in myosin HC, there is a clear functional correlation with a given phenotype. Myosin HC is a large subunit of the key contractile protein, myosin, which is present in multiple molecular forms and appears to be the major determinant of myosin ATPase activity.[16] Because ATPase activity is correlated with contractile velocity,[17] the significance for different HC isoforms is generally attributed to their role in mediating different speeds of muscle shortening. In mammalian ventricles, three myosin isoforms labeled as V_1, V_2, and V_3 that were identified by electrophoresis have the following stoichiometry of their HCs: $(HC_{alpha})_2$, $(HC_{alpha}HC_{beta})$, and $(HC_{beta})_2$, respectively. In contrast to myosin HC, the light chains of the three isomyosins are identical. The ATPase activity of V_1 isomyosin is about three times that of V_3, whereas V_2 has an intermediate enzymatic activity.

Ventricular isomyosins have been detected in all mammals examined. The relative ratio of individual types of myosins, however, differs depending on the animal species.[1] In contrast to mammals, the avian heart contains only one myosin HC form in the ventricles, whereas the atria have another type.[18] The isomyosin complement of the

TABLE 1. Major Isoforms of Myofibrillar Proteins

Myosin	
Heavy chain	Fast (IIa, IIb); slow = beta (mammals); cardiac[a] (alpha, beta); embryonic; neonatal
Light chain-1[b]	Fast; slow = ventricular; atrial; embryonic
Light chain-2	Fast; slow = ventricular; atrial
Light chain-3	Fast
Actin	Alpha-skeletal; alpha-cardiac
Tropomyosin	Alpha-fast = ventricular (mammals); alpha-slow; Alpha-cardiac (birds)
Troponin	
C	Fast; slow = cardiac
I	Fast; slow; cardiac
T	Fast; slow; cardiac
Protein C	Fast; slow; cardiac

[a] In mammals, both atria and ventricle contain alpha and beta-HCs. In birds, the ventricular isoform is not identical to the slow isoform.

[b] Regarding the fast isoforms, the LC-1 and LC-3 are also referred to as alkali chain 1 and 2, respectively. The LC-2 undergoes phosphorylation and is sometimes abbreviated as LC-P. The fast isoform of LC-2 is also called regulatory or DTNB-chain.[1]

heart, although typical of a given species, is not fixed but depends upon a variety of factors such as developmental stage, hemodynamic load of the heart, and hormonal and nutritional status.[19] Of the factors so far identified, thyroid hormone seems to have the most dramatic effect. The hypothyroid state favors the expression of V_3 isomyosins, whereas thyroid hormone is required for synthesis of V_1.[18,20] By immunofluorescence, some cells have been found to react exclusively to anti-V_1 or anti-V_3 antibodies, although others reacted to both.[21] It is particularly interesting that different isomyosins have been found in cells connected directly by an intercalated disc.[22] This observation poses a provocative question about the factors that determine cardiac phenotype in those neighboring cells of the myocardium that are electrically coupled and similar in their mechanical properties and microenvironment.

In the case of other myofibrillar proteins, the functional role of different isoforms is less evident. For example, the alpha-skeletal and cardiac isoactins differ in only 4 out of 375 amino acid residues,[23] and their genes are highly homologous, not only in the coding regions but also in their intron-exon organization and in the promoter region.[24] So far no differences in the role of isoactins in activation of myosin ATPase have been reported.

One interesting phenomenon concerning the relationship among myofibrillar protein isoforms is that the cardiac isoforms are often identical to those expressed in slow muscles. In the case of myosin, this is true for mammalian (but not avian) myosin HCs as well as the two light chains present in "slow" myosin. The calcium-binding subunit of troponin also shows this identity. The two other troponin subunits, however, are distinct among all three major classes of muscles (fast, slow, and cardiac). Tropomyosin is different too, because in mammals the ventricular isoform is identical to that expressed in fast muscles.

There is a generalization about the multiplicity of myofibrillar proteins where each gene family has its own repertoire to generate different isoforms. For example, in the case of cardiac isomyosins, the three isoforms result from a combination of two different heavy chains, whereas the light chains are identical among all three isomyosins. By contrast, in fast muscles the situation is reversed. Here, the combination of two distinct light chains (LC-1 and LC-3) with identical heavy chains produces three fast isomyosins. Only two cross-striated isoforms of actin, however, are known in muscles of adult animals that are expressed exclusively in either cardiac or skeletal muscles. There are no slow or fast isoforms present. The mammalian tropomyosin is found to exist in (alpha$_{slow}$-beta) isoform in slow muscles and (alpha$_{fast}$-beta) and (alpha$_{fast}$)$_2$ in fast muscles.

Considerably more information has to be obtained before we will be able to understand the meaning of isoform diversity. For example, comparison of genomic organization will undoubtedly provide some important clues about the evolutionary relationship among the isoforms. Furthermore, functional studies such as the *in vitro* expression of cDNA[25] will allow production of large quantities of different isoforms and generation of mutants in order to determine precisely their role in contractility. In this respect, the target gene modification of embryonic stem cells with recombinant DNA constructs and subsequent analysis of transgenic animals[26] holds great promise for answering some of the above puzzling aspects of muscle protein diversity.

DEVELOPMENTAL SHIFTS IN THE EXPRESSION OF MYOFIBRILLAR PROTEINS

A very interesting aspect of muscle development is that many of the myofibrillar protein isoforms expressed in the earliest stage of myogenesis are either identical to or indistinguishable from those present in adult cardiac muscle, using the existing methodologies. For example, both presumptive avian fast and slow skeletal muscles of the myotome and limb muscle masses express ventricular-like myosin HC, together with an embryonic (fast-like) type.[27] With the onset of functional innervation the ventricular-like isoform disappears first, followed by the embryonic that is gradually replaced by neonatal and adult forms.[28,29] The ventricular-like myosin HC has been also noticed in cultured cells derived from skeletal muscle[30,31] and in regenerating muscles.[32] Both are known to recapitulate the sequential expression of myosin HC seen in normally developing muscles.

Similarly, mRNA analysis with ventricular HC-specific cDNA probe has shown that the ventricular myosin HC gene is expressed in bulk limb muscle obtained from

18-day rat fetus.[33] This early stage is often followed by sequential expression of embryonic, neonatal, and adult myosin HC.[34]

Why the myofibrillar phenotype of all cross-striated muscle primordia is cardiac-like is not understood. It is of interest, however, that at the earliest stage of development, both the myocardium, myotome, and limb bud muscle masses have epithelial characteristics, being attached to each other by means of specialized apical junctions.[35] The myocardium retains this organization throughout its entire life span. By contrast, skeletal muscle primordia lose their epithelial characteristics as they differentiate into multinucleated myotubes. The cardiac-like phenotype of muscle primordia thus could be histotypic of striated muscle in its epithelial stage.[36]

There are other examples of cardiac isoforms of muscle proteins being expressed during early myogenesis of skeletal muscles. These include the coexpression of cardiac and skeletal alpha-actins in avian[37,38] and mammalian[39] muscles and the initial expression of cardiac troponin T,[40] protein C,[41] and mammalian (but not avian) myosin light chains.[42] Eventually, all of them are eliminated and replaced by skeletal isoforms.

The embryonic development of the heart is as complex as that of skeletal muscle. In the case of myosin HC, both the embryonic ventricular and atrial myocardium initially express isoforms that are immunologically indistinguishable from the adult ventricular myosin HC. The ventricle remains reactive with this antibody throughout life, whereas in the atrium, it is replaced gradually by an atrial-specific isoform that is never expressed in the ventricle, neither in the embryo nor in the adult.[43] Using different sets of antibodies, additional isoforms have been found in the developing heart, some of them gradually becoming restricted to the conducting system.[44]

The developmental transition of myosin light chains follows a different path.[45] In the ventricle, the embryonic (skeletal) isoform of LC-1 is coexpressed with the ventricular one, and after birth the embryonic form disappears. This is in contrast to the atria where the embryonic isoform remains throughout life. As far as actins are concerned, the skeletal alpha-isoform is coexpressed with the cardiac one in the early stage of cardiac development.[46] With maturation, however, the former actin becomes repressed, and only alpha-cardiac actin is present in both chambers of the adult heart.

CONTROL OF GENE EXPRESSION IN SKELETAL AND CARDIAC MUSCLES

Regulation of gene expression may occur at multiple levels, such as transcription, processing and degradation of the mRNA, efficiency of mRNA translation, and protein degradation.[47] Generally, transcription by RNA polymerase II plays the principal role, and the degree of transcriptional activation is determined by multiple sequence-specific DNA-protein interactions that occur in distinct regulatory regions of the gene.[48] The cis-acting elements composed of promoter and enhancer sequences mediate a basal or an inducible transcription level and contain overlapping target sites for sequence-specific transacting factors.[49] Specific DNA binding protein alone or in complex with accessory proteins may bind to these nucleotide sequences. In muscle, multiple cis-acting elements have been identified in genes encoding the alpha-actin family,[50,51] in embryonic[52] and slow/cardiac myosin HCs,[53] and in creatine kinase.[54]

An example of a promoter function analysis is shown in FIGURE 1.[53] Here, deletions of the rabbit myosin HC-beta promoter region were examined using a transient transfection assay. Selected promoter sequences were fused to the chloramphenicol acetyltransferase (CAT) reporter gene, and the construct DNA was transfected into myogenic cells that were allowed to differentiate or where the differentiation was prevented by the addition of 5-bromodeoxyuridine (BudR). When the promoter is active, the reporter CAT gene is transcribed and the message translated. The assay of CAT enzymatic activity thus provides a measure of promoter function.

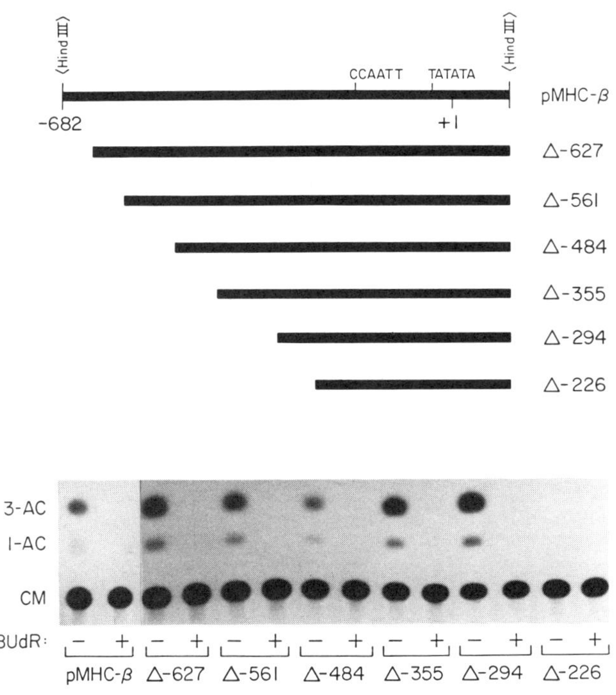

FIGURE 1. Functional assay of 5' deletions of the myosin HC-beta promoter region. Top: A plasmid containing the 781 bp of the myosin HC-beta promoter region, pMHC-beta, spans from −682 to +99 relative to cap (transcription initiation) site at +1. Basic promoter elements, CCAATT and TATATA boxes, are indicated at respective sites. The plasmid was linearized near the 5' end of the HC-beta insert, and progressive deletions were generated with Bal31 exonuclease. Deletion end points relative to +1 were confirmed by sequencing and are shown on the right. Bottom: Mutant plasmids were transfected into primary avian myoblast cultures in either the presence (+) or absence (−) of BudR. Cell extracts were incubated with [14C]chloramphenicol (CM), and the acetylated products of the enzymatic reaction (1-AC and 3-AC) were separated by chromatography. (Cribbs *et al.*[53] With permission from the *Journal of Biological Chemistry*.)

By creating progressive 5' deletions of the promoter, we showed that only the region extending 294 base pairs upstream from the transcription initiation site[53] is necessary for the muscle-specific expression. Linker-scanner mutagenesis indicated that the positive regulation in differentiated skeletal muscle is mediated by at least two distinct elements within the 5'-flanking region of the myosin HC-beta gene.

This study will serve as a basis for future isolation and characterization of transcription factors involved in muscle-specific expression of the beta-myosin HC gene.

REFERENCES

1. SWYNGHEDAUW, B. 1986. Developmental and functional adaptation of contractile proteins in cardiac and skeletal muscles. Physiol. Rev. **66:** 710-749.

2. KONIECZNY, S. F. & C. P. EMERSON JR. 1984. 5-Azacytidine induction of stable mesodermal stem cell lineages from 10T1/2 cells. Evidence for regulatory genes controlling determination. Cell **38:** 791-800.

3. DAVID, R. L., H. WIENTRAUB & A. B. LASSAR. 1987. Expression of a single transfected cDNA converts fibroblast to myoblast. Cell **51:** 987-1000.

4. WRIGHT, W. E., D. A. SASSOON & V. K. LIN. 1989. Myogenin, a factor regulating myogenesis, has a domain homologous to MyoD. Cell **56:** 607-617.

5. PINNEY, D. F., S. H. PEARSON-WHITE, S. F. KONIECZNY, K. E. LATHEM & C. P. EMERSON JR. 1988. Myogenic lineage determination and differentiation, evidence for a regulatory gene pathway. Cell **53:** 781-793.

6. BRAUN, T., G. BUSCHHAUSEN-DENKER, E. BOBER, E. TANNICH & H. H. ARNOLD. 1989. A novel human muscle factor related to but distinct from MyoD induces myogenic conversion in 10T1/2 fibroblast. EMBO J. **8:** 701-709.

7. MANASEK, F. J. 1970. Histogenesis of the embryonic myocardium. Am. J. Cardiol. **25:** 149-168.

8. ZAK, R. 1974. Developmental and proliferation capacity of cardiac muscle cells. Circ. Res. (Suppl. II). **34-35:** 17-26.

9. CUTILLETA, A. F., M.-C. AUMONT, A. C. NAG & R. ZAK. 1977. Separation of muscle and non-muscle cells from adult rat myocardium: An application to the study of RNA polymerase. J. Mol. Cell. Cardiol. **9:** 399-407.

10. MANASEK, F. J. 1968. Mitosis in developing cardiac muscle. J. Cell Biol. **37:** 191-196.

11. HUMPHRIES, S. E., R. WHITTALL, A. MINTY, M. BUCKINGHAM & R. WILLIAMSON. 1981. There are approximately 20 actin genes in the human genome. Nucleic Acids Res. **9:** 4895-4908.

12. NGUYEN, H. T., R. M. GUBITS, R. M. WYDRO & B. NADAL-GINARD. 1982. Sarcomeric myosin heavy chain is coded by a highly conserved multigene family. Proc. Natl. Acad. Sci. USA **79:** 5230-5234.

13. BREITBARD, R. E., H. T. NGUYEN, R. M. MEDOFRD, A. T. DESTREE, V. MAHDAVI & B. NADAL-GINARD. 1985. Intricate combinatorial patterns of exon splicing generate multiple regulated troponin-T isoforms from a single gene. Cell **41:** 67-82.

14. NABESHIMA, Y., Y. FUJII-KURIYAMA, M. MURAMATSU & K. OGATA. 1984. Alternative transcription of two models of splicing results in two myosin light chains from one gene. Nature **308:** 333-338.

15. ROBBINS, J., T. HORAN, J. GULICK & K. KROPP. 1986. The chicken myosin heavy chain family. J. Biol. Chem. **261:** 6606-6612.

16. SIVARAMAKRISHNAN, M. & M. BURKE. 1982. The free heavy chain of vertebrate skeletal myosin subfragment 1 shows full enzymatic activity. J. Biol. Chem. **257:** 1102-1105.

17. BARANY, K. M. 1967. ATPase activity of myosin correlated with speed of muscle shortening. J. Gen. Physiol. **50:** 197-218.

18. HOH, J. F. Y., P. A. MCGRATH & P. T. HALE. 1978. Electrophoretic analysis of multiple forms of rat myosin: effect of hypophysectomy and thyroid replacement. J. Mol. Cell. Cardiol. **10:** 1053-1075.

19. ZAK, R. 1981. Contractile function as a determinant of muscle growth. Cell Muscle Motil. **1:** 1-33.

20. EVERETT, A. W., W. A. CLARK, R. A. CHIZZONITE & R. ZAK. 1983. Change in synthesis of rate of alpha- and beta-myosin heavy chains in rabbit heart after treatment with thyroid hormone. J. Biol. Chem. **258:** 2421-2425.

21. SAMUEL, J. L., I. RAPPAPORT, J. J. MERCADIER, A. M. LOMPRE, S. SARTORE, C. TRIBANI, S. SCHIAFFINO & K. SCHWARTZ. 1983. Distribution of myosin isozymes within single cardiac cells: An immunohistochemical study. Circ. Res. **52:** 200-209.

22. SARTORE, S., L. GORZA, S. P. BORMIOLI, S. D. LIBERA & S. SCHIAFFINO. 1981. Myosin types and fiber types in cardiac muscle. J. Cell Biol. **88:** 226-233.

23. VANDEKERCKHOVE, J. & K. WEBER. 1979. The complete amino acid sequence of actins from bovine aorta, bovine heart, bovine fast skeletal muscle, and rabbit slow skeletal muscle. Differentiation **14:** 123-133.

24. CHANG, K. S., K. N. ROTHBLUM & R. J. SCHWARTZ. 1985. The complete sequence of the chicken alpha-cardiac actin gene: A highly conserved vertebrate gene. Nucleic Acids Res. **13:** 1223-1237.

25. KNECHT, D. A. & W. F. LOOMIS. 1987. Antisense RNA inactivation of myosin heavy chain gene expression in *Dictyostelium discoideum*. Science **236:** 1081-1086.

26. THOMAS, K. R. & M. R. CAPECCHI. 1987. Site-directed mytagenesis by gene targeting in mouse embryo-derived stem cells. Cell **51:** 503-512.

27. SWEENEY, L. J., J. M. KENNEDY, R. ZAK, K. KOKJOHN & S. W. KELLEY. 1989. Evidence for expression of a common myosin heavy chain phenotype in future fast and slow skeletal muscles during initial stages of avian embryogenesis. Dev. Biol. **133:** 361-374.

28. GAUTHIER, G. F., S. LOWEY, P. A. BENFIELD & A. W. HOBBS. 1982. Distribution and properties of myosin isozymes in developing avian and mammalian skeletal muscle fibers. J. Cell Biol. **92:** 471-484.

29. UMEDA, P. K., C. J. KAVINSKY, A. M. SINHA, H-J. HSU, S. JAKOVCIC & M. RABINOWITZ. 1983. Cloned mRNA sequences for two types of embryonic myosin heavy chains from chick skeletal muscle. II. Expression during development using S1 nuclease mapping. J. Biol. Chem. **258:** 5206-5214.

30. CANTINI, M., S. SARTORE & S. SCHIAFFINO. 1980. Myosin types in cultured muscle cells. J. Cell. Biol. **85:** 903-909.

31. GORZA, L., S. SARTORE, C. TRIBAN & S. SCHIAFFINO. 1983. Embryonic-like myosin heavy chain in regenerating chicken muscle. Exp. Cell Res. **143:** 395-403.

32. STEWART, A. F. R., J. M. KENNEDY, E. BANDMAN & R. ZAK. 1989. A myosin isoform repressed in hypertrophied ALD muscle of the chicken reappears during regeneration following cold injury. Dev. Biol. **135:** 367-375.

33. NARUSAWA, M., R. B. FITZSIMONS, S. IZUMO, B. NADAL-GINARD, N. A. RUBINSTEIN & A. M. KELLY. 1987. Slow myosin in developing rat skeletal muscle. J. Cell Biol. **104:** 447-459.

34. WHALEN, R. G., S. M. SELL, G. S. BUTLER-BROWNE, K. SCHWARTZ, P. BOUVERET & I. PINSET-HARSTROM. 1981. Three myosin heavy-chain isozymes appear sequentially in rat muscle development. Nature **292:** 805-809.

35. MANASEK, F. J. 1968. Embryonic development of the heart. I. A light and electron microscopic study of myocardial development in the early chick embryo. J. Morphol. **125:** No. 3, July.

36. SWEENEY, L. J., W. A. CLARK JR., P. K. UMEDA, R. ZAK & F. J. MANASEK. 1984. Immunofluorescence analysis of the primordial myosin detectable in embryonic striated muscle. Proc. Natl. Acad. Sci. USA **81:** 797-800.

37. PATERSON, B. M. & J. D. ELDRIDGE. 1984. Alpha-cardiac actin is the major sarcomeric isoform expressed in avian skeletal muscle. Science **224:** 1436-1438.

38. HAYWARD, L. & R. J. SCHWARTZ. 1986. Sequential expression of chicken actin genes during myogenesis. J. Cell Biol. **102:** 1485-1493.

39. MINTY, A. J., S. ALONSO, M. CARAVATTI & M. E. BUCKINGHAM. 1982. A fetal muscle actin mRNA in the mouse and its identity with cardiac actin mRNA. Cell **30:** 185-192.

40. TOYOTA, N. & Y. SHIMADA. 1981. Differentiation of troponin in cardiac and skeletal muscles in chicken embryos as studied by immunofluorescence microscopy. J. Cell Biol. **91:** 497-504.

41. BAHLER, M. H., H. MODER, M. EPPENBERGER & T. WALLIMAN. 1985. Heart C-protein is transiently expressed during skeletal muscle development in the embryo, but persists in cultured myogenic cells. Dev. Biol. **112:** 345-352.

42. WHALEN, R. G., S. M. SELL, A. ERICKSON & L. E. THORNELL. 1982. Myosin subunit

types in skeletal and cardiac tissues and their developmental distribution. Dev. Biol. **91:** 478-484.

43. SWEENEY, L. J., R. ZAK & F. J. MANASEK. 1987. Transitions in cardiac isomyosin expression during differentiation of the embryonic chick heart. Circ. Res. **61:** 287-295.

44. EVANS, D., J. B. MILLER & F. E. STOCKDALE. 1988. Developmental patterns of expression and coexpression of myosin heavy chains in artia and ventricles of the avian heart. Dev. Biol. **127:** 376-383.

45. BARTON, P. J. & M. E. BUCKINGHAM. 1985. The myosin alkali light chain proteins and their genes. Biochem. J. **231:** 249-262.

46. SHIMIZU, N., S. KAMEL-REID & R. ZAK. 1988. Expression of actin mRNAs in denervated chicken skeletal muscle. Dev. Biol. **128:** 435-440.

47. DARNELL, J. E. 1982. Variety in the level of gene control in eukaryotic cells. Nature **297:** 365-370.

48. DYNAN, W. S. & R. TJIAN. 1985. Control of eukaryotic messenger RNA synthesis by sequence-specific DNA-binding proteins. Nature **316:** 774-778.

49. MANIATIS, T., S. GOODBURN & J. A. FISHER. 1987. Regulation of inducible and tissue-specific gene expression. Science **236:** 1237-1245.

50. BERGSMA, D. J., J. M. GRICHNIK, L. M. A. GORSSETT & R. J. SCHWARTZ. 1986. Delimitation and characterization of cis-acting DNA sequences required for the regulated expression and transcriptional control of the chicken skeletal alpha-actin gene. Mol. Cell. Biol. **6:** 2462-2475.

51. MINTY, A. & L. KEDES. 1986. Upstream regions of the human cardiac actin gene that modulate its transcription in muscle cells: Presence of an evolutionarily-conserved repeated motif. Mol. Cell. Biol. **6:** 2125-2136.

52. BOUVAGNET, P. F., E. E. STREHLER, G. E. WHITE, M. A. STRECHLER-PAGE, B. NADAL-GINARD & V. MAHDAVI. 1987. Multiple positive and negative 5' regulatory elements control the cell-type specific expression of the embryonic skeletal myosin heavy chain gene. Mol. Cell. Biol. **7:** 4377-4389.

53. CRIBBS, L. L., N. SHIMIZU, C. E. YOCKEY, J. E. LEVIN, S. JAKOVCIC, R. ZAK & P. K. UMEDA. 1989. Muscle-specific regulation of a transfected rabbit myosin heavy chain beta-gene promoter. J. Biol. Chem. **264:** 10672-10678.

54. JAYNES, J. B., J. E. JOHNSON, J. N. BUSKIN, C. L. GARTSIDE & S. D. HAUSCHKA. 1988. The muscle creatine kinase gene is regulated by multiple upstream elements, including a muscle-specific enhancer. Mol. Cell. Biol. **8:** 62-70.

Precocious Expression of NAPA-73, an Intermediate Filament-Associated Protein, during Nervous System and Heart Development in the Chicken Embryo

GARY CIMENT

Department of Cell Biology and Anatomy
Vollum Institute
Oregon Health Sciences University
Portland, Oregon 97201

MONOCLONAL ANTIBODIES AGAINST THE NAPA-73 ANTIGEN

In order to generate probes recognizing markers expressed during early peripheral nervous system development, monoclonal antibodies were generated against various early neural crest derivatives. In one set of studies, freshly dissected 7 day embryonic chicken dorsal root ganglia were injected into mice, and then splenocytes from these mice were used to generate hybridoma cell lines.[1,2] The resultant hybridomas were screened using indirect immunocytochemistry for their production of antibodies recognizing neurons, but not non-neuronal cells. One of the antibodies generated in this fashion was found to recognize an antigen within the axons and, to a somewhat lesser degree, cell bodies of neurons (FIGURES 1A and 1B). Interestingly, this antibody also recognized a subpopulation of neuronal precursor cells in neural crest cell cultures (FIGURES 1C and 1D). This antibody was initially designated by the arbitrary moniker E/C8, but was later termed NAPA-73, which is an acronym for neurofilament-associated protein, avian-specific, 73,000 daltons (see below).

PRECOCIOUS EXPRESSION OF NAPA-73 IMMUNOREACTIVITY DURING NERVOUS SYSTEM AND HEART DEVELOPMENT

To examine the appearance of NAPA-73 during early embryogenesis, we performed immunocytochemical localization studies using cryostat tissue sections through chicken embryos of various ages. We found that NAPA-73 immunoreactivity first appeared during the second and third days of development in the central nervous system, in migrating neural crest cell subpopulations, as well as in the heart.

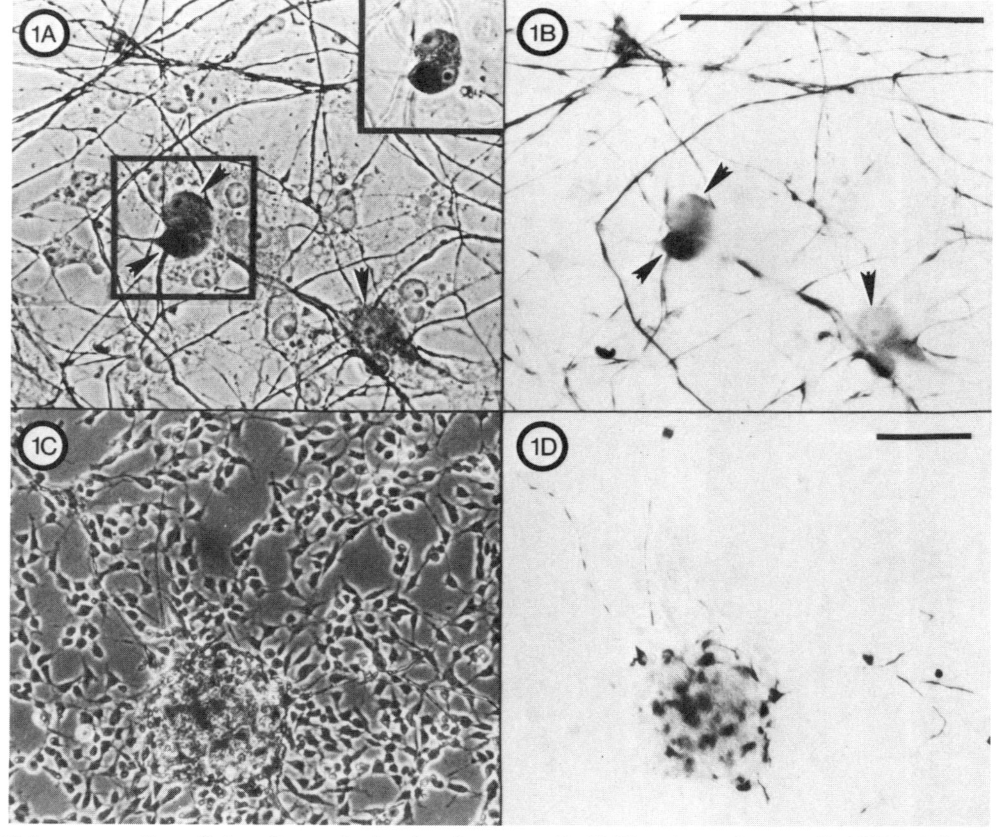

FIGURE 1. NAPA-73 immunoreactive cells in cultures of avian dorsal root ganglia (A,B) and neural crest cells (C,D). Cells were cultured for 68-72 hours, fixed with paraformaldehyde, and then treated with a horseradish peroxidase conjugate of the NAPA-73 antibody, as described.[2] Peroxidase activity was visualized using the Hanker-Yates reagent,[23] and then the cultures were photographed using either phase-contrast optics (A,C) or bright field illumination (B,D). Note in panel B the immunostaining of the axons and cell bodies of neuronal cells, but not non-neuronal cells. Note in panel D the immunostaining of a subpopulation of neural crest cells. Bars = 100 μm. (G. Ciment & J. A. Weston.[2] With permission from Academic Press.)

In the central nervous system, NAPA-73[+] cells were observed as early as the 16 somite stage in cranial regions of the neural tube. FIGURE 2B shows immunoreactive cells in the marginal zone[3] of both dorsal and ventral regions of the rhombencephalon. In addition, local concentrations of NAPA-73[+] cells could also be found along the ventral surface of the midbrain (not shown), corresponding to sites at which neurons of the oculomotor and trigeminal motor nuclei later begin to differentiate.[4,5] The possibility that NAPA-73 immunoreactivity is expressed prior to terminal mitosis in these cells is supported by observations that all of the cells within the neural tube are mitotic at these developmental stages.[6,7] In contrast to early embryos, however, NAPA-73 seems to be expressed exclusively by postmitotic neuroblasts in older chicken embryos.[8]

NAPA-73 immunoreactivity is also expressed by a subpopulation of migrating neural crest cells *in vivo*.[9] FIGURE 2B shows that at the 16 somite stage, antigen-positive cells can be seen at the level of the anterior rhombencephalon, but are only rarely seen at more rostral or caudal levels (FIGURES 2C and 2D), even at slightly earlier or later developmental stages (not shown). The NAPA-73[+] neural crest cells migrate lateral to the pharynx and eventually populate the various branchial arches (FIG. 3) (see also ref. 10). From their location in the posterior branchial arches, some NAPA-73[+] neural crest-derived cells may migrate into the adjacent gut to give rise to the enteric nervous system.[11–13] Other branchial arch cells lose expression of NAPA-73 immunoreactivity and have been hypothesized to give rise to various connective tissue elements of the face and neck. Interestingly, the period when these cells lose NAPA-73 immunoreactivity is the same period in which these cells lose their developmental ability to give rise to neurons.[9] These observations would also suggest, therefore, that expression of NAPA-73 by these neural crest-derived cells may be a marker of their neurogenic potential.

In the heart, NAPA-73 immunoreactivity can be seen as early as the 10 somite stage,[2] when the heart primordium first starts beating. By the 16 somite stage (FIG. 4), NAPA-73[+] cells can be found within the epimyocardial layer of the truncus arteriosus, bulbus cordis and ventricles, but not by epimyocardial cells of the atrium or sinus venosus. Although neural crest-derived cells have been observed in some of these same general regions of the heart,[14] it is unlikely that all of the NAPA-73[+] cells seen in FIGURE 4 are neural crest-derived. For one thing, neural crest cells localize to a relatively small region within the truncus arteriosus, whereas the NAPA-73[+] cells are found within large areas of the epimyocardium (see FIG 4B). In contrast to the high proportion of immunoreactive cells at early developmental stages, only a subpopulation of cells within the myocardium of the hatchling express NAPA-73 immunoreactivity (FIG. 5). This subpopulation of cells may correspond to a diffuse conduction system within the avian myocardium. In any case, it seems likely that the NAPA-73[+] cells in the heart have very different developmental properties as compared to the NAPA-73[+] neuronal precursor cells in the central nervous system.

NAPA-73 IS AN INTERMEDIATE FILAMENT-ASSOCIATED PROTEIN THAT BINDS TO VARIOUS FILAMENT TYPES AT DIFFERENT STAGES OF DEVELOPMENT

Ultrastructural studies show that the NAPA-73 antigen is associated with bundles of intermediate (10 nanometer) filaments in cultured neurons.[15] In these experiments,

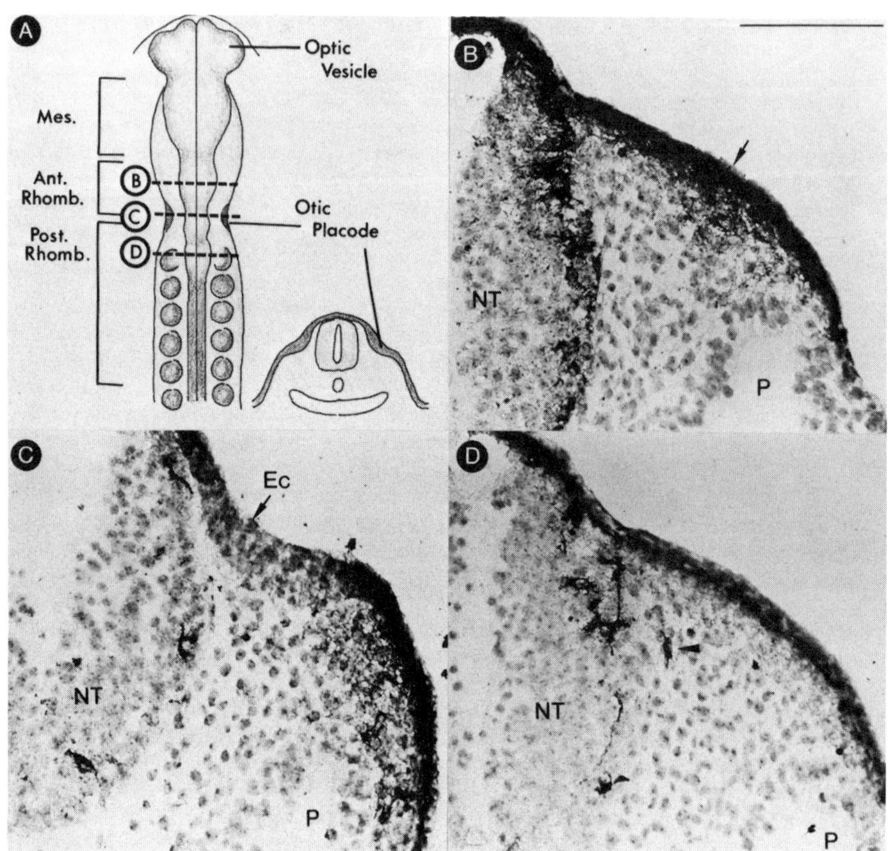

FIGURE 2. NAPA-73 immunoreactivity in tissue sections through the rhombencephalon of a 16 somite chicken embryo. Cryostat sections were made through an unfixed embryo, dried onto microscope slides overnight, and then incubated with the horseradish conjugate of NAPA-73. Peroxidase activity was visualized as described in the legend for FIG. 1. **A:** An illustration of a 16 somite embryo, showing axial levels corresponding to B–D. **B:** A section through the anterior rhombencephalon, approximately 42 μm rostral to the otic placode. **C:** A section through the center of the otic placode. **D:** A section through the posterior rhombencephalon, approximately 50 μm caudal to the otic placode. Note the many NAPA-73 immunoreactive neural crest cells under the unstained ectoderm (arrow) in **B,** and the single NAPA-73 immunoreactive neural crest cell in **D** (arrowhead). Ant. Rhomb., anterior rhombencephalon; Ec, ectoderm; Mes, mesencephalon; NT, neural tube; P, pharynx; Post. Rhomb., posterior rhombencephalon; Bar = 100 μm. (G. Ciment & J. A. Jackson.[9] With permission from Academic Press.)

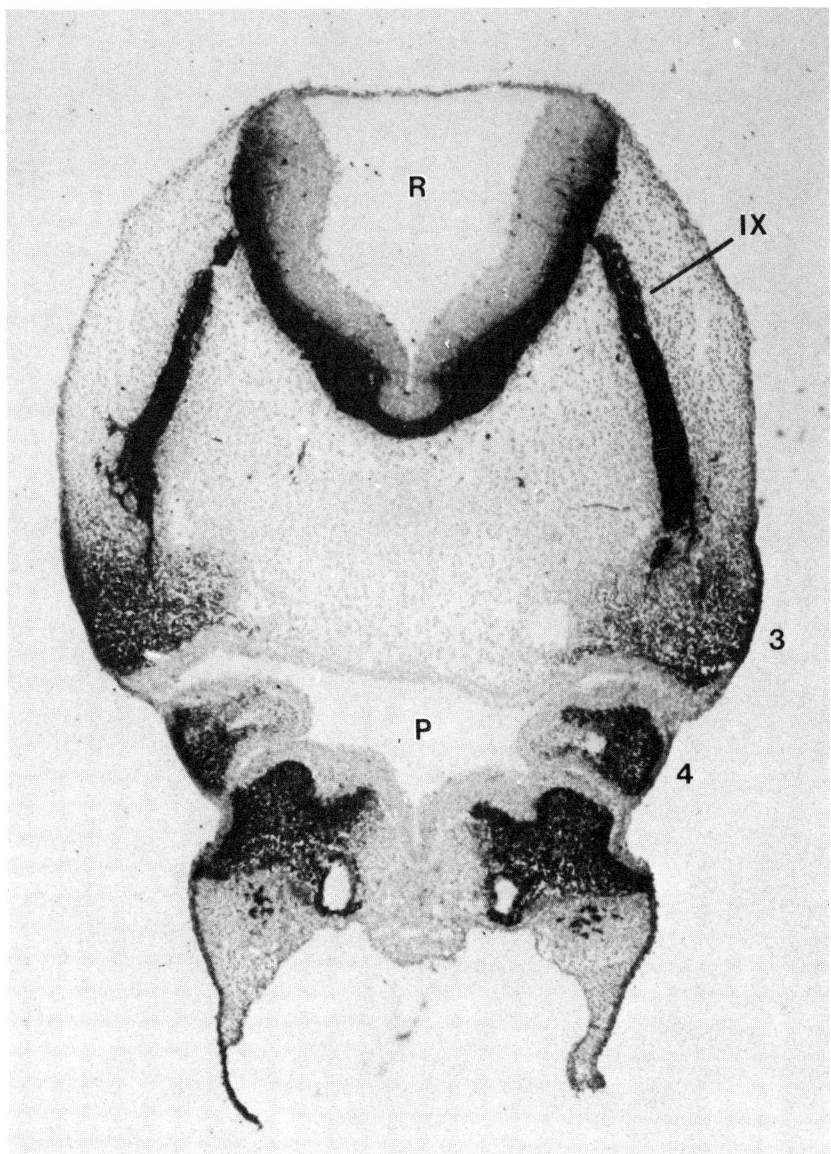

FIGURE 3. NAPA-73 immunoreactivity in a cryostat tissue section through the posterior branchial arches of a 4 day chicken embryo, as described in the legend for FIG. 2. Note the NAPA-73 immunoreactive neural crest-derived cells of the marginal zone of the rhombencephalon (R), the ninth cranial nerve (IX), the third branchial arch (3), and the fourth branchial arch (4). P, pharynx.

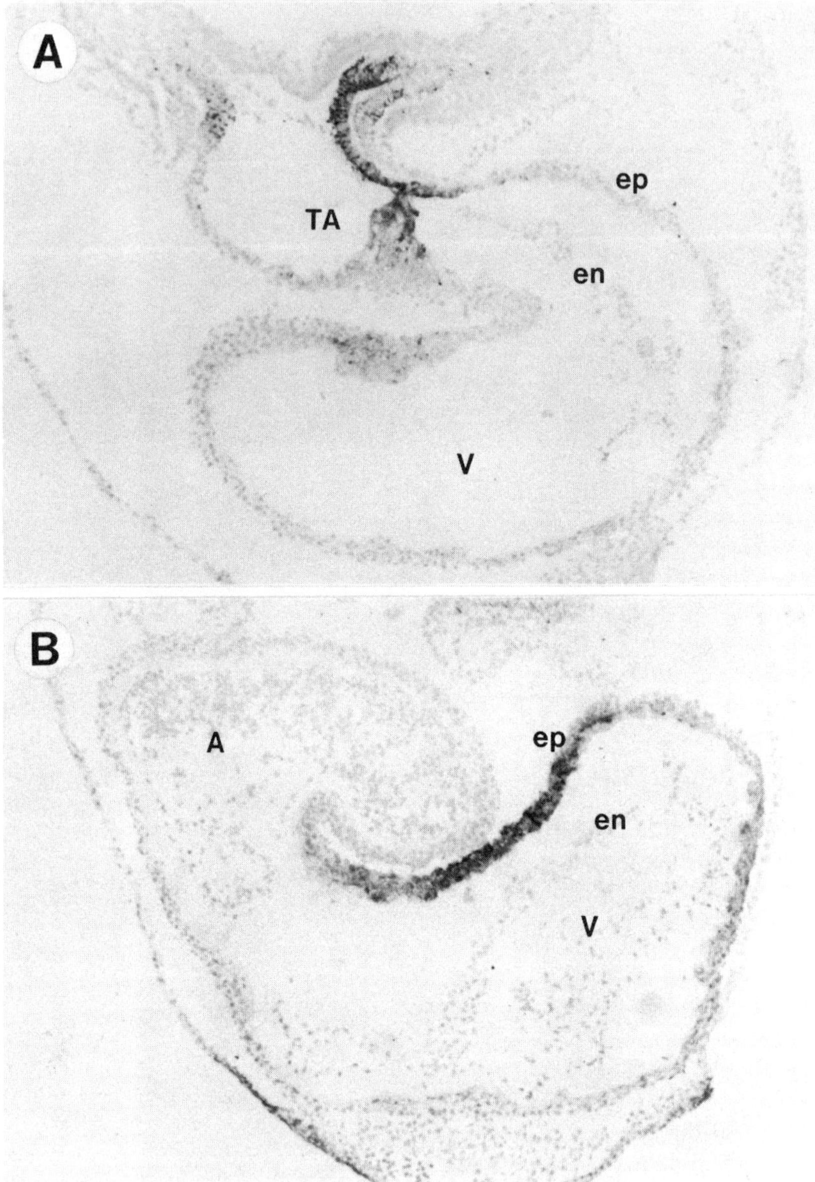

FIGURE 4. NAPA-73 immunoreactivity in cryostat tissue sections through the heart of a 16 somite chicken embryo, as described in the legend for FIG. 2. Note the immunostaining of the epimyocardial cell layer (ep) of the truncus arteriosus (TA) and ventricle (V), but lack of immunostaining in the atrium (A) or in the endocardial cell layer (en).

dorsal root ganglia were dissociated and cultured, fixed, treated with NAPA-73 antibody, processed for indirect colloidal gold immunocytochemistry, and then examined under the electron microscope. FIGURES 6A and 6B show that NAPA-73 immunoreactivity was associated with bundles of neurofilaments in these cells but did not seem to decorate individual neurofilament profiles. By contrast, control experiments using an antibody against NF-M, the middle subunit of neurofilament, associated with both individual intermediate filament profiles (FIG 6C) as well as bundles (not shown). These and other data suggest that NAPA-73 is not a core protein of the neurofilament complex, but may be involved with the bundling of these cytoskeletal elements.

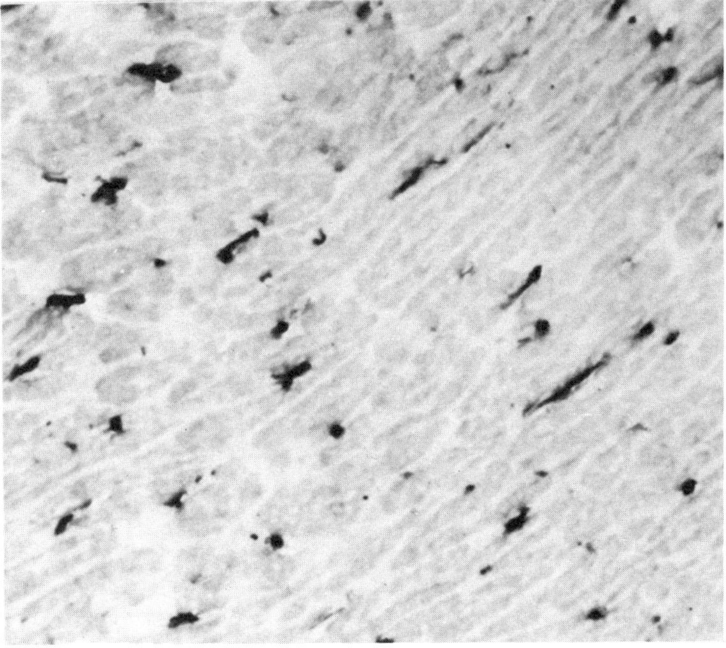

FIGURE 5. NAPA-73 immunoreactivity in a cryostat tissue section through the myocardium of a hatchling chicken embryo, as described in the legend for FIG. 2. Note the immunostaining of a subpopulation of cells.

Biochemical studies are consistent with the notion that NAPA-73 is an intermediate filament-associated protein. Early studies of the stability of NAPA-73 immunoreactivity showed, for example, that treatment with various proteases destroyed this antigen in fixed neuronal cell cultures,[2] suggesting that the epitope recognized by the NAPA-73 antibody was either a protein or was associated with a protein. More recent studies[15] using immunoprecipitation and immunoabsorption show that the NAPA-73 antibody binds to a protein that has a mobility corresponding to about 73,000 daltons on sodium dodecyl sulfate (SDS)-polyacrylamide gels (FIG. 7, lanes 1 and 4). Interestingly, such immunopurified preparations of NAPA-73 were always found to be "contaminated" with two other protein bands.[15] FIGURE 7 shows that when NAPA-73 was immu-

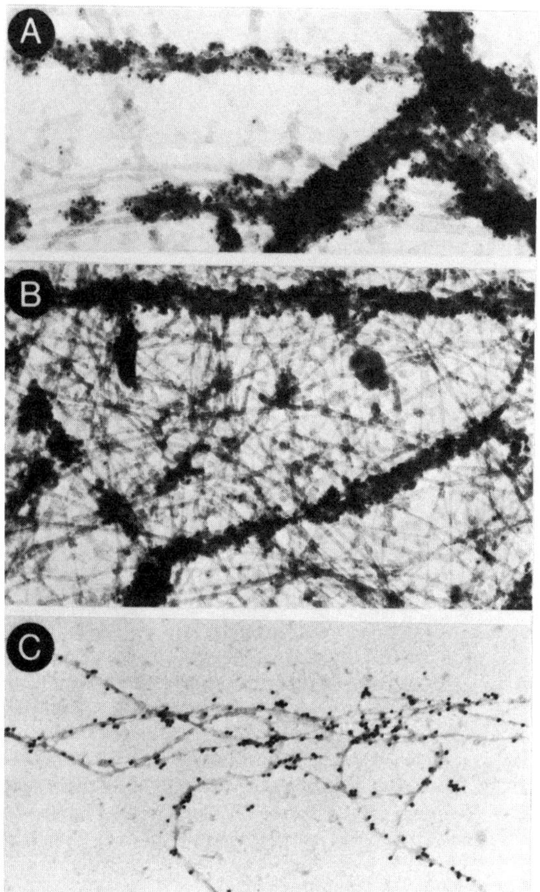

FIGURE 6. Immunoelectron microscopic localization of NAPA-73 immunoreactive material in cultures of chicken dorsal root ganglion neurons. Cultures were fixed and incubated with NAPA-73 antibody; then this mouse antibody was detected using indirect immunocolloidal gold localization methods. **A:** NAPA-73-mediated decoration of a neuron, showing the presence of immunoreactivity in bundles, but not individual neurofilament profiles. **B:** NAPA-73-mediated decoration of a neuron atop a non-neuronal cell. Note the absence of colloidal gold labeling of the individual filament strands (presumably glial filaments). **C:** Anti-NF-M-mediated decoration of a neuron, showing labeling of individual neurofilament profiles.

nopurified from 4 day chicken heads (in which brain is the only immunoreactive tissue), a second protein band at about 54,000 daltons was also present (lane 1). Immunoblotting studies revealed that this second band was vimentin (compare lane 2 with lane 3), another intermediate filament protein. When NAPA-73 was purified from 20 day chicken brains, however, vimentin was not present; another "contaminating" band of about 160,000 daltons appeared, however, and this band was identified as NF-M (compare lane 6 with lane 5). These studies would suggest that NAPA-73 is an intermediate filament-associated protein with a relatively promiscuous specificity.

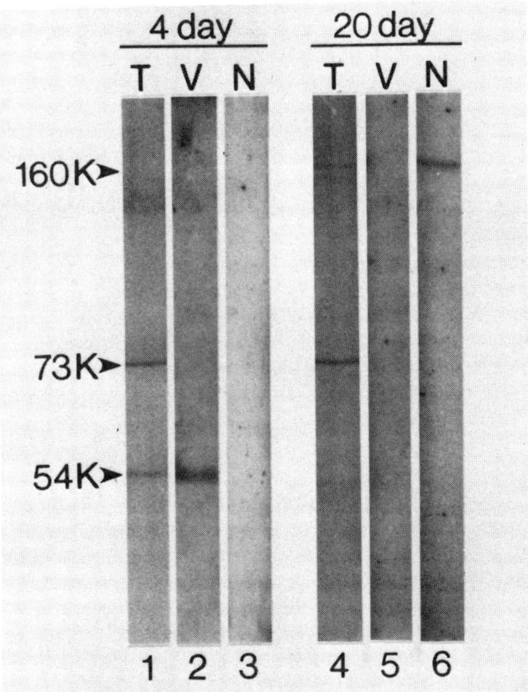

FIGURE 7. NAPA-73 is associated with vimentin in homogenates of 4 day embryonic chicken heads and with NF-M in homogenates of 20 day embryonic chicken brains. Lanes T are silver-stained protein bands in sodium dodecylsulfate-polyacrylamide gels. Lanes V are radioautographs of immunoblots of corresponding lanes incubated with antichicken vimentin antiserum, followed by secondary labeling with [125I]protein A. Lanes N are radioautographs of immunoblots of corresponding lanes incubated with antichicken NF-M antiserum, followed by secondary labeling with [125I]protein A. Immunopurification of NAPA-73 was performed as described.[15] Note vimentin immunoreactivity in material immunopurified from 4 day embryonic tissue and NF-M immunoreactivity in material immunopurified from 20 day brain tissue. (Ciment et al.[15] With permission from the Journal of Cell Biology.)

This ability to associate with different intermediate filament types may indicate a possible function for NAPA-73. It has been suggested that the intermediate filaments themselves function as the internal scaffolding of cells, which contributes to cell shape and may permit or hinder cellular movements.[16,17] Presumably, the expression of different intermediate filament proteins by different cell types would confer different structural properties to these cells. Perhaps the various identified intermediate filament-associated proteins,[18–22] including NAPA-73, function to modulate these structural properties by influencing the extent of intermediate filament bundling, the extent of association with other cellular elements, and other structural properties of this scaffolding. This would suggest that the regulation of expression of various intermediate filament-associated proteins contributes directly to the diversity of cellular shapes and other cellular properties observed during development.

SUMMARY

A monoclonal antibody was generated, against early neural crest-derived cells, which recognizes an epitope present on a novel intermediate filament-associated protein. This protein has been named NAPA-73 and is expressed by progenitor cells of the nervous system and heart. Biochemical and ultrastructural studies indicate that this protein associates with bundles of intermediate filaments and therefore may play a role in the determination of cell shape.

REFERENCES

1. CIMENT, G. & J. A. WESTON. 1981. Immunochemical studies of avian peripheral neurogenesis. *In* Monoclonal Antibodies to Neural Antigens. R. McKay, M. C. Raff & L. F. Reichardt, Eds.: 73-89. Cold Spring Harbor Press. Cold Spring Harbor, New York.
2. CIMENT, G. & J. A. WESTON. 1982. Early appearance in neural crest and crest-derived cells of an antigenic determinant present in avian neurons. Dev. Biol. **93:** 355-367.
3. Boulder Committee. 1970. Embryonic vertebrate central nervous system: Revised terminology. Anat. Rec. 166: 257-262.
4. HEATON, M. B. & S. A. MOODY. 1980. Early development and migration of the trigeminal motor nucleus in the chick embryo. J. Comp. Neurol. **189:** 61-99.
5. HEATON, M. B. 1981. The development of the oculomotor nuclear complex in the Japanese quail embryo. J. Comp. Neurol. **198:** 633-648.
6. FUJITA, S. 1963. The matrix cell and cytogenesis in the developing central nervous system. J. Comp. Neurol. **120:** 37-42.
7. FUJITA, S. 1964. Analysis of neuron differentiation in the central nervous system by tritiated thymidine autoradiography. J. Comp. Neurol. **122:** 311-328.
8. WU, D. K. & J. DE VELLIS. 1987. The expression of the intermediate filament-associated protein (NAPA-73) is associated with the stage of terminal differentiation of chick brain neurons. Brain Res. **421:** 186-193.
9. CIMENT, G. & J. A. WESTON. 1985. Segregation of developmental abilities in neural-crest-derived cells: Identification of partially restricted intermediate cell types in the branchial arches of avian embryos. Dev. Biol. **111:** 73-83.
10. NODEN, D. W. 1975. An analysis of the migratory behavior of avian cephalic neural crest cells. Dev. Biol. **42:** 106-130.
11. LE DOUARIN, N. M. & M.-A. TEILLET. 1973. The migration of neural crest cells to the wall of the digestive tract in avian embryos. J. Embryol. Exp. Morphol. **30:** 31-48.
12. CIMENT, G. & J. A. WESTON. 1983. Enteric neurogenesis by neural crest-derived branchial arch mesenchymal cells. Nature **305:** 424-427.
13. TUCKER, G. C., G. CIMENT & J. P. THIERY. 1986. Pathways of avian neural crest cell migration in the developing gut. Dev. Biol. **116:** 439-450.

14. KIRBY, M. L., T. F. GALE & D. E. STEWART. 1983. Neural crest cells contribute to normal aorticopulmonary septation. Science **220:** 1059-1061.
15. CIMENT, G., A. RESSLER, P. C. LETOURNEAU & J. A. WESTON. 1986. A novel intermediate filament-associated protein, NAPA-73, that binds to different filament types at different stages of nervous system development. J. Cell Biol. **102:** 246-251.
16. LAZARIDES, E. 1980. Intermediate filaments as mechanical integrators of cellular space. Nature **283:** 249-256.
17. FUCHS, E. & I. HANUKOGLU. 1983. Unraveling the structure of the intermediate filaments. Cell **34:** 332-334.
18. STEINERT, P. M., J. S. CANTIERI, D. C. TELLER, J. D. LONGSDALE-ECCLES & B. A. DALE. 1981. Characterization of a class of cationic proteins that specifically interact with intermediate filaments. Proc. Natl. Acad. Sci. USA **78:** 4097-4101.
19. LAWSON, D. 1983. Epinemin: A new protein associated with vimentin filaments in non-neural cells. J. Cell Biol. **97:** 1891-1905.
20. WANG, E., J. G. CAIRNCROSS, W. K. A. YUNG, E. A. GARBER & R. K. H. LIEM. 1983. An intermediate filament-associated protein, p50, recognized by monoclonal antibodies. J. Cell Biol. **97:** 1507-1514.
21. NAPOLITANO, E. W., J. S. PACHTER, S. S. M. CHIN & R. K. H. LIEM. 1985. Beta-internexin, a ubiquitous intermediate filament-associated protein. J. Cell Biol. **101:** 1323-1331.
22. PACHTER, J. S. & R. K. H. LIEM. 1985. Alpha-internexin, a 66-kD intermediate filament-binding protein from mammalian central nervous tissues. J. Cell Biol. **101:** 1316-1322.
23. HANKER, J. S., P. E. YATES, C. B. METZ & A. RUSTIONI. 1977. A new, specific, sensitive and noncarcinogenic reagent for the demonstration of horseradish peroxidase. Histochem. J. **9:** 789-792.

Origins and Assembly of Avian Embryonic Blood Vessels[a]

DREW M. NODEN

Department of Anatomy
New York State College of Veterinary Medicine
Cornell University
Ithaca, New York 14853

INTRODUCTION

In contrast to most participants in this volume, my interests are in the development of endothelial and perivascular tissues outside of the heart. These endothelial populations arise temporally concomitant with the onset of cardiogenesis, but they present a very different morphological appearance. I believe that our understanding of both cardiogenesis and peripheral vasculogenesis will be enhanced by comparing how these two components of a functionally integrated system develop.

The development of embryonic vessels begins in advance of and independent of the morphogenesis of most internal organs. This process occurs both integrated with and independent of a functional circulation, depending upon the precise region and stage being considered. Embryonic vessels lack morphological features characteristic of arteries or veins, and indeed often switch their roles frequently during the early stages of vascular remodeling. The remodeling of local vascular plexuses is intimately coordinated with the individual patterns of organ development.

There is an extensive descriptive literature on embryonic blood vessel development in avian[1-4] and mammalian embryos.[1,5-9] Surprisingly, many of the elegant and entirely correct observations contained in these studies have been overlooked by contemporary investigators and reviewers. For example, a frequently repeated mistake is to describe the embryonic pulmonary arteries as branches of the sixth aortic arches.[10-13] Several studies, however, have shown that the pulmonary arteries arise as two independent components: branches off the fourth aortic arches and a plexus of endothelial vesicles that develop within pulmonary mesenchyme. Later, these components fuse together and are contacted by outgrowths (sixth aortic arch roots) from the dorsal aortae; one of these branches will become the ductus arteriosus.[14-18] (See, however, reference 19.) By contrast—and very enigmatic given the dependence of all other embryonic tissues upon an intact, functional vascular network—there have been few experimental analyses of how endothelial and perivascular tissues develop.

My research is directed towards two problems associated with the early aspects of blood vessel formation: When and where do endothelial and perivascular smooth muscle and connective tissues arise? and How do these precursor populations assemble

[a]This research was supported by NIH (NIDR) Grant DEO6632.

into vascular channels located in precise locations? This second question has two components; one is the local assembly of angiogenic cells into endothelial tissue, and the other is the assembly of endothelial tissue into definitive, patent blood vessels.

This review presents the results of recent analyses on the development of craniofacial blood vessels in the avian embryo. The choice of regions is based on many years of familiarity with the development of other craniofacial tissues (*e.g.,* neural crest, myogenic precursors, paraxial and lateral mesoderm, epibranchial placodes; reviewed in references 20 and 21). As will be discussed, however, these results are applicable to most parts of the embryo. The choice of organisms, quail and chick embryos, reflects first the accessibility of these embryos to experimental manipulation and also the availability of antibodies that recognize quail endothelial cells, as will be discussed in detail later.

WHEN AND WHERE DO ENDOTHELIAL CELLS ARISE?

Blood vessel development is morphologically first evident outside the embryo on the yolk sac, where focal aggregations of mesenchymal cells form *blood islands* adjacent to extraembryonic endoderm within splanchnic mesoderm. This process begins concomitant with the onset of neural plate and somite formation. The number of these blood islands increases rapidly throughout the area vasculosa. Within each blood island the cells located marginally transform into endothelial cells and form a vesicle. The isolated central cells soon exhibit cytochemical features characteristic of embryonic hemoblasts. It is not known when the genetic programming for these transformations occurs.

Extraembryonic vascular channels are established as a result of fusion of adjacent vesicles; subsequently, these primitive channels branch and elongate towards the embryo. Noting this pattern, His[22] proposed that all blood vessels within the embryo develop from extraembryonic precursors. New blood vessel formation by budding and branching of existing endothelium is called *angiogenesis.* This occurs in the adult during vascularization of tumors[23,24] and neovascularization of wounds.[25-27]

The theory of extraembryonic origins was challenged by several workers, in particular Florence Sabin,[1] who saw the appearance of endothelial vesicles in intraembryonic splanchnic mesoderm (*e.g.,* references 28-30). These intraembryonic endothelial vesicles are most evident at the endoderm-mesoderm interface. They do not arise as mesenchymal aggregates, and in most cases their formation is not associated with the generation of blood cell precursors (see, however, ref. 31.) Some observers argued that isolated intraembryonic endothelial vesicles were, in fact, transiently separated tips of elongating extraembryonic-derived vessels,[32] but this view had few supporters.

Experimental support of intraembryonic vascular origins came from the experiments of Hahn,[33] Stockard,[34] and Reagan.[35] Reagan surgically isolated parts of the prevascular chick embryo and found that primitive blood vessels still form within the embryo. More recently Rosenquist[36] found many labeled aortic arch endothelial cells following transplantation of [3H]thymidine-labeled head mesodermal precursors. This has been confirmed by Johnston *et al.*[37] using a replicating nuclear marker. Neither the distribution of these angiogenic precursors nor their mode of assembly into endothelial tissue has been established, however.

The development of intraembryonic blood vessels, particularly those such as the dorsal aortae that elongate at the mesoderm:endorderm interface,[38,39] has been examined using scanning electron microscopy. These studies confirm the presence of endothelial vesicles located spatially and temporally adjacent to elongating blood vessels. But, again, the origin of endothelial cells in these clusters is unresolved in these studies.

Thus, the prevailing view of peripheral blood vessel formation is that vesicles arising within splanchnic mesoderm fuse and grow throughout the embryo,[40,41,25] as summarized schematically in FIGURE 1. The actual proportion of endothelial cells derived by *in situ* vesicle formation and angiogenesis is not known.

Our ability to analyze the early stages of blood vessel formation, especially the issue of embryonic endothelial cell origins has improved tremendously as a result of the generation of monoclonal and polyclonal antibodies that bind to a species-specific epitope found on embryonic and adult endothelial cells of the Japanese quail (monoclonals;[42-46] polyclonals[21,47-49]).

Applying these antibodies to quail embryos reveals the presence in very young (early somite) embryos of single endothelial cell precursors (*i.e.,* angioblasts) as well

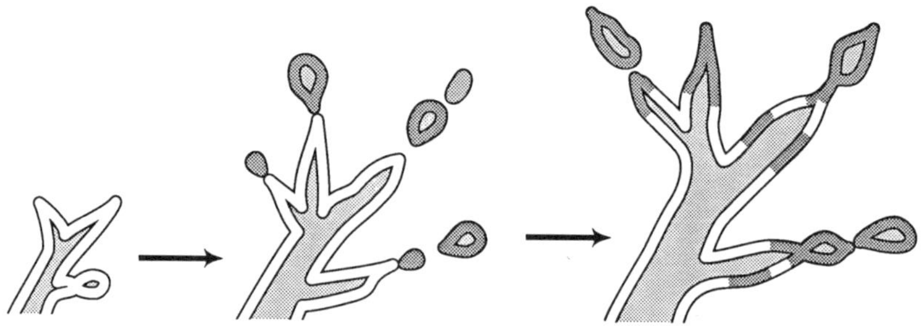

FIGURE 1. The classical model of intraembryonic blood vessel development. Both angiogenesis (growth by sprouting and branching from existing vessels) and *in situ* formation of endothelial vesicles, which fuse with existing branches, participate in new blood vessel formation.

as compact endothelial clusters that subsequently contribute to vesicle and vessel formation and elongation.[44-46] In some parts of the body, (*e.g.,* formation of intersomitic vessels) no such precursors are seen, suggesting that deeper vessels develop exclusively by budding and branching from early-formed vessels.

Unavailable from these descriptive studies is an understanding of where these angioblasts and cells within endothelial clusters originate. Do they arise *in situ* at the sites where first immunologically detectable, or do their precursors form elsewhere and move to these sites? To resolve this problem, each mesenchymal tissue and some epithelial tissues were transplanted from quail embryos into chick embryos, as shown schematically in FIGURE 2. Except for lateral splanchnic mesoderm, these grafts, which contain fewer than 500 cells, are made before the appearance of any intraembryonic endothelial cells. Polyclonal antibodies that bind only quail endothelial cells were applied to sections from chimeric embryos fixed several days after tissue transplantation. The presence of immunopositive cells in host embryos (FIG. 3) indicates that the grafted tissue contained committed endothelial precursors.

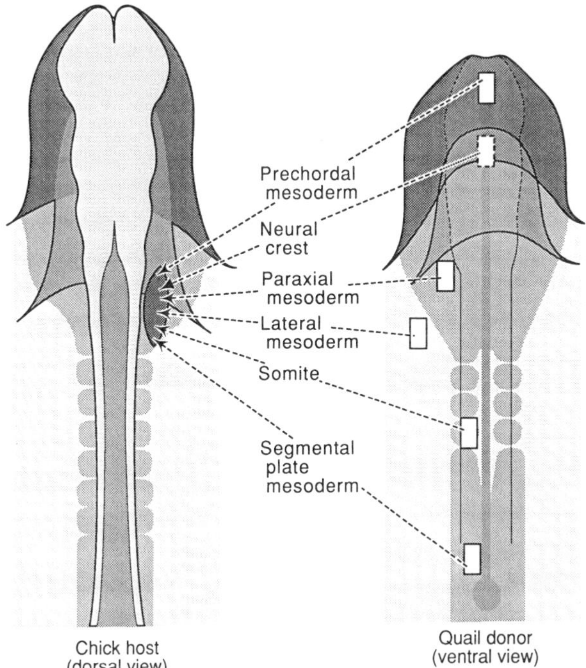

FIGURE 2. Scheme of embryonic transplantations designed to identify embryonic tissues that contain angioblasts. Several quail tissues from head and trunk regions were implanted into chick hosts close to the site at which the otic placode develops.

The results, summarized in TABLE 1, indicate that most mesodermal populations contain cells committed to the endothelial lineage, with only the prechordal plate mesoderm lacking these precursors. Neither the neural crest nor neural tube tissues form vascular endothelium. Thus, even within limb buds, somites, and somitomeres, all tissues that have been thought to become vascularized by ingrowth of branches from adjacent blood vessels, there are cells capable of expressing the endothelial phenotype. Conversely, there are other tissues, for example the central nervous system and those areas of the face and jaw formed by neural crest-derived mesenchyme, that must become vascularized by ingrowth of exogenous endothelial tissues or precursors.

TABLE 1. Distribution of Endogenous Angioblasts in Embryonic Tissues

Cephalic tissues		Trunk tissues	
paraxial mesoderm	+	whole somites	+
lateral mesoderm	+	dorsal half somites	+
prechordal mesoderm	−	segmental plate	+
notochord	−	lateral somatic mesoderm	+
neural crest	−	lateral splanchnic mesoderm	+
brain	−	spinal cord	−

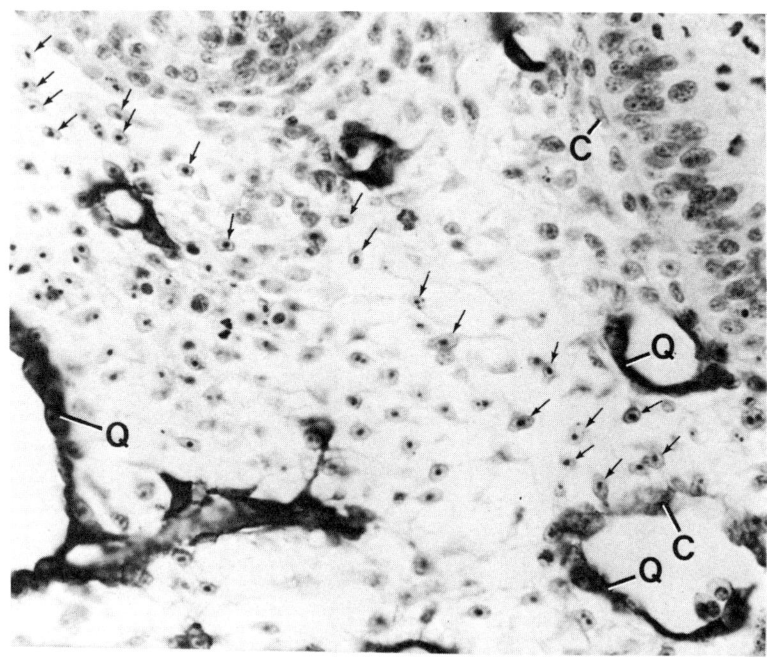

FIGURE 3. Tissue from a quail-chick chimeric embryo showing that quail (Q) but not chick (C) endothelial cells are recognized by the antibody (black staining). Quail nonendothelial mesenchymal cells (small arrows) can be identified by the presence of a condensed nucleolar heterochromatin marker. Note that some vessels contain both quail and chick endothelial cells; × 280.

ASSEMBLY OF ENDOTHELIAL TISSUE

How do these nearly ubiquitous endothelial precursors come together to form a confluent endothelium? This is an assembly problem that focuses on the movements of individual angioblasts and the establishment of contacts between them that results in the histogenesis of endothelial tissue.

Most grafted quail cells remain near the site of implantation. The presence of this mesenchymal mass is easily detected because quail cells have a nucleolar heterochromatin marker not found in chick (host) cells.[50] These cells proliferate and give rise to a variety of muscle[51,52] and connective tissues.[53,54] Not surprisingly the greatest density of labeled endothelial cells is found in those vessels located closest to the site of implantation. Many labeled endothelial cells were found far from the site of implantation, however, as single cells, clusters, vesicles, and parts of definitive vessels (FIG. 4), often interspersed with chick (host) endothelial cells. Thus, there is a massive emigration of endothelial cells from the transplanted mesoderm, and many of these emigrés join with host endothelial cells in the formation of craniofacial arteries and veins. Because some aortic arches are entirely formed by endothelial cells from the transplant while other are chimeric, it is evident that angiogenesis (budding and branching), local vesicle formation, and emigration of individual endothelial precursors have all occurred.

This exodus of endothelial precursors from the graft is unlike the patterns of movement exhibited by any other mesenchymal cell population in that it is omnidirectional; labeled cells move dorsally to the brain, caudally to the future cardiac and thoracic regions (FIG. 5), and rostrally into future facial tissues. No region of the embryo within several hundred micrometers of the implant site is spared!

Because most tissue implants were made beneath or beside the otic placode, there was little expectation that grafted cells would contribute to endocardial or coronary endothelial tissues. In some embryos, however, focal or clonal patches of outflow tract endocardium were labeled (FIG. 6). Also, from this implant site some angioblasts invaded the future pulmonary, myocardial, and hepatic regions, although the fate of these endothelial cells has not yet been determined.

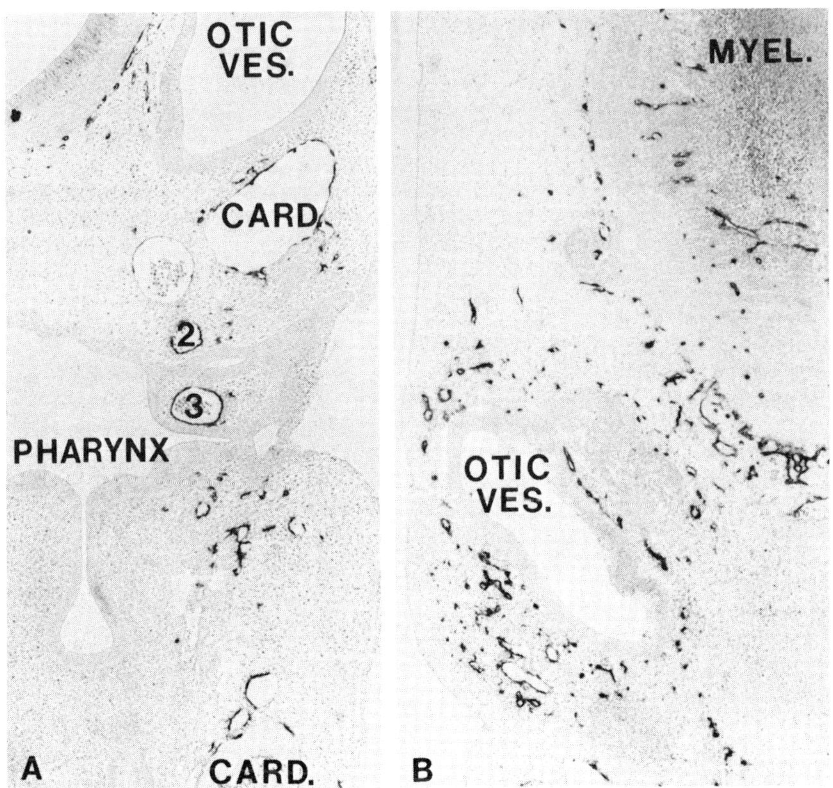

FIGURE 4. Distribution of quail endothelial cells in two embryos, 2 (**A**) or 3 (**B**) days following transplantation. From an implantation site near the base of aortic arch 3, quail angioblasts have migrated in all directions, including dorsally to the myelencephalon (MYEL.), cranial cardinal venous plexus (CARD.), and periotic regions; ventrally to the cardiac region (see FIG. 5); and rostrally and caudally to the areas where aortic arches 2 and 3 (2, 3) develop; × 68.

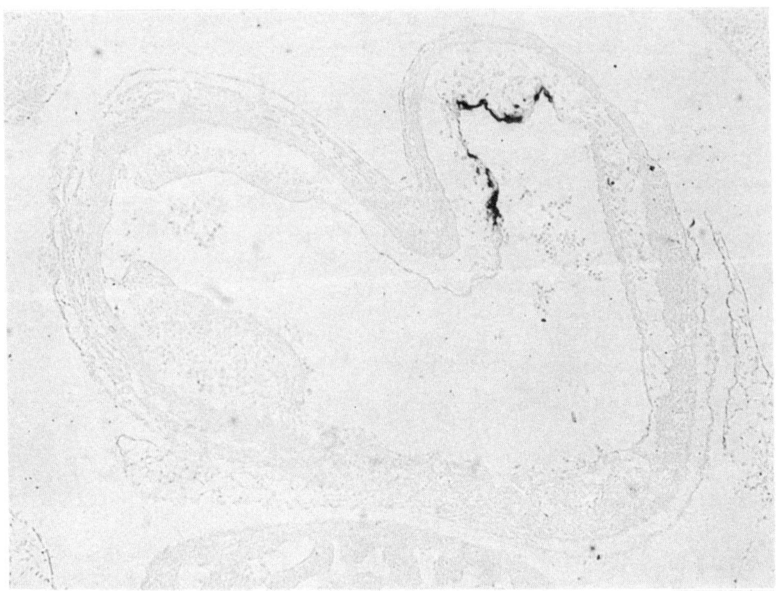

FIGURE 5. Section through the atrioventricular and outflow tract regions of the heart from a chimeric embryo. Transplanted quail angioblasts participated together with host endocardial precursors in assembly of outflow tract endocardium; × 108.

These results define three concurrent processes by which blood vessels form (FIG. 7). The initial formation and elongation of some vessels occurs by interstitial proliferation of endothelial cells concomitant with budding and branching. This mode of development, angiogenesis, is most apparent in the aortic arches. It is also the exclusive means of blood vessel formation in the central nervous system. In addition, there is extensive local formation of endothelial vesicles throughout head mesodermal mesenchyme. In our chimeras, some of these vesicles are exclusively host or donor in

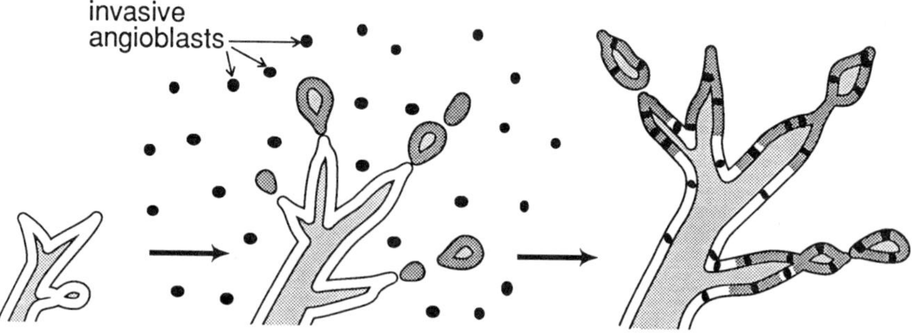

FIGURE 6. Revised model embryonic blood vessel development. Three processes are involved: angiogenesis (sprouting and branching), *in situ* formation of endothelial vesicles, and invasion of migrating angioblasts (shown in black).

derivation; others are mixed. Finally, there is a subpopulation of committed endothelial precursors that exhibit extensive invasive migrations, a process that seeds all intraembryonic mesenchyme with endothelial precursors even if such precursors are already present.

FORMATION OF DEFINITIVE BLOOD VESSELS

As all anatomists know, the positions at which specific blood vessels are located are not random, although there are many variations. Some of these quail-chick trans-

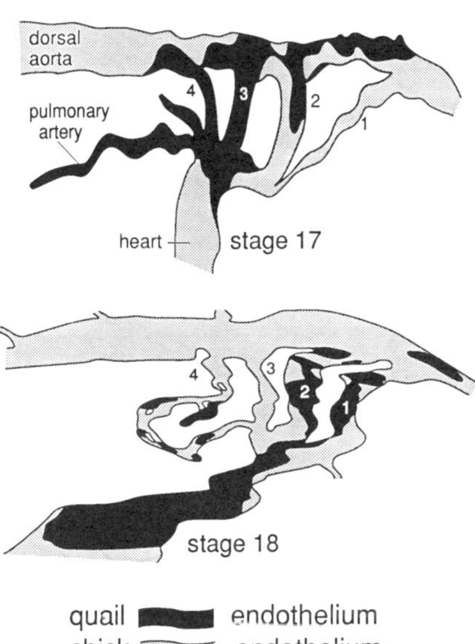

FIGURE 7. Computer reconstructions of two chimeric embryos illustrating the locations of transplant-derived quail and host chick endothelial cells in the outflow tract, aortic arches, and dorsal aorta. Labeled veins and capillaries are not shown. In these embryos the sites of graft excision and implantation were identical.

plants, particularly those in which trunk angioblasts were grafted into the head, indicate how embryonic endothelial tissue is caused to form definitive patent channels in specific locations. Transplanted endothelial precursors invade craniofacial mesenchymal and neural epithelial tissues and subsequently participate in the formation and remodeling of blood vessels appropriate for and unique to the head (FIG. 8). In assessing these results, one must remember that the grafted precursors normally would not form aortic arches or a cranial cardinal venous plexus, nor would they encounter neural crest-derived mesenchymal tissue. Thus, cues directing the spatial assembly of developing blood vessels reside within the cellular environment surrounding them, not within endothelial cells. In this respect developing blood vessels behave similarly to voluntary muscles,[52] the integument,[54,55] and many other tissues, each of which derives pattern-generating cues from local connective tissue-forming mesenchyme (reviewed in references 21 and 56).

ORIGINS OF PERIVASCULAR TISSUES

Prior to the expression of distinct cytological features, perivascular mesenchymal cells express smooth muscle-specific α-actin. Later, this population condenses adjacent to endothelium. The interactions underlying these events have not been defined.

Except with respect to the myocardium, evidence regarding the origin of perivascular mesenchyme is anecdotal. In several studies in which quail neural crest[57–60] or paraxial mesoderm[51] has been transplanted, quail perivascular smooth muscle tissue has been identified. These few studies suggest that whichever mesenchyme is adjacent to each vascular channel when it initially forms will coalesce and later differentiate as smooth muscle and adventitia.

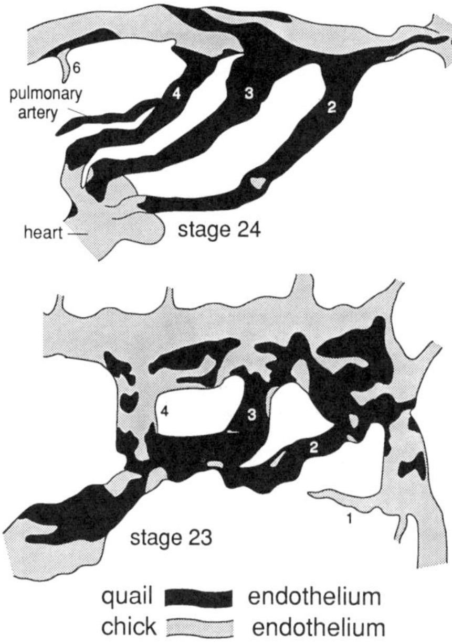

FIGURE 8. Similar reconstructions illustrating the ability of trunk angioblasts to form normal craniofacial blood vessels following their implantation beneath the otic placode. The patterns of blood vessel assembly in these embryos are similar to those seen following orthotopic transplantation (FIG. 7).

UNRESOLVED ISSUES

An essential but poorly understood feature of the developing vascular system is the generation of cell heterogeneity. This is an obligate feature of the vascular system and includes the acquisition of distinct histological and functional characteristics of arteries, arterioles, capillaries, veins, and lymphatics, and the programming of tissue- and organ-specific vascular characteristics. These heterogeneities are evident both in endothelial and perivascular tissues.

Embryonic endothelial tissues appear morphologically identical. Except for the heart, blood vessels lack enveloping mesenchymal envelopes characteristic of mature vessels and distinct to arteries, veins, and capillaries. The identification of embryonic arteries and veins is based solely upon function criteria—primarily the direction of blood flow—and this frequently reverses through a particular vessel during vascular remodeling. Developing tissues, however, typically initiate programming for regional- and tissue-specific phenotypic expressions prior to their overt differentiation, and often the histological signs of such expression are among the last to be manifest.

Endothelial populations express several unique regional and organ-specific features[61-64] (reviewed by Auerbach[65]); however, except for the development of brain-specific endothelial properties,[66] little is known about the generation of these key regional differences. Mature endothelial cells are sensitive and responsive to altered microenvironments, especially changes in the extracellular matrix.[64,67] Based on the known critical roles of matrix components on the development of other tissues, it is likely that interactions among endothelium, matrix, and surrounding mesenchyme will be critical in blood vessel wall assembly and histodifferentiation. Could the regional differences, or possibly the microheterogeneity documented in some endothelial populations, be attributable to the disparate patterns of endothelial lineage in the embryo?

It has been proposed that endodermal cells underlying some early angiogenic populations may play a role in their assembly[68,69] and, in the case of endocardial cells, their cytodifferentiation.[70,71] Recent scanning electron microscopic analyses have identified a layer of mesenchymal cells that forms a thin but confluent monolayer interposed between endoderm and angiogenic mesoderm in the quail embryo.[72] The formation of this layer immediately preceding the development of the dorsal aortae and vitelline network suggests, but does not prove, that it has a role in vasculogenesis.

Embryonic endothelial precursors are activated to divide rapidly. As shown by the quail-chick chimera studies, a subset of these endothelial precursors also exhibits an invasive migratory behavior. The mechanisms initiating and effecting these dramatic changes in behavior are not known. The down-regulation of endothelial proliferation and migration is equally enigmatic but must be carefully controlled or else the embryo will become a hemangioma. Thus, in contrast to the quiescent nature of mature endothelial cells, extreme changes in endothelial cell behavior are routine during development.

SUMMARY

Two processes by which embryonic blood vessels develop are well-known: angiogenesis (growth by budding and branching of existing vessels) and local formation of endothelial vesicles that coalesce with elongating vessels. The former process appears to be more prevalent, with the latter restricted to vessels that form near the endoderm-mesoderm interface. The contributions of endothelial cells formed by each of these processes to specific blood vessels has not been defined, however, nor have the origins of precursors (angioblasts) of intraembryonic endothelial populations been established.

To identify the origins of endothelial cells, precursor populations from quail embryos were transplanted into chick embryos. Antibodies that recognize quail endothelial cells were applied to sections from chimeric embryos fixed 2-5 days after surgery. These experiments reveal that all intraembryonic mesodermal tissues, except the notochord and prechordal plate, contain angiogenic precursors. Many angioblasts emigrate from the grafted tissue, invading surrounding mesenchyme and contributing to the formation of arteries, veins, and capillaries in a wide area. The invasive behavior of these angioblasts is unlike that of any other embryonic mesenchymal cell type and represents a third process operating during embryonic blood vessel formation.

Transplanted angioblasts, even those excised from quail trunk regions, form normal craniofacial vascular channels, including the cardiac outflow tract. These results demonstrate that the control over blood vessel assembly resides within the connective tissue-forming mesenchyme of the embryo, not within endothelial precursors.

ACKNOWLEDGMENTS

The technical assistance of M. Shimamura, J. Oyer, and E. Koehn, and the clerical support by J. Reed are gratefully acknowledged.

REFERENCES

1. SABIN, F. R. 1917. Origin and development of the primitive vessels of the chick and the pig. Carnegie Contrib. Embryol. **6:** 61-124.
2. HUGHES, A. F. W. 1934. On the development of the blood vessels in the head of the chick. Philosoph. Trans. R. Soc. Lond. B. Biol. Sci. **224:** 75-144.
3. LANOT, R. 1980. Formation of the early vascular network in chick embryo: Microscopical aspects. Arch. Biol. **91:** 423-438.
4. LEVINSOHN, E. M., D. S. PACKARD JR., E. M. WEST & D. R. HOOTNICK. 1984. Arterial anatomy of chicken embryo and hatching. J. Anat. **169:** 377-405.
5. BREMER, J. L. 1914. The earliest blood vessels in man. Am. J. Anat. **16:** 447-475.
6. HEUSER, C. H. 1923. The branchial vessels and their derivatives in the pig. Carnegie Contrib. Embryol. **15:** 121-139.
7. REAGAN, F. P. 1929. A century of study upon the development of the eutherian vena cava inferior. Q. Rev. Biol. **IV:** 179-212.
8. PADGET, D. H. 1948. The development of the cranial arteries in the human embryo. Carnegie Contrib. Embryol. **32:** 206-261.
9. PADGET, D. H. 1957. The development of the cranial venous system in man, from the viewpoint of comparative anatomy. Carnegie Contrib. Embryol. **36:** 80-140.
10. MOORE, K. L. 1982. The Developing Human. 3rd edit. W. B. Saunders Co. Philadelphia, PA.
11. NODEN, D. M. & A. DE LAHUNTA. 1985. The Embryology of Domestic Animals. Williams & Wilkins. Baltimore, MD.
12. SADLER, T. W. 1985. Langman's Medical Embryology, 5th edit. Williams & Wilkins. Baltimore, MD.
13. CARLSON, B. M. 1988. Patten's Foundations of Embryology, 5th edit. McGraw-Hill. New York.
14. BREMER, J. L. 1909. On the origin of the pulmonary arteries in mammals. Anat. Rec. **3:** 334-340.
15. FEDOROW, V. 1910. Uber die Entwickelung der Lungenvene. Anta. Hefte **40:** 529-603.
16. BUELL, C. E. 1922. Origin of the pulmonary vessels in the chick. Carnegie Contrib. Embryol. no. 66.
17. CONGDON, E. D. 1922. Transformation of the aortic-arch system during the development of the human embryo. Carnegie Contrib. Embryol. **14:** 47-110.
18. AUER, J. 1948. The development of the human pulmonary vein and its major variations. Anat. Rec. **101:** 581-594.

19. EFFMANN, E. L., S. A. WHITMAN & B. R. SMITH. 1986. Aortic arch development. RadioGraphics **6:** 1065-1089.

20. NODEN, D. M. 1984. Craniofacial development: new views on old problems. Anat. Rec. **208:** 1-13.

21. NODEN, D. M. 1988. Interactions and fates of avian craniofacial mesenchyme. Development **103:** 121-140.

22. HIS, W. 1900. Lecithoblast und Angioblast der Wirbeltiere. Abhandl. Math.-Naturw. Kl., K. sachs Ges. **22.**

23. FOLKMAN, J. 1980. Angiogenesis *in vitro.* Nature **288:** 551-556.

24. FOLKMAN, J. 1985. Toward an understanding of angiogenesis: Search and discovery. Perspect. Biol. Med. **29:** 10-36.

25. WAGNER, R. C. 1980. Endothelial cell embryology and growth. Adv. Microcirc. **9:** 45-75.

26. SHOLLEY, M. M., G. P. FERGUSON, H. R. SEIBEL, J. L. MONTOUR & J. D. WILSON. 1984. Mechanisms of neovascularization. Lab. Invest. **51**(6): 624-634.

27. D'AMORE, P. A. & R. W. THOMPSON. 1987. Mechanisms of angiogenesis. Ann. Rev. Physiol. **49:** 453-464.

28. BALFOUR, F. N. 1873. The development of the blood vessels in the chick. Q. J. Micr. Sci. **13:** 607-720.

29. EVANS, H. M. 1909. On the development of the aorta, cardinal and umbilical veins, and other blood vessels of embryos from capillaries. Anat. Rec. **3:** 498-518.

30. SABIN, F. R. 1916. The origin and development of the lymphatic system. John Hopkins Hosp. Rep. **17:** 347-440.

31. OLAH, I., J. MEDGYES & B. GLICK. 1988. Origin of aortic cell clusters in the chicken embryo. Anat. Rec. **222:** 60-68.

32. HUNTINGTON, G. S. 1914. The development of the mammalian jugular lymph sac. Am. J. Anat. **16:** 259-316.

33. HAHN, H. 1909. Exoerimentelle Studien uber die Entstehung des Blutes und der ersten Gefasse beim Huhnchen. Roux's Arch. Dev. Biol. **27:** 337-433.

34. STOCKARD, C. R. 1915. The origin of blood and vascular endothelium in embryos without a circulation of the blood and in the normal embryo. Am J. Anat. **18:** 227-327.

35. REAGAN, F. P. 1915. Vascularization phenomena in fragments of embryonic bodies completely isolated from yolk-sac entoderm. Anat. Rec. **9:** 329-241.

36. ROSENQUIST, G. C. 1970. Aortic arches in the chick embryo: Origin of the cells as determined by radioautographic mapping. Anat. Rec. **168:** 351-359.

37. JOHNSTON, M. C., D. M. NODEN, R. D. HAZELTON, J. L. COULOMBRE & A. J. COULOMBRE. 1979. Origins of avian ocular and periocular tissues. Exp. Eye Res. **29:** 27-43.

38. MEIER, S. 1980. Development of the chick embryo mesoblast: pronephros, lateral plate, and early vasculature. J. Embryol. Exp. Morphol. **55:** 291-306.

39. HIRAKOW, R. & T. HIRUMA. 1981. Scanning electron microscopic study on the development of primitive blood vessels in chick embryos at the early somite stage. Anat. Rec. **163:** 299-306.

40. McCLURE, C. F. W. 1921. The endothelial problem. Anat. Rec. **22:** 219-237.

41. SABIN, F. R. 1922. Direct growth of veins by sprouting. Carnegie Contrib. Embryol. **14:** 1-10.

42. PEAULT, B. M., J-P. THIERY & N. M. LE DOUARIN. 1983. Surface marker for hemopoietic and endothelial cell lineages in quail that is defined by amonoclonal antibody. Proc. Natl. Acad. Sci. USA **80:** 2976-2980.

43. LABASTIE, M-C., T. J. POOLE, B. M. PEAULT & N. M. LE DOUARIN. 1986. MB1, a quail leukocyte-endothelium antigen: Partial characterization of the cell surface and secreted forms in cultured endothelial cells. Proc. Natl. Acad. Sci. USA **83:** 9016-9020.

44. PARDANAUD, L., C. ALTMAN, P. KITOS, F. DIETERLEN-LELIEVRE & C. A. BUCK. 1987. Vasculogenesis in the early quail blastodisc as studied with a monoclonal antibody recognizing endothelial cells. Development **100:** 339-349.

45. COFFIN, J. D. & T. J. POOLE. 1988. Embryonic vascular development: Immunohistochemical identification of the origin and subsequent morphogenesis of the major vessel primordia in quail embryos. Development **102:** 735-748.

46. POOLE, T. J. & J. D. COFFIN. 1988. Developmental angiogenesis: Quail embryonic vasculature. Scanning Microsc. **2**(1): 443-448.
47. LANCE-JONES, C. L. & C. F. LAGENAUR. 1987. A new marker for identifying quail cells in embryonic avian chimeras: a quail-specific antiserum. J. Histochem. Cytochem. **35:** 771-780.
48. NODEN, D. M. 1987. Immunocytochemical analysis of avian craniofacial angiogenesis. Anat. Rec. **218:** 99A.
49. NODEN, D. M. 1989. Embryonic origins and assembly of blood vessels. Am. Rev. Respir. Dis. **140:** 1097-1103.
50. LE DOUARIN, N. M. 1973. A biological labeling technique and its use in experimental embryology. Dev. Biol. **30:** 217-222.
51. NODEN, D. M. 1983b. The embryonic origins of avian cephalic and cervical muscles and associated connective tissues. Am. J. Anat. **168:** 257-276.
52. NODEN, D. M. 1986. Patterning of avian craniofacial muscles. Dev. Bio. **116:** 347-356.
53. CHEVALLIER, A. 1979. Role of somitic mesoderm in the development of the thorax in bird embryos. J. Embryol. Exp. Morphol. **49:** 73-88.
54. MCLOUGHLIN, C. B. 1963. Mesenchymal influences on epithelial differentiation. Symp. Soc. Exp. Biol. **17:** 359-388.
55. NODEN, D. M. 1983. The role of the neural crest in patterning of avian cranial skeletal, connective, and muscle tissues. Dev. Biol. **96:** 144-165.
56. NODEN, D. M. 1987. Interactions between cephalic neural crest and mesodermal populations. *In* Developmental and Evolutionary Aspects of the Neural Crest. P. F. A. Maderson, Ed.: 89-119. John Wiley & Sons. New York.
57. NODEN, D. M. 1975. An analysis of the migratory behavior of avian cephalic neural crest cells. Dev. Biol. **42:** 106-130.
58. NODEN, D. M. 1978. The control of avian cephalic neural crest cytodifferentiation. I. Skeletal and connective tissues. Dev. Biol. **67:** 296-312.
59. LELIEVIRE, C. S. & N. M. LE DOUARIN. 1975. Mesenchymal derivatives of the neural crest: analysis of chimaeric quail and chick embryos. J. Embryol. Exp. Morphol. **34**(1): 125-154.
60. KIRBY, M. L. & D. E. BOCKMAN. 1984. Neural crest and normal development: A new perspective. Anat. Rec. **209:** 1-6.
61. FUJIMOTO, T. & S. J. SINGER. 1986. Immunocytochemical studies of endothelial cells *in vivo*. I. The presence of desmin only, or of desmin plus vimentin, or vimentin only, in the endothelial cells of different capillaries of the adult chicken. J. Cell Biol. **103:** 2775-2786.
62. MICHALAK, T., F. P. WHITE, A. L. GARD & G. R. DUTTON. 1986. A monoclonal antibody to the endothelium of rat brain microvessesls. Brain Res. **379:** 320-328.
63. GUMKOWSKI, F., G. KAMINSKA, M. KAMINSKI, L. W. MORRISSEY & R. AUERBACH. 1987. Heterogeneity of mouse vascular endothelium. *In vitro* studies of lymphatic, large blood vessel and microvascular endothelial cells. Blood Vessels **24:** 11-23.
64. PAULI, B. U. & C-L. LEE. 1988. Organ preference of metastasis—the role of organ-specifically modulated endothelial cells. Lab. Invest. **58:** 379-387.
65. AUERBACH, R. 1988. Patterns of tumor metastasis: Organ selectively in the spread of cancer cells. Lab. Invest. **58:** 361-364.
66. RISAU, W., R. HALLMANN & U. ALBRECHT. 1986. Differentiation-dependent expression of proteins in brain endothelium during development of the blood-brain barrier. Dev. Biol. **117:** 537-545.
67. MARTINEZ-HERNANDEZ, A. 1985. The hepatic extracellular matrix. Lab. Invest. **53:** 166-186.
68. WILT, F. W. 1965. Erythropoiesis in the chick embryo: The role of endoderm. Science **147:** 1588-1590.
69. LINASK, K. K. & J. W. LASH. 1986. Precardiac cell migration: Fibronectin localization at mesoderm-endoderm interface during directional movement. Dev. Biol. **114:** 87-101.
70. JACOBSON, A. G. 1960. Influences of ectoderm and endoderm on heart differentiation in the newt. Dev. Biol. **2:** 138-154.

71. LEMANSKI, L. F., D. J. PAULSON & C. S. HILL. 1979. Normal anterior endoderm corrects the heart defect in cardiac mutant salamanders (Ambystoma mexicanum). Science **204:** 860-862.
72. REISS, K. Z. & D. M. NODEN. 1989. SEM characterization of a novel cellular layer separating splanchnic and somitic mesoderm from endoderm in quail embryos. Anat. Rec. **225:** 165-175.

Cardiac Mapping of Regional Glucose Utilization in Fetal Cats, Rabbits, and Chicks Using [^{14}C]2-Deoxyglucose[a]

DAVID R. KOSTREVA [b]

Departments of Anesthesiology and Physiology
Medical College of Wisconsin
and
Research Service
Zablocki Veterans Administration Medical Center
Milwaukee, Wisconsin 53295

INTRODUCTION

The heart and cardiovascular system constitute the first fully functioning embryonic organ complex. Because this system is developed early in embryonic life, much of its differentiation takes place directly from the most primitive of germ layers. For example, most of the heart has been thought to be derived primarily from mesoderm and perhaps some mesenchyme.[1] Recent studies by Kirby and co-workers,[2–20] however, have demonstrated that a region of the neural crest called the cardiac neural crest contributes to the actual formation of the heart, forming the outflow septa.[3,5,18] This area of neural crest extends from the midotic placode to the caudal limit of somite 3,[3] and it also populates pharyngeal arches 3, 4, and 6.[18] If this portion of the neural crest is ablated in the early chick embryo prior to neural crest migration, the outflow septa of the heart does not develop,[17] resulting in a cardiac defect known as persistent truncus arteriosus. Other cardiac defects that have resulted from ablation of the cardiac or cranial neural crest in the developing chick include double outlet right ventricle, ventricular septal defect, transposition of great vessels, defects similar to tetralogy of Fallot, double inlet left ventricle, straddling right AV valve, right AV valve atresia, persistent AV canal, and defects of the aortic arch.[3,8,10,15,17,20,21] It has also been reported that the cardiac neural crest supplies ectomesenchymal cells to the developing heart.[3,5] If these ectomesenchymal cells are not available specifically from the cardiac neural crest, cardiac malformations may develop.[3,5]

[a] These studies were supported by the Department of Anesthesiology of the Medical College of Wisconsin and by the Research Service of the VA.

[b] Address for correspondence: David R. Kostreva, Research Service/151, VA Medical Center, Milwaukee, Wisconsin 53295.

The very same cardiac neural crest that forms part of the heart also gives rise to the parasympathetic ganglia and efferent nerves that innervate the heart.[3,7,13,22,23] The parasympathetic afferent innervation of the heart arises from the nodose placode, which is located lateral to the cardiac neural crest.[4,22,24] The distinction between the origin of the cardiac parasympathetic afferents versus the efferents is not absolute, however. For instance, Kirby[4] has shown that if the cardiac neural crest is ablated, in addition to the resulting cardiac malformations mentioned above, 30% of the efferent parasympathetic innervation to the heart will be eliminated. In order for the chick heart to be made completely parasympathetically aneural, both the cardiac neural crest and the nodose placode must be ablated.

Sympathetic innervation of the chick heart arises from the truncal neural crest just medial to somites 10 through 20.[9,12,13,15,21] If this portion of the neural crest is ablated bilaterally, the heart is rendered sympathetically aneural without any known cardiac malformations as depicted diagrammatically in FIGURE 1. In a recent study,

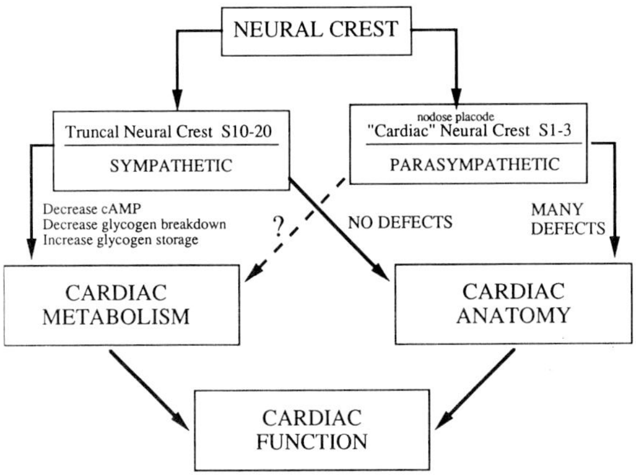

FIGURE 1. Diagramatic representation of the relationship between neural crest, cardiac metabolism, cardiac anatomy, and cardiac function.

Faith *et al.*[2] demonstrated that ablation of the premigratory truncal neural crest over somites 10 through 20 produced chick hearts that not only lacked sympathetic innervation, but that also had a marked decrease in cyclic AMP. In addition, a decrease in glycogen breakdown and an increase in glycogen storage was also observed. These data suggest that metabolism of the developing heart is directly influenced by its sympathetic innervation, although no cardiac anatomical effects have been observed with truncal neural crest (sympathetic) ablation. The metabolic effects of parasympathetic ablation of the developing heart, however, have not been studied. It is precisely these recently discovered facts that formed the rationale for the preliminary studies conducted in our laboratory.

One of the basic underlying assumptions of our studies is that both cardiac anatomy and cardiac metabolism are the major determinants of cardiac function. Without normal cardiac metabolism or normal cardiac structure, cardiac function will be abnormal. This is diagramatically depicted in FIGURE 2. During development, the energy requirements of the heart are channeled in two directions. The first being the energy used in growth and maturation of the structure of the heart. The second being the energy required for normal functioning of the developing heart, because as the heart is being knit together it is also working, that is, it is beating rhythmically, contracting and ejecting blood as it is being formed. Therefore, a significant amount of energy is expended to maintain the work done by the developing heart. It should also be emphasized that cardiac metabolism and anatomy are reciprocally dependent during both development and adulthood. Cardiac metabolism certainly plays a role in the normal anatomical growth of the heart even after birth. In addition, metabolism also affects the structure of the heart during the repair of any cardiac injury. Conversely, any alteration in cardiac anatomy may also affect cardiac metabolism. For instance, an area of infarct or injury will not only affect the metabolism of the site of altered anatomy, but the adjacent areas of healthy myocardial tissue will also be affected due to the abnormal stresses and strains resulting from the altered anatomy. Therefore the interdependence of metabolism and structure has a considerable effect on normal cardiac function.

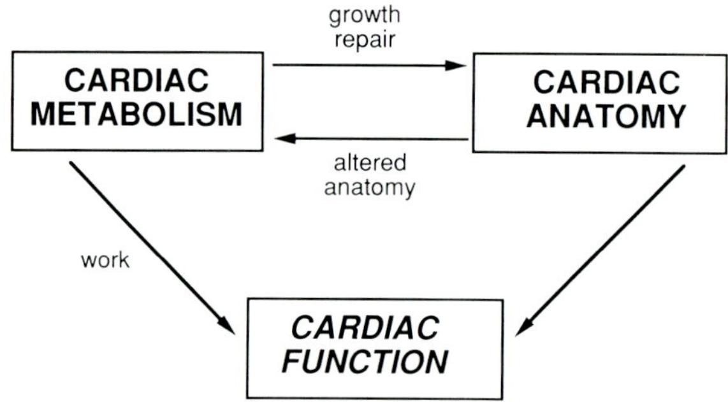

FIGURE 2. Diagram displaying the reciprocal relationships between cardiac metabolism, cardiac anatomy, and cardiac function.

A second basic assumption is that cardiac metabolism in the embryo and fetus is essentially glycolytic. It is well-known that the adult heart uses a variety of metabolic substrates to meet its energy requirements, as shown in FIGURE 3. In general, there is a well-established concept that cardiac metabolism in the embryo starts out primarily glucose-dependent and then switches to become primarily free fatty acid-dependent sometime during postnatal development,[25–27] as summarized in FIGURE 4. In general, most studies indicate that the metabolic requirements of the developing heart are met primarily by glucose and stored glycogen.[28–34,36] Several excellent reviews of the literature on the metabolism of the developing heart have been written by Battaglia and Meschia,[29] Harary[31] and Jones and Rolph.[32] Some of the experimental evidence indicating the predominance of glucose metabolism by the developing heart is derived from studies like those of Breuer *et al.*[30] who demonstrated that glucose accounted for all of the metabolic requirements of the heart in newborn puppies. Comparison of the newborn puppy and adult glucose/O_2 quotients yielded values of 1.1 and 0.3, respectively. In addition, myocardial uptake of free fatty acids could not be demonstrated in the newborn puppies. A relatively small rate of free fatty acid utilization

ADULT HEART

- FREE FATTY ACIDS (primary)
  GLUCOSE (secondary)
  LACTATE
  SHORT CHAIN FATTY ACIDS
  KETONES
  ACETATE
  PYRUVATE

EMBRYONIC & FETAL HEART

- GLUCOSE

FIGURE 3. Myocardial substrates.

has also been demonstrated in *in vitro* studies of the newborn rat[35] and fetal bovine[33] heart as compared with the adults. It is also well-known that fetal and neonatal hearts are both relatively resistant to hypoxia. One of the hypotheses used to explain this phenomenon is that the fetal myocardium stores glycogen in high concentrations, which can then be used to meet the needs of the heart during hypoxia. The importance of glucose utilization as the primary metabolic substrate for the myocardium during gestation and in the newborn is reinforced by reports indicating that hypoglycemia in newborn infants may lead to heart failure.[28,36]

There are several reasons why free fatty acid metabolism is not a primary energy source for the fetal heart. First, it has been shown that fetal heart mitochondria are immature because they have low cristae density.[37] Second, the activities of tricarboxylic acid cycle enzymes and electron-transport chain enzymes range from 10 to 50% and 25 to 70% of the adult levels, respectively, over the last third of gestation.[32] Third, the capacity of the fetal heart to oxidize fatty acids like palmitate or palmityl-CoA is on the order of 10-30% of their newborn and adult counterparts.[32] Fourth, there is extensive evidence that carnitine-dependent utilization of fatty acids is low in fetal animals.[35,38] Fifth, fatty acid concentrations appear to be very low in fetal serum.[39] This limited capacity for fatty acid oxidation is demonstrated further by the inability of the newborn pig heart to maintain a physiological work load when perfused with palmitate or octanoate alone.[40]

Although slight changes in glucose uptake can be detected during cardiac development in the chick, Ureta[41] has shown that the relative activity for the hexokinase enzyme and its primary isozymes does not change in the chick from the 10 day embryo

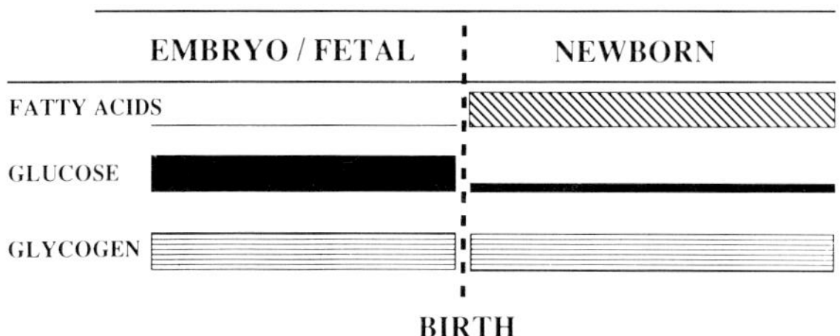

FIGURE 4. Temporal changes in cardiac substrate utilization.

through hatching and into adulthood. In addition, the adult chicken hexokinases 2 and 3 remain dominant throughout life. In the mammal, Stave[42] has demonstrated that changes in glycolytic enzyme activities in rabbit heart muscle during development are minor. This suggests a rather constant glucose metabolism during cardiac development in the rabbit. The only major fluctuation that occurs at birth is a temporal elevation of hexokinase and phosphoglucomutase. Shortly after birth these levels return to the fetal range.

It is well-understood that a number of humoral factors, including thyroid hormone, insulin, and epinephrine can influence the metabolism of the adult heart. Foa et al.[43] have shown that in the early life of the chick embryo there is no demonstrable effect of insulin on glucose uptake; however, during the seventh day of embryonic development, an insulin-sensitive glucose transport system develops and becomes the rate-limiting factor of glucose uptake. They also proposed that the entry of glucose into the early embryonic heart is by simple diffusion. As development proceeds, the high permeability of the plasma membrane to glucose is lost, and the carrier-mediated transport system appears. Kutchai et al.[44] compared cardiac uptake of glucose with 2-deoxyglucose at 5, 10, 15, and 20 days of development. They found that insulin could stimulate 2-deoxyglucose uptake, but not glucose in 5-6 day embryonic hearts. They also showed that both glucose and 2-deoxyglucose uptake decreased between 5 and 15 days with no further decrease in uptake between 15 and 20 days.

Glucose is the primary metabolic substrate for the heart during development. Because glucose and free fatty acid utilization are known to be directly related to cardiac work, myocardial oxygen consumption, and increased energy requirements,[25,45-52] measurements of localized changes in myocardial glucose utilization could greatly increase our understanding of the metabolic events that encompass cardiac development. The [14C]2-deoxyglucose utilization technique is an ideal method for these kinds of studies, because glucose utilization is an important indicator of cardiac function, the technique is noninvasive during the experiment, the quantitative resolution is such that even the smallest of embryonic hearts can be studied carefully, and changes in regional glucose utilization compared to controls will clearly indicate either physiological and pathological significance inasmuch as glucose is the major substrate for cardiac metabolism in the embryo and fetus. The [14C]2-deoxyglucose technique is a noninvasive, high spatial resolution, autoradiographic, metabolic mapping technique that allows assessment of both brain and cardiac glucose utilization in the same animal preparation. Studies by Sokoloff et al.[53] have clearly demonstrated that brain function and brain metabolism, that is, [14C]2-deoxyglucose utilization, are equivalent.

Takala and Hassinen[51,52] have shown in the Langendorf perfused rat heart that there is a direct relationship between [3H]deoxyglucose uptake and the mechanical work load of the heart. Studies by L'Abbate et al.[54] in dogs, Matsunami[55] in monkeys, Yonekura et al.[56] in rats, and our own studies in dogs, rats, cats, monkeys, rabbits, ferrets, and unhatched chicks[57-60] have demonstrated that the [14C]2-deoxyglucose technique can be used to assess cardiac function in a wide variety of species. We have also shown that regional cardiac metabolism can be altered significantly by stimulation of specific cardiac nerves and reflexes.[57,58,60] The neural influences on cardiac function are well-known.[61-67] A reasonable question regarding the [14C]2-deoxyglucose method is: What does a glucose utilization map of the heart demonstrate? First of all, because this technique is a good indicator of glucose utilization with excellent resolution, it can indicate whether or not there is a uniformity of glucose metabolism across the heart. Second, it can determine if there are regional differences in glucose utilization. For instance, the endocardial regions of the left ventricle can be compared precisely with the epicardial regions of the same ventricle. Third, inasmuch as glucose is the primary metabolic fuel in the developing heart, and inasmuch as metabolism is directly related to the work of the heart, one can estimate the relative work of specific regions of the heart and accordingly make assumptions concerning relative changes in contractility in those specific regions. Fourth, the inotropic effects of neural and or neurohumoral influences on the whole or specific regions of the heart can be assessed in a noninvasive manner. This last point is difficult to reproduce using other techniques because most of them are invasive. Overall the [14C]2-deoxyglucose method provides a unique imaging technique to assess cardiac function in the adult and developing heart *in vivo* and *in ovo*.

REGIONAL GLUCOSE UTILIZATION BY THE FETAL AND ADULT FELINE HEART

Our initial study on the developing heart was designed to quantitatively assess the regional glucose utilization of the developing fetal feline heart during three stages of gestation and to compare these values with each other as well as with the maternal regional heart values. The specific aims of this study were to determine if glucose utilization by the whole heart in the developing feline fetus changes from early to late gestation, if there are differences in the amount of glucose utilization by specific regions of the heart, and if these regional differences in glucose utilization are consistent throughout gestation or if they are characteristic of a particular stage of development. This is the first study to quantitatively assess regional myocardial glucose utilization in the developing fetus using the high spatial resolution autoradiographic [14C]2-deoxyglucose technique.

Regional differences in myocardial glucose utilization by the fetal and adult cat heart were studied using the [14C]2-deoxyglucose autoradiographic technique in anesthetized pregnant and nonpregnant adult cats. Three pregnant adult cats (3-3.8 kg), at 25, 35, and 49 days of pregnancy, were anesthetized with pentobarbital sodium (35 mg/kg i.v.). Supplemental doses of anesthetic were given as needed to insure an adequate anesthetic state. The animals were intubated and placed on positive pressure ventilation with 100% oxygen mixed with room air using a Bird respirator. Arterial blood pressure was measured from a femoral catheter, and samples of arterial blood were analyzed for blood gas concentrations. The respirator was adjusted to keep blood gases within normal physiological ranges (PO_2 > 100 Torr, PCO_2 22-30 Torr, and pH 7.18-7.4). Systemic blood pressure and a lead II electrocardiogram were recorded using a polygraph. The contralateral femoral artery and vein were both cannulated for blood sampling throughout the experiment. A single bolus of [14C]2-deoxyglucose, 100 μCi/kg (American Radiolabelled Chemical, St. Louis, MO; specific activity 50-60 mCi/mmol), suspended in sterile saline was injected intravenously. Periodic arterial blood samples were obtained to determine blood glucose concentrations and scintillation counts during the 45 minute experiment.[53] At the end of the 45 minutes, the abdomen was surgically opened and the exposed fetuses were rapidly removed and frozen in −40 °C isopentane along with the maternal hearts. The fetuses and the maternal hearts were then frozen-sectioned at 20 μm increments using an AO cryostat. The frozen sections were placed on glass coverslips and dried on a warming tray. Each serial section was mounted on hardboard and numbered along with a set of [14C] standards. The tissue sections and the standards were then covered with a sheet of Kodak MR-1 film and placed in an X-ray cassette for 12 days. After the exposure, the film was developed, and selected corresponding tissue sections were stained with hematoxylin and eosin. The autoradiographs were then scanned using a computerized scanning densitometer with an aperture setting of 150 μm square for the adult hearts and 50 μm for the fetal hearts. The autoradiographs of the [^{14}C] standards on each sheet of film were used for calibrating the autoradiographic densities. Each standard was read with the same aperture setting, and these values, along with the blood glucose values, scintillation counts, and the lumped constant for the cat brain[53] were used to transform the densitometer readings of optical density into glucose utilization using the Sokoloff equation.[53] Because the lumped constant for cardiac muscle has not been calculated for the cat, the measurements presented here are considered to be relative rather than absolute. This, however, does not prohibit the interpretation of relative changes in regional cardiac glucose utilization presented in TABLE 1. The average glucose utilization of specific regions for each of the fetal and adult hearts were

TABLE 1. Regional Feline Cardiac Glucose Utilization[a]

	Global	RV	Septum	LV	Apex
25 day fetuses N = 6	$75 \pm 4^{b,c}$	$75 \pm 10^{b,c}$	$75 \pm 10^{b,c}$	$84 \pm 14^{b,c}$	$65 \pm 14^{b,c}$
35 day fetuses N = 3	$51 \pm 1^{b,c}$	$50 \pm 9^{b,c}$	54 ± 11^{b}	53 ± 10^{b}	48 ± 9^{b}
49 day fetuses N = 2	38 ± 4^{b}	$48 \pm 8^{b,c}$	39 ± 3^{b}	29 ± 3	36 ± 3
maternal N = 3	15 ± 4	13 ± 2	16 ± 4	14 ± 5	16 ± 5
control adults N = 13	30 ± 7	16 ± 5	35 ± 8	36 ± 8^{d}	34 ± 8^{d}

[a] Values are mean glucose utilization expressed in μmol/100 g/min $\pm$ SEM. RV = right ventricle; LV = left ventricle; N = number of animals. Significant differences were determined using the unpaired t test when $p < 0.05$.
[b] Significant difference between control adult hearts and fetal hearts.
[c] Significant difference between maternal hearts and fetal hearts.
[d] Significant difference between control adult hearts and maternal hearts.

compared with each other using the nonpaired t test on the mean values obtained from each animal.

Regional glucose utilization was examined in 11 fetal hearts and 16 adult hearts. Two of the fetuses were at 49 days of gestation, having a crown-rump length of 10 cm; three were at 35 days of gestation, having a crown-rump length of 4-4.5 cm; and six were at 25 days, having a crown-rump length of 2 cm. The gestational period for the cat is 62 days. Global, right ventricular, septal, left ventricular and apical myocardial glucose utilization were compared using the unpaired t test. It was found that all regions of the 25 day fetal heart had significantly greater glucose utilization ($p < 0.05$) than the control and maternal hearts. The 35 day fetal hearts have quantitatively less glucose utilization, per unit area, for all regions of the heart as compared with the 25 day fetal hearts; however, this was still significantly more than that utilized by the same regions of the adult control hearts. Similar results were obtained for the global, right ventricular, and septal regions of the 49 day fetal hearts; however, the left ventricular and apical values were not significantly different from the control adult values. It should also be noted that there is a progressive decrease in glucose utilization by all regions of the heart with increasing fetal age. FIGURES 5, 6, and 7 are representative examples of the computer scanned autoradiographs of the feline fetal and maternal heart. FIGURE 5 depicts the glucose utilization of an entire sagittal section of a 25 day feline fetus. The left ventricle of the heart is outlined by the white box. The fetus was scanned using an aperture of 100 μm square. The glucose utilization scale on the right side of the FIGURE is for the whole fetal scan. The left ventricle of the heart was rescanned using an aperture setting of 50 μm square and is shown in the box at the bottom of the FIGURE. A separate glucose utilization scale is displayed on the left side using a different scale (10-150 μmol/100 g/min). It should be noted that the posterior wall of the left ventricle has a glucose utilization that is almost two times that of the anterior wall. This suggests that the amount of work done by the posterior versus the anterior wall of the left ventricle is significantly greater because glucose is the primary metabolic substrate for the developing heart. FIGURE 6 represents an autoradiographic section of the 25 day maternal heart, where glucose utilization is displayed on the same scale as that for the fetal hearts. This demonstrates that glucose utilization is rather uniform throughout the adult beating heart with the exception of the papillary muscles, which always have a very high glucose metabolism. It is interesting to note that the papillary muscles, which have a high metabolic demand, are also known to have quite a few stretch or length receptors with either vagal or sympathetic afferent neurons. This suggests that the papillary muscles are contractile regions of the heart that must be carefully regulated through reflex neural mechanisms. FIGURE 7 consists of representative sections taken through the hearts from the three different fetal age groups. All three of these examples were scanned using an aperture of 100 μm; therefore the change in size of the heart during development is to scale for all three hearts. First of all, the change in average glucose utilization for the 25, 35, and 49 day fetal hearts should be noted. Specific regional differences in glucose utilization are also evident in the 35 and 49 day hearts. The 35 day heart is inverted with its apex at the top. The right ventricle is shown on the left with a rather medium range glucose utilization. The basal half of the septum, however, has a very high glucose utilization as does the base of the left ventricle shown on the right side of the figure. The 49 day feline fetal heart also has marked regional differences in glucose utilization, with the left ventricle having a greater glucose utilization than either the septum or the right ventricle. One thing that should be kept in mind, however, is that we are looking at the metabolism of only a single 20 μm thick section of tissue, and that the shape and distribution of glucose utilization can sometimes change over even several millimeters of distance, as depicted in FIGURE 8. Therefore, similar regions of the heart can only be compared with the same spatially defined areas in other hearts that are studied. These results demonstrate that regional differences exist even within the developing heart. In addition, this study also clearly demonstrates that the developing heart uses significantly more ($p < 0.05$) glucose in early stages of development than in late cardiac development.

RATIONALE AND EXPERIMENTAL EVIDENCE FOR USING MATERNAL PLASMA AND SCINTILLATION COUNTS FOR THE DETERMINATION OF FETAL GLUCOSE UTILIZATION VALUES

Because the [^{14}C]2-deoxyglucose technique is quantitative, several measurements from each animal are essential. These include measurements of plasma glucose and

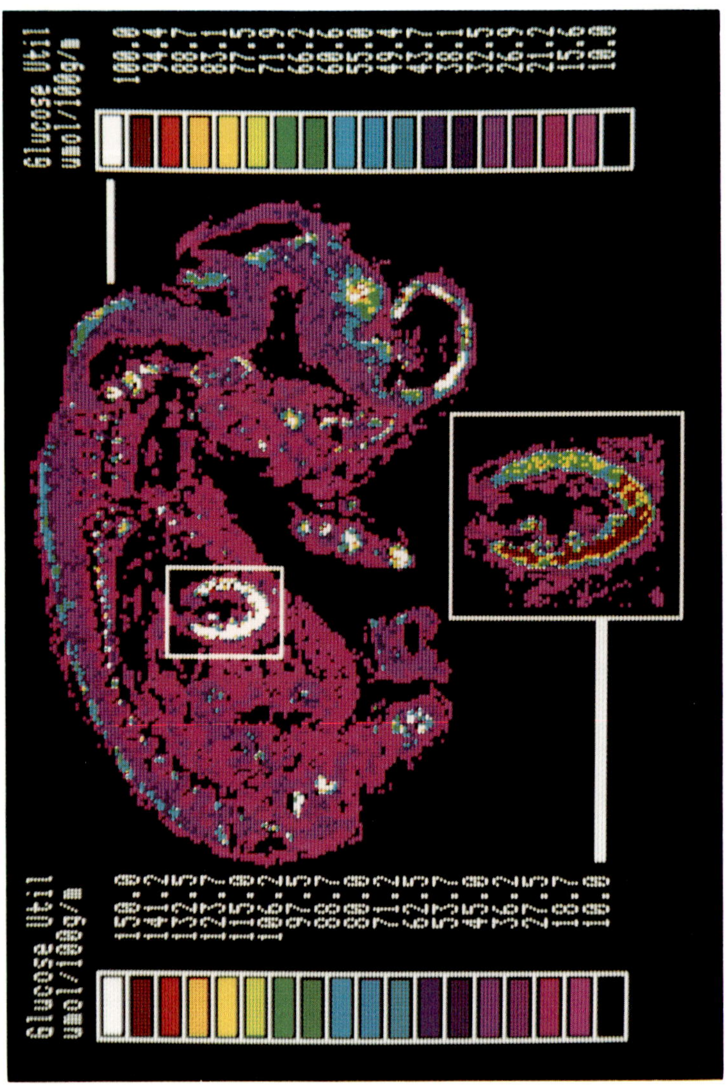

FIGURE 5. Computerized scan of a [^{14}C]2-deoxyglucose autoradiograph from a 25 day feline fetus.

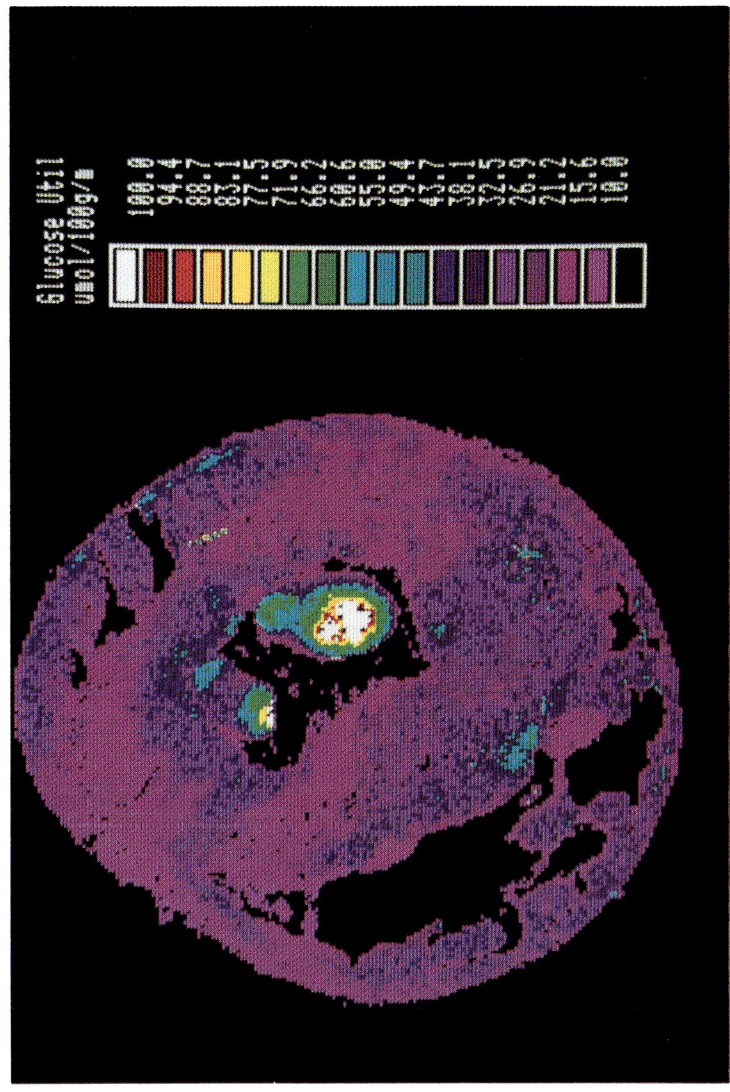

FIGURE 6. Glucose utilization of a 25 day pregnant maternal feline heart sectioned transversely.

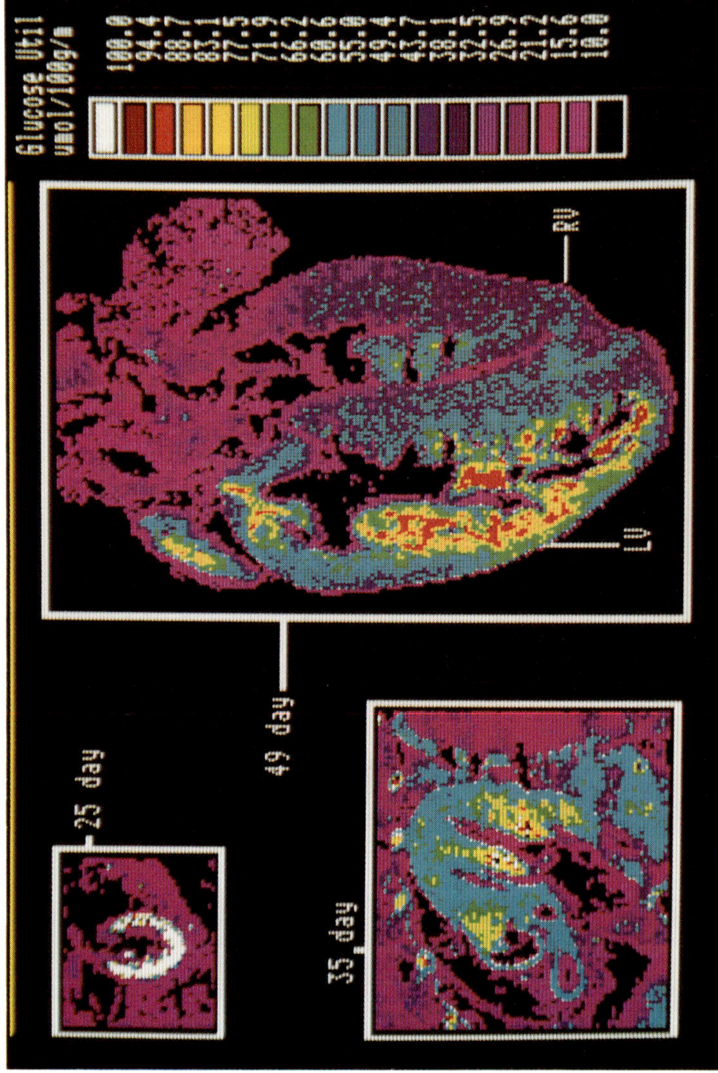

FIGURE 7. Comparative changes in feline fetal myocardial glucose utilization during three stages of gestation.

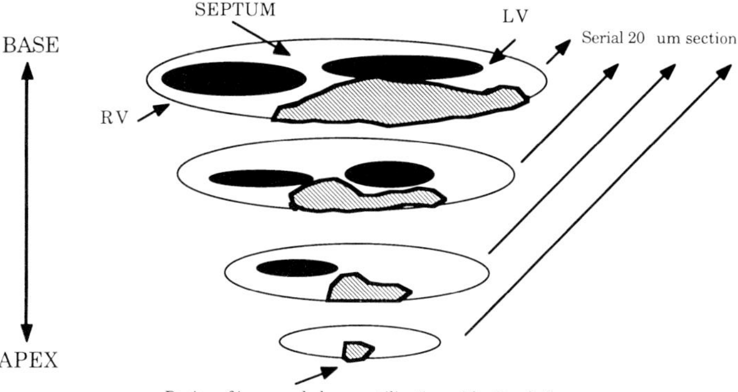

FIGURE 8. Three-dimensional analysis of the heart.

plasma scintillation counts. The third measurement from each animal comes from the autoradiographic images after sacrifice and sectioning of the organ to be studied. This is based on the operational equation of the [^{14}C]2-deoxyglucose method,[53] shown in FIGURE 9, which consists of several components. The letter A in FIGURE 9 represents the autoradiographic optical density measurements expressed in absolute units of radioactivity per gram of tissue; B approaches 0 if the experiment is maintained for 45 minutes; C is the value for the lumped constant, which is species specific; D represents the plasma glucose and scintillation counts that must be measured from each experimental animal; and E represents the calculated value for glucose utilization (μmol/100 g/min). Based on this information, the integral is the only measured data during the experiments that will influence the interpretation of the autoradiographic data. Because it is very difficult as well as being very invasive to obtain 14 (0.3 mL) samples from the fetuses of small mammals, a study in pregnant rabbits was designed

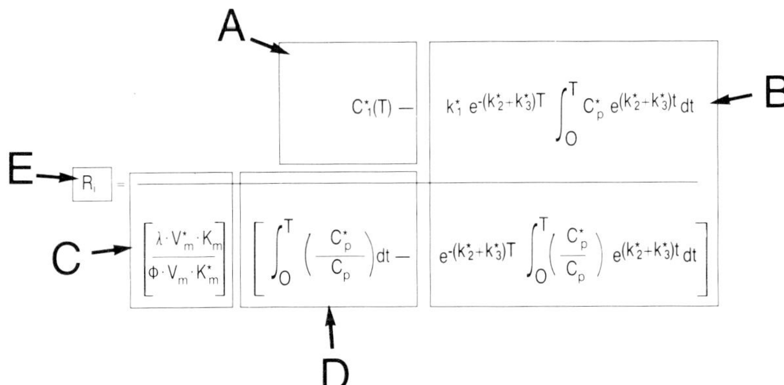

$$R_i = \frac{C_i^*(T) - k_1^* \, e^{-(k_2^*+k_3^*)T} \int_0^T C_p^* \, e^{(k_2^*+k_3^*)t} \, dt}{\left[\dfrac{\lambda \cdot V_m^* \cdot K_m}{\phi \cdot V_m \cdot K_m^*}\right]\left[\int_0^T \left(\dfrac{C_p^*}{C_p}\right)dt - e^{-(k_2^*+k_3^*)T} \int_0^T \left(\dfrac{C_p^*}{C_p}\right) e^{(k_2^*+k_3^*)t} \, dt\right]}$$

FIGURE 9. The Sokoloff equation for determination of regional glucose utilization using [^{14}C]2-deoxyglucose autoradiography.

to determine if there was a significant difference between the integrals of the maternal versus the fetal measurements of plasma glucose and scintillation counts. A series of four pregnant rabbits at 28 days of gestation were anesthetized, intubated, and ventilated, and the abdomen was opened to expose the uterus. A connecting branch of the uterine vein was cannulated with tubing, and the cannula was directed to a single fetal-placental unit for sampling of venous blood. The maternal femoral artery and vein were also cannulated for sampling and administering of supplemental anesthetic. A single bolus of [^{14}C]2-deoxyglucose 100 μCi/kg was injected i.v. into the maternal circulation, and the timed sampling procedure for plasma glucose levels and scintillation counting was initiated. The following integrals of the operational equation for the [^{14}C]2-deoxyglucose method were calculated from both the maternal arterial blood samples and the fetal-placental blood samples.

Maternal	Fetal
9639	11228
11001	10836
8674	9226
6540	6660

A percent difference between each corresponding maternal and fetal integral was also calculated. For three of the four maternal animals, the percent error in measurement of glucose utilization between using the maternal versus the fetal blood samples was between 2 and 6 percent. In the fourth animal the percent error was 16 percent. These errors of measurement of glucose certainly fall within the range of error for any biological study. Using the paired t test no significant difference was found between the integrals from the maternal and fetal samples. It was therefore concluded that calculations of local fetal glucose utilization can be made using the maternal plasma glucose and scintillation count values.[68] This information now provides us with a means of using the [^{14}C]2-deoxyglucose method to noninvasively study the regional metabolism of the developing heart and brains in small mammals, including the rabbit, cat, and rat.

PRELIMINARY QUANTITATIVE ASSESSMENT OF GLUCOSE UTILIZATION IN THE *IN VIVO* DEVELOPING RABBIT FETUS

The rabbit is a good and reliable mammalian model to study the developing heart, because precise timing of conception can be assured and multiple fetuses make this animal model cost-effective. Preliminary experiments conducted in our laboratory, using the identical procedure as that described for the pregnant cats, have shown that the fetal rabbit heart like the fetal cat heart has regional differences in glucose utilization. FIGURE 10 is a representative example of the pattern and distribution of regional glucose utilization in all areas of the 18 day developing rabbit fetus, including the heart, using high spatial resolution autoradiography. The whole fetal autoradiographic section was scanned at 150 μm square per pixel point. The heart was then rescanned at 25 μm square per pixel point. It is obvious from this data that there are distinct regional differences in glucose utilization within the normal fetal myocardium. These differences may reflect regional differences in cardiac work. The developing rabbit heart like the developing cat heart exhibits an overall lessening of glucose metabolism with maturation of the fetus. One of the subtle differences between the developing rabbit and cat hearts noted in these preliminary studies was a greater utilization of

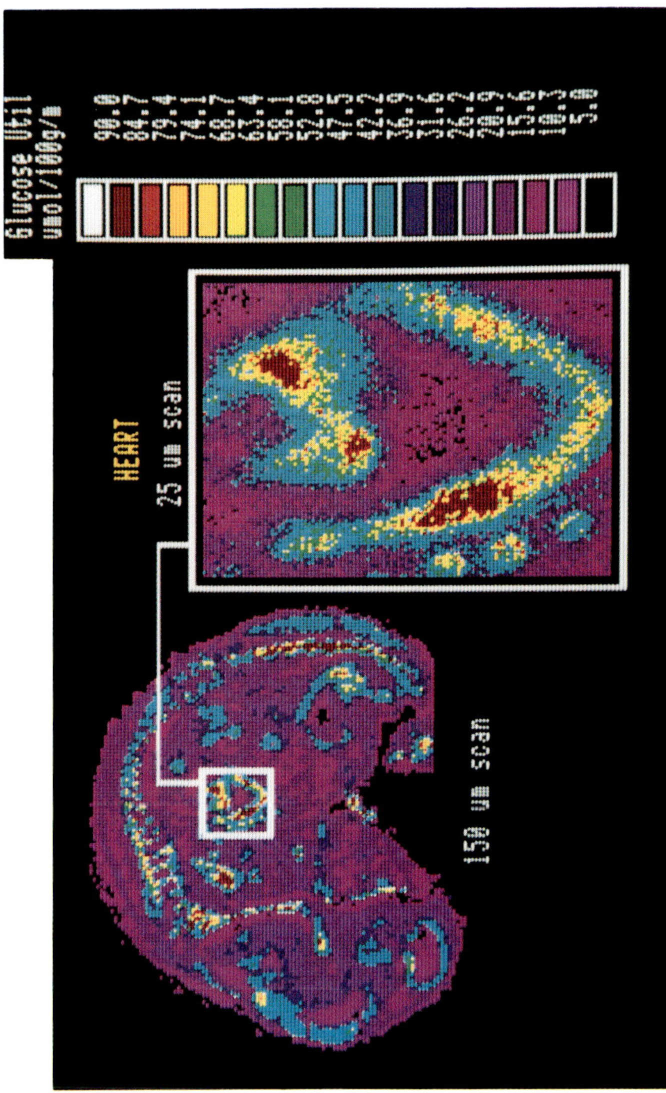

FIGURE 10. Glucose utilization of an 18 day rabbit fetus sectioned through the left ventricle of the heart.

glucose by the myocardial layers of the rabbit heart than by the epicardial or endo/ subendocardial regions.

REGIONAL DISTRIBUTION OF GLUCOSE UTILIZATION IN THE DEVELOPING CHICK HEART AT 11 DAYS OF INCUBATION

The species most widely used as a model for cardiac development is the chick. In addition to the wealth of information already available, as demonstrated by the material covered in this volume, it was noted that the metabolism of the developing chick heart was never studied using an autoradiographic technique. This kind of study could yield new information concerning the regional metabolism of the developing heart as well as its control by the autonomic nervous system. Therefore a series of preliminary studies was implemented using the [^{14}C]2-deoxyglucose technique in the chick to specifically study the developing chick heart. Fourteen developing chicks at 11 days of incubation were administered a single bolus of 6 μCi of [^{14}C]2-deoxyglucose (specific activity 55 mCi/mmol) suspended in saline, through the vitelline vein. After 45 minutes at 37 °C, the chicks were rapidly removed from the eggs and frozen in -40 °C isopentane. The chicks were then frozen-sectioned sagittally at 20 μm, and placed on glass coverslips. They were then dried, covered with film, and stored in X-ray cassettes with a set of [^{14}C] standards for 12 days. An example of a computer scanned auto-radiograph of glucose utilization in the 11 day chick heart is shown in the left panel of FIGURE 11. Red represents the greatest [^{14}C]2-deoxyglucose utilization, followed by yellow and then by green. The blues and white represent the least amount of glucose utilization. The autoradiographic data revealed that glucose utilization is not uniform across the walls of the 11 day developing chick heart, nor from the base of the heart to the apex. The apex uses considerably less glucose than the base, and the right ventricle and septum uses more glucose than the left ventricle. There are some additional well-defined regions of the left ventricular wall, however, that have relatively high glucose utilization. This study demonstrates that glucose utilization by the 11 day developing heart is not uniform.

REGIONAL DISTRIBUTION OF MYOCARDIAL BLOOD FLOW IN THE DEVELOPING CHICK HEART USING THALLIUM-201

One question that immediately arises when one looks at the regional differences in glucose utilization by the developing heart is: Does regional myocardial blood flow have the same directional changes as regional myocardial glucose utilization? The only way to answer this question is to use an autoradiographic method that has the same spatial resolution as the [^{14}C]2-deoxyglucose technique. Thallium-201 was selected as the preferred method over radioactive microspheres inasmuch as the microspheres require that chunks of tissue be counted in a scintillation counter, or if used autoradiographically, the microspheres would appear as a few spots of intense activity on the autoradiographs. Thallium-201 autoradiography, however, is an index of blood flow because it binds to the myocardium in proportion to regional myocardial blood flow.[56,69,70] Thallium-201 is therefore distributed within the autoradiographs in

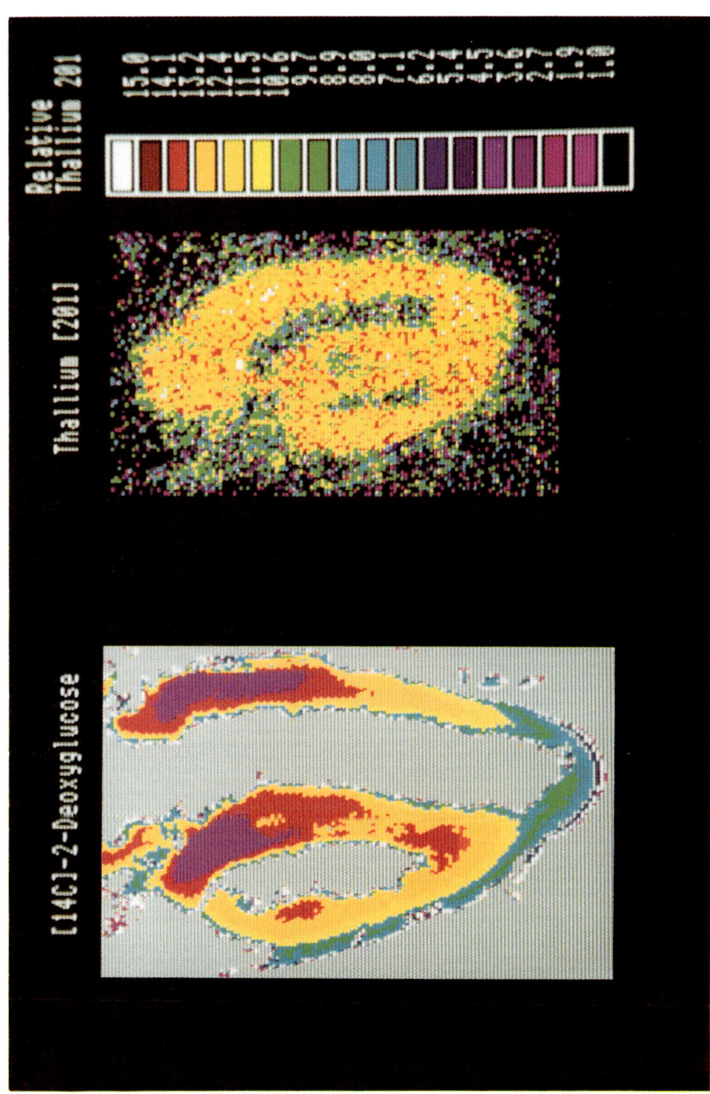

FIGURE 11. Myccardial glucose utilization and blood flow in an 11 day incubated chick heart.

proportion to myocardial blood flow. The distribution of blood flow in the developing chick heart was studied autoradiographically in four chicks at 11 days of incubation, and in four chicks at 17 days of incubation. The purpose of this study was to determine if the regional changes in glucose utilization that were observed in the developing chick hearts, of the same age, were due to regional differences in myocardial blood flow. These two ages were selected for both the [^{14}C]2-deoxyglucose utilization studies and the thallium-201 studies because the coronary arteries are not fully functional at 11 days of incubation, whereas at 17 days, experimental evidence suggests that they may be fully functional. Therefore, glucose delivery to the myocardium is accomplished by diffusion for most of the developmental period. Thallium-201 was injected into the vitelline vein, 2.2 μCi/g fetal weight, in a volume of 1 mL of saline using a 30 gauge needle. After 5 minutes, the viability of the chick was determined by observing a regular heartbeat and spontaneous movements of the fetus. The unhatched chick was then removed from the egg and frozen in $-40\,°$C isopentane. The chicks were then frozen-sectioned at 20 μm increments using a cryostat, and prepared for autoradiography on the same day as the experiment, because thallium-201 has a half life of 74 hours. After 6 hours of exposure to mammography film and developing, the autoradiographs were scanned using a computerized densitometer. Representative examples of the thallium-201-scanned autoradiographs from the 11 day and 17 day chick hearts are shown in FIGURES 11 and 12. In the 11 day chick hearts, the blood flow across the heart was uniform. This was in contrast to the marked regional differences in glucose utilization across the same regions of the heart. Yonekura[56] demonstrated in hypertensive Dahl rats that regional myocardial blood flow was homogeneous using thallium-201. Simultaneous autoradiographic measurements of free fatty acid uptake, however, demonstrated that there were marked regional decreases in free fatty acid in the same regions where blood flow was measured to be uniform. This suggests, as does our preliminary data from the developing chick, that regional myocardial blood flow may not always be coupled with regional changes in myocardial metabolism. In the 17 day chick hearts, regional differences in glucose utilization were observed; however, these were coupled with changes in blood flow as indicated by the thallium-201 autoradiographs.

REGIONAL DISTRIBUTION OF GLUCOSE UTILIZATION IN THE DEVELOPING CHICK HEART AT 17 DAYS OF INCUBATION

Using the identical procedure described above, we studied the distribution of glucose utilization in chick hearts at 17 days of incubation. In this pilot study one major change was made. Rather than injecting the [^{14}C]2-deoxyglucose on the basis of the egg weight, the amount injected was based on the weight of the fetus. The reason for this change was twofold; first, it was more accurate to base the dose injected on the fetal weight; and second, many of the 11 day autoradiographs were quite dark, indicating that the original dose of [^{14}C]2-deoxyglucose was in excess of what was really needed. Therefore, in the present study and in all future studies, the amount of [^{14}C]2-deoxyglucose to be injected is to be based on 100 μCi/kg of fetal weight. FIGURE 12 is an example of the pattern of glucose utilization in the chick heart at 17 days of incubation. The right ventricle is located on the left side of the FIGURE and the left ventricle is shown on the right. In general, the glucose utilization of the 17 day chick heart seems to be rather uniform with occasional pockets of increased

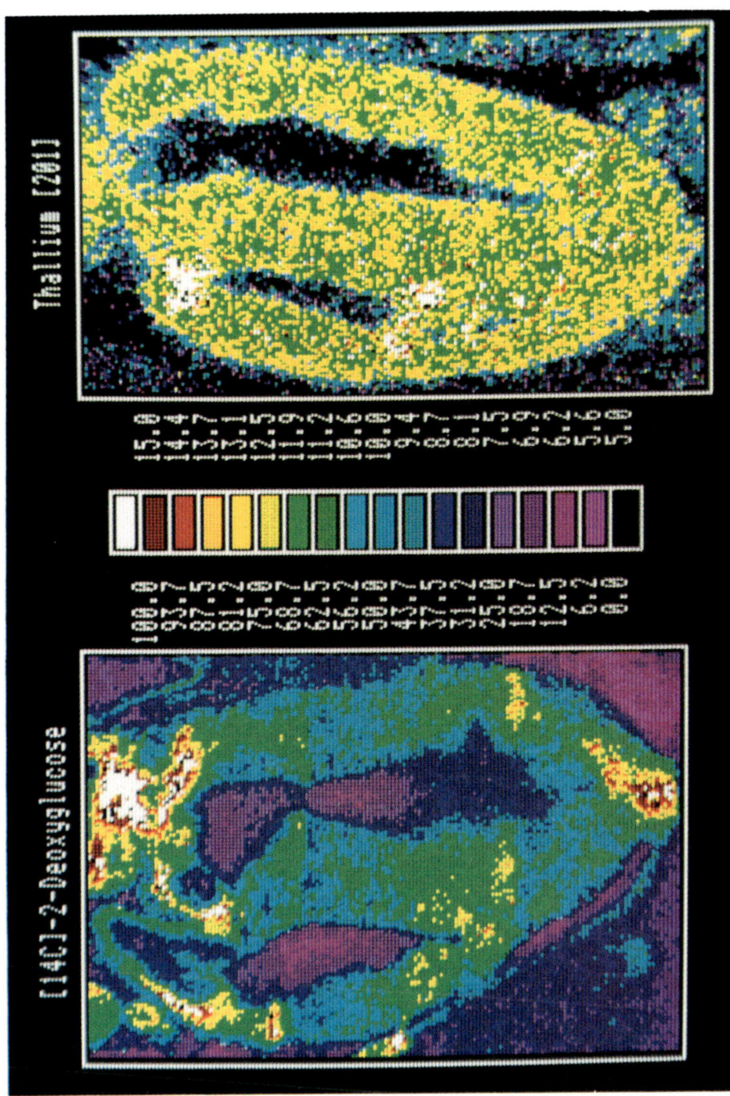

FIGURE 12. Myocardial glucose utilization and blood flow in a 17 day incubated chick heart.

glucose utilization primarily at the base of the heart and a small pocket of activity at the apex. The increased activity at the base seems to agree with that seen in adult mammalian hearts.[57–60] The pocket of increased glucose utilization at the apex, however, does not have a correlate in the mammalian model. The blood flow pattern shown on the right panel of FIGURE 12 is similar to the glucose utilization pattern with the exception of the apex. It should be remembered, however, that this is preliminary data that will be clarified in further studies of the developing chick and rabbit hearts using these techniques.

SUMMARY AND DISCUSSION

The scope of these preliminary studies has been directed toward a more thorough understanding of the fundamental metabolic processes of the developing avian and mammalian heart. Our data strongly suggest that glucose utilization of the developing avian and mammalian hearts is not uniform. In fact, regional differences exist in all of the species studied to date. Regional myocardial blood flow does remain rather uniform during most of the gestation period. This suggests that there is an uncoupling of myocardial blood flow and metabolism within the developing chick heart. Regional blood flow distribution has not been studied autoradiographically in the developing mammalian heart.

The question arises, therefore: What does all of this have to do with embryonic origins of cardiac development? The answer to this question is given partially in FIGURE 1, which was presented near the beginning of this chapter. Specific regions of the neural crest give rise to the sympathetic or parasympathetic components of cardiac innervation. Ablations of the truncal neural crest S10-20, which give rise to the sympathetic component of cardiac innervation, do not seem to give rise to any known defects in cardiac anatomy. Significant defects in cardiac metabolism related to cAMP and glycogen metabolism are produced, however. On the other hand, ablations of cardiac neural crest S1-3, which give rise to the parasympathetic innervation of the heart, also produce many cardiac defects including persistent truncus arteriosus. The metabolic effects of this cardiac parasympathetic ablation, however, have not been studied. As discussed earlier we know that normal cardiac metabolism and normal cardiac anatomy are required for normal cardiac function and that cardiac metabolism and anatomy are reciprocally dependent upon one another. It is the neural influences on both cardiac anatomy and metabolism that are of particular interest, because these effects not only influence the developing heart, but they are prominent throughout adult life as well. The importance of understanding the metabolism of the developing heart is also underscored in the management of the neonate with a diabetic mother. As we begin to more fully understand the metabolic processes of the developing heart and the obvious changes that occur in cardiac metabolism at birth, as the heart switches metabolic fuels from glucose to free fatty acids, it may be possible someday to devise metabolic treatments that will render a better quality of life for newborns with compromised cardiac function.

There are many windows through which one can view the developing heart. Windows of anatomy, physiology, molecular biology, genetics, pharmacology, and ion channels. What has been presented in this chapter is just a hazy glimpse of the developing heart through the window of cardiac metabolism. The view is not clear because the data presented are preliminary and require a concentrated effort to evaluate and integrate this new metabolic information with that derived from the other disciplines contributing to our understanding of cardiac development in health and disease. It will be the marriage of this information that will ultimately enable us to fully understand and possibly manipulate the course of events that will eradicate abnormal cardiac development of all causes. These studies should yield new and important information that will further our understanding of the underlying mechanisms of congenital heart disease, providing a basis for the development of enhanced diagnostic and therapeutic strategies for the prevention and treatment of congenital cardiac defects.

ACKNOWLEDGMENT

The technical help and expertise of Mr. James Wood was greatly appreciated.

REFERENCES

1. BOYD, J. D. 1965. Development of the heart. *In* Handbook of Physiology; Section 2: Circulation. W. F. Hamilton, Ed. **III:** 2511-2543. American Physiological Society. Washington, D.C.
2. FAITH, D. S., M. L. KIRBY & D. W. SICKLES. 1987. Carbohydrate, lipid and oxidative metabolism in the sympathetically aneural chick heart. J. Mol. Cell. Cardiol. **19:** 349-355.
3. KIRBY, M. L. 1987. Cardiac morphogenesis - recent research advances. Pediatr. Res. **21:** 219-224.
4. KIRBY, M. L. 1988. Nodose placode contributes autonomic neurons to the heart in the absence of cardiac neural crest. J. Neurosci. **8:** 1089-1095.
5. KIRBY, M. L. 1988. Nodose placode provides ectomesenchyme to the developing chick heart in the absence of cardiac neural crest. Cell Tissue Res. **252:** 17-22.
6. KIRBY, M. L. & R. S. ARONSTAM. 1983. Atropine-induced alterations of normal development of muscarinic receptors in the embryonic chick heart. J. Mol. Cell. Cardiol. **15:** 685-696.
7. KIRBY, M. L., R. S. ARONSTAM & J. J. BUCCAFUSCO. 1985. Changes in cholinergic parameters associated with failure of conotruncal septation in embryonic chick hearts after neural crest ablation. Circ. Res. **56:** 392-401.
8. KIRBY, M. L. & D. E. BOCKMAN. 1984. Neural crest and normal development: a new perspective. Anat. Rec. **209:** 1-6.
9. KIRBY, M. L., D. C. CONRAD & D. E. STEWART. 1987. Increase in the cholinergic cardiac plexus in sympathetically aneural chick hearts. Cell. Tissue Res. **247:** 489-496.
10. KIRBY, M. L., T. F. GALE & D. E. STEWART. 1983. Neural crest cells contribute to normal aorticopulmonary septation. Science **220:** 1059-1061.
11. KIRBY, M. L., J. W. MCKENZIE & T. A. WEIDMAN. 1980. Developing innervation of the chick heart: a histofluoresence and light microscopic study of sympathetic innervation. Anat. Rec. **196:** 333-340.
12. KIRBY, M. & D. STEWART. 1984. Adrenergic innervation of the developing chick heart: Neural crest ablations to produce sympathetically aneural hearts. Am. J. Anat. **171:** 295-305.
13. KIRBY, M. L. & D. E. STEWART. 1983. Neural crest origin of cardiac ganglion cells in the chick embryo: identification and extirpation. Dev. Biol. **97:** 433-443.
14. KIRBY, M. L. & D. E. STEWART. 1986. *In* Developmental neurobiology of the autonomic nervous system. P.M. Gootman, Ed.: 135-158. The Human Press, Inc. Clifton, N.J.

15. KIRBY, M. L., K. L. TURNAGE, III & B. M. HAYS. 1985. Characterization of conotruncal malformations following ablation of "cardiac" neural crest. Anat. Rec. **213:** 87-93.

16. KIRBY, M. L., T. A. WEIDMAN & J. W. McKENZIE. 1980. An ultrastructural study of the cardiac ganglia in the bulbar plexus of the developing chick heart. Dev. Neurosci. **3:** 174-184.

17. NISHIBATAKE, M., M. L. KIRBY & L. H. S. VAN MIEROP. 1987. Pathogenesis of persistent truncus arteriosus and dextraposed aorta in the chick embryo after neural crest ablation. Circulation **75:** 255-264.

18. PHILLIPS, M. T., M. L. KIRBY & G. FORBES. 1987. Analysis of cranial neural crest distribution in the developing heart using quail-chick chimeras. Circ. Res. **60:** 27-30.

19. PHILLIPS, M. T., M. L. KIRBY & D. E. STEWART. 1986. Cyclic AMP in normal and sympathetically aneural chick hearts during development. J. Mol. Cell. Cardiol. **18:** 827-835.

20. STEWART, D. E., M. L. KIRBY & K. K. SULIK. 1986. Hemodynamic changes in chick embryos precede heart defects after cardiac neural crest ablation. Circ. Res. **59:** 545-550.

21. BESSON, WILLIAM T., III, M. L. KIRBY et al. 1986. Effects of cardiac neural crest lesion size at various embryonic ages on incidence and type of cardiac defects. Circulation **73:** 360-364.

22. MARTEL, A. D'AMICO & D. M. NODEN. 1983. Contributions of placodal and neural crest cells to avian cranial peripheral ganglia. Am. J. Anat. **166:** 445-468.

23. TOSNEY, K. W. 1982. The segregation and early migration of cranial neural crest cells in the avian embryo. Dev. Biol. **89:** 13-24.

24. NARAYANAN, C. H. & Y. NARAYANAN. 1980. Neural crest and placodal contributions in the development of the glossopharyngeal-vagal complex in the chick. Anat. Rec. **196:** 71-82.

25. NEELY, J. R. & H. E. MORGAN. 1974. Relationship between carbohydrate and lipid metabolism and the energy balance of heart muscle. Annu. Rev. Physiol. **36:** 413-459.

26. WATSHAW, J. B. 1979. Fatty acid metabolism during development. Semin. Perinatol. N.Y. **3:** 131-139.

27. WERNER, J. C., R. E. SICARD & H. G. SCHULER. 1989. Palmitate oxidation by isolated working fetal and newborn pig hearts. Am. J. Physiol. **256:** E315-E321.

28. AMATAYAKUL, O., G. R. CUMMING & J. C. HAWORTH. 1970. Association of hypoglycemia with cardiac enlargement and CHF in newborn infants. Arch. Dis. Child. **45:** 717-720.

29. BATTAGLIA, F. C. & G. MESCHIA. 1978. Principal substrates of fetal metabolism. Physiol. Rev. **58:** 499-527.

30. BREUER, E., E. BARTA, E. PAPPOVA & L. ZLATOS. 1967. Developmental changes of myocardial metabolism. I. Peculiarities of cardiac carbohydrate metabolism in the early post-natal period in dogs. Biol. Neonat. **11:** 367-377.

31. HARARY, I. 1979. Biochemistry of cardiac development: *in vivo* and *in vitro* studies. *In* Handbook of Physiology, Section 2: The Cardiovascular System. R. M. Berne & N. Sperelakis, Eds.: 43-60. Williams and Wilkins Co. Baltimore, MD.

32. JONES, C. T. & T. P. ROLPH. 1985. Metabolism during fetal life: a functional assessment of metabolic development. Physiol. Rev. **65:** 357-430.

33. WARSHAW, J. B. 1969. Cellular energy metabolism during fetal development. I. Oxidation phosphorylation in the fetal heart. J. Cell Biol. **41:** 651-657.

34. WILDENTHAL, K. 1973. Studies of foetal mouse hearts in organ culture: metabolic requirements for prolonged function *in vitro* and the influence of cardiac maturation on substrate utilization. J. Mol. Cell Cardiol. **5:** 87-99.

35. WITTELS, B. & R. BRESSLER. 1965. Lipid metabolism in the newborn heart. J. Clin. Invest. **44:** 1639-1646.

36. WYLER, F., F. ROHNER, A. OLAFSSON, H. CHRISTEN & C. FLIEGEL. 1976. Cardiomegaly in neonatal hypoglycemia. Eur. J. Pediatr. **121:** 119-124.

37. SMITH, H. E. & E. PAGE. 1977. Ultrastructural changes in rabbit heart mitochondria during the perinatal period. Dev. Biol. **57:** 109-117.

38. WERNER, J. C., V. WHITMAN, R. R. FRIPP, H. G. SCHULER, J. MUSSELMAN & R. L. SHAM. 1983. Fatty acid and glucose utilization in isolated working fetal pig hearts. Am. J. Physiol. **245:** E19-E23.

39. POND, W. G. & K. A. HOUPT. 1978. The Biology of the Pig. 82-101. Cornell Univ. Press. Ithaca, N.Y.
40. WERNER, J. C., V. WHITMAN, T. C. VARY, R. R. FEIPP, J. MUSSELMAN & H. G. SCHULTER. 1983. Fatty acid and glucose utilization in isolated, working newborn pig hearts. Am. J. Physiol. **244:** E19-E23.
41. URETA, T. 1982. The comparative isozymology of vertebrate hexokinases. Comp. Biochem. Physiol. **71B:** 549-555.
42. STAVE, U. 1964. Age-dependent changes of metabolism. I. Studies of enzyme patterns of rabbit organs. Biol. Neonat. **6:** 128-147.
43. FOA, P. P., M. MELLI, C. K. BERGER, D. BILLINGER & G. G. GUIDOTTI. 1965. Action of insulin on chick embryo heart. Fed. Proc. **24:** 1046-1050.
44. KUTCHAI, H., S. L. KING, M. MARTIN & E. D. DAVES. 1977. Glucose uptake by chicken embryo hearts at various stages of development. Dev. Biol. **55:** 92-102.
45. GIBBS, C. L. 1978. Cardiac Energetics. Physiol. Rev. **58:** 174-254.
46. LIEDTKE, A. J., S. H. NELLIS & O. D. MJOS. 1984. Effects of reducing fatty acid metabolism on mechanical function in regionally ischemic hearts. Am. J. Physiol. **247:** H387-H394.
47. OPIE, L. H. 1968. Metabolism of the heart in health and disease. Part I. Am. Heart J. **76:** 685-698.
48. OPIE, L. H. 1969. Metabolism of the heart in health and disease. Part II. Am. Heart J. **77:** 100-122.
49. OPIE, L. H. 1969. Metabolism of the heart in health and disease. Part III. Am. Heart J. **77:** 383-410.
50. TAEGETMEYER, H. 1986. *In* Positron Emission Tomography and Autoradiography: Principles for the Brain and Heart. M. Phelps, J. Mazziotta & H. Schelbert, Eds.: Chapter 4. Raven Press. New York.
51. TAKALA, T. E. S. & I. E. HASSINEN. 1981. Effects of mechanical work load on the transmural distribution of glucose uptake in the isolated perfused rat heart, studied by regional deoxyglucose trapping. Circ. Res. **49:** 62-69.
52. TAKALA, T. E. S., H. J. RUSKOAHO & I. E. HASSINEN. 1983. Transmural distribution of cardiac glucose uptake in rat during physical exercise. Am. J. Physiol. **244:** H131-H137.
53. SOKOLOFF, L. *et al.* 1977. The [^{14}C]deoxyglucose method for the measurement of local cerebral glucose utilization: theory, procedure, and normal values in the albino rat. J. Neurochem. **28:** 897-916.
54. L'ABBATE, A., P. CAMICI, M. G. TRIVELLA, G. PELOSI, L. TADDEI, G. VALLI & G. F. PLACIDI. 1979. Uneven myocardial glucose utilization as determined by [^{14}C]deoxyglucose uptake. J. Nucl. Med. Allied Sci. **23:** 167-172.
55. MATSUNAMI, K. 1982. Radioactive deoxyglucose uptake into the heart muscle of the monkey. Jn. J. Physiol. **32:** 321-325.
56. YONEKURA, Y. *et al.* 1985. Regional myocardial substrate uptake in hypertensive rats: a quantitative autoradiographic measurement. Science **227:** 1494-1496.
57. KOSTREVA, D. R. 1983. Functional mapping of cardiovascular reflexes and the heart using 2-[^{14}C]deoxyglucose. Physiologist **26:** 333-350.
58. KOSTREVA, D. R., J. A. ARMOUR & Z. J. BOSNJAK. 1985. Metabolic mapping of a cardiac reflex mediated by sympathetic ganglia in dogs. Am. J. Physiol. **249:** R317-R322.
59. KOSTREVA, D. R., J. D. WOOD & M. M. OLSEN. 1987. High spatial resolution autoradiographic assessment of regional myocardial glucose utilization in the fetal and adult feline heart. Fed. Proc. **46:** 4682.
60. HERMAN, N. L. & D. R. KOSTREVA. 1986. Alterations in cardiac [^{14}C]deoxyglucose uptake induced by two renal afferent stimuli. Am. J. Physiol. **251:** R867-R877.
61. ARMSTRONG, P. B. 1931. Functional reactions in the embryonic heart accompanying the ingrowth and development of the vagus innervation. J. Exp. Zool. **58:** 43-61.
62. KUNTZ, A. 1910. The development of the sympathetic nervous system in mammals. J. Comp. Neurol. Psychol. **20:** 211-258.
63. KUNTZ, A. 1910. The development of the sympathetic nervous system in birds. J. Comp. Neurol. Psychol. **20:** 283-308.
64. LE GRANDE, M. C., G. H. PAFF & R. J. BOUCEK. 1966. Initiation of vagal control of heart rate in the embryonic chick. Anat. Rec. **155:** 163-166.

65. PAPPANO, A. 1977. Ontogenetic development of autonomic neuroeffector transmission and transmitter reactivity in embryonic and fetal hearts. Pharm. Rev. **29:** 3-33.
66. RANDALL, W. C., Ed. 1977. Neural Regulation of the Heart. Oxford University Press. New York.
67. RANDALL, W.C., Ed. 1984. Nervous Control of Cardiovascular Function. Oxford University Press. New York.
68. KOSTREVA, D. R. 1989. Fetal glucose utilization using maternal plasma glucose and scintillation values. Brain Res. **487:** 384-387.
69. SCHELBERT, H. R. & M. SCHWAIGER. 1986. PET studies of the heart. *In* Positron Emission Tomography and Autoradiography: Principles and Applications for the Brain and Heart. M. Phelps, J. Mazziotta & H. Schelbert, Eds.: 581-666. Raven Press. New York.
70. STRAUSS, H.W., K. HARRISON, J. K. LANGAN, E. LEBOWITZ & B. PITT. 1975. Thallium-201 for myocardial imaging: relation of thallium-201 to regional myocardial perfusion. Circulation **51:** 641-645.

The Instructive Role of Fibronectins in Cell Migrations during Embryonic Development

JEAN-LOUP DUBAND, SYLVIE DUFOUR, AND
JEAN PAUL THIERY

*Laboratoire de Physiopathologie du Développement du Centre
National de la Recherche Scientifique
Ecole Normale Supérieure
75230 Paris Cedex 05, France*

Migration and coalescence of cells originating from different territories of the embryo play a key role in morphogenesis in pluricellular organisms. These processes are also particularly essential for induction, and therefore govern the differentiative capacities of cells. In some favorable exceptions cell migrations can be visualized directly, but in most cases only the labeling of progenitors permits us to define precisely the pattern of translocation of cells.[1] These techniques in association with light and electron microscopy have revealed that the great majority of embryonic cell migrations occur within or in contact with a fibrillar extracellular matrix containing glycosaminoglycans and proteoglycans, collagens, fibronectins, cytotactin or tenascin, and thrombospondin. Particular attention was focused on fibronectins, because they were shown to promote adhesion and migration of cells *in vitro*,[2,3] and therefore could play a role in cell migrations *in vivo*. In this brief review, we first describe the major structural and functional properties of fibronectins; then we examine their role in the migration of neural crest cells, a cell population that is well-known for its striking migratory properties. Finally, we compare the mode of migration of neural crest cells with other motile cells and more particularly with those that contribute to the heart anlage.

STRUCTURE AND FUNCTIONS OF FIBRONECTINS AND OF THEIR INTEGRIN RECEPTORS

Fibronectins constitute a family of large heterodimeric multifunctional glycoproteins present in most extracellular matrices, in the plasma, and in other body fluids.[4] Structural and functional studies have clearly established that all fibronectin molecules contain distinct domains that interact with various extracellular glycoproteins and proteoglycans including collagen, fibrin, and heparin. On the other hand, fibronectins possess binding properties for cell surface receptors. One critical advance has been to identify in fibronectin molecules a unique tetrapeptide sequence (RGDS) as a crucial adhesive recognition signal for cells.[5] Fibronectins have been implicated in a variety of cell behaviors, including adhesion, spreading, morphology, and migration. They are also thought to play an important role in thrombosis, wound healing, and in cancer invasion and metastasis.[6] It is now generally accepted that most if not all biological properties of fibronectins derive from their adhesive functions.

Different fibronectin forms arise by an alternative splicing mechanism operating in three distinct regions of the primary transcript. Two exons called extra domain 1 (ED1 or EIIIA) and extra domain 2 (ED2 or EIIIB) can be spliced independently except in the liver where the plasma form of fibronectins lacks these two sequences.[7,8] Another region associated with the last type III homology and designated as type III homology connecting segment (IIICS) or variable region (V) undergoes a differential alternative splicing leading to two to five different messages depending on the species examined.[9–11]

An important recent discovery is that fibronectins contain several cell-adhesion sites aside from the RGDS sequence. The first indication for this derives from the observation that, although short fragments of fibronectins containing the RGDS sequence retain some adhesive functions, their estimated affinity for the receptor is decreased by one to two orders of magnitude if they are below a certain size. Using wild type and mutated fusion proteins of different sizes in the RGDS region, it was possible to map a new adhesion site located approximately 200 amino acids towards the amino terminus from the RGDS sequence.[12] This site in synergy with the RGDS site provides full affinity, and together these sites constitute the major adhesion domain. A second important domain is located in the IIICS region.[13] This domain is also composed of two distinct, independent sites that were found to promote selectively, and in an additive manner, adhesion of melanoma cells. Interestingly, because these two sites are located in the IIICS region, they can be alternatively spliced, and consequently they are not present in all fibronectin molecules. Finally, a third adhesion domain located in the heparin-binding domain adjacent to IIICS has been shown to play a critical role in adhesion of tumor and nerve cells.[14,15]

Surface receptors for fibronectins belong to a family of receptors called integrins. They are heterodimeric transmembrane glycoproteins that have been classified according to their β subunits.[16,17] So far, three different β subunits have been found, and each of them can be associated with several distinct α subunits. There are several fibronectin-binding integrins, the best characterized of which is $\alpha5 \beta1$, also termed VLA-5. The binding of $\alpha5 \beta1$ fibronectin receptors to fibronectins can be inhibited by soluble RGDS peptides, whereas none of the other members sharing the same $\beta1$ subunit are sensitive to this tetrapeptide.

One of the most important features of the fibronectin receptor is its potential ability to transduce the adhesive signal intracellularly because it provides a physical link between the external ligand and the cytoskeleton. Indeed, there is evidence that the short cytoplasmic domain of the α or β subunits can interact with talin. Talin can also associate with vinculin, which is known to interact with other cytoskeletal proteins including tensin and α-actinin. All these proteins are concentrated at specific adhesion sites in stationary cells spread on fibronectin substrates.[18] Furthermore, binding of fibronectins to their receptors can induce the clustering of these elements and local reorganization of the cytoskeleton, subsequently affecting cell shape and cell behavior. Conversely, at least in Rous sarcoma transformed cells, phosphorylation on a tyrosine residue of the β subunit of the fibronectin receptor can alter binding to fibronectins and prevent the proper assembly of the cortical cytoskeleton, leading to the rounding up of the transformed cells.[19]

Fibronectins and integrins have been detected in all the vertebrates examined so far where they were found to appear very early during development. For example, in the mouse embryo, fibronectin molecules are first detected as early as the 16-cell stage.[20] In birds and in fish, they are present in the blastoderm just prior to the movements involved in gastrulation and epiboly.[21] In amphibians, fibronectins are already present in the oocyte; they are also synthesized during the cleavage stage from maternally derived mRNA.[22] In all species, fibronectins are later predominantly associated with the extracellular matrices of mesenchymes and with most if not all basement membranes of epithelia. A great majority of embryonic cells in vertebrates express β1-containing integrins;[23–25] however, the prevalence of each member of the β1 class of receptors during development has not been determined yet.

ROLE OF FIBRONECTINS IN THE MIGRATION OF NEURAL CREST CELLS

The neural crest provides a powerful paradigm for cell migration in the early vertebrate embryo.[26] The development of crest cells is a multistep process where cells may be found alternatively in a cohesive or a dispersed state. It starts with the loss of the epithelial arrangement of premigratory neural crest cells at the apex of the closing neural tube followed by extensive migration along well-characterized pathways through adjacent structures. After reaching their sites of arrest in various areas of the embryo, neural crest cells often coalesce into cohesive compact cells and undergo differentiation into a large variety of cell types, ranging from neurons and glial cells of the peripheral nervous system to connective tissues in the head and neck. Among the reasons that make the neural crest attractive to study cell migration are the ability to culture crest cells and somewhat mimic their *in vivo* translocations in an *in vitro* system, and the possibility of directly perturbing their migration *in vivo*.

Requirement of Fibronectins for Neural Crest Cell Migration

Evidence for a prominent role of fibronectins in neural crest cell migration has come from *in vitro* experiments in which it was found that crest cells preferentially attach, spread, and migrate onto matrices or amorphous substrates containing fibronectins rather than onto other extracellular matrix components including collagen, glycosaminoglycans, and laminin.[27–29] Many perturbation experiments performed with RGDS-containing synthetic peptides and with antibodies directed either to fibronectins or to the β1 subunits of integrins have demonstrated that direct interaction between fibronectins and the surface of neural crest cells is required for their adhesion and motility both *in vivo* and *in vitro*.[23,28,30–32]

Mode of Interaction of Neural Crest Cells with Fibronectins

If neural crest cells require fibronectins for their migration, it should be remembered that nonmotile cells also depend on fibronectins for their anchorage to the substratum. How can a single molecule promote both the permanent anchorage of an immobile cell and the labile adhesion of a motile cell to their substrates? This apparent dual function of fibronectins may result in part from differences in the modes of interaction between locomoting and stationary cells and fibronectin molecules.

The primary condition required for cell locomotion is that the cell should not adhere too strongly to the substratum to avoid paralysis. This has been demonstrated using silicone-rubber sheets as a substrate for migration.[33] There appears to be an inverse correlation between the degree of motility of a cell and its ability to induce distortions in the rubber sheet, suggesting that motile cells are not attached firmly to the substratum or that they do not generate sufficient forces for wrinkling. The importance of weak transient adhesion to the substratum in cell locomotion has been further demonstrated by culturing neural crest cells onto high affinity antibodies to the fibronectin receptor.[23] Under these conditions, fibronectin receptors bind almost irreversibly to the antibodies and, consequently, the rate of migration of neural crest cells is considerably reduced.

Differences in the strength of interaction with the substratum are presumably reflected in the organization of both the substratum contact sites and cytoskeleton. The primary mode of anchorage to the substratum of a stationary cell is by way of restricted sites called focal and close contacts where the ventral membrane is in close proximity to the substratum. Much of the rest of the ventral plasma membrane is further away from the substratum.[34] By contrast, locomotory cells interact more uniformly with the substratum at broad close contacts and develop only a limited number of focal contacts.[23,35] In stationary cells, actin microfilaments are bundled into stress fibers that terminate in focal contacts. In these regions, actin bundles are attached to the membrane by way of the cytoskeletal proteins talin, vinculin, and tensin.[18] In motile cells, actin microfilaments are not extensively bundled and are mainly distributed as a network in the cellular cortex,[23,33] whereas talin and vinculin remain primarily diffuse throughout the cytoplasm. Fibronectin receptors are distributed as a nearly homogeneous pattern over the entire surface of motile cells, in striking contrast to stationary cells where they are concentrated in clusters around focal contacts and in fibrillar streaks that align with fibronectin fibrils externally and actin microfilament bundles internally.[36,37]

Thus, the immobilization and concentration of fibronectin receptors at focal contacts and fibrillar streaks in coincidence with actin bundles may increase locally the binding strength between the receptor, fibronectins, and the cytoskeleton, providing a strong and stable attachment to the substratum and inducing complete immobilization of the cell. By contrast, the absence of concentration of receptors at specific sites on the cell surface together with a poorly organized cytoskeleton would enable the cell to change shape rapidly and allow labile adhesions to the substratum required for motility.

Aside from differences in the subcellular distribution of molecules involved in substratum adhesion, the specificity of the locomotory behavior of crest cells may also reside at a more discrete level, that is, in the mode of recognition of fibronectin molecules by fibronectin receptors. Indeed, advances in the cell-binding domains of fibronectins have revealed a far more intricate way of interaction between a cell and fibronectins than thought before. Recent experiments have suggested that the various cell-binding sites along fibronectins show specificity not only for the cells they bind (see above), but also for the function they mediate. Thus, it was found that neural crest cells recognize for their attachment and spreading the RGDS sequence in association with its synergistic site, but they are also able to bind for their attachment the CS1-adhesion site of the IIICS region. In addition, neither the RGDS site nor the CS1 site alone is able to promote independently the migration of neural crest cells. This process requires at least the presence of both sites, but it cannot be excluded that other sequences within fibronectins may also be involved. This study clearly indicates that the various adhesion sites of fibronectins possess functional specificities and can act synergistically, resulting in the acquisition by cells of complex, coherent behavior.[38] An important consequence may arise from this observation. Because the CS1 binding site can be alternatively spliced in fibronectin molecules, it is of interest to know whether fibronectin variants containing this domain would be differentially distributed in embryos. *In situ* hybridization studies carried out at stages of development when neural crest cells are migrating did not reveal, however, specific sites of mRNA production of the different variants.[39]

Regulation of Interactions between Fibronectin Receptors and their Ligands

Direct binding of the fibronectin receptor with fibronectins, on one hand, and talin, on the other hand, has been described with the isolated molecules,[40] thus confirming *in situ* observations that the receptor provides a transmembrane linkage between the extracellular matrix and the cytoskeleton. Differences in the distribution of fibronectin receptors on the surface of motile and stationary cells then suggest that the links between the receptor and its ligands would differ in the two states. The use of the fluorescence recovery after photobleaching technique appeared particularly suitable for examining the dynamics of the interaction between the receptor and its ligands. Indeed, the lateral mobility of integral membrane proteins within the plane of the plasma membrane is indicative of the degree of association of the molecule with peripheral structures such as the extracellular matrix and the cytoskeleton.[41,42] It was found that the population of fibronectin receptors is mobile in locomotory cells, whereas it is almost totally immobile when it is concentrated in focal contacts and fibrillar streaks in stationary cells.[43] Thus, the high lateral mobility of the receptor in motile cells suggests that a large majority of receptors are bound to fibronectins and cytoskeletal components, but these interactions are very transient; the receptors rapidly dissociate from their ligands to establish new associations with other peripheral molecules. Increase in the number of peripheral ligands simultaneously bound to the receptor would increase the immobile fraction of receptors. This multivalent, immobilized receptor state would provide stable anchorage to the substratum. It will be important in the future to examine how the receptor is transported and localized to sites appropriate for locomotion, inasmuch as the numbers and types of these sites presumably regulate the locomotory state of a cell.

What could be the regulatory mechanism of the interaction between the receptor and its ligands? A diffuse distribution of fibronectin receptors has been reported in virally transformed cells.[44] In such cells, it has also been shown that the receptor is phosphorylated on tyrosine residues,[19] which could possibly modify its binding properties. No receptor phosphorylation, however, could be detected in embryonic motile cells, indicating that the process of regulation of receptor binding differs considerably in these cells and in transformed cells.[45] Alternatively, regulation of receptor binding would preferentially involve rapid internalization of the receptor. When living cells are labeled with a rhodamine-conjugated monoclonal antibody directed to the receptor, fluorescence is rapidly seen in vesicles in the cytoplasm of motile cells but not in stationary cells. Whether the receptor is internalized with fibronectin molecules and cytoskeletal elements, however, remains to be determined.

CONCLUDING REMARKS

The example of the neural crest provides strong evidence for a direct interaction between embryonic migratory cells and fibronectins. It remains to establish, however, whether other migratory cells and, more particularly, cells that contribute to the heart also require fibronectins for their displacement.

In the chicken embryo, two waves of migration of cells have been described during the genesis of the heart. The first one occurs during gastrulation and involves a subset of mesodermal cells that regroup in a particular region of the embryo to form the precardiac cells. These cells subsequently move anteriorly to reach the midline of the embryo, where they differentiate into two endocardial tubes, which fuse later to form the beating tubular heart. An increasing concentration of fibronectins has been detected along the migratory route of the precardiac mesoderm, suggesting a haptotactic mechanism, that is, a gradient of adhesiveness on the substrate involved in the directionality of migration of these cells.[46] *In vitro,* a culture of whole embryos at the stage of precardiac cell migration in the presence of a variety of antibodies clearly demonstrated that only antifibronectin antibodies were able to arrest migration of precardiac cells before reaching the midline; consequently, heart tissues form in several separate regions of the embryo. In agreement with these results, RGDS peptides also induced abnormal development of the heart primordium with a partial cardia bifida. Antibodies to the $\beta1$ chains of integrins, however, were unable to perturb these morphogenetic events.[47]

The second wave of migration takes place later, when the heart tube has formed. The inner endocardium layer becomes separated from the myocardium by an expanded extracellular matrix, namely the cardiac jelly. A number of endocardiac cells from the atrioventricular zone soon break away from the endocardium and migrate into the cardiac jelly to form the heart septa and the valves. In this region, the cardiac jelly contains a gradient of fibronectins, suggesting again a haptotactic mechanism for migration of cells.[48] No perturbation experiments have been designed, however, to establish the precise function of fibronectins during this process.

Therefore, cell migrations during genesis of the heart may also require fibronectins as a substrate. Many questions, however, remain to be solved. First, Do the various migrating embryonic cells share common mechanisms to use fibronectin molecules for their displacement? Because embryonic cell migration can often be blocked by RGDS peptides, it is likely that, in most cases, the fibronectin receptor involved is $\alpha5\ \beta1$. One cannot exclude that certain cell types use other receptors for translocation, however; one of the candidates is the $\alpha3\ \beta1$ receptor that binds fibronectin by way of an RGDS-insensitive mechanism. Such would be the case of the precardiac cells, the migration of which is apparently not perturbed by antibodies to $\alpha5\beta1$. Second, What are the factors that induce cells to become endowed with motile properties? Fibronectins per se cannot trigger this process *in vivo,* because they are frequently present in the cells' environment prior to onset of migration. Third, What are the directional cues that permit cells to reach their target sites, inasmuch as migratory pathways are not the only sites of fibronectin expression?

Parts of the answers may lie in the properties of fibronectins themselves. Other functional domains of fibronectins could possibly participate in migratory events. For example, there is evidence for a potential role for the extra domain 1 in wound healing (ffrench-Constant, personal communication), as well as in neural crest migration where fibronectin variants containing this domain are particularly abundant (our unpublished results). Another explanation may be found in the inability of migrating cells to synthesize or retain fibronectins at their surface. Such is the case for primordial germ cells and neural crest cells, but not for endocardial cells migrating in the cardiac jelly.[39,49,50] It is therefore important to determine the possible role of fibronectins produced by migratory cells and whether they remain associated at the cell surface.

REFERENCES

1. LE DOUARIN, N. M. 1984. Cell **38:** 353-360.
2. ALI, I. U. & R. O. HYNES. 1978. Cell **14:** 439-446.
3. YAMADA, K. M., K. OLDEN & I. PASTAN. 1978. Ann. N.Y. Acad. Sci. **312:** 256-277.
4. HYNES, R. O. & K. M. YAMADA. 1982. J. Cell Biol. **95:** 369-377.
5. RUOSLAHTI, E. & M. D. PIERSCHBACHER. 1986. Cell **44:** 517-518.
6. MOSHER, D. F., Ed. 1989. Fibronectin. Academic Press. New York.
7. GUTMAN, A. & A. R. KORNBLHITT. 1987. Proc. Natl. Acad. Sci. USA **84:** 7179-7182.
8. SCHWARZBAUER, J. E., R. S. PATEL, D. FONDA & R. O. HYNES. 1987. EMBO J. **6:** 2573-2580.
9. KORNBLIHTT, A. R., K. UMEZAWA, K. VIBE-PEDERSEN & F. E. BARALLE. 1985. EMBO J. **4:** 1755-1759.
10. SCHWARZBAUER, J. E., J. W. TAMKUN, I. R. LEMISCHKA & R. O. HYNES. 1983. Cell **35:** 421-431.
11. NORTON, P. A. & R. O. HYNES. 1987. Mol. Cell. Biol. **7:** 4297-4307.
12. OBARA, M., M. KANG & K. M. YAMADA. 1988. Cell **53:** 649-657.
13. HUMPHRIES, M. J., A. KOMORIYA, S. K. AKIYAMA, K. OLDEN & K. M. YAMADA. 1987. J. Biol. Chem. **262:** 6886-6892.
14. MCCARTHY, J. B., S. T. HAGEN & L. T. FURCHT. 1986. J. Cell Biol. **102:** 179-188.
15. ROGERS, S. L., P. C. LETOURNEAU, B. A. PETERSON, L. T. FURCHT & J. B. MCCARTHY. 1987. J. Cell Biol. **105:** 1435-1442.
16. HYNES, R. O. 1987. Cell **48:** 549-554.
17. BUCK, C. A. & A. F. HORWITZ. 1987. Annu. Rev. Cell Biol. **3:** 179-205.
18. BURRIDGE, K., K. FATH, T. KELLY, G. H. NUCKOLLS & C. TURNER. 1988. Annu. Rev. Cell Biol. **4:** 487-525.
19. HIRST, R., A. HORWITZ, C. BUCK & L. ROHRSCHNEIDER. 1986. Proc. Natl. Acad. Sci. USA **83:** 6470-6474.
20. WARTIOVAARA, J., I. LEIVO & A. VAHERI. 1979. Dev. Biol. **69:** 247-257.
21. DUBAND, J.-L., T. DARRIBÈRE, H. BOULEKBACHE, J.-C. BOUCAUT & J. P. THIERY. 1987. *In* Cell Membranes: Methods and Reviews. E. L. Elson, W. A. Frazier & L. Glaser, Eds. Vol 3: 1-53. Plenum Press. New York.
22. LEE, G., R. O. HYNES & M. KIRSCHNER. 1984. Cell **36:** 729-740.
23. DUBAND, J.-L., S. ROCHER, W.-T. CHEN, K. M. YAMADA & J. P. THIERY. 1986. J. Cell Biol **102:** 160-179.
24. DARRIBÈRE, T., K. M. YAMADA, K. E. JOHNSON & J.-C. BOUCAUT. 1988. Dev. Biol. **126:** 182-194.
25. DE SIMONE, D. W. & R. O. HYNES. 1988. J. Biol. Chem. **263:** 5333-5340.
26. LE DOUARIN, N. M. 1982. The Neural Crest. Cambridge University Press. Cambridge, U.K.
27. NEWGREEN, D. F., I. L. GIBBINS, J. SAUTER, B. WALLENFELS & R. WÜTZ. 1982. Cell Tiss. Res. **221:** 521-549.
28. ROVASIO, R. A., A. DELOUVÉE, R. TIMPL, K. M. YAMADA & J. P. THIERY. 1983. J. Cell Biol. **96:** 462-473.
29. TUCKER, R. P. & C. A. ERICKSON. 1984. Dev. Biol. **104:** 390-405.
30. BOUCAUT, J.-C., T. DARRIBÈRE, T. J. POOLE, H. AOYAMA, K. M. YAMADA & J. P. THIERY. 1984. J. Cell Biol. **99:** 1822-1830.
31. BRONNER-FRASER, M. 1985. J. Cell Biol. **101:** 610-617.
32. POOLE, T. J. & J. P. THIERY. 1986. *In* Progress in Developmental Biology. H. C. Slavkin, Ed.: 235-238. A. R. Liss. New York.
33. TUCKER, R. P., B. F. EDWARDS & C. A. ERICKSON. 1985. Cell Motility **5:** 225-237.

34. CHEN, W.-T. & S. J. SINGER. 1982. J. Cell Biol. **95:** 205-222.
35. COUCHMAN, J. R. & D. A. REES. 1979. J. Cell Sci. **39:** 149-165.
36. CHEN, W.-T., E. HASEGAWA, T. HASEGAWA, C. WEINSTOCK & K. M. YAMADA. 1985. J. Cell Biol. **100:** 1103-1114.
37. DAMSKY, C. H., K. A. KNUDSEN, D. BRADLEY, C. A. BUCK & A. F. HORWITZ. 1985. J. Cell Biol. **100:** 1528-1539.
38. DUFOUR, S., J.-L. DUBAND, M. J. HUMPHRIES, M. OBARA, K. M. YAMADA & J. P. THIERY. 1988. EMBO J. **7:** 2661-2671.
39. FFRENCH-CONSTANT, C. & R. O. HYNES. 1988. Development **104:** 369-382.
40. HORWITZ, A. F., K. DUGGAN, C. A. BUCK, M. C. BECKERLE & K. BURRIDGE. 1986. Nature **320:** 531-532.
41. AXELROD, D. 1983. J. Membr. Biol. **75:** 1-10.
42. JACOBSON, K., A. ISHIHARA & R. INMAN. 1987. Annu. Rev. Physiol. **49:** 163-175.
43. DUBAND, J.-L., G. H. NUCKOLLS, A. ISHIHARA, T. HASEGAWA, K. M. YAMADA, J. P. THIERY & K. JACOBSON. 1988. J. Cell Biol. **107:** 1385-1397.
44. CHEN, W.-T., J. WANG, T. HASEGAWA, S. S. YAMADA & K. M. YAMADA. 1986. J. Cell Biol. **103:** 1649-1661.
45. DUBAND, J.-L., S. DUFOUR, K. M. YAMADA & J. P. THIERY. 1988. FEBS Lett. **230:** 181-187.
46. LINASK, K. K. & J. W. LASH. 1986. Dev. Biol. **114:** 87-101.
47. LINASK, K. K. & J. W. LASH. 1986. Dev. Biol. **129:** 315-323.
48. MJAATVEDT, C. H., R. C. LEPERA & R. R. MARKWALD. 1987. Dev. Biol. **119:** 59-67.
49. NEWGREEN, D. F. & J. P. THIERY. 1980. Cell Tissue Res. **211:** 269-291.
50. HEASMAN, J., R. O. HYNES, A. P. SWAN, V. THOMAS & C. C. WYLIE. 1981. Cell **27:** 437-447.

Cardiovascular Defects Associated with Alcohol, Retinoic Acid, and Other Agents

ROGER N. RUCKMAN[a]

Department of Pediatrics
George Washington University
School of Medicine and Health Sciences
Washington, D.C.
and
Department of Cardiology
Children's Hospital National Medical Center
Washington, D.C. 20010

INTRODUCTION

Study of agents that are potentially teratogenic depends on human epidemiologic data and findings from animal models. Several factors are important in the choice of an animal model. First, the conditions of the experiments must be appropriate. For example, the mother animal must be properly nourished and in good health. The animal model chosen should have relative freedom from spontaneous malformation patterns. There should be an opportunity to examine dose-reponse relationships in order to delineate the full range of potential malformations. Ideally, the model should allow measurement of key physiologic parameters that help delineate the mechanism of action of the agent.[1]

In the study of mechanism, stage sensitivity is a major consideration. Three broad periods need to be understood: the time from fertilization to postimplantation, the steps of organogenesis, and the final histogenesis. An agent may act at all three of these stages, possibly causing death of the embryo with spontaneous abortion in the first stage, production of a cardiac defect in the second stage, and fetal growth failure in the third stage.[2]

Several other factors are important in understanding of the mechanism of action. Some agents have no observable effect at a certain dose. As the dose is increased, a point is reached where an effect is first noted. This is referred to as a threshold effect. With further increases of dose, a whole range of effects may then appear. It is important to look at several species or different strains within a species because genetic variability affects susceptibility to a given agent. One species or strain may show no response, whereas another may develop complex cardiac anomalies. Finally, where possible, the

[a] Address for correspondence: Department of Cardiology, Children's Hospital National Medical Center, 111 Michigan Ave., N.W., Washington, D.C. 20010.

specific action of the agent should be defined. The agent may stimulate a mutation, cause a chromosomal aberration, interrupt a biochemical process, or have direct cytotoxic effects.[2] In the case of alcohol, we will examine its actions that affect cell growth and migration, look at the role of its metabolite acetaldehyde, and review its effects on amino acid transport and handling of key nutrients. Retinoic acid, by contrast, has direct cytotoxicity and has interactions with DNA. Differentiation is delayed, and protein synthesis is altered.[2] In this review of alcohol, retinoic acid, and related agents, the range of cardiac defects and associated anomalies will be examined in the human and several animal species.

ALCOHOL

After the initial observations by Lemoine[3] and by Jones and Smith,[4] a human malformation syndrome related to alcohol exposure in pregnancy was identified. The term fetal alcohol syndrome was applied to the constellation of growth deficiency, developmental delay, craniofacial abnormality, and other organ defects, including cardiac.[5] The human findings were confirmed in multiple subsequent reports. It became evident that pregnancies involving chronic alcohol consumption were as frequent as 24-29 per 1000 births with an associated perinatal mortality of 17%, observed growth deficiency of 97%, and mental deficiency in nearly half (44%).[6] Other malformations typically found involved the eye, limb, heart, and palate.[6] A set of diagnostic criteria for the human fetal alcohol syndrome evolved to include retarded growth, CNS/psychomotor disturbance, abnormal facies, and increased frequency of malformations.[3] These findings plus increased mortality rates were noted in several species.[7]

As experience grew, the range of cardiac anomalies was noted to vary in severity. Simple atrial septal defect has shown the highest incidence, much more common than ventricular septal defects.[8] Other anomalies have included tetralogy of Fallot, pulmonary artery stenosis or aplasia, mitral stenosis, idiopathic hypertrophic subaortic stenosis (IHSS), and caval anomalies. It should be noted that complete documentation of the extent and severity of cardiac anomalies may be incomplete due to the lack of echo, cardiac catheterization, or autopsy data in some of the reported cases. One study,[8] which did document cardiac defects by cardiac catheterization or pathologic exam, demonstrated an incidence of 29%, rising to 50%, in the more severe forms of the syndrome.

When the fetal alcohol syndrome is examined overall, a dose-response relationship is noted. Chronic exposure to 1 ounce of ethanol is associated with a low incidence, 1-2 ounces with a 10% incidence, and greater than two ounces with a 19% incidence.[6] Studies in animals have shown that survival is related to dose. Chick embryos exposed acutely at 72-80 hours and observed at 14 days showed 87% survival when a dose of 0.20 mL 50% ethanol was employed, ranging to 27% survival when the exposure used was 0.40 mL 50% ethanol.[9] In a model of chronic ethanol exposure, chick embryos were exposed every 24 hours to 100% ethanol. There was 67% survival at 71 hours and 21% survival at 97 hours when conditions of .075 mL ethanol were used. With a recurring dose of 0.1 mL ethanol, survival fell to 44% and 17% at 71 and 97 hours, respectively.[10]

The recurrence of specific cardiac anomalies varies with dose. In the chick model with acute exposure, lower doses such as 0.20 mL 50% ethanol are associated with a 43% incidence of ventricular septal defect.[9] As the dose is increased, for example to 0.36 mL, an overriding aorta is noted as well as a ventricular septal defect in 74 percent. At that same dose, some examples of double outlet right ventricle are noted. The frequency of the latter rises from 7% at 0.36 mL exposure to 12% after 0.40 mL exposure.[9]

Studies in the mouse have given some clues concerning the specific mechanism of cardiac injury. After acute ethanol exposure, the specific components of cardiac tissue that are injured, when examined under the electron microscope, are the atrioventricular (AV) endocardial cushions, the AV canal, conal tissue, and the membranous septum.[11] The extent of the injury relates to or is partly regulated by the timing of exposure, the involvement of endocardial cells, deficiencies in the cardiac tube, altered flow, and alterations of neural crest. Three of the key developmental steps in cardiac development have been examined closely. At the point of looping, a small abnormal contour is noted. The primitive left ventricle has been found to have an abnormal shape. The conoventricular flange has been found to be absent.[9]

When several of the organs affected by ethanol are examined, species overlap is noted between the mouse and the human.[11-13] Vessel tortuosity is noted in the eyes, and microcephaly is common to both species. Midface and jaw abnormalities are common. The hearts of both show ventricular septal defects and atrial septal defects.

In the chick exposed chronically to ethanol, survival varies according to both stage and dose. Specifically, viability decreases with increasing dose and with increasing stage.[10] When heart rate is examined in this model, a dose-related increase in heart rate is noted at 71 and 73 hours. Those embryos observed at 95 and 97 hours, however, do not show a dose-related change in heart rate compared to sham. Similarly, there is a loss of function as measured by shortening fraction when dose is increased in the 73 hour chick embryo, but not in older embryos. It is noteworthy that the 73 hour chick embryo is in the process or active cardiogenesis. Ethanol appears to have an immediate effect on cardiac contractility at this stage. Observations of electron micrographs of myocardial tissue exposed under these conditions support the concept that alterations of form are associated with changes in function. The electron micrographs show loss of myofibril integrity, swelling of mitochondria with breakdown of cristae, and changes in nuclear chromatin. Such changes are not noted in older embryos. Accordingly, the embryo appears to have some capacity for repair. Vascular abnormalities, however, are noted to persist in the 95 and 97 hour chick.[10]

Further examination of the chick model reveals that vascular abnormalities are common. The range of abnormalities includes hemorrhages, hematoma formation, and even bleeding into the pericardial space. If a hematoma were to occur and persist adjacent to a developing organ, abnormal morphology of that organ may occur. Overall flow of blood and stream patterns within the developing heart are also important. Atrial septation is noted to occur at the point of lowest blood flow. A temporary disturbance in flow, such as by loss of contractility due to alcohol exposure, could be the basis for the frequently observed atrial septal defect noted in several species.[11,14-16]

Vascular injury is important because it may alter blood pressure relationships within the embryo, which, in turn, can influence function and flow within the heart.[17] Hematoma formation adjacent to a blood vessel can also modulate flow patterns. The passage of nutrients required for protein synthesis is dependent on integrity of the vasculature. It has been shown that alcohol can directly interfere with protein synthesis.[13] Altered protein synthesis, in turn, can affect modeling of the heart.

To summarize, in the chronic ethanol-exposed chick model, several pathophysiologic concerns are important. It should be noted that early cardiogenesis is occurring independently of significant autonomic nervous system influence. Embryos at 71 and 73 hours have no functioning sympathomimetic receptors, making them unresponsive to direct nerve stimuli or to the effects of circulating catecholamines.[18] Ethanol is observed to be associated with depressed contractility, which, in turn, can be associated with an increase in heart rate, which may be compensatory. Direct examination of myofibrils by electron microscopy confirms alteration of cellular and subcellular morphology. The combined effects of altered myofibril integrity and change in function can produce altered blood streaming, which may be a factor in the development of atrial and ventricular septal defects. Such defects are the most frequently noted cardiac anomalies in both animal models and the human fetal alcohol syndrome. Specific developmental processes have been noted in the mouse.[11] In this model, several key events occur on days 12 and 13 of development. On day 12, the AV cushions fuse, the conal cushions develop, and there is a shift of the AV conus. In the ethanol exposed mouse, however, cushion tissue is noted to be deficient. Furthermore, the shift of the AV canal is abnormal such that the AV canal is related to the left ventricle (LV). On day 13, the normal developmental stages include completion of the interventricular septum, fusion of conal ridges, and appropriate contact of tissue from the conal ridge, the septum, and the cushions. After ethanol exposure, the defect in the interventricular septum fails to close, there is lack of fusion of conal ridges, and the needed contact of component tissues fails to occur.

Studies looking at specific tissues that comprise the morphologic components of the heart have demonstrated a significant role for the mesoderm.[13] Cardiac mesoderm has anterior midline origins. Migration of cells to the developing heart is altered after exposure to ethanol. Furthermore, the proliferation rate of mesodermal cells is noted to decrease. The overall result from these processes is deficiency of key cell populations needed for the normal development of the heart.

If one considers additional sources of migrating cells, the neural crest should be emphasized. Deficiency of neural crest cell activity and migration leads to a pattern of anomalies. Specifically, the face, pharyngeal pouch, and heart are dependent on neural crest cells. The observed defects are conotruncal anomalies of the heart; micrognathia, hypertelorism, and clefts of the face; and deficiency or absence of the thymus and parathyroids during pharyngeal pouch development. Furthermore, neural crest deficiencies are associated with malformation clusters or syndromes, including DiGeorge syndrome, fetal alcohol syndrome, and the CHARGE association.[19,20]

It is noteworthy that the neural crest role in anomalous development varies according to timing. Specifically, with early exposure to ethanol, there is deficiency of neural crest cell production. With later exposure, however, there is direct damage to the neural crest. If exposures are repeated, multiple defects involving multiple systems are noted.[12]

Some additional understanding of dose-response has been noted in studies in the mouse. Considering multiple organ systems, a differing set of anomalies is noted at low dose versus those noted at high dose. Low dose is associated with an abnormal supraoccipital bone, and hemopericardium is also observed. At somewhat higher doses, ventricular septal defects are noted. At still higher doses, missing sternebra and rib anomalies are found.[21]

Studies in the mouse have also clarified issues of stage dependence. Variations in timing of exposure to ethanol cause a reproducible spectrum of anomalies. Specifically, exposure on day 7 to 8 causes defects of the brain and eyes, whereas exposure on day 9 to 10 causes abnormal limb development. If the exposure is delayed to day 12 to 13, the heart develops abnormally, and ventricular septal defects or atrioventricular defects are found.[11,12]

Metabolic considerations are also important. It appears that ethanol or its metabolites influence multiple organ systems throughout development. Ethanol is highly lipid-soluble and may act as early as the blastocyst stage. Alcohol is cleared from the system according to metabolic rate, which varies in different strains of mice, thus helping to explain the varying sets of anomalies seen in different strains. Fundamental to our understanding of these observations is the enzymatic activity in the liver. In both the mouse and the human, two enzyme systems are responsible for the metabolism of ethanol. Alcohol dehydrogenase is found in the cytosol fraction, and in the microsomal fraction is the ethanol oxidizing system. The latter is inducible. It appears that enzyme activity varies from one strain to the next.

If one examines the cellular and subcellular changes within the developing heart after ethanol exposure, some quantitation can be applied to changes within the myofibrils and the mitochondria. If quantitative electron microscopy is performed, the principal changes in the mouse mitochondria, which are the earliest changes noted, can be classified into three stages. In the earliest changes noted, the primary (1°) stage, the mitochondria are small and condensed with electron-dense matrices. In the secondary (2°) stage, the mitochondria are enlarged and show electron-lucent matrices and evidence for break up of cristae. The most advanced (3°) set of changes include significantly enlarged mitochondria with electron-lucent matrices, vacuolization, and loss of inner membrane integrity. With alcohol exposure, nearly half of exposed mice show the 3° set of changes. In addition, there is increased density of matrix volume.[22] The observations of morphologic changes in mitochondria are important also from the standpoint of function. Located on the inner mitochondrial membrane are the electron transport and oxidative phosphorylation-related enzymes. Disruption of the inner membrane can, therefore, be associated with abnormal oxidative metabolism.[22]

Cardiac myofibrils undergo a series of changes after exposure to ethanol. Myofibrils appear fragmented. There is a lack of congruence of fibrils. A phenomenon called streaming occurs in which the linearity of the Z-line, A band, and I band is lost. The usual number of myofibrils is reduced. If one compares a ratio of myofibril volume to cytoplasmic volume, the number is reduced. In addition, ethanol is associated with loss of the sarcoplasmic reticulum.[22]

The final expression of phenotype in the human appears to be related to the dose of ethanol to which the embryo is exposed, the timing of exposure, and the genetic background and susceptibility of a given embryo.[23] Given such a set of conditions, the typical pattern of human cardiac defects is seen in fetal alcohol syndrome with an incidence of 29 percent. In those with more severe exposure, the incidence of defects rises to 50 percent. In either situation, the most common cardiac defect is the atrial septal defect, noted much more frequently than the ventricular septal defect.[8] Looking at other species, the most common abnormality in the rat is the atrial septal defect. Aberrant pulmonary vein is also noted.[16] In the mouse, septal defects in combination with other anomalies are common. Specifically, double outlet right ventricle, tetralogy of Fallot, and atrioventricular canal are noted in addition to simple ventricular septal defect. Furthermore, anomalies of the distal great vessels are common.[11] In the chick, intracardiac and aortic arch abnormalities of a similar spectrum are noted. In addition, the subclavian artery is often abnormal.[9]

Animal studies, similar to the human data, demonstrate that the final form of cardiac defects will vary according to the timing of the dose of ethanol, the various developmental processes that are occurring simultaneously, and the occurrence of linkages. Specifically, developmental processes vary in the length of time needed for completion. The start of one process can depend on the proper completion of an antecedent series of steps.[16] Different strains within a species or different species can show variable susceptibility. Within the series of developmental steps required to define the finished heart, certain biochemical precursors are required. For example, glycoproteins, glycosaminoglycans, and proteoglycans, which may be inhibited by ethanol, are needed for the steps in atrial septation.[16]

Another consideration in our understanding of the mechanism of ethanol effect is its action on the placental circulation. In the monkey, ethanol exposure causes collapse of the umbilical vasculature. Consequently, an indirect mechanism of injury can occur through impaired blood flow and fetal hypoxia. The occurrence of hypoxia can, in turn, be associated with acidosis. The developing central nervous system is especially sensitive to hypoxia and acidosis. Consequently, some of the CNS abnormalities noted in the fetal alcohol syndrome may be explained by this mechanism.[24]

Another line of investigation has involved study of the relative action of ethanol and its metabolite, acetaldehyde. In the rat, clearance of ethanol occurs equally as rapidly in the pregnant rat and the virgin rat. The placenta presents a minimal barrier to circulation in the fetus. If one then examines the rat in early pregnancy (12 days) versus later pregnancy (21 days), concentrations of ethanol and acetaldehyde in the pregnant rat are essentially the same. The rates of ethanol oxidation in the fetus are, however, different at these two times. Acetaldehyde metabolism is more complex, involving the placenta as well as the liver. Equilibration of ethanol in the fetus is rapid inasmuch as passage across the placenta is rapid with no alcohol dehydrogenase activity in the rat placenta. It is important to note that, in the rat at 17 days of pregnancy, there is no fetal liver alcohol dehydrogenase activity. At 21 days, the activity is very low, on the order of 20% of adult liver capacity. Similar findings in the human raise concerns about the ability of the fetal liver to clear ethanol. It has been suggested, assuming that ethanol can pass back across the placenta, that the main route for ethanol metabolism is by the maternal liver. Acetaldehyde, accordingly, is found in the maternal circulation. The metabolite does not cross the placenta unless it reaches high concentrations. Observations of low acetaldehyde levels in fetal blood after high ethanol intake support the concept that placenta and fetal liver are able to oxidize most of the acetaldehyde that comes from the maternal circulation. There appears to be an acetaldehyde threshold above which the capacity of the fetoplacental unit for acetaldehyde metabolism is exceeded. It further appears that the threshold is lower in early pregnancy because aldehyde dehydrogenase is absent from the fetal liver. Overall, the major route for elimination of alcohol from the fetus is through the maternal liver.[25]

RETINOIC ACID AND OTHER AGENTS

Vitamin A is a naturally occurring retinoid. In an attempt to find compounds with a better therapeutic index in treating dermatologic conditions, synthetic analogues were derived. From the naturally occurring *all-trans*-retinoic acid, the geometric isomer 13-*cis*-retinoic acid was manufactured.[26] The various vitamin A congeners are retinol, or vitamin A itself, retinoic acid (tretinoin), 13-*cis*-retinoic acid (isotretinoin), and etretinate (ETR).[27] Isotretinoin (ITR) was first marketed in 1982 under the brand name Accutane. Because of knowledge of vitamin A toxicity and teratogenicity of retinoic acid in laboratory animals, appropriate warnings were issued, advising that the drug not be used by pregnant women. Reports began to appear, however, related to its use during pregnancy. An isotretinoin dysmorphic syndrome was described in 1984.[28] The components of the syndrome involved anomalies of the ears, face, central nervous system, and heart. Specifically, the ears were noted to be rudimentary and low set. An abnormal facial appearance due to a depressed nasal bridge was noted. The brain was edematous with changes in the cerebellum and hippocampus, and dilatation of the ventricles. The heart had transposition of the great arteries, ventricular septal defect, and an anomalous right subclavian artery. Rats exposed to isotretinoin were also found to have defects of the ears and central nervous system. Cleft palate has been described. In the human, as case experience has grown, a typical cluster of anomalies includes the central nervous system, ears, and heart.[27] Other commonly noted human malformations have included abnormalities of the thymus. If one compares experience with ITR, retinol, and ETR, the greatest range of anomalies is associated with ITR. All three compounds have potent effects on the developing central nervous system. Cardiac defects have been described with ITR and retinol but not ETR. When the range of cardiac defects is examined, simple septal defects are less common than in the fetal alcohol syndrome. More complex lesions such as double outlet right ventricle, transposition of the great arteries, tetralogy of Fallot, and truncus arteriosus are noted. In addition, the aortic arch is often affected with coarctation, arch hypoplasia, or complete interruption. The right subclavian artery has been found to have an anomalous origin.[29] When multiple organ systems are affected, certain associations are common, particularly cardiac and thymic or central nervous system and thymic anomalies. The pattern of malformations has raised speculation concerning the mechanism of teratogenesis. For both retinoic acid and vitamin A, the action appears to be on the cephalic neural crest. Considering the heart specifically, this action on neural crest leads to deficiency of branchial arch mesenchyme, which, in turn, contributes to the observed cardiac defects.[29]

Some interesting species variations have been noted. Mice have been found to have ventricular septal defects and conotruncal anomalies. Both mice and rats have a frequent incidence of heterotaxy syndrome.[27] In animal species as well as the human, a critical period for exposure is important, that is, between 2–5 weeks postconception in the human. In the case of ITR, the drug itself has a half-life of less than one day. The compound, however, is metabolized to a toxic metabolite, 4-oxo-isoretinoin, which has a half-life of several days. ETR has a half-life of several months. Accordingly, there is more of an opportunity for these compounds to act during the critical period of the embryo.[27]

CONCLUSION

In summary, developmental steps in cardiogenesis in several species show dose and stage sensitivity to potential teratogens. Alcohol, retinoic acid, and its congeners exert both direct and indirect effects on the developing heart. Direct effects from the agent or a metabolite can occur on cells and subcellular components, such as mitochondria and metabolic processes. Indirect effects include alteration of neural crest cell migration to the developing heart and blood vessels, disruption of the fetoplacental circulation, and changes in flow through the heart itself due to alterations in function or geometry. Careful investigation of the action of these teratogens has given us clues concerning the processes that control the development of anomalies. Clearly, more studies are needed not only to better predict the potential adverse effects of drugs and chemicals but also to define the critically sensitive steps in cardiogenesis.

REFERENCES

1. BRENT, R. L. 1985. *In* Prevention of Physical and Mental Congenital Defects. M. Marois, Ed.: 191–195. Alan R. Liss. New York.

2. BECKMAN, D. A. & R. L. BRENT. 1986. Clin. Perinatol. **13:** 649-687.
3. LEMOINE P. H., H. HAROUSSEAU, J. P. BORTEYRU & J. C. MENUET. 1968. Ouest Med. **25:** 477-482.
4. JONES, K. L. & D. W. SMITH. 1973. Lancet **2:** 999-1001.
5. JONES, K. L., D. W. SMITH, C. N. ULLELAND & A. P. STREISSGUTH. 1973. Lancet **1:** 1267-1271.
6. HANSON, J. W., K. L. JONES & D. W. SMITH. 1976. J. Am. Med. Assoc. **235:** 1458-1460.
7. STREISSGUTH, A. P., S. LANDESMAN-DWYER, J. C. MARTIN & D. W. SMITH. 1980. Science **209:** 353-361.
8. LOSER, H. & F. MAJEWSKI. 1977. Br. Heart J. **39:** 1374-1379.
9. FANG, T., H. J. BRUYERE, S. A. KARGAS, T. NISHIKAWA, Y. TAKAGI & E. F. GILBERT. 1987. Teratology **35:** 95-103.
10. RUCKMAN, R. N., D. J. MESSERSMITH, S. A. O'BRIEN, P. R. GETSON, R. L. BOECKX & D. E. MORSE. 1988. Teratology **37:** 317-327.
11. DAFT, P. A., M. C. JOHNSTON & K. K. SULIK. 1986. Teratology **33:** 93-104.
12. WEBSTER, W. S., D. A. WALSH, S. E. McEWEN & A. H. LIPSON. 1983. Teratology **27:** 231-243.
13. SULIK, K. K. 1984. *In* Mechanisms of alcohol damage *in utero.* Ciba Found. Symp. **105:** 124-141. London.
14. HENDRIX, M. J. C. & D. E. MORSE. 1977. Dev. Biol. **57:** 345-363.
15. RANDALL, C. L. & W. J. TAYLOR. 1979. Teratology **19:** 305-312.
16. BEAUCHEMIN, R. R., L. P. GARTNER & D. V. PROVENZA. 1984. Anat. Anz. Jena **155:** 17-28.
17. RAJALA, G. M., J. H. KALBFLEISCH & S. KAPLAN. 1976. J. Embryol. Exp. Morphol. **36:** 685-695.
18. PAFF, G. H. & T. P. GLANDER. 1958. Anat. Rec. **160:** 405.
19. BOCKMAN, D. E. & M. L. KIRBY. 1984. Science **223:** 498-500.
20. SIEBERT, J. R. 1983. Science **221:** 908.
21. CHERNOFF, G. F. 1977. Teratology **15:** 223-230.
22. UPHOFF, C., C. NYQUIST-BATTIE & R. TOTH. 1984. Teratology **30:** 119-129.
23. CLARREN, S. K. & D. W. SMITH. 1978. N. Engl. J. Med. **298:** 1063-1067.
24. MUKHERJEE, A. B. & G. D. HODGEN. 1982. Science **218:** 700-702.
25. ZORZANO, A. & E. HERRERA. 1989. Pediatr. Res. **25:** 102-106.
26. PECK, G. L., T. G. OLSEN, F. W. YODER, J. S. STRAUSS, D. T. DOWNING, M. PANDYA, D. BUTKUS & J. ARNAUD-BATTANDIER. 1979. N. Engl. J. Med. **300:** 329-333.
27. ROSA, F. W., A. L. WILK & F. O. KELSEY. 1986. *In* Teratogen Update: Environmentally Induced Birth Defect Risks. J. L. Sever & R. L. Brent, Eds.: 61-70. Alan R. Liss. New York.
28. BRAUN, J. T., R. A. FRANCIOSI, A. R. MASTRI, R. M. DRAKE & B. L. O'NEILL. 1984. Lancet **1:** 506-507.
29. LAMMER, E. J., D. J. CHEN, R. M. HOAR, N. D. AGNISH, P. J. BENKE, J. T. BRAUN, C. T. CURRY, P. M. FERNHOFF, A. W. GRIX, I. T. LOTT, J. M. RICHARD & S. C. SUN. 1985. N. Engl. J. Med. **313:** 837-841.

Alteration of Cardiogenesis after Neural Crest Ablation[a]

MARGARET L. KIRBY

Department of Anatomy
Medical College of Georgia
Augusta, Georgia 30912-2000

For many years studies of congenital heart defects were stymied because of the lack of reliable models for studying cardiac dysmorphogenesis. The last ten years have seen a dramatic increase in the availability of models for studying abnormal heart development. These now include genetic models of trisomies and situs inversus as well as several teratogenic models, one of which has been presented by Roger Ruckman in the previous chapter. Many of these models of genetic or teratogenic cardiac dysmorphogenesis are suspected to alter heart development by interfering with neural crest development.

Neural crest cells are essential for normal development of the heart.[1] Cells from the region of neural crest located between the midotic placode and the caudal limit of somite 3 migrate through pharyngeal arches 3, 4, and 6 where they provide support for the aortic arch arteries.[1-3] Some of the neural crest cells continue their migration into the aortic sac where they form the aorticopulmonary septum and extend from there into the truncal region where they participate in truncal septation.[4] Other cells derived from the same region of the neural crest differentiate into the neural anlage of the parasympathetic ganglia that mediate the decreased chronotropic response of the mature heart.[5,6] The region of the neural crest between the midotic placode and somite 3 has been referred to as cardiac neural crest, for convenience[7] (FIG. 1). Chimeric experiments using quail donors and chick hosts have shown that most of the neural crest cells involved in truncal septation are derived from neural crest that populates arch 4, with lesser contributions from neural crest populating arches 3 and 6.[8]

A variety of heart malformations can be produced by removal of all or part of the cardiac neural crest by extirpation or ablation.[7,9,10] Ablation of the cardiac neural crest in its entirety results in failure of the aorticopulmonary and truncal septa to form.[1,4] When these septa do not form, the outflow region of the heart remains undivided, resulting in persistent truncus arteriosus (PTA). Paradoxically, even though the cardiac neural crest has been removed completely to produce the persistent truncus arteriosus, parasympathetic ganglia develop in the heart.[11]

Removal of lesser quantities of cardiac neural crest results in a variety of outflow tract malalignments that have been classified as dextroposed aorta (DPA). The mal-

[a] This work was supported by NIH Grants HD 17063 and HL 36059 and was done during the tenure of an Established Investigatorship from the American Heart Association with funds contributed in part by the Georgia affiliate.

alignment defects that have been seen after neural crest ablation include double outlet right ventricle, tetralogy of Fallot, overriding aorta, and Eisenmenger's complex.

Because malalignment occurs in both PTA as well as DPA, the development of the outflow septa is thought to be independent from the process that produces malalignment.[12] At present, it is thought that malalignment is the result of hemodynamic abnormalities in the pharyngeal region.

Recently, studies in my lab have focused on the specificity of the ectomesenchymal and neural components of the cardiac neural crest. These studies were prompted by the apparent paradox in the findings that removal of the cardiac neural crest resulted in PTA (indicating an absence of the cardiac neural crest in the heart), with an almost

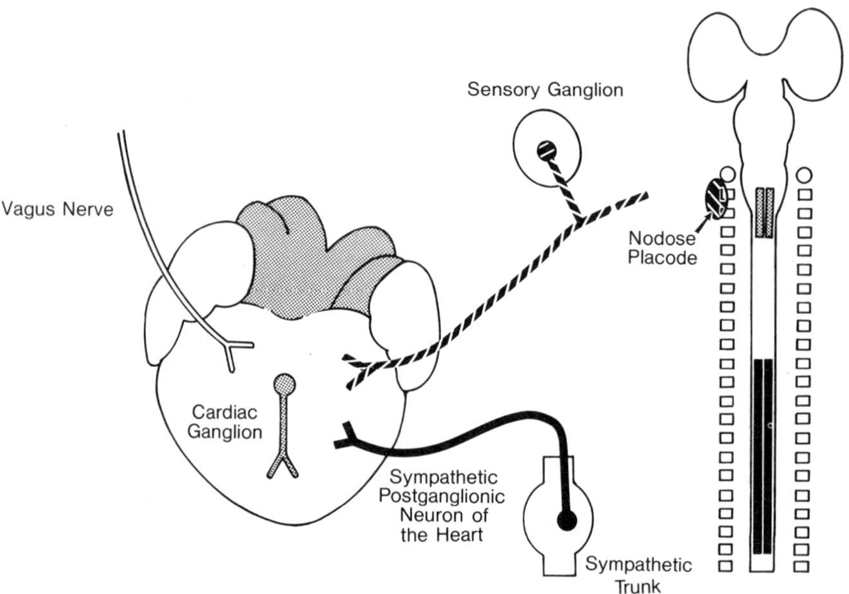

FIGURE 1. Diagram illustrating the various components of the cardiac neural crest. The aorticopulmonary and truncal septa are formed from ectomesenchymal cells derived from the cardiac neural crest, as are the parasympathetic postganglionic neurons. The sensory innervation of the heart is from the inferior ganglion of the vagus, which is derived from the nodose placodes. (M. L. Kirby.[1] With permission from *Pediatric Research.*)

normal level of parasympathetic innervation (indicating the presence of the cardiac neural crest).[11] Originally it was thought that this demonstrated a regeneration or compensation of the neural component of cardiac neural crest without a concomitant regeneration of the ectomesenchymal component. The first set of experiments described herein were designed to explain this phenomenon.

In the trunk, the neural crest gives rise to all of the peripheral neurons, as well as supporting cells and Schwann cells.[13,14] In the head, the derivation of the cranial sensory ganglionic neurons is divided between the neural crest and a series of placodes that form lateral to the neural tube.[15] The neural crest provides all of the autonomic neurons, supporting and Schwann cells for the cranial ganglia and autonomic ganglia regardless of the origin of the neurons.[16]

Using ablation of various combinations of the surface ectoderm, including neural tube, cardiac and noncardiac neural crest, and nodose placodes, it was determined that regeneration of the neural component of cardiac neural crest was prevented only when cardiac neural crest and nodose placodes were removed simultaneously.[17] Hearts from embryos with combined ablations of caridac neural crest and nodose placodes showed a wider variety of abnormalities than hearts from embryos with ablations of cardiac neural crest alone (FIG. 2). In order to show directly that cells of the nodose placodes were capable of seeding the cardiac ganglia in the absence of the cardiac neural crest, two types of chimeric embryos were produced.

A right or left nodose placode from stage 9 quail embryos was transferred to stage 9 chick hosts whose complementary nodose placode had been removed. After the grafted ectoderm had become adherent, the cardiac neural crest was ablated using microcautery. In order to determine whether cells from the nodose placode seed cardiac ganglia in the presence of an intact neural crest, the controls for this experiment were embryos with the nodose placode graft but without the cardiac neural crest ablation.

In control embryos, the nodose ganglion consisted of quail neurons with chick supporting cells on the side of the transplant. On the contralateral side, the ganglion consisted of chick neurons with chick supporting cells. No quail cells could be found in the heart or near the outflow vessels, nor were any quail cells found in any of the other cranial ganglia. In experimental embryos, the ipsilateral nodose ganglion consisted mostly of quail neurons with a few chick supporting cells. The contralateral nodose ganglion was usually small or absent. The cardiac ganglia consisted of quail neurons with a sparse population of chick supporting cells. An unexpected finding in these experiments was the presence of quail cells clustered in the truncal cushions in a pattern reminiscent of neural crest-derived ectomesenchyme but not as well-organized.[18] These condensations were surrounded by a large number of chick mesenchymal cells showing a similar but not identical pattern of segregation, as do neural crest ectomesenchymal cells from mesenchyme derived from the endocardium. The truncal cluster was not organized in a whorl pattern as is the neural crest when it is present. By 8-9 days of incubation, quail cells could be found in the tunica media of the base of the common outflow vessel emanating from the heart. By contrast, no quail cells were found in any of the great vessels or hearts in the control embryos.

An atrial field stimulation study was undertaken, in order to determine whether the cardiac ganglion neurons derived from the nodose placodes are functional. Under the conditions of the field stimulation, neurons derived from the nodose placodes responded identically to neurons derived from the neural crest in producing a decrease in heart rate.[19] It is not known at present whether these neurons are connected appropriately to the central nervous system.

These experiments show that the neural component of the cardiac neural crest can be generated from other areas of the neurogenic ectoderm, whereas an ectomesenchymal component derived from another area of the ectoderm is not successful in closing the outflow septa.

In another series of experiments, the degree of plasticity of the ectomesenchymal and neural components of other regions of the neural crest was assessed.[20] In these experiments, quail donor embryos provided cardiac, trunk, or mesencephalic neural crest to replace or add to the chick host cardiac neural crest.

When cardiac neural crest was replaced by trunk or mesencephalic neural crest, the majority of hearts developed PTA, indicating that ectomesenchyme from these other regions was not competent to effect truncal septation (TABLE 1). Quail-derived ectomesenchyme was found in the truncal and aorticopulmonary regions in the mes-

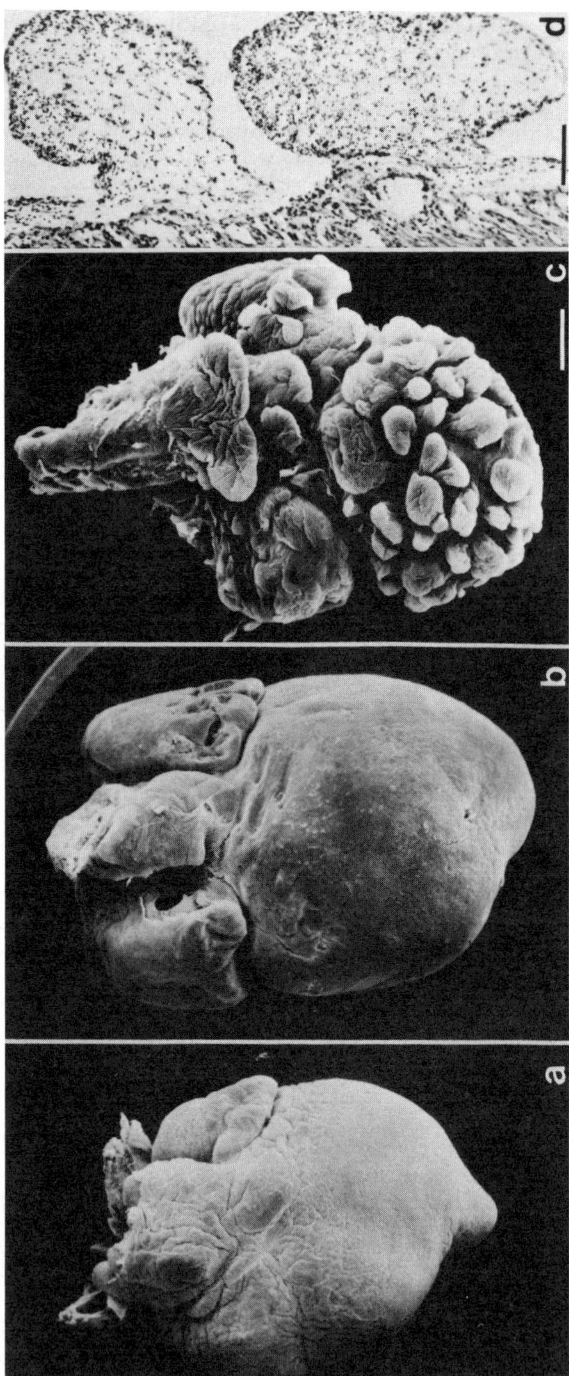

FIGURE 2. Scanning electron micrographs of hearts from embryos after sham surgery (a), cardiac neural crest ablation (b), or cardiac neural crest and nodose placode ablation (c). The hearts in b and c show a persistent truncus arteriosus. The histological appearance of blebs on the surface of a heart with combined ablation is shown in d. (M. L. Kirby.[18] With permission from *Cell and Tissue Research.*)

encephalic grafts but not in the trunk neural crest grafts. The majority of these hearts did have quail-derived neurons and supporting cells in the cardiac ganglia.

Cardiac neural crest addition did not cause any significant alterations in the development of the heart or its innervation. Mesencephalic neural crest addition resulted in PTA with normal innervation (TABLE 1). The quail-derived ectomesenchyme in the hearts was ectopically placed, and in one embryo, the quail cells had formed a nodule of cartilage. Le Douarin and Teillet[21] and Le Lièvre et al.[22] also found cartilage in intermediate cell mass derivatives when mesencephalic neural crest

TABLE 1. Comparison of Ectomesenchyme and Cardiac Ganglia Derived from Different Regions of Neural Crest

	N	Morphology	Number of Animals with Quail Cells			
			Truncal/AP Septum	Vessel Walls	Neurons	Non-neuronal Support Cells
Replacement						
M[a]/C	7	6 PTA 1 Normal	2(ectopic)	2	5	5
C[b]/C	11	10 Normal 1 PTA	11	11	11	11
T[c]/C	12	5 PTA 3 DORV[g] 2 Not determined 2 Normal	0	0	6	6
Addition						
M+[d]	7	6 PTA 1 Normal	6(5 ectopic) 1 cartilage)	3	7	7
C+[e]	13	8 Normal 4 VSD[h] 1 DORV	13	13	12	12
T+[f]	11	9 Normal 2 VSD	1	1	0	8

[a] M = mesencephalic neural crest.
[b] C = cardiac neural crest.
[c] T = trunk neural crest.
[d] Mesencephalic neural crest addition.
[e] Cardiac neural crest addition.
[f] Trunk neural crest addition.
[g] Double outlet right ventricle.
[h] Ventricular septal defect.

was transplanted to the trunk region. After trunk neural crest addition, the majority of hearts were structurally normal (TABLE 1). Virtually no trunk-derived ectomesenchyme was found in the outflow tract. None of the hearts had neurons in the cardiac ganglia that were derived from trunk neural crest; the majority had non-neuronal support cells derived from the added trunk neural crest.

Inasmuch as the trunk additions were made from quail embryos at the same age as their chick hosts, the trunk neural crest would be several hours less mature than the cardiac neural crest, which might favor earlier migration and differentiation of the cardiac neural crest. For this reason, another set of experiments was undertaken using quail donors several hours older (stages 12-14) than their chick hosts (stage 9). In these experiments, the older quail trunk neural crest was able to compete more successfully with the cardiac neural crest in production of neurons in the cardiac ganglia (TABLE 2). The trunk neural crest still did not provide a significant population of ectomesenchymal cells to the outflow tract, however.

These experiments support the idea that the ectomesenchymal component of the cardiac neural crest performs a unique function in the embryo that is not duplicated by other cells. Furthermore the ectomesenchymal derivatives of the cranial neural crest are determined early in development and differentiate according to a predetermined fate even when transplanted to a new environment as early as the neural fold stage of development. The neurons derived from the cardiac neural crest are less specifically determined, as these can be replaced by either cells derived from the nodose placodes or other regions of the neural crest.

TABLE 2. Cardiac Ganglia after Trunk Neural Crest Addition

Neural Crest Adjacent to Somites	N	Number of Animals with Quail Cells in Cardiac Ganglia			
		Neurons	(Percent)	Non-neuronal Support Cells	(Percent)
5-10	4	4	(100)	4	(100)
10-15	4	2	(50)	2	(50)
15-20	5	2	(40)	5	(100)
20-25	3	0	(0)	1	(30)

REFERENCES

1. KIRBY, M. L. 1987. Cardiac morphogenesis—recent research advances. Pediatr. Res. **21:** 219-224.
2. LE LIÈVRE, C. S. & N. M. LE DOUARIN. 1975. Mesenchymal derivatives of the neural crest: analysis of chimeric quail and chick embryos. J. Embryol. Exp. Morphol. **34:** 123-154.
3. NODEN, D. M. 1980. The migration and cytodifferentiation of cranial neural crest cells. *In* Current Trends in Prenatal Craniofacial Development. Pratt and Christiansen, Eds.: 3-25. Elsevier. North Holland, The Netherlands.
4. KIRBY, M. L., T. F. GALE & D. E. STEWART. 1983. Neural crest cells contribute to aorticopulmonary septation. Science **220:** 1059-1061.
5. KIRBY, M. L. & D. E. STEWART. 1983. Neural crest origin of cardiac ganglion cells in the chick embryo: identification and extirpation. Dev. Biol. **97:** 433-443.
6. PAPPANO, A. J. 1977. Ontogenetic development of autonomic neuroeffector transmission and transmitter reactivity in embryonic and fetal hearts. Pharmacol. Rev. **29:** 3-33.
7. KIRBY, M. L., K. L. TURNAGE & R. M. HAYS. 1985. Characterization of conotruncal malformations following ablation of cardiac neural crest. Anat. Rec. **13:** 87-93.
8. PHILLIPS, M. T., M. L. KIRBY & G. FORBES. 1987. Analysis of cranial neural crest distribution in the developing heart using quail-chick chimeras. Circ. Res. **60:** 27-30.

9. BESSON III, W. T., M. L. KIRBY, L. H. S. VAN MIEROP & J. R. TEABEAUT II. 1986. Effects of cardiac neural crest lesion size at various embryonic ages on incidence and type of cardiac defects. Circulation **73:** 360-364.

10. NISHIBATAKE, M., M. L. KIRBY & L. H. S. VAN MIEROP. 1987. Pathogenesis of persistent truncus arteriosus and dextroposed aorta in the chick embryo after neural crest ablation. Circulation **75:** 255-264.

11. KIRBY, M. L., R. S. ARONSTAM & J. J. BUCCAFUSCO. 1985. Changes in cholinergic parameters associated with failure of conotruncal septation in embryonic chick hearts after neural crest ablation. Circ. Res. **56:** 392-401.

12. KIRBY, M. L. 1988. Role of extracardiac factors in heart development. Experientia **44:** 944-950.

13. HORSTADIUS, S. 1950. The Neural Crest. Oxford University Press. London.

14. LE DOUARIN, N. M. 1982. The Neural Crest. Cambridge University Press. London.

15. LE DOUARIN, M. M., J. FONTAINE-PERUS & G. COULY. 1986. Cephalic ectodermal placodes and neurogenesis. Trends Neurosci. **9:** 175-180.

16. D'AMICO-MARTEL, A. & D. M. NODEN. 1983. Contributions of placodal and neural crest cells to avian cranial peripheral ganglia. Am J. Anat. **166:** 445-468.

17. KIRBY, M. L. 1988. Nodose placode contributes autonomic neurons to the heart in the absence of cardiac neural crest. J. Neurosci. **8:** 1089-1095.

18. KIRBY, M. L. 1988. Nodose placode provides ectomesenchyme to the developing chick heart in the absence of cardiac neural crest. Cell Tissue Res. **252:** 17-22.

19. KIRBY, M. L., T. L. CREAZZO & J. L. CHRISTIANSEN. 1989. Chronotropic responses of chick hearts to field stimulation following various neural crest ablations. Circ. Res. **65:** 1547-1554.

20. KIRBY, M. L. 1989. Plasticity and predetermination of mesencephalic and trunk neural crest transplanted into the region of the cardiac neural crest. Dev. Biol. **134:** 402-412.

21. LE DOUARIN, N. M. & M.-A. M. TEILLET. 1974. Experimental analysis of the migration and differentiation of neuroblasts of the autonomic nervous system and of neurectodermal mesenchymal derivatives, using a biological cell marking technique. Dev. Biol. **41:** 162-184.

22. LE LIÈVRE, C. S., C. G. SCHWEIZER, C. M. ZILLER & N. M. LE DOUARIN. 1980. Restrictions of developmental capabilities in neural crest cell derivatives as tested by *in vivo* transplantation experiments. Dev. Biol. **77:** 362-378.

Altered Development of Pharyngeal Arch Vessels after Neural Crest Ablation[a]

DALE E. BOCKMAN, MARY E. REDMOND, AND
MARGARET L. KIRBY

*Department of Anatomy
Medical College of Georgia
Augusta, Georgia 30912-2000*

INTRODUCTION

When probing the embryonic origins of defective heart development, it is important to keep in mind that when congenital defects are encountered, they usually are multiple. They commonly are cardiovascular defects. In many cases, systems in addition to the cardiovascular system are affected. Ablation of neural crest causes defects in the heart, great vessels, and other organs.[1–3]

Another factor to be kept in mind is that the heart and vessels develop as a system. The dorsal aorta joins the heart and ventral aorta very early by way of the first pharyngeal arch vessel. From that time, the parts of the system function together. An alteration in one part would reasonably be expected to have an effect on one or more of the remaining parts. Alteration in flow in one region during the early stages of development might be expected to affect not only flow in another region, but also the morphogenesis of another region.

The mechanisms by which cardiovascular defects are produced are incompletely understood. Certainly a variety of agents produce impaired developments. The similarities in the defects produced by different agents, and the similarity of these with defects of unknown etiology, suggest that it might be fruitful to search for common pathways upon which these multiple agents may operate. The contributions of cranial neural crest are intimately involved with the development of the cardiovascular system; thus they would seem to be legitimate candidates for a common pathway.

We have focused recently on the interrelationship of the heart and pharyngeal arch vessels, with emphasis on the role played by contributions from cranial neural crest. Our studies[4,5] have led us to concentrate more and more on the early stages of cardiovascular development.

[a] This work was supported by NIH Grant HL36095.

296

In order to outline the pertinent relationships of neural crest, major vessels, and the heart, we will present, in turn, some of the critical aspects of normal cardiovascular development, observations made after neural crest ablation, and conclusions that may be drawn from these experiments.

ANGIOGENESIS OF HEART, AORTAE, AND PHARYNGEAL ARCH VESSELS

Angiogenesis with the embryo occurs first as presumptive endothelial cells aggregate, and the vascular endothelial cells express a defined program of events to generate a capillary network.[6] Main channels oriented in the longitudinal axis on either side of the embryo approach the center to fuse into the primitive heart and ventral aorta. A similar process produces the dorsal aorta. The channels extend anteriorly, where fusion of extensions from dorsal and ventral aortae causes the system to be united.[7] The heart and ventral aorta are closely associated with the ventral surface of the foregut (developing pharynx), whereas the dorsal aorta is closely associated with the dorsal surface of the foregut. The anterior connections (the primitive first arch vessels) loop around either side of the anterior extent of the foregut.

After the first *in situ* fusion of primitive endothelial cells, much of the remaining angiogenesis is a result of budding from existing vascular channels. Buds from the dorsal and ventral aortae approach each other, unite, and form paired channels that become the second pair of arch vessels, traversing the second pharyngeal arch. This process is repeated, in time, for each of the pairs of arch vessels: the third, fourth, and sixth. The controlling events that trigger budding in each of these locations remain to be determined.

Soon, the first and second pairs of arch vessels regress. They revert to a capillary plexus and cease to exist as main channels. In the chick, the left fourth arch vessel disappears. The paired dorsal aortae, in the interval between their junction with the third and fourth arch vessels, also disappear with time. The mechanism by which vascular regression occurs is not known. It may be presumed, however, that altered flow is at least part of the trigger for this regression.

A primary association seems to be that between endothelium and endoderm. Secondarily, mesenchyme is inserted between them.

COMPONENTS OF PHARYNGEAL ARCHES

Pharyngeal arches are populated mainly by ectomesenchyme. Much of the mesenchyme within the arches and the walls of arteries that develop from arch vessels are derived from ectomesenchyme. Exceptions include the muscular plate and endothelium, which are mesodermal in origin.[8-10] Therefore, much of the extracellular matrix in this region derives from ectomesenchyme. The extracellular matrix in the developing heart is continuous with that of the pharyngeal arches.

The locations of components of the pharyngeal arches normally are predictable. A moderate size vessel, whose wall consists solely of endothelium, occupies the central area. Mesenchyme surrounds the vessel, separating it from epithelium. The epithelium is ectoderm externally and endoderm internally. The muscular plate is located lateral to the vessel. Thus the mesenchyme of the pharyngeal arch serves as the wall of the vessel. The characteristics of this mesenchyme determine, in part, some of the functional characteristics of the cardiovascular system during early development. It follows that if the mesenchyme is altered, the characteristics of the cardiovascular system might be altered.

NEURAL CREST ABLATION

Experimental ablation of neural crest has been carried out at stage 9-10.[11] The tops of the neural folds from the level of the otic placode to the fifth somite are ablated bilaterally by microcautery or microsurgery. Shams are subjected to all the processes needed to gain access to the embryos, including making a hole in the shell and shell membrane, staining the embryo with neutral red, and tearing the vitelline membrane. Controls are incubated without treatment.

When the cardiovascular system is evaluated at late stages of incubation after this experimental protocol, defects in the heart and in the great vessels are observed.[1,12] In order to understand how the experimental animals were deviating from the normal developmental pattern, we undertook a study that compared normal development of the heart and great vessels with development after neural crest ablation, over an extended period of incubation times.

ESTABLISHING A LONGITUDINAL PROFILE

In this study,[4] neural crest was ablated at stage 9-10, and the results were evaluated at stages 13 through 32. The morphology of the heart and outflow tract were evaluated by scanning electron microscopy. The arch vessels were evaluated microscopically after intravital injection of India ink followed by clearing of the embryo to allow direct visualization and measuring of the arch vessel apparatus.

Ablation of neural crest caused most hearts to be abnormal. There appeared to be a combination of delayed development and abnormal location and/or proportions. Aberrations became more obvious with increasing age. Localized enlargements and uncoordinated growth of different regions were commonly observed.

It was significant that alterations in the heart were present in stages before the derivatives of neural crest normally participated in the partitioning of the outflow tract of the heart. We concluded from this fact that a factor in addition to partitioning, such as altered blood flow, contributes to aberrant heart development.

Neural crest ablation caused failure of arch vessels three, four, and six to develop to the proper size in some animals. Ablation led to a great heterogeneity of vessel size.

Clear evidence of early alteration of cardiovascular development led us to concentrate on the stages in which the earliest development of the arch vessel apparatus is taking place.

VERY EARLY VESSEL DEVELOPMENT

In this study,[5] developing vessels were studied on days three through five of incubation after neural crest ablation at stage 9-10. Vascular development was assessed by (1) scanning electron microscopic study of plastic casts made by injecting the vascular system and then removing the tissue, (2) cleared specimens injected intra-

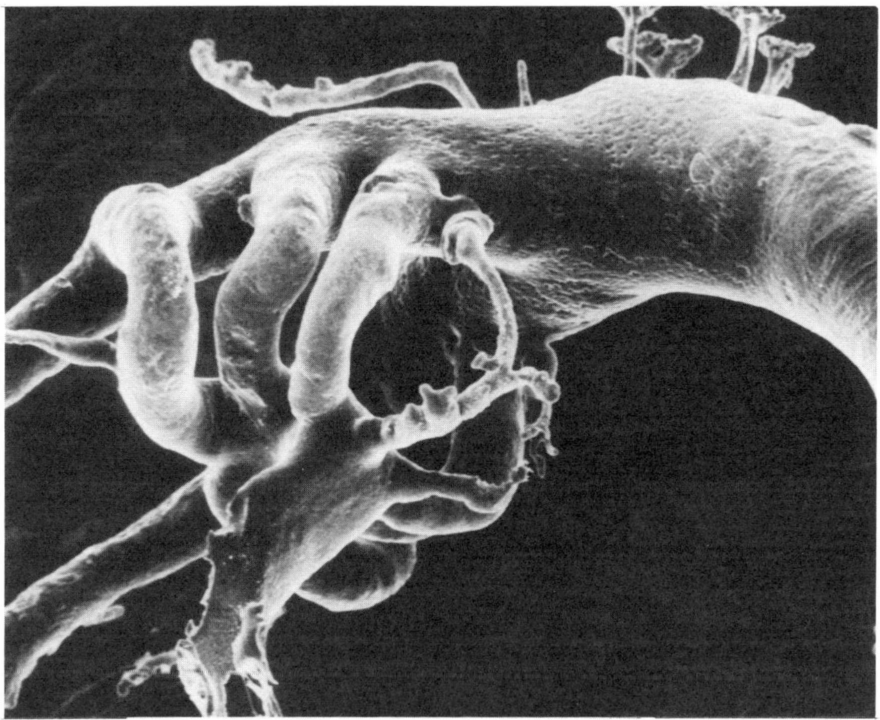

FIGURE 1. Scanning electron micrograph of a cast from a control embryo injected at four days of incubation, viewed from the left and behind. Arch vessels two, three, and four are fully formed and symmetrical. Arch vessel six is forming in the caudal part of the complex. (Bockman *et al.*[5] With permission from *Anatomical Record.*)

vascularly with India ink, and (3) serial histological sections. Early results led us to concentrate on the earliest stages (approximately stage 18) because alterations were already present then.

A notable finding was the early loss of bilateral symmetry. Whereas the normal pattern of arch vessel development is of a symmetrical "basket" of vessels surrounding the developing pharynx to join the aortic sac and dorsal aortae (FIG. 1), experimentally ablated animals displayed moderate to severe deviation from this pattern (FIG. 2). Furthermore the size of the individual arch vessels on a single side tended to vary a

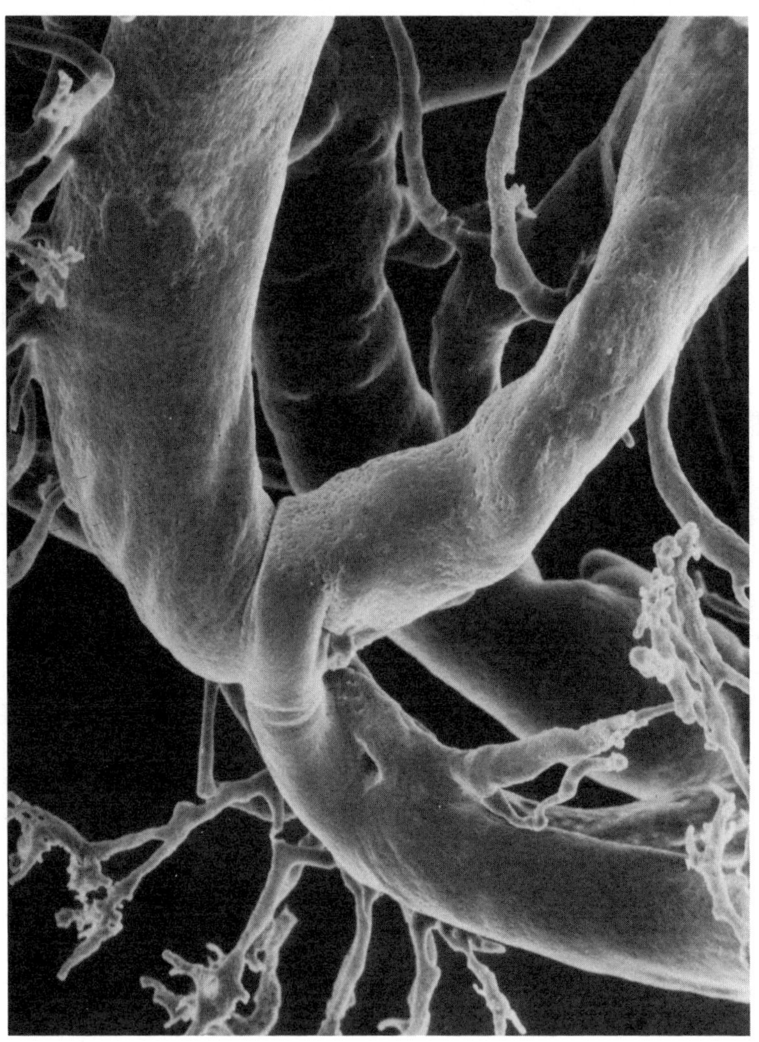

FIGURE 2. Scanning electron micrograph of a cast from an embryo after neural crest ablation. The embryo was injected at four days of incubation. The head region is toward the left. A single, large outflow tract joins with the dorsal aorta and primitive carotid vessels. There is remarkable deviation from the symmetrical "basket" pattern of controls. (Bockman et al.[5] With permission from Anatomical Record.)

great deal from each other. Rather than having a reasonably uniform diameter, there were apt to be very large or very small vessels in any given arch. This is consistent with the variability observed in the previously described study.

Vessels frequently were missing. The flow pattern was thus altered significantly. A common pattern was for a single, large vessel to continue directly from the outflow tract to the aorta, with small vessels representing part of the remaining arch apparatus. Blood flow into some arches was solely derived from the dorsal aorta, rather than the normal pattern of flow from aortic sac to dorsal aorta through that region. Irregular vessels and flow patterns are obvious in the artist's reconstruction shown in FIGURE 3.

Embryos were oriented in the embedding medium to allow cross sections through arch vessels to be cut, and to allow assessment of the relationships and quantities of

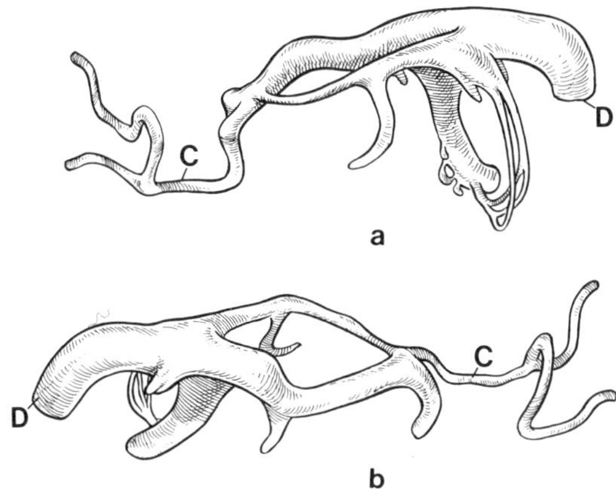

FIGURE 3. Artist's rendering of a three-dimensional reconstruction from a neural crest-ablated embryo on the fourth incubation day. A large outflow tract on the right side connects with the dorsal aorta (D), which bifurcates irregularly. Left arch vessels are represented only by tiny vessels. An irregular circular anastomosis is formed by the joining of vessels continuing from the aortic bifurcation anteriorly. A single primitive carotid vessel (C) supplies the head region. Ventrally projecting vessels from the aorta supply the arches. (Bockman *et al.*[5] With permission from *Anatomical Record.*)

arch components. There was a significant decrease (approximately 50%) in the quantity of mesenchyme present in the arches of experimental animals.

Furthermore, the relationship of the arch vessels to the epithelium of the pharynx was markedly different. The endothelium was directly apposed to the epithelium of the pharynx in animals with neural crest ablation (FIG. 4). The mesenchyme, which normally intervenes between endothelium and epithelium, was missing around much of the perimeter of the endothelium. In experimental animals, a mean of approximately 50% of the endothelium was directly apposed to epithelium, without intervening mesenchyme.

The changes observed in these early stages of development persisted through the study period so as to preclude the possibility of recovery in later developmental periods.

CONCLUSIONS

The described studies lead us to several conclusions that seem consistent with the observations, and with principles established by other investigations. After neural crest ablation, there is a selective failure of some arch vessels to develop. Vessels may be absent, too large, too small, or aberrant in their connections. There is a loss of bilateral symmetry, a condition that is quite characteristic in normal development of the arch

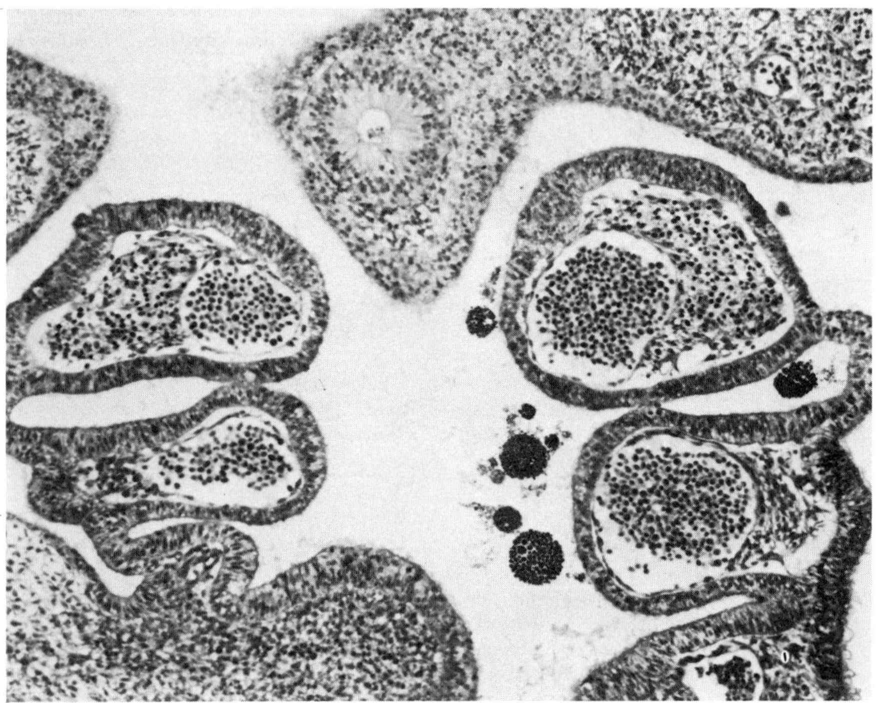

FIGURE 4. Cross section through arches from an experimental animal on the third incubation day. Arch mesenchyme is reduced and oriented laterally. The vessels tend to be more medially placed; in many places no mesenchyme intervenes between endothelium and epithelium. (Bockman *et al.*[5] With permission from *Anatomical Record.*)

vessel apparatus. With altered vessel diameter and connections, the channels through which blood flows are different, and the flow through them is altered. Even the direction of flow through certain segments may be altered.

After neural crest ablation, there is a significant decrease in the quantity of mesenchyme present in the arches, and its pattern of distribution is different. The mesenchyme intervening between the inner aspect of the arch vessels and the pharyngeal epithelium tends to be missing, with direct apposition of endothelium and epithelium.

These alterations occur very early. They are already present at stage 18, well before the period when septation of the outflow tract of the heart normally occurs.

Several possible mechanisms for the observed alterations may be suggested. It is possible that the failure of mesenchyme derived from neural crest to arrive at the proper time and in the proper quantities precludes its normal interaction with the developing vessels. There may even be enhanced regression of some vessels due to the absence of ectomesenchyme.

Ectomesenchyme is an important component of the functional "wall" of each arch vessel. Decreased quantities of this component may lead to defective development.

It would seem important to pursue the constitution of extracellular matrix in the arch areas subsequent to neural crest ablation. It is a reasonable extension that altered ectomesenchymal cells lead to altered ectomesenchymal matrix.

A BROADER PERSPECTIVE OF NEURAL CREST CONTRIBUTIONS

The alterations in cardiovascular development discussed above are, of course, not unique to experimental ablation of the neural crest. Naturally occurring conditions, such as the DiGeorge syndrome, typically involve not only the heart and great vessels but also other organs, such as parathyroids and thymus.[13–15] The known association of cranial neural crest with development of all these organs has been an important reason to suggest that they may be due to defective contributions from neural crest.[2,3,16]

Similar syndromes have been observed after other agents were administered accidentally or experimentally. Defects in the heart, great vessels, and thymus were observed after an analogue of vitamin A was taken by pregnant women.[17] Maternal alcohol abuse leads to similar syndromes.[15] These effects have been duplicated experimentally.[18,19]

The derivatives of neural crest may be a common pathway upon which different agents, including genetic programs, may have an effect. The timing, severity of the attack, and other agents present or absent at the time may modulate the initial damage, and the final results that then may appear as congenital defects, single or in a cluster.

The principles of interaction of neural crest derivatives with developing blood vessels probably will be transferable, to some extent, in understanding the defects of any of the organs affected in these syndromes.

ACKNOWLEDGMENTS

We gratefully acknowledge the medical illustration by Ms. Karen Waldo, and the technical assistance of Ms. Penny Roon, Ms. Harriett Stadt, and Mr. Hal Gauldin.

REFERENCES

1. KIRBY, M. L., T. F. GALE & D. E. STEWART. 1983. Neural crest cells contribute to normal aorticopulmonary septation. Science **220:** 1059-1061.

2. BOCKMAN, D. E. & M. L. KIRBY. 1984. Dependence of thymus development on derivatives of the neural crest. Science **223:** 498-500.

3. KIRBY, M. L. & D. E. BOCKMAN. 1984. Neural crest and normal development: A new perspective. Anat. Rec. **209:** 1-6.

4. BOCKMAN, D. E., M. E. REDMOND, K. WALDO, H. DAVIS & M. L. KIRBY. 1987. Effect of neural crest ablation on development of the heart and arch arteries in the chick. Am. J. Anat. **180:** 332-341.

5. BOCKMAN, D. E., M. E. REDMOND & M. L. KIRBY. 1989. Alteration of early vascular development after ablation of cranial neural crest. Anat. Rec. **225:** 209-217.

6. FOLKMAN, J. 1985. Tumor angiogenesis. Adv. Cancer Res. **43:** 175-203.

7. COFFIN, J. D. & T. J. POOLE. 1988. Embryonic vascular development: Immunohistochemical identification of the origin and subsequent morphogenesis of the major vessel primordia in quail embryos. Development **102:** 735-748.

8. JOHNSTON, M. C. 1966. A radioautographic study of the migration and fate of cranial neural crest cells in the chick embryo. Anat. Rec. **156:** 143-156.

9. LE LIÉVRE, C. S. & N. M. LE DOUARIN. 1975. Mesenchymal derivatives of the neural crest: Analysis of chimeric quail and chick embryos. J. Embryol. Exp. Morphol. **34:** 125-154.

10. LE DOUARIN, N. M. 1982. The Neural Crest. Cambridge University Press. London.

11. HAMBURGER, V. & H. HAMILTON. 1951. A series of normal stages in the development of the chick embryo. J. Morphol. **88:** 49-92.

12. NISHIBATAKE, M., M. L. KIRBY & L. H. S. VAN MIEROP. 1987. Pathogenesis of persistent truncus arteriosus and dextroposed aorta in the chick embryo after neural crest ablation. Circulation **75:** 225-264.

13. HUBER, J., P. CHOLNOKY & H. E. SOETHOUT. 1967. Congenital aplasia of parathyroid glands and thymus. Arch. Dis. Child. **42:** 190-192.

14. KRETSCHMER, R., B. JAY, D. BROWN & F. S. ROSEN. 1968. Congenital aplasia of the thymus gland (DiGeorge's Syndrome). N. Eng. J. Med. **297:** 1295-1301.

15. AMMANN, A. J., D. W. WARA, M. J. COWAN, D. J. VARRETT & E. R. STIEHM. 1982. The DiGeorge syndrome and the fetal alcohol syndrome. Am. J. Dis. Child. **136:** 906-908.

16. COULY, G., A. LAGRUE & C. GRISCELLI. 1983. Le syndrome de DiGeorge, neurocristopathie rhombencephalique exemplaire. Rev. Stomatol. Chir. Maxillofac. **84:** 103-108.

17. LAMMER, E. J., D. T. CHEN, R. M. HOAR, N. D. AGNISH, P. J. BENKE, J. T. BRAUN, C. J. CURRY, P. M. FERNHOFF, A. W. GRIX, I. T. LOTT, J. M. RICHARD & S. C. SUN. 1986. Retinoic acid embryopathy. A new human teratogen and a mechanistic hypothesis. N. Eng. J. Med. **313:** 837-841.

18. JOHNSTON, M. C., K. K. SULIK, W. S. WEBSTER & B. L. JARVIS. 1985. Isotretinoin embryopathy in a mouse model: Cranial neural crest involvement. Teratology **32:** 26A-27A.

19. DAFT, P. A., M. C. JOHNSTON & K. K. SULIK. 1986. Abnormal heart and great vessel development following acute ethanol exposure in mice. Teratology **33:** 93-104.

Hemodynamic Changes

Wall Stresses and Pressure Gradients in Neural Crest-Ablated Chick Embryos

LINDA LEATHERBURY,[a] DAVID S. BRADEN,[a]
HITOSHI TOMITA,[b] HAROLD E. GAULDIN,[b] AND
WILLIAM F. JACKSON [c]

[a]*Department of Pediatric Cardiology*
[b]*Department of Anatomy*
[c]*Department of Physiology and Endocrinology*
Medical College of Georgia
Augusta, Georgia 30912

INTRODUCTION

The developing chick embryo has been shown to be an acceptable model for studying human cardiac morphogenesis. Ablation of premigratory neural crest in these embryos results in a variety of cardiac malformations with the type of defect seen dependent upon the location and the size of the neural crest ablation.[1,2] For example, loss of neural crest cells destined for the third and fourth aortic arches specifically interferes with aorticopulmonary and truncal septation as well as aortic arch development, yielding an estimated 95% cardiovascular anomaly rate. This includes a 65% incidence of persistent truncus arteriosus and a 50% incidence of aortic arch anomalies.[3]

By using a microcinephotography system of filming the developing chick embryo, we have previously demonstrated dilated ventricular chambers and altered conotruncal dimensions in 3.5-day-old, neural crest-ablated chick embryos.[4] These changes occurred in early cardiogenesis long before septation of the outflow tracts began.[1,2] These embryos also had depressed ventricular function as evidenced by a decreased shortening fraction: 53% in ablated embryos versus 76% in nonablated embryos.[5] Embryos with neural crest ablation also demonstrated an increased incidence of absence of the right fourth aortic arch artery. Loss of an aortic arch artery might lead to an increase in the resistance to blood flow across this vascular network. Therefore, it was hypothesized that such an increase in resistance would increase the afterload experienced by the heart, which in turn would elevate ventricular wall stress and might lead to altered ventricular dimensions and depressed indices of ventricular performance. The purpose of the present study was to test this hypothesis by estimating ventricular wall stress from ventricular pressure and dimension measurements, and by assessing the pressure gradient across the arch arteries, as an index of their vascular resistance in control and neural crest-ablated embryos.

MATERIAL AND METHODS

Neural Crest Ablation

Fertilized Arbor Acre chicken eggs (Seaboard Hatchery, Athens, Georgia) were incubated in forced draft incubators at 38°C in 97% relative humidity. After 25 to 30 hours of incubation, they were "windowed" and prepared for microsurgery as reported by Narayanan.[6] The stage of development of the embryos was determined according to Hamburger and Hamilton.[7] The overlying vitelline membrane was torn, and the embryo was stained with neutral red. Surgical ablation by microcautery was performed on the embryonic neural folds at stages 9 or 10. In these experiments, neural crest was ablated bilaterally between the midotic placode and somite two. This region corresponds to presumptive cardiac neural crest for pharyngeal arches three and four.[3]

After microsurgery, the eggs were sealed with plastic tape and reincubated in the same high-humidity incubator for an additional 24 hours, after which they were transferred to a second incubator at 37°C and 70% relative humidity. Control eggs were transferred to incubators in parallel with the experimental eggs. The control embryos were windowed prior to microcinephotographic filming and were replaced in incubators to be sure that they were at the appropriate temperature. Twenty-one control and fifteen experimental embryos were analyzed after further incubation to Hamburger-Hamilton stage 18 of development (approximately 3 days).

Microcinephotography Technique

Experimental and control eggs were transferred to a heated sand bath. A microthermocouple probe was placed on the surface of the yolk adjacent to the embryo to monitor temperature, which was maintained at 37.5°C. In the stage 18 chick embryo, the heart formed a looped cardiac tube with bilateral aortic arches 2, 3, and 4 normally present.[7] A stage 18 embryos lies on the yolk sac such that the right-sided cardiovascular structures are delineated by red blood streams that are seen through the transparent embryonic tissue. Left-sided structures are visible only if the embryo is turned over on the yolk sac surface. Limb and wing buds do not obscure the cardiac tube or aortic arch arteries until later in development.

Microcinephotography was performed on 14 control and 12 experimental embryos with a high speed Redlake Lowcam II camera mounted on an Olympus stereo microscope. Lighting for filming was provided by a stroboscopic source (Strobex Model 236) that was triggered by the opening of the camera shutter and by two continuous fiberoptic light sources. Each embryo was filmed for five seconds at a film rate of 100 frames per second. Each egg was positioned in the sand bath the same distance from the microscope lens, giving a 30 times magnification factor onto the film. A micrometer was filmed with each embryo to allow exact calculation of the magnification factor.

The processed film was projected onto a digitizing pad for analysis. For each chick analyzed, three end-diastolic and three end-systolic frames were selected for measurement. Primitive right ventricular dimensions were measured directly. Ventricular width was measured at end-systole and end-diastole at the widest point of the ventricle. Ventral and dorsal wall thicknesses were measured in end-systole and end-diastole at the same point. Ventricular length was calculated in both end-systole and end-diastole from the apex of the primitive right ventricle to the junction of the primitive ventricle and the conotruncal cushions. The point of measurement at the region of the conotruncal cushions was chosen as the point where lines drawn from the ventral and dorsal walls intersected. These ventricular dimensions and wall thicknesses were used for the calculation of ventricular wall stresses.

Pressure Measurements

Intraventricular and dorsal aortic pressures were measured using glass microelectrodes (5 μm tip) filled with 2 M NaCl and a WPI 900 Servo-Null pressure system.[8] The signal from the Servo-Null transducer was digitized (12 bit, 100 Hz) by an IBM AT-based data acquisition system and stored on disk for later analysis. Peak systolic, end-diastolic, and mean pressures were then determined from these digitized signals. Pressure measurements were made immediately after completion of microcinephotography. Any embryo that bled on insertion of an electrode was discarded from the study. The order of measurement of ventricular and dorsal aortic pressures was randomized. Heart rates were determined from the digitized pulsatile pressure records.

Calculation of Ventricular Wall Stresses

Using the digitized ventricular dimensions and wall thicknesses and the measured ventricular pressures at end-systole and peak systole, wall stresses were calculated by use of the formulas presented in TABLE 1.[9-11] It is recognized that in calculating peak systolic stress, the assumption is made that peak stress occurs at peak pressure and that neither wall thickness nor ventricular width change markedly during isovolumic contraction or early ejection. In stage 18 chick embryos, there is no true isovolumic contraction phase because blood is going into the truncus in late diastole. Therefore, inasmuch as these assumptions are not entirely accurate, these estimates are useful only to compare the experimental and control groups and not to attempt to provide absolute values for these variables.

Statistical Analysis

Statistical analysis was performed using a one-tailed Student's *t* test or a one-factor ANOVA. Statistical significance was assessed at the 95% confidence level.

TABLE 1. Calculation of Ventricular Wall Stress[a]

1. End-systolic Meridional Stress (g/cm^2)
   = Pes $\times$ Dex $\times$ 1.35/4 hes (1 + hes/Des)
2. End-systolic Circumferential Stress (g/cm^2)
   = Pes $\times$ Des $\times$ 1.35 $\times$ (1 − (Des^2/2 Les^2))/2 hes
3. Peak Systolic Meridional Stress (g/cm^2)
   = PSVP $\times$ Ded $\times$ 1.35/4 hed (1 + hed/Ded)
4. Peak Systolic Circumferential Stress (g/cm^2)
   = PSVP $\times$ Ded $\times$ 1.35 $\times$ (1 − (Ded^2/2 Led^2))/2 hed

[a] Pes = end-systolic pressure (mm Hg); Des = ventricular width (mm) at end-systole; hes = ventral wall thickness (mm) at end-systole; Les = ventricular length (mm) at end-systole; PSVP = peak systolic ventricular pressure (mm Hg); Ded = ventricular width (mm) at end-diastole; hed = ventral wall thickness (mm) at end-diastole; Led = ventricular length (mm) at end-diastole; 1.35 = conversion factor from mm Hg to g/cm^2.

RESULTS

Aortic Arch Artery Abnormalities

Review of the microcineangiograms revealed that 58% of the embryos studied exhibited evidence of markedly hypoplastic right fourth aortic arch arteries. Thirty-three percent revealed total absence of blood flow in the right fourth aortic arch artery, and 25% revealed minimal blood flow in this vessel. Concomitantly, the same 58% revealed evidence of dilatation of the right third aortic arch artery.

Ventricular Dimensions and Wall Thicknesses

Ventricular dimensions are presented in TABLE 2. Experimental embryos displayed altered ventricular dimensions. Ventricular width at its widest location was increased in experimental embryos but not to a statistically significant level. Ventricular length, however, was significantly greater in experimental embryos. Thus, the ventricles of

TABLE 2. Ventricular Dimensions in Stage 18 Chick Embryos (mm; $\bar{x}$ ± SEM)

	Width		Length	
	Systole	Diastole	Systole	Diastole
Control (N = 14)	0.37 ± 0.02	0.62 ± 0.02	0.62 ± 0.01	0.80 ± 0.03
Experimental (N = 12)	0.43 ± 0.03	0.66 ± 0.02	0.77 ± 0.04	0.99 ± 0.06
Percent Change	+16	+6	+24	+24
p Value	0.04	NS	0.001	0.004

TABLE 3. Ventricular Wall Thicknesses in Stage 18 Chick Embryos
(mm; $\bar{x} \pm$ SEM)

	Ventral Wall		Dorsal Wall	
	Systole	Diastole	Systole	Diastole
Control (N = 14)	0.24 ± 0.01	0.17 ± 0.01	0.17 ± 0.01	0.13 ± 0.01
Experimental (N = 12)	0.18 ± 0.01	0.13 ± 0.01	0.14 ± 0.01	0.11 ± 0.01
Percent Change	−25	−24	−18	−15
p Value	0.001	0.003	0.015	0.013

experimental embryos were shown to be dilated compared to controls but with the maintenance of a somewhat ellipsoid shape.

Ventricular wall thicknesses in experimental and control embryos are shown in TABLE 3. The ventricles of experimental embryos had significantly thinner ventral and dorsal walls. Both experimental and control embryos exhibited an increase in ventricular wall thickness in systole as compared to diastole. The experimental embryos, however, had significantly thinner ventricular walls in both phases of the cardiac cycle.

Ventricular Pressures and Heart Rate

TABLE 4 illustrates ventricular pressures and heart rates in stage 18 chick embryos. Peak systolic ventricular pressures were not significantly different between the two groups. Despite the previously described incidence of ventricular dilatation seen in experimental embryos at this stage, the end-diastolic pressures in these experimental embryos were not significantly different from those found in control embryos. There were also no significant differences in heart rates obtained during pressure measurements in control and experimental embryos.

TABLE 4. Ventricular Pressures and Heart Rates in Stage 18 Chick Embryos
($\bar{x} \pm$ SEM)

	Peak Systolic (mm Hg)	End-Diastolic (mm Hg)	Heart Rate (min^{-1})
Control (N = 21)	1.64 ± 0.07	0.34 ± 0.02	152.9 ± 3.2
Experimental (N = 15)	1.69 ± 0.05	0.39 ± 0.02	152.6 ± 4.0
Percent Change	+4	+18	0
p Value	NS[a]	NS	NS

[a] Not significant.

TABLE 5. Ventricular Wall Stress in Stage 18 Chick Embryos (g/cm^2; $\bar{x} \pm$ SEM)

	End-Systolic		Peak Systolic	
	Meridional	Circumferential	Meridional	Circumferential
Control (N = 14)	0.13 ± 0.02	0.35 ± 0.05	1.59 ± 0.18	2.75 ± 0.25
Experimental (N = 12)	0.22 ± 0.08	0.51 ± 0.04	2.47 ± 0.23	4.39 ± 0.25
Percent Change	+69	+46	+55	+60
p Value	0.013	0.017	0.006	0.001

Ventricular Wall Stresses

Ventricular wall stress values are shown in TABLE 5. As hypothesized, ventricular wall stresses were significantly greater in the experimental embryos both at end-systole and peak systole. Values found were consistent with those described in human studies:[9–12] circumferential stresses were almost two times the meridional stresses both at end-systole and at peak systole.

Dorsal Aortic Pressures

Dorsal aortic pressures are shown in TABLE 6. Systolic, diastolic, and mean pressures were essentially the same in both control and experimental embryos. Although pulse pressures were slightly greater in experimental embryos, this difference did not achieve statistical significance ($p > 0.10$). Pressure measurements made in ventricles and in dorsal aortas revealed evidence of a systolic pressure gradient across the aortic arch artery network. There was no significant difference, however, in this gradient between control and experimental embryos.

TABLE 6. Dorsal Aortic Pressures in Stage 18 Chick Embryos (mm Hg; $\bar{x} \pm$ SEM)

	Systolic	Diastolic	Pulse Pressure	Mean	V sys − DA sys[a]
Control (N = 21)	0.91 ±0.05	0.51 ±0.04	0.40 ±0.02	0.72 ±0.05	0.73 ±0.08
Experimental (N = 15)	0.91 ±0.05	0.43 ±0.04	0.48 ±0.05	0.66 ±0.04	0.79 ±0.06
Percent Change	0	−16	+20	−8	−8
p Value	NS	NS	NS	NS	NS

[a] V sys − DA sys = Ventricular-Dorsal Aortic systolic pressure.

DISCUSSION

The goal of this research is to study abnormal cardiac development that leads to structural heart disease. Ablation of cardiac neural crest produces relatively predictable types of congenital heart defects, with a high anomaly rate.[1,2] This model serves as a useful tool to study the morphology and hemodynamics associated with congenital heart disease early in cardiac development.[1,2] A previous study, in which all of the cardiac neural crest was ablated, showed that there were abnormalities in hemodynamics in early cardiac development prior to the stage when any structurally abnormal heart disease was present.[8] Also, a microcinephotographic study of chick embryos with neural crest ablation at the looped cardiac tube stage (Hamburger-Hamilton stage 18) showed alterations in cardiac morphology as well as function: ventricles were dilated and displayed evidence of depressed contractility.[4] Subsequent quantification of hemodynamic variables showed that the primitive ventricle had a decreased shortening fraction with ventricular dilatation as a compensatory mechanism that allowed the embryo to maintain a normal cardiac output.[5] It was speculated that these altered hemodynamics were secondary to abnormalities in the aortic arch arteries.

Neural crest ablation produces structural heart disease, including a high incidence of aortic arch anomalies in chick embryos whose cardiovascular system is developed.[3] At earlier points in development, neural crest ablation produces great variability in the size of the aortic arch arteries when viewed in fixed specimens.[13] Furthermore, cinephotographic studies of living embryos demonstrated frequent occurrences of absent or severely decreased blood flow in the right fourth aortic arch artery, the vessel that would become the definitive aorta in the mature chick.[4] Therefore, it was proposed that there may be an increased resistance to blood flow across the total sum of the aortic arch arteries, which might lead to the previous observations of a decreased shortening fraction and ventricular dilatation.

As one means to evaluate this hypothesis, we calculated ventricular wall stresses. In other systems, singular increases in meridional wall stresses are usually associated with hypertrophy associated with increases in afterload,[12] such as what would be produced by an increase in the blood flow resistance offered by the aortic arch arteries. In the present study, however, we found that both circumferential and meridional wall stresses were significantly elevated in neural crest-ablated embryos. These findings are more suggestive of volume overload or ventricular dilatation due to myocardial dysfunction.[12] Simple volume overload, unaccompanied by changes in the myocardium, appears unlikely, as end diastolic pressures were not elevated. Wall stresses, however, in the ventricles of the experimental embryos may have been increased due to some primary myocardial defect and inadequate compensatory myocardial hypertrophy.

To address the hypothesis of an increased resistance to blood flow across the aortic arch arteries more directly, peak systolic pressures were measured in the primitive right ventricle and in the descending aorta. Ventricular and dorsal aortic pressures were similar in control and experimental embryos, and the values recorded agree with pressures measured by Van Mierop[14] and Clark[15] in embryos at the same stage of development. Previously we have provided evidence that although dilated, the hearts in neural crest-ablated embryos deliver a normal cardiac output.[5,16] If arch artery vascular resistance was increased after neural crest ablation, then the pressure drop across the arches would have to be elevated, as the flows are the same. In control and experimental embryos, peak systolic ventricular pressures, peak systolic dorsal aortic pressures, and their differences were identical. Thus, although there is hypoplasia or aplasia[3,13] and altered blood flow patterns (see RESULTS) in the arch arteries of embryos with neural crest ablation, it appears that blood flow resistance through this vascular network is unchanged. These observations imply that the embryos can compensate for altered arch artery structure. Consistent with this hypothesis is the observation that loss of blood flow in the right fourth aortic arch artery was invariably accompanied by evidence of increased flow in the right third aortic arch artery.

Thus, there is no evidence that the increased wall stress and dilatation observed in neural crest-ablated embryos results from an increased afterload due to an increase in blood flow resistance through the aortic arch arteries at this point in development. It is possible that at an earlier point in development after neural crest ablation, the resistance offered by the arch arteries was elevated and subsequently caused myocardial dysfunction. An alternative hypothesis, however, is that primary myocardial dysfunction is induced by neural crest ablation, which leads to the observed alterations in hemodynamics.

REFERENCES

1. KIRBY, M. L. 1987. Cardiac morphogenesis—Recent research advances. Pediatr. Res. **21:** 219-224.
2. KIRBY, M. L. 1988. Role of extracardiac factors in heart development. Experientia **44:** 944-951.
3. NISHIBATAKE, N., M. L. KIRBY & L. H. S. VAN MIEROP. 1987. Pathogenesis of persistent truncus arteriosus and dextroposed aorta in the chick embryo after neural crest ablation. Circulation **75:** 255-264.
4. LEATHERBURY, L., H. E. GAULDIN, K. WALDO & M. L. KIRBY. 1990. Microcinephotography of the developing heart in neural crest-ablated chick embryos. Circulation. In press.
5. LEATHERBURY, L., H. E. GAULDIN, H. A. STADT & M. L. KIRBY. 1988. Depressed myocardial function precedes development of persistent truncus arteriosus in neural crest-ablated chick embryos. Am. College Cardiol. **11:** 9A.
6. NARAYANAN, C. H. 1970. Apparatus and current techniques in the preparation of avian embryos for microsurgery and for observing embryonic behavior. Bioscience **20:** 868-871.
7. HAMBURGER, V. & H. L. HAMILTON. 1951. A series of normal stages in the development of the chick embryo. J. Morphol. **88:** 49-92.
8. STEWART, D. E., M. L. KIRBY & K. K. SULIK. 1986. Hemodynamic changes in chick embryos precede heart defects after cardiac neural crest ablation. Circ. Res. **59:** 545-550.
9. GAULT, J. H., J. ROSS JR. & E. BRAUNWALD. 1968. Contractile state of the left ventricle in man: Instantaneous tension-velocity-length relations in patients with and without disease of the left ventricular myocardium. Circ. Res. **22:** 451-459.
10. GROSSMAN, W., P. JONES & L. P. MCLAURIN. 1975. Wall stress and patterns of hypertrophy in the human left ventricle. J. Clin. Invest. **56:** 56-64.
11. BORROW, K. M., A. NEUMAN & J. WYNE. 1982. Sensitivity of end-systolic pressure-dimension and pressure-volume relations to the inotropic state in the human. Circulation **65:** 988-997.
12. GOULD, K. L., K. LIPSCOMB, G. W. HAMILTON & E. EDWARD. 1974. Relation of left ventricular shape, function and wall stress in man. Am. J. Cardiol. **34:** 627-634.
13. BOCKMAN, D. E., M. E. REDMOND, K. WALDO, H. DAVIS & M. L. KIRBY. 1987. Effect of neural crest ablation on development of the heart and arch arteries in the chick. Am. J. Anat. **180:** 332-341.
14. VAN MIEROP, L. H. S. & C. J. BERTUCH. 1976. Development of arterial blood pressure in the chick embryo. Am. J. Physiol. **212**(1): 43-48.

15. CLARK, E. B., N. HU, J. L. DUMMETT, O. K. VANDEKRIEFT, C. OLSON & J. R. TOMAENK. 1986. Ventricular function and morphology in chick embryo from stages 18 to 29. Am. J. Physiol. **250:** H409–H413.
16. JACKSON, W. F., H. E. GAULDIN, H. TOMITA & L. LEATHERBURY. 1990. Neural crest ablation does not alter ventricular pressure or estimated cardiac output despite altered morphology. Ann. N.Y. Acad. Sci. This volume.

Experimentally Induced Long QT Syndrome in the Chick Embryo[a]

JAMES L. CHRISTIANSEN[b] AND
MARGARET L. KIRBY[c]

[b]*Department of Pediatrics*
Section of Pediatric Cardiology
University of Iowa
Iowa City, Iowa 52242

[c]*Heart Development Group*
Department of Anatomy
Medical College of Georgia
Augusta, Georgia 30912-2000

INTRODUCTION

The long QT syndrome is an idiopathic congenital disorder in which affected individuals have abnormal prolongation of the QT interval of the electrocardiogram, signifying delayed repolarization.[1] Prolongation of the QT interval may be associated with ventricular arrhythmias, syncope, and sudden death.[2] Although acquired conditions of QT prolongation have been categorized as secondary to drugs, electrolyte imbalance, hypothermia, cerebral vascular disease, and neck surgery, the idiopathic or congenital types, with or without heritable features, remain the major focus of interest.[1] Heritable long QT conditions include the autosomal recessive Jervell and Lange-Nielsen syndrome linked with congenital deafness and the Romano-Ward syndrome, which is characterized by QT prolongation and normal hearing.[3–5]

Although the etiology remains elusive, several pathogenetic mechanisms have been proposed to explain the idiopathic long QT syndrome and its risk of ventricular tachyarrhythmias. The most popular hypothesis supports the concept of an imbalance in the sympathetic innervation to the heart, with a lower than normal right-sided cardiac sympathetic activity, allowing "dispersion" of repolarization and a propensity for ventricular tachycardia and fibrillation.[6] This hypothesis is derived from animal studies showing that stimulation of the left-sided sympathetic nerves or ablation of the right-sided stellate ganglion was associated with QT prolongation and a lowered threshold for ventricular arrhythmias.[7,8] Other theories have stressed a primary "neuropathology" as playing a central role, with certain affected individuals showing inflammatory or degenerative changes in the cardiac conduction system or cardiac

[a]This study was supported by a Grant-in-Aid from the American Heart Association, Georgia affiliate, and NIH Grants HL 36059 and HD 17063. Dr. Kirby is an Established Investigator of the American Heart Association, with funds contributed in part by the Georgia affiliate.

sympathetic ganglia.[6,9] Furthermore, there is growing evidence to implicate a defect of the cardiac cell membrane involving abnormalities of ionic current flow and its regulation, especially with regard to potassium and calcium. Recently, investigators were able to mimic several features of the long QT syndrome in canines using toxic doses of cesium, which produced QT prolongation and enhanced after-depolarization.[10] Study of these hypotheses has been hampered by the unavailability of an animal model that allows investigation of developmental aspects of this disease and its potential mechanism. In addition, little is known about interactions of autonomic terminals during development that result in an appropriate balance of neural input to the heart.

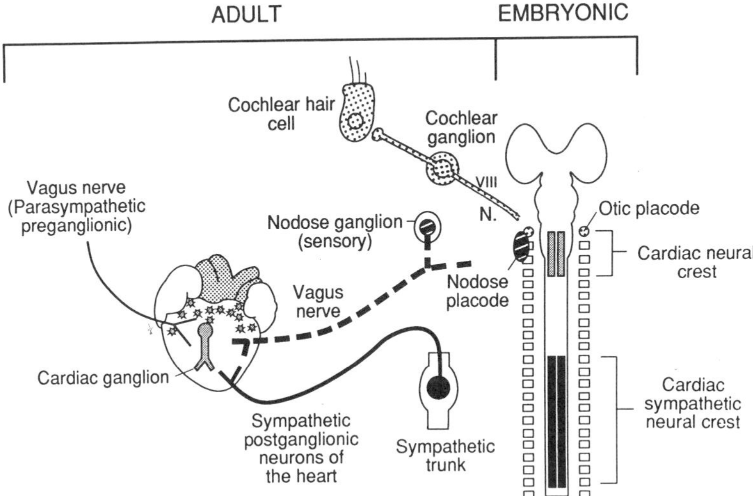

FIGURE 1. Illustration of the relationship of cardiac innervation and its derivation in the chick embryo. The parasympathetic postganglionic neurons are derived from neural crest adjacent to somites 1-3 (cardiac neural crest) (gray shading). The cardiac sympathetic postganglionic neurons (sympathetic trunk) arise from trunk neural crest adjacent to somites 10-20 (highlighted in black). The sensory innervation of the heart is derived from cells that arise from the nodose placode, forming neurons in the inferior ganglion of the vagus (nodose ganglion). Note the proximity of the nodose placode to the otic placode (speckled area), from which are derived structures of the inner ear.

Recent studies on the development and interactions of cardiac innervation in the chick embryo present an opportunity to test pathogenetic mechanisms of the long QT syndrome from an embryological standpoint. At least three sets of nerves form the innervation to the chick heart as shown in FIGURE 1.[11,12] Postganglionic cardiac sympathetic nerves are located in the first thoracic sympathetic ganglia of the paravertebral sympathetic trunks. The parasympathetic postganglionic cardiac nerves (cardiac ganglia) are found on the surface of the heart. Sensory innervation to the heart arises from neurons located in the inferior or thoracic ganglia of the vagus, the precursor of which is the nodose placode. Neural crest is the source of the parasympathetic and sympathetic innervation of the heart. Parasympathetic cardiac ganglia are derived from neural crest adjacent to somites 1-3. Sympathetic postganglionic neurons arise from the neural crest adjacent to somites 10-20. The nodose placode is an ectodermal thickening lying on the dorsal embryonic surface adjacent to the otic placode from which inner ear structures develop.[11] The proximity of the otic and nodose placodes in early development offers an attractive hypothesis to developmentally link the association of deafness and electrocardiographic abnormalities found in the congenital long QT syndrome, as injury to this area has the potential of causing hearing loss with perturbations of cardiac innervation.

As one phase of a study to assess the effects of alterations of cardiac innervation on electrocardiographic activity, we sought to determine whether selective perturbation of sensory innervation to the developing chick heart could alter the QT interval of the embryonic chick electrocardiogram.

METHODS

Fertile chicken eggs were obtained fresh and stored at 15-20°C until incubation. After incubation at 38°C and 97% humidity for 32-35 hours, eggs were windowed using a disc sander and prepared for microsurgery according to the method reported by Narayanan.[13] Embryonic structures were made visible by lightly staining with the vital dye, neutral red. The vitelline membrane was then torn to expose the embryonic structures of interest. All microsurgical procedures were performed on embryos at Hamburger-Hamilton stage 10 of development as determined by published criteria.[14]

Microsurgery

Premigratory surface ectoderm in the area of the right nodose placode (FIG. 1) was removed by microcautery with the aid of a dissecting microscope. A unilateral ablation was performed in part to limit mortality associated with surgical manipulation. Eggs were then resealed and returned to the 38°C incubator. When the circulation was established (about 72 hours of incubation), eggs were moved to an incubator maintained at 37°C and 70% humidity until ready for use. Sham-operated controls were prepared in parallel, undergoing identical preparatory procedures without microcautery.

Electrocardiography

After functional autonomic innervation was established,[12,15,16] three lead electrocardiograms were obtained using stainless steel electrodes placed through the shell at incubation day 17, 18, or 19 in an electrically grounded, controlled temperature environment. Lead orientation was kept constant to allow comparison of results between embryos. Bipolar electrograms were obtained using lead pairs and a grounded reference electrode. A thermistor was placed within the egg to monitor temperature, which was kept constant at 37 ± 0.2°C. Electrocardiographic leads were connected to a switching box to allow sequential recording of lead pairs. This in turn was connected with an isolated preamplifier and amplifier with a frequency response of 0.05 to 100 hz. Electrocardiograms were recorded at paper speeds of 50 and 100 mm/s using a standard chart recorder. The best quality lead tracing was used to measure the RR and QT intervals, as indices of heart rate and repolarization, respectively. The QT interval was then corrected for heart rate using formula $QT_c = QT/(RR)^{1/2}$ and averaged for ten complexes. Measurement of intervals was accomplished using hand-held calipers without knowledge of embryo grouping. Embryos were excluded from analysis if high-quality electrocardiograms could not be obtained.

Pathologic Analysis

Following electrocardiography, embryos were sacrificed, analyzed for gross defects, and staged for maturity using published criteria.[14] The heart was rapidly perfused with Carnoy's fixative, and the embryo was postfixed by immersion in 10% neutral buffered formalin. The heart and great vessels were examined grossly for abnormalities. Then detailed dissection was undertaken with particular attention paid to the orientation and course of the cardiac outflow to detect abnormalities of the aortic arch or its branches, as well as to catalogue intracardiac defects, if any. Additional note was made of the presence and size of the nodose ganglia (inferior ganglia of the vagus). Embryos with severe gross defects were excluded from analysis.

Statistical Methods

Results of electrocardiographic analysis for RR and QT_c for sham and experimental groups were compared using ANOVA and the unpaired one-tailed t test. A p value of <0.05 was considered to reflect a significant difference between the two groups.

RESULTS

A total of 114 embryos were subjected to microcautery or sham operation (84, right nodose placode ablation; 30, sham operation). Viability ranged from 24% in the experimental group to 40% in the sham-operated controls. These rates compared favorably with viability rates in previous studies using the same techniques.[17,18] There were 32 embryos that survived for study. Seventeen embryos were excluded from analysis: 12 because of poor quality electrocardiographic tracings, 5 because of severe malformations.

Fifteen embryos were selected for analysis, as shown in TABLE 1. Embryos subjected to right nodose placode ablation had longer mean rate corrected QT intervals than sham-operated embryos ($p = 0.001$). Further comparison of the experimental group to a larger reference population of embryos not subjected to microsurgery

TABLE 1. Results of Electrocardiogram Analysis[a]

Group	N	HR (bpm)[b]	QT_c[c]
Experimental	7	207 ± 0.3	.341 ± .004
Sham	8	222 ± 0.4	.316 ± .005
		$p = .02$	$p = .001$

[a] Data presented as mean ± SEM.
[b] HR, heart rate in beats per minute.
[c] QT_c, rate corrected QT interval.

yielded similar results ($p < 0.001$) (TABLE 2). Additionally, experimental embryos had lower average heart rates than sham-operated controls ($p = 0.02$). No arrhythmias were detected during electrocardiographic monitoring. Gross and pathological analysis of both groups is depicted in TABLE 3. Embryos from both groups were affected. Three embryos in the experimental group and two in the sham-operated control group had cardiac or other structural defects. Cardiac defects were confined to the area of the membranous interventricular septum where a small ventricular septal defect was present in four embryos. Analysis of the outflow region and aortic arch vessels of these embryos revealed no abnormalities. The right and left nodose ganglia were located in all embryos. A qualitative size comparison between the two showed mild hypoplasia of the right nodose ganglion (ipsilateral to microcautery ablation) in the three embryos with more marked QT prolongation. Extracardiac defects were more frequently seen in the experimental group, but rate-corrected QT prolongation did not appear to be related to the presence of extracardiac defects.

DISCUSSION

The association of congenital deafness, syncope, and electrocardiographic prolongation of the QT interval has intrigued investigators since its first clinical description by Jervell and Lange-Nielsen in 1957.[3] The strong association between syncopal episodes and physical or emotional stress implied a critical role of the sympathetic nervous system in the genesis of arrhythmias typical of the syndrome.[2-4] The basic premise that the increased risk of ventricular arrhythmias was a consequence of an

TABLE 2. Distribution of Heart Rate-Corrected QT Interval Related to Age in Embryos Not Subjected to Nodose Placode Ablation[a]

Embryo age	N	QT_c
Day 17	9	.304 ± .004
Day 18	16	.307 ± .005
Day 19	9	.304 ± .006
Day 20	10	.308 ± .004

[a] Data presented as mean ± SEM.

imbalance in the sympathetic innervation to the heart, with an underactivity of the right-sided sympathetic cardiac nerves, was supported by circumstantial evidence from both human and animal studies. Findings that implicated an abnormality of right-sided sympathetic cardiac nerves included data showing that (1) interruption of the right cardiac sympathetic activity in dogs mimics the characteristic electrocardiographic changes,[7] (2) sympathetic control of heart rate is almost exclusively mediated through right-sided cardiac nerves, with most affected patients manifesting a low resting heart rate and impaired chronotropic response to exercise,[19,20] and (3) right stellate ganglion destruction in dogs lowers the threshold for ventricular fibrillation.[8] Whereas various acute[6–8,10] and chronic[21] animal preparations have been proposed as

TABLE 3. Pathological Analysis of Embryos

Experimental animal No.	Observed Defects			QT$_c$
	Heart	Nodose ganglion	Other	
1	VSD[a]	normal	hypoplastic maxilla encephalocele	.333
2	normal	normal	none	.323
3	VSD	normal	mild abdominal wall defect	.342
4	normal	normal	none	.332
5	normal	R[b] hypoplastic	none	.339
6	normal	R hypoplastic	mild abdominal wall defect mild ectopia cordis	.354
7	normal	R hypoplastic	none	.363

Sham-operated animal No.	Observed defects			QT$_c$
	Heart	Nodose ganglion	Other	
1	normal	normal	none	.314
2	normal	normal	none	.300
3	normal	normal	none	.320
4	VSD	normal	none	.310
5	normal	normal	none	.299
6	normal	normal	none	.326
7	normal	normal	none	.329
8	VSD	normal	encephalocele	.326

[a] VSD, ventricular septal defect.
[b] R, right.

models because they have findings mimicking those of the long QT syndrome, there is as yet no suitable animal model from which to study developmentally the mechanisms that may underlie the evolution of these conditions.

Recent studies in the chick embryo and mouse have advanced knowledge of the interactions of parasympathetic, sympathetic, and sensory nerves. The production of sympathetically aneural chick hearts by removing neural crest cell precursors of sympathetic innervation has enabled study of the effects of removing only one division of the autonomic input to the heart.[22,23] When the sympathetic innervation to the developing heart was removed, parasympathetic innervation was increased by

50-100% due to both hypertrophy and hyperplasia of the ganglion cells as well as their terminals.[24] Studies in the adult mouse iris have further demonstrated the reciprocal modulation of sensory, sympathetic, and parasympathetic terminals in the target organ.[25,26] Removal of any one set of nerves allowed reciprocal increases in growth of the remaining nerves, possibly by altering the availability of growth factors produced by the target organ.

The chick embryo is an easily manipulated animal in which to study interactions of the autonomic nervous system as they might relate to pathogenesis of the idiopathic long QT syndrome. As compared to murine systems, the development and functional activity of autonomic innervation to the heart in avians occurs early.[15,16] This feature allows study of possible perturbations of neural input to the heart in a functionally intact system prior to hatching. It has been established that cholinergic neuroeffector transmission begins on day 12 of incubation, although functional adrenergic transmission is not demonstrable until embryonic day 16.[12] Therefore, characterization of electrocardiographic changes at embryonic day 17 or later has the potential for extrapolation to possible autonomic interactions later in life as the sympathetic and parasympathetic nervous systems mature.

Perturbation of the anlage of cells destined to provide sensory innervation to the heart, prior to their migration, results in prolongation of the QT interval of the embryonic chick electrocardiogram. Additionally, the mean heart rate of affected embryos was lower than that of sham-operated controls. These findings mimic those of children with the idiopathic form of the long QT syndrome.[27] The mechanism of these changes is not known. Whether they represent a direct result of deficient sensory innervation, or are secondary to an induced imbalance of sympathetic or parasympathetic innervation, remains to be determined by future studies. Improvements in surgical technique and studies to characterize and measure changes in autonomic and sensory innervation are important for answering questions regarding the role of symmetry and the potential for neural regeneration in this model.

In our opinion, the occurrence of heart and other structural defects in these embryos does not weaken the utility of this model. Spontaneous occurrence of ventricular septal defects has been known to occur in White Leghorn chick embryos.[28] The absence of associated aortic arch and conotruncal anomalies in the experimental group is an important finding for excluding an additional effect of microcautery on migrating cardiac neural crest. In addition to its role in supplying all of the postganglionic parasympathetic innervation to the heart, cardiac neural crest supplies mesenchymal elements to the aorticopulmonary septum and aortic arches.[12,29] Similarly, the more frequent occurrence of midline and chest wall defects in the experimental groups may reflect the extensive manipulation required to successfully perform microcautery. In addition, the first surgical procedure, tearing the vitelline membrane, performed on embryos in both experimental and control groups, may cause significant lateral tension resulting in partial separation of the neural tube. This may explain the occasional occurrence of encephalocele in each group. Finally, the finding of maxillary hypoplasia (upper beak shorter than lower beak) in one experimental animal may imply some effect on migrating cranial neural crest, as these cells form the skeleton of the upper and lower jaws in addition to other skeletal structures in the head.[30] Although cephalic to the nodose placode, neural crest cells in this region may have been inadvertently damaged by manipulation or microsurgical procedures.

The value of this model as currently developed[31] lies in its potential to provide new insights into autonomic interactions that may be involved in the pathogenesis of the idiopathic long QT syndrome. Our speculation that this syndrome may be related to perturbations of sensory innervation to the heart is important in that the contiguity of the otic and nodose placodes early in embryonic development, in humans[32] as well as in avians, provides a developmental link to the poorly understood association of hearing abnormalities that characterize one presentation of the syndrome.

REFERENCES

1. SURAWICZ, B. & S. B. KNOEBEL. 1984. Long QT: good, bad, or indifferent? J. Am. Coll. Cardiol. **4:** 398-413.
2. SCHWARTZ, P. J., M. PERITI & A. MALLIANI. 1975. The long QT syndrome. Am. Heart J. **89:** 378-390.
3. JERVELL, A. & F. LANGE-NIELSEN. 1957. Congenital deaf-mutism, functional heart disease with prolongation of the Q-T interval and sudden death. Am. Heart J. **54:** 59-68.
4. ROMANO, C., G. GEMME & R. PONGIGLIONE. 1963. Aritmie cardiache rare dell'eta pediatrica. La Clinic Paediatrica **45:** 656-683.
5. WARD, O. C. 1964. A new famial cardiac syndrome in children. J. Irish Medical Assoc. **54:** 103-106.
6. SCHWARTZ, P. J. 1985. Idiopathic long QT syndrome: Progress and questions. Am. Heart J. **109:** 399-411.
7. YANOWITZ, R., J. B. PRESTON & J. A. ABILDSKOV. 1966. Functional distribution of right and left stellate innervation to the ventricles: production of neurogenic electrocardiographic changes by unilateral alternation of sympathetic tone. Circ. Res. **18:** 416-428.
8. SCHWARTZ, P. J., N. G. SNEBOLD & A. M. BROWN. 1976. Effects of unilateral cardiac sympathetic denervation on the ventricular fibrillation threshold. Am. J. Cardiol. **37:** 1034-1040.
9. JAMES, T. N., D. P. ZIPES, R. E. FINEGAN, J. W. EISELE & J. E. CARTER. 1979. Cardiac ganglionitis associated with sudden unexpected death. Ann. Intern. Med. **91:** 727-734.
10. LEVINE, J. H., J. F. SPEAR, T. GUARNIERI, M. L. WEISFELDT, C. D. J. DE LANGEN, L. C. BECKER & E. N. MOORE. 1985. Cesium chloride-induced long QT syndrome: demonstration of afterdepolarizations and triggered activity *in vivo.* Circulation **72:** 1092-1103.
11. D'AMICO-MARTEL, A. & D. M. NODEN. 1983. Contributions of placodal and neural crest cells to avian cranial peripheral ganglia. Am. J. Anat. **166:** 445-468.
12. KIRBY, M. L. & D. E. STEWART. 1986. Development of the ANS innervation to the avian heart. *In* Developmental Neurobiology of the Autonomic Nervous System. P. Gootman, Ed.: 135-158. Humana Press. Clifton, NJ.
13. NARAYANAN, C. H. 1970. Apparatus and current techniques in the preparation of avian embryos for microsurgery and for observing embryonic behavior. Bioscience **20:** 868-871.
14. HAMBURGER, V. & H. C. HAMILTON. 1951. A series of normal stages in the development of the chick embryo. J. Morphol. **88:** 49-62.
15. PAPPANO, A. 1975. Development of autonomic neuroeffector transmission in the chick embryo heart. *In* Developmental and Physiological Correlates of Cardiac Muscle. M. Lieberman & T. Sano, Eds.: 235-247. Raven Press. New York.
16. MARVIN, W. J., K. HERMSMEYER, R. I. McDONALD, L. M. ROSKOSKI & R. ROSKOSKI. 1980. Ontogenesis of cholinergic innervation in the rat heart. Circ. Res. **46:** 690-695.
17. KIRBY, M. L., R. S. ARONSTAM & J. J. BUCCAFUSCO. 1985. Changes in cholinergic parameters associated with failure of conotruncal septation in embryonic chick hearts after neural crest ablation. Circ. Res. **56:** 392-401.
18. NISHIBATAKE, M., M. L. KIRBY & L. H. S. VAN MIEROP. 1987. Pathogenesis of persistent truncus arteriosus and dextroposed aorta in the chick embryo after neural crest ablation. Circulation **75:** 255-264.
19. RANDALL, W. C. & W. G. ROHSE. 1956. The augmentor action of the sympathetic cardiac nerves. Circ. Res. **4:** 470-475.
20. SCHWARTZ, P. J. & H. L. STONE. 1976. Role of right stellate ganglion during exercise. Eur. J. Clin. Invest. **6:** 328 (abstract).
21. SCHWARTZ, P. J. 1978. Experimental reproduction of the long QT syndrome. Am. J. Cardiol. **41:** 374-379.

22. KIRBY, M. L. & D. E. STEWART. 1984. Adrenergic innervation of the developing chick heart. Neural crest ablations to produce sympathetically aneural hearts. Am. J. Anat. **171:** 295-305.
23. PHILLIPS, M. T., M. L. KIRBY & D. E. STEWART. 1986. Cyclic AMP in normal and sympathetically aneural hearts during development. J. Mol. Cell. Cardiol. **18:** 827-835.
24. KIRBY, M. L., D. C. CONRAD & D. E. STEWART. 1987. Increase in the cholinergic cardiac plexus in sympathetically aneural chick hearts. Cell Tissue Res. **247:** 489-496.
25. KESSLER, J. A. 1985. Parasympathetic, sympathetic, and sensory interactions in the iris: Nerve growth factor regulates cholinergic ciliary ganglion innervation *in vivo.* J. Neurosci. **5:** 2719-2725.
26. KESSLER, J. A., W. O. BELL & I. B. BLACK. 1983. Interactions between sympathetic and sensory innervation of the iris. J. Neurosci. **3:** 1301-1307.
27. VINCENT, G. M. 1986. The heart rate of Romano-Ward syndrome patients. Am. Heart J. **112:** 61-64.
28. KUHLMANN, R. S. & G. L. KOLESARI. 1984. The spontaneous occurrence of aortic arch and cardiac malformations in the White Leghorn chick embryo (Gallus domesticus). Teratology **30:** 55-59.
29. KIRBY, M. L. 1987. Cardiac morphogenesis—recent research advances. Pediatr. Res. **21:** 219-224.
30. LE DOUARIN, N. 1982. The Neural Crest. pp. 54-90. Cambridge University Press. Cambridge.
31. CHRISTIANSEN, J. L., H. A. STADT, M. J. MULROY & M. L. KIRBY. 1989. Electrocardiographic QT prolongation after ablation of the nodose placode in the chick embryo: a developmental model of the idiopathic long QT syndrome. Pediatr. Res. **26:** 11-15.
32. KISSEL, P., J. M. ANDRE & A. JACQUIER. 1981. The Neurocristopathies. pp. 1-14. Masson Publishing. New York.

Effect of Adrenergic Innervation on Growth of SHR Myocytes

DIANNE L. ATKINS, THOMAS R. LLOYD,
WILLIAM J. MARVIN JR., AND
JANE K. ROSENTHAL

*University of Iowa
Department of Pediatrics
Iowa City, Iowa 52242*

We have previously presented data demonstrating the trophic effect of adrenergic innervation on the growth of cultured ventricular cells.[1] Following the onset of *in vitro* adrenergic innervation, myocardial cells from normotensive Wistar-Kyoto (WKY) rats had increased cell, sarcoplasm, nuclear, mitochondrial, and sarcomere volumes. The spontaneously hypertensive genetic counterstrain of WKY, the SHR, develops cardiomegaly and hypertrophy prior to the onset of hypertension, implying that factors other than blood pressure regulate myocardial growth.[2,3] Cardiomegaly can be caused by an increase in myocardial cell size or number. This study was undertaken to measure the size of single neonatal SHR cultured myocytes after *in vitro* adrenergic innervation to determine if the trophic effect of innervation can explain the development of cardiomegaly in the SHR prior to the onset of systemic hypertension. The results were compared to the response of WKY cells.

Ventricular myocyte cultures were prepared from both WKY and SHR neonatal rat hearts by mechanical and enzymatic dispersion. Simultaneous thoracolumbar sympathetic ganglion explants were added to half the cultures. In this system, neuroeffector transmission is present by 48 hours.[4,5] Isolated and innervated SHR and WKY myocytes were randomly selected after 96 hours in culture and were fixed, stained, and serially sectioned (90 nm) for transmission electron microscopy. Photomicrographs ($\times 3000$ and $\times 24,000$) were prepared of every fifth section. Absolute cell volume, μ^3, and sarcoplasmic, sarcomere, and mitochondrial volumes were stereologically analyzed using overlying grids of 10 nm and 20 nm; the data were entered into a computerized point counting system. Significant differences were identified by one- and two-way ANOVA, accepting $p < 0.05$ as significant.

SHR and WKY total cell volume were not different prior to *in vitro* adrenergic innervation (1472 ± 308, n = 6, and 1555 ± 778, n = 7, $p > 0.05$). Sarcoplasmic, nuclear, and mitochondrial volumes were also similar between the two cell types. SHR sarcomere volume was half WKY sarcomere volume ($p < 0.05$). Adrenergic innervation significantly increased total cell volume of both cell types (3053 ± 466, n = 5, and 4566 ± 1097, n = 5, $p < 0.001$), but the percentage increase was less in the SHR (107% and 194% $p < 0.01$). Significant increases were also observed in sarcoplasmic, mitochondrial, and sarcomere volumes. Although significant increases in sarcomere and mitochondrial volumes occurred after adrenergic innervation ($p < 0.05$), sarcomere volume/mitochondrial volume was less in SHR than WKY (0.69 and 1.34) and did not change after innervation.

Cross-strain innervation experiments demonstrated that the increase in cell volume after adrenergic innervation is greater in WKY cells regardless of the source of neurons. When innervated with WKY or SHR neurons the percent increase in mean cell volume of WKY is the same (196% vs 194%, $p > 0.05$). In marked contrast, SHR myocytes innervated with WKY neurons are no larger than SHR myocytes innervated with SHR neurons (130% vs. 107% $p > 0.05$). Thus the size difference in response to innervation is due to differences in the myocardial cells rather than differences in the neurons. Adrenergic innervation alone is not sufficient to explain the cardiomegaly present in SHR while still normotensive.

REFERENCES

1. ROSENTHAL, J. K. & W. J. MARVIN, JR. 1988. Anat. Rec. **220:** 82A.
2. CLUBB, F. J., JR. & S. P. BISHOP. 1984. Lab. Invest. **50:** 571-577.
3. TOMANEK, R. J. 1979. Lab. Invest. **40:** 428-433.
4. MARVIN, W. J., JR., D. L. ATKINS, V. L. CHITTICK, D. D. LUND & K. HERMSMEYER. 1984. Circ. Res. **55:** 49-58.
5. ATKINS, D. L. & W. J. MARVIN, JR. 1989. Circ. Res. **64:** 1051-1067.

Degradation of Hyaluronic Acid Enhances Myocardial Performance of the Postlooped Rat Heart *in Situ*

H. SCOTT BALDWIN,[a] THOMAS R. LLOYD,[b] AND
MICHAEL SOLURSH[c]

[a]*Department of Pediatrics*
[c]*Department of Biology*
University of Iowa
Iowa City, Iowa 52242
and
[b]*Department of Pediatrics*
University of Arizona
Tucson, Arizona 85724

The primitive heart tube is composed of endocardium and myocardium separated by extracellular matrix or "cardiac jelly." During the initial stages of looping this extracellular matrix is composed primarily of hyaluronic acid (HA). Although the structural contribution made by hyaluronic acid during early heart development has been the subject of intense investigation, no information exists about its role in the ontogeny of embryonic myocardial function. The purpose of our study was to quantify the effect of hyaluronate degradation on the myocardial performance of prelooped and early postlooped embryonic rat hearts *in situ*.

METHODS

Wistar rat embryos were explanted on gestational day 9.5 (positive vaginal smear = day 0) and cultured under a gas phase of 5% O_2, 5% CO_2, and 90% N_2 in rat serum alone (controls) or rat serum containing 20 turbidity-reducing units (TRU)/mL of Streptomyces hyaluronidase (SH), an enzyme that specifically degrades hyaluronate. Myocardial function was determined by video motion analysis at each edge of the bulbus cordis and primitive ventricle in prelooped (24 h in culture) and postlooped embryos (36 h in culture). Alcian blue staining at pH 2.5 was used to document the extent of HA degradation.

RESULTS

Despite extensive degradation of HA throughout the initial stages of looping, all treated, as well as control embryos, developed an "S" looped configuration. There was no difference in cardiac function between control and treated embryos prior to looping. Immediately following looping, however, there was a significant ($p < 0.05$) increase in shortening fraction ($20 \pm 2\%$, n = 10 vs. $30 \pm 2\%$, n = 20), maximum velocity of contraction ($591 \pm 76\ \mu/s$ vs. $952 \pm 90\ \mu/s$), and maximum velocity of relaxation ($594 \pm 79\ \mu/s$ vs. $921 \pm 80\ \mu/s$) in SH-treated embryos when compared with controls measured at the bulbus cordis. Similar increases were seen in postlooped-treated embryos when measured at the primitive ventricle.

CONCLUSIONS

These observations suggest that (1) hyaluronic acid is not essential for looping of the mammalian heart, *in situ*, and that (2) HA does play a role, however, in the maintenance of normal embryonic myocardial function.

Congenital Cardiac Malformations and Chronic Alcoholism in Rat Fetuses

A. BALLESTEROS, M. A. MARCO, E. R. FRIZELL,
J. A. F. LÓPEZ DE OCHOA, M. FRESNILLO, AND
I. VILLA ELÍZAGA

Department of Pediatrics
University of Navarra
Navarra, Spain

INTRODUCTION

The fetal alcohol syndrome (FAS) is a well-defined clinical consequence with a rate of between 1 and 2 for every 1000 born alive.[1] The complete syndrome includes a slowing down of pre- and postnatal growth, microcephalia with mental retardation, an abnormal facial aspect, as well as a high incidence of other malformations, particularly those that affect the heart.[2]

Due to the lack of experimental studies orientated towards analyzing congenital cardiac malformations in rats induced by chronic gestational exposure to ethanol, we intend to develop the present research.

MATERIAL AND METHODS

We used 40 albino rats of the Sprague-Dawley variety; they were distributed into four groups: control (group C), non-alcoholic *ad libitum;* embryonic (group E), alcoholic *ad libitum;* fetal (group F), alcoholic, pair-fed to E; and pair-fed (group P), nonalcoholic, pair-fed to E.

Once the gestational period had begun, the embryonic group continued receiving elevated quantities of alcohol in its diet until the end of gestation, in such a way that their blood ethanol levels remained within the critical area, specifically during organogenesis. The ethylic concentrations in the diets of the fetal group diminished drastically at the beginning of the gestation only to be gradually increased later on in the first 14 days of gestation, so that the litters would not be exposed to critical levels of alcohol during the embryonic period, although they would be during the fetal development period. Alcohol blood levels were determined on the 42d day in the pregestational period and on the 3d, 7th, 14th, and 19th gestational days, also. A cesarian section was performed on the 20th day and three fetuses were randomly chosen and serially cut (10 μm) and examined through a light microscope. We were looking for cardiac malformations as well as studying the ventricular muscular mass.[3] Similarly two fetuses were randomly chosen; their fetal weight and cardiac weight were obtained as well as the relationship between cardiac weight and fetal weight.

RESULTS AND DISCUSSION

As far as cardiopathies in general are concerned, the rate was 47.83, 6.66, 6.66, and 3.33% for the fetuses in the E, F, P, and C groups, respectively (FIG. 1). The ventricular septal defect was the only cardiopathy detected in all of the groups.

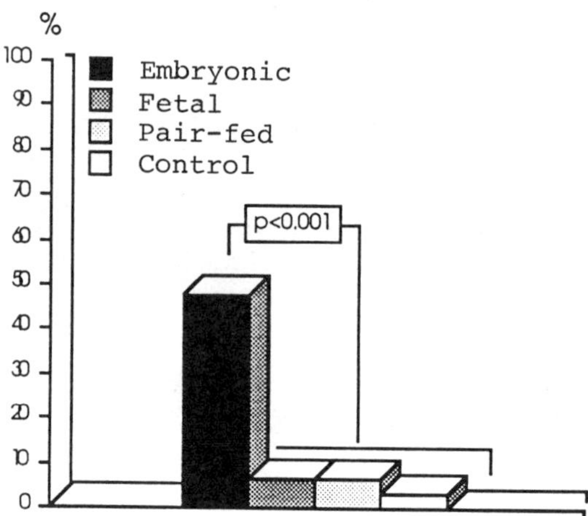

Moreover, four overriding aorta appeared, and two biventricular agenesia appeared exclusively in the E group (FIG. 2). We found similar results, insofar as the type of malformations described in mice.[4] The median of the fetal cardiac weights was 18.9, 23, 29.55, and 30.27 mg for the E, F, P, and C groups, significant difference existing among all the groups ($p < 0.05$). Nonetheless, when comparing the percentage of fetal weight corresponding to cardiac weight, the comparison was similar in the fetuses of the different groups, remaining around 0.80%, values similar to those of other authors with rats 3 days old and similar to those in our group F.[5] In reference to the total ventricular and net muscular areas of section, the P and C groups were significantly greater with respect to the alcoholic groups (E and F) (FIG. 3).

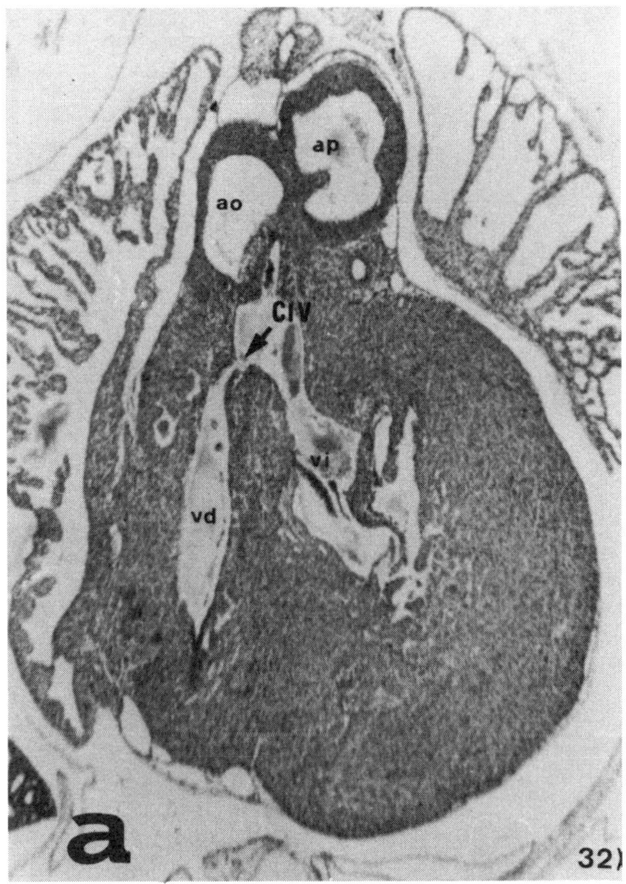

FIGURE 2. Ventricular septal defects and overriding aorta. **a:** Ventricular septal defect; **b:** overriding aorta; **c:** ventricular septal defect and overriding aorta. **ao:** aorta; **ap:** pulmonary trunk; **acao:** overriding aorta; **civ:** ventricular septal defect; **vd:** right ventricle; **vi:** left ventricle.

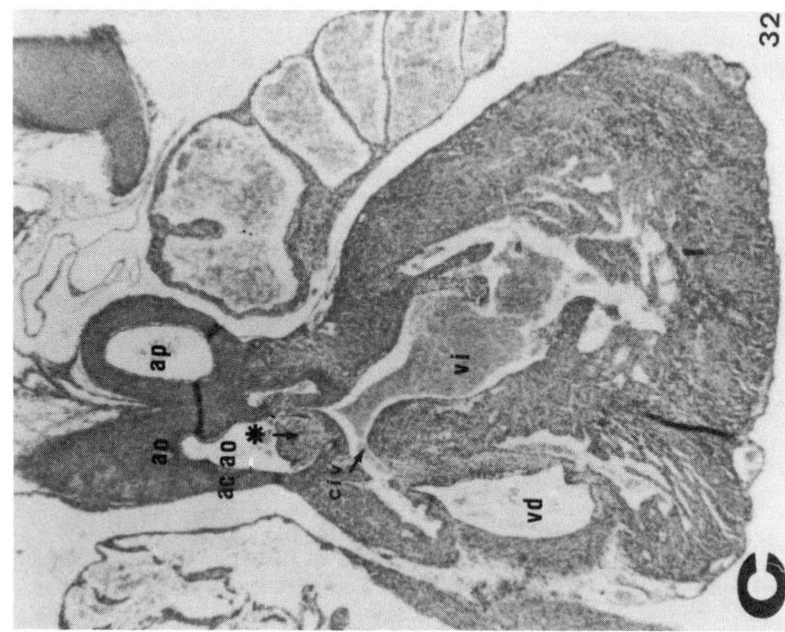

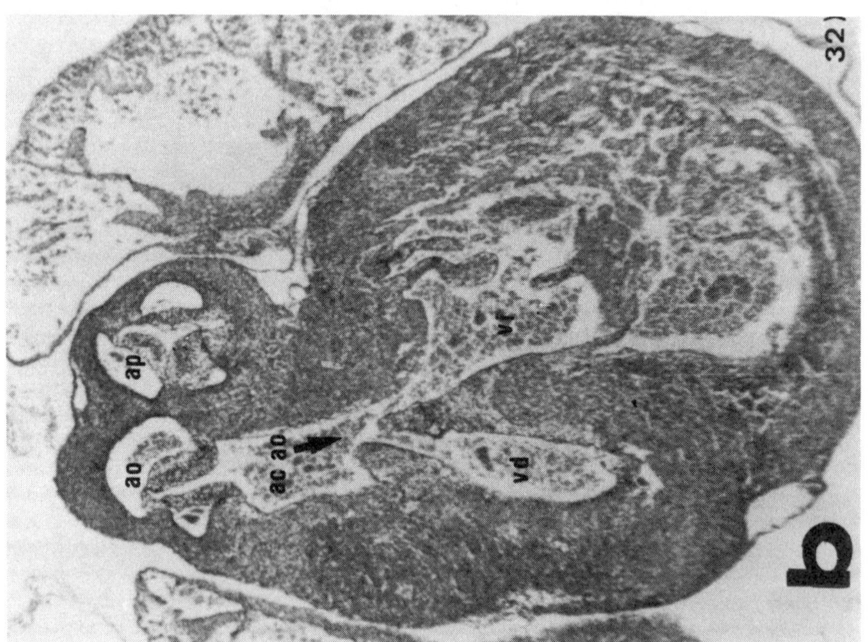

FIGURE 2b and c. See legend on p. 329.

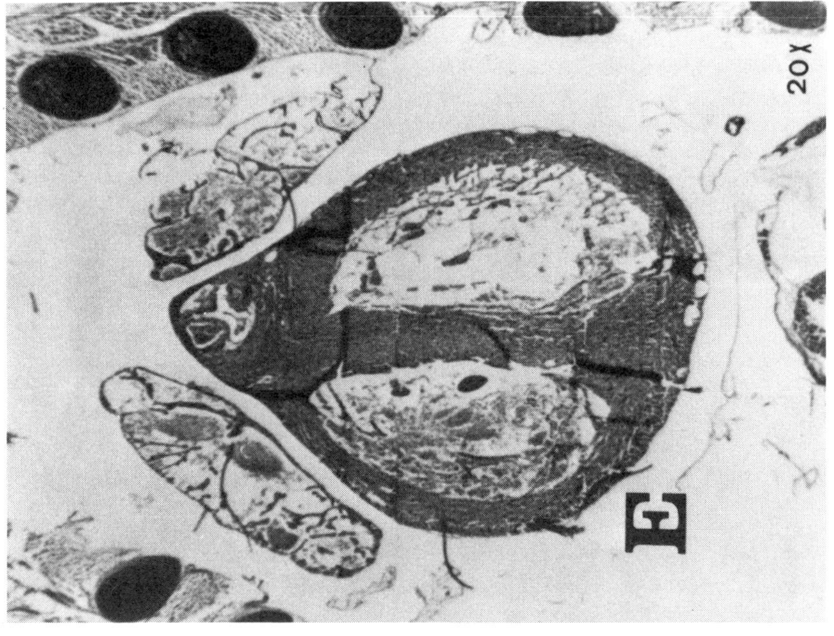

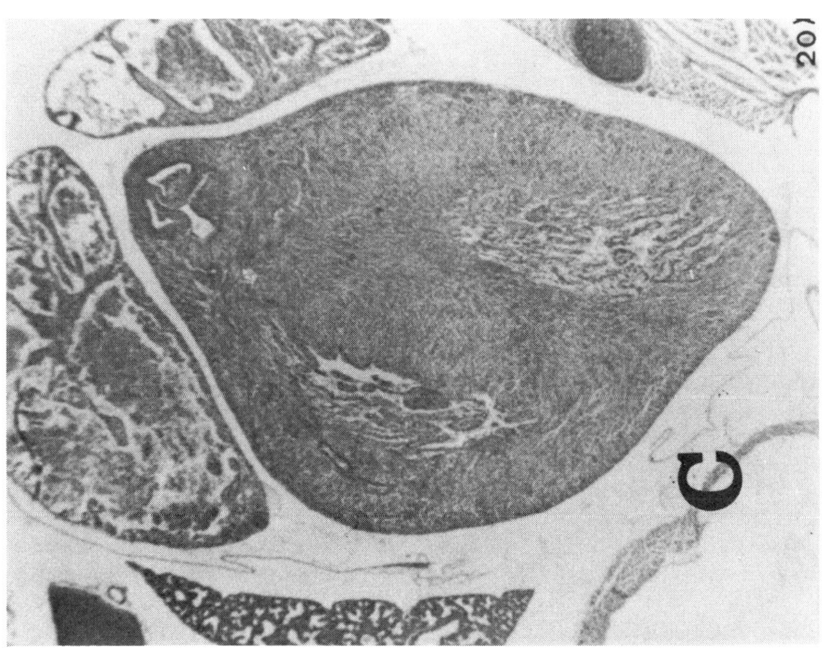

FIGURE 3. Cardiac size in the different groups (C, E, F, P).

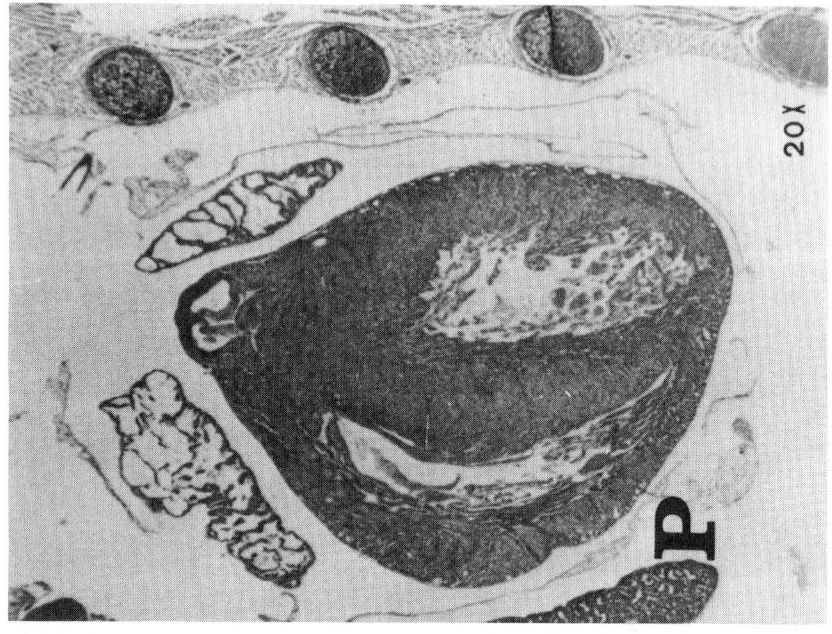

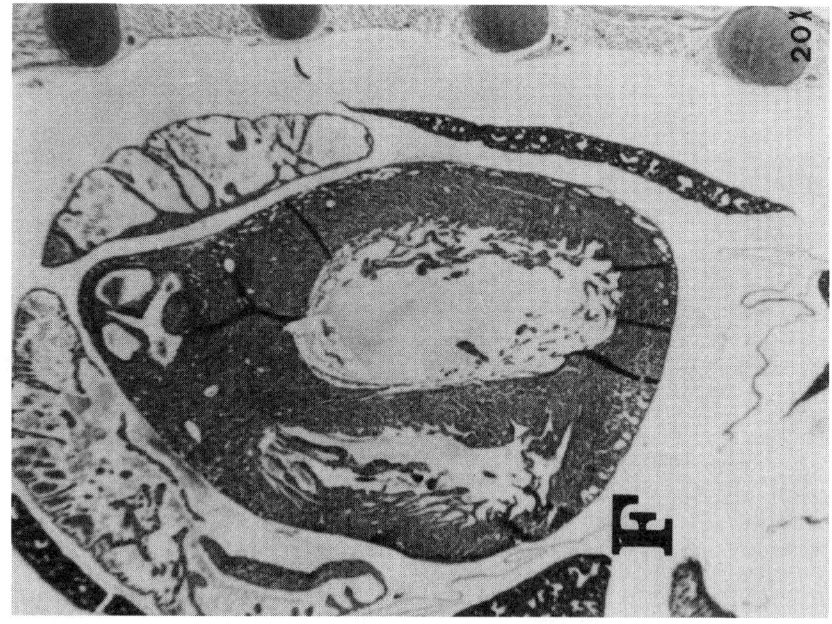

FIGURE 3. (*Continued*)

CONCLUSIONS

(1) The development in Sprague-Dawley rats of the alcoholic embryopathy requires the establishment of chronic alcoholic intoxication prior to gestation and throughout it, in levels of alcoholemia greater than 100 mg/dL; a relationship exists between these levels during the embryonic period and the frequency of cardiac malformations. (2) The alteration of heart growth induced by alcohol is related to that of body weight. (3) Gestational exposure to alcohol induces a cardiac hypoplasia and hypotrophy, whereas denutrition is only associated with cardiac hypotrophy.

REFERENCES

1. CLARREN, S. K. & D. W. SMITH. 1978. The FAS: Experience with 65 patients and a review of the world literature. N. Engl. J. Med. **298:** 1063-1067.
2. MAJEWSKI, F. 1981. Alcohol embryopathy: Some facts and speculations about pathogenesis. Neurobehav. Toxicol. Teratol. **3:** 129-144.
3. SANDOR, G. S., D. F. SMITH & P. M. MAC LEOD. 1981. Cardiac malformations in the fetal alcohol syndrome. J. Pediatr. **98:** 771-773.
4. RANDALL, C. L. & W. J. TAYLOR. 1979. Prenatal ethanol exposure in mice: Teratogenic effects. Teratology **19:** 305-312.
5. HENDERSON, G. I. & S. SCHENKER. 1977. The effect of maternal alcohol consumption on the viability and visceral development of the newborn rat. Res. Commun. Chem. Pathol. Pharmacol. **16**(1): 15-32.

Consequences of Early Identification
of the Arterial Orifices

MARGOT M. BARTELINGS AND
ADRIANA C. GITTENBERGER-DE GROOT

Department of Anatomy and Embryology
University of Leiden
2300 RC Leiden, the Netherlands

Conventional theories of morphogenesis,[1-3] dealing with the separation of the great arteries and their outflow tracts, suggest the intricate involvement of several septal structures. Early identification of the arterial orifice level reveals a quite different mechanism with regard to these separation processes.[4-6] The arterial orifice level is represented, in the early human embryo, by the borderline between the mesenchymal wall of the aortic sac and the myocardial wall of the outlet segment. In a preseptation embryonic stage (Carnegie 14), this borderline shows a remarkable curved configuration, reaching up to the level of origin of the fourth and sixth arch arteries, which is also the level where septation, by the compact mesenchyme of the aortopulmonary septum (APS), starts. This implies that septation by the APS starts at the arterial orifice level and immediately involves the outlet segment as well. At stage 15, the aortic orifice, connecting to the ascending aorta, becomes separated from the pulmonary orifice. The pulmonary trunk is initially extremely short, as the sixth arch arteries and pulmonary arteries originate immediately above the orifice level. Thus the great arteries are not separated over a considerable length (FIG. 1). At stage 16, the arterial orifice level has an even more remarkable configuration, being curved and twisted. The aortic orifice is situated right dorsally and caudally with respect to the pulmonary orifice (FIG. 2). The two columns of compact mesenchyme of the APS extend far proximally into the right ventricular outlet, whereas they reach hardly below the aortic orifice. This implies that the position of the arterial orifices as well as the relative dimensions of their outflow tracts are, in a very early stage, similar to those in the fully developed heart. With further development the columns of the APS, being in contact with the myocardial wall, will mobilize the myocardium to form the "outlet septum," which because of the caudal position of the aortic orifice is not a true septum between the outflow tracts, but rather the posterior wall of the right ventricular outflow tract. Thus separation of the great arteries, their orifices and infundibula can be attributed to a single structure, the APS.

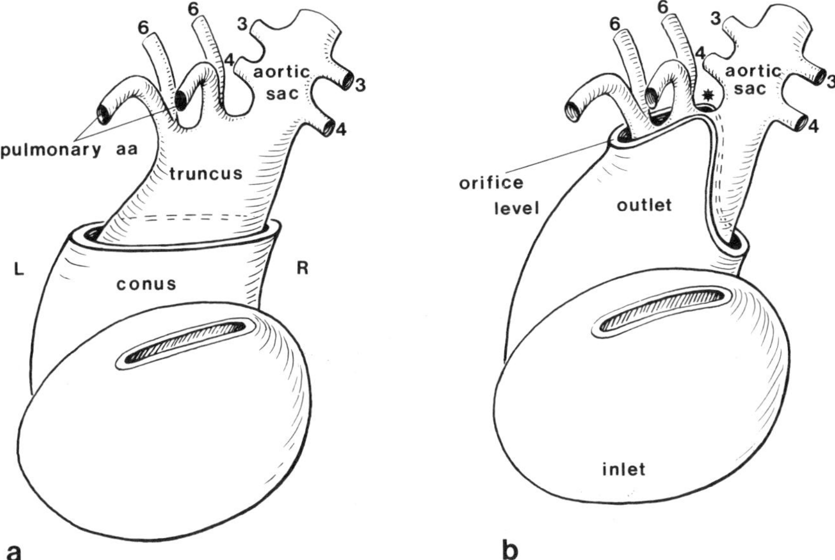

FIGURE 1. (a). Conventional theories suggest the involvement of several septal structures in the separation process of the aortic sac (APS), the truncus (truncal septum), and the conus (conal septum). (b). The configuration of the arterial orifice level implies that septation by the APS starts at the arterial orifice level (*) and immediately involves the outlet segment, and that the great arteries are not separated over a considerable length.

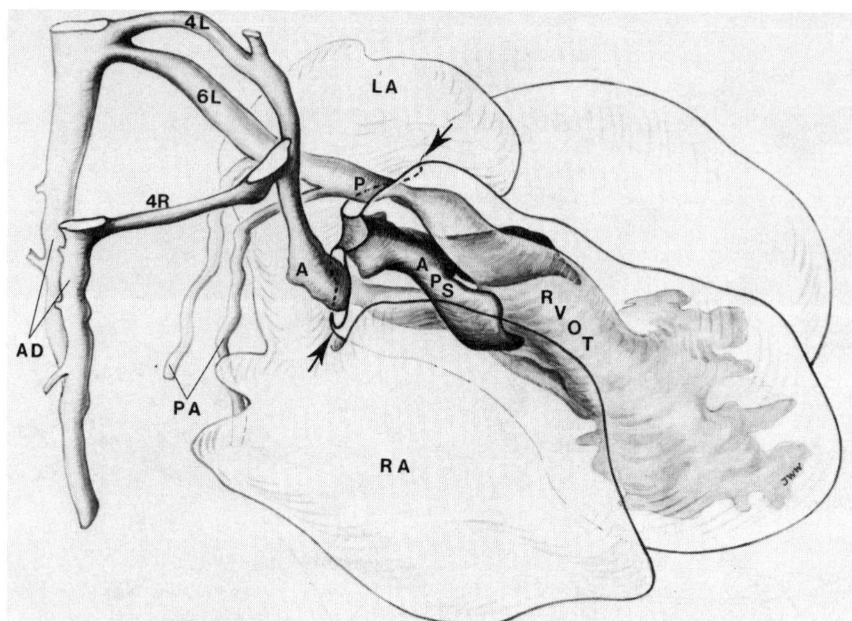

FIGURE 2. Graphic reconstruction of the heart of a human embryo (stage 16). View from the right. RA: right atrium; LA: left atrium; PA: pulmonary arteries; AD: aortae dorsales; 4R, 4L, 6L: 4th right, 4th left and 6th left arch arteries. Please note the position of the arterial orifices (arrows) and the APS. The long right ventricular outflow tract (RVOT) leads to the short pulmonary trunk (P), whereas the ascending aorta (A) is rather long. (Bartelings & Gittenberger-de Groot.[6] With permission from the *International Journal of Cardiology.*)

REFERENCES

1. KRAMER, T. C. 1942. Am. J. Anat. **3:** 343–370.
2. VAN MIEROP, L. H. 1979. Morphological development of the heart. *In* Handbook of Physiology. R. M. Berne, Ed. Williams & Wilkins. Baltimore.
3. ASAMI, I. 1980. Partitioning of the arterial end of the embryonic heart. *In* Etiology and Morphogenesis of Congenital Heart Disease. R. van Praagh & A. Takao, Eds. Futura. New York.
4. BARTELINGS, M. M. & A. C. GITTENBERGER-DE GROOT. 1988. Anat. Embryol. **177:** 537–542.
5. BARTELINGS, M. M., A. C. G. WENINK, A. C. GITTENBERGER-DE GROOT & A. OPPENHEIMER-DEKKER. 1986. Acta Morphol. Neerl-Scand. **24:** 181–192.
6. BARTELINGS, M. M. & A. C. GITTENBERGER-DE GROOT. 1989. Int. J. Cardiol. **22:** 289–300.

Age-Dependent Heart Rate Response to Phenylephrine in Chick Embryos

D. WOODROW BENSON JR. AND SHARON HUGHES

Children's Memorial Hospital
Northwestern University
Chicago, Illinois 60614

The chick embryo appears to have precise heart rate requirements during cardiovascular development, as increases in heart rate parallel increases in body mass. The factors determining heart rate control during development have not been well-defined, however. Whether alpha adrenergic receptors may elicit a positive chronotropic response in the developing heart has been controversial.[1-5] In order to evaluate this possibility, we determined the heart rate response to intravenous phenylephrine (alpha-1-adrenergic agonist) in the developing chick embryo at 4, 8, 12, and 16 days of incubation (Hamburger-Hamilton stages 24, 34, 38, and 42, respectively).

METHODS

Studies were performed in ovo on 50 white Leghorn chick embryos. Heart rate was determined continuously from an arterial velocity recording (20 mHz pulsed-Doppler velocity meter), which was digitally sampled at 2 ms intervals, stored on a Bernulli disc, and analyzed with a software package from RC Physiocorder. Phenylephrine was dissolved in chick Ringers solution (0.120 mol/L NaCl, 0.005 mol/L KCl, 0.001 mol/L CaCl) and administered intravenously in a vitelline vein as 1000, 100, 10, or 0 mg/kg. The volume injected was 5, 32, 46, or 46 microliters for 4, 8, 12, or 16 day embryos, respectively. These volumes were chosen to be less than 6% of circulating embryo volumes. The fluid was injected over 5 to 10 seconds. Heart rate was monitored continuously for 2 minutes following injection. A positive response was considered to be a heart rate change of more than 15 percent.

RESULTS

No embryo had a heart rate increase to phenylephrine. FIGURE 1 illustrates typical heart rate decrease during a recording from a 12-day embryo that received a dose of

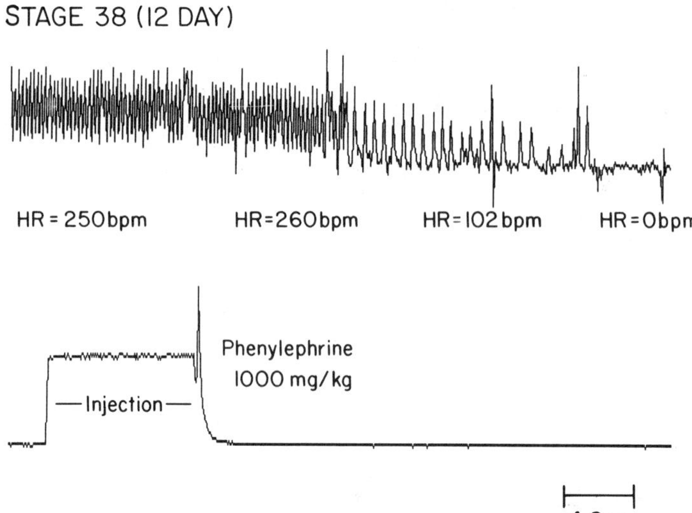

FIGURE 1. Heart rate response to phenylephrine. The upper trace is an arterial Doppler velocity tracing from a stage 38 embryo. The time of injection is shown on the marker trace below.

1000 mg/kg. Within 15 seconds of initiation of injection, the heart rate begins to slow, and by 30 seconds asystole has occurred. TABLE 1 shows the ratio of the number of embryos with a heart rate decrease following phenylephrine to the numbers of embryos studied.

DISCUSSION

In the developing chick embryo, there is an age and dose-dependent heart rate response to phenylephrine. There is no heart rate response in young embryos to high dose phenylephrine. All older embryos responded to high-dose phenylephrine, and some responded to lower doses. No embryo had a heart rate increase to phenylephrine. We speculate that the observed heart rate decrease may be due to a developing baroreceptor reflex rather than a direct alpha-1 adrenergic receptor effect on cardiac automaticity.

TABLE 1. Ratio of Number with Rate Decrease to Number Studied

| | Age | | | |
Phenylephrine Dose	4 d	8 d	12 d	16 d
(Control)	0/6	0/3	0/3	0/3
1000 mg/kg	0/4	3/6	3/3	3/3
100 mg/kg		0/5	0/6	2/5
10 mg/kg				0/3

REFERENCES

1. GIRARD, H. 1973. Adrenergic sensitivity of circulation in the chick embryo. Am. J. Physiol.
    224: 461-469.
2. ST. PETERY, L. B. JR., L. H. S. VAN MIEROP. 1974. Evidence for the presence of adrenergic
    receptors in the six-day-old chick embryo. Am. J. Physiol. **227:** 1406-1410.
3. ST. PETERY, L. B., JR., L. H. S. VAN MIEROP. 1977. Evidence for the presence of adrenergic
    receptors in the three-day-old chick embryo. Am. J. Physiol. **232:** H250-H254.
4. ROSEN, M. R., A. J. HORDOF, J. P. ILVENTO & P. DANILO JR. 1977. Effects of adrenergic
    amines on electrophysiologic properties and automaticity of neonatal and adult canin
    Purkinje fibers. Circ. Res. **40:** 390-400.
5. MCCORMACK, J., J. VILLAFANE, H. XU, H. GELBAND, A. STOLFI & A. S. PICKOFF. 1986.
    Alpha adrenergic receptors are excitatory in the neonatal canine myocardium. Am. Heart
    J. **112:** 643.

Coronary Vessel Vasculogenesis[a]

DAVID L. BOLENDER, MARK D. OLSON,[b] AND
ROGER R. MARKWALD

Department of Anatomy and Cellular Biology
Medical College of Wisconsin
Milwaukee, Wisconsin 53226
and
[b]*Department of Anatomy and Cell Biology*
University of North Dakota School of Medicine
Grand Forks, North Dakota

INTRODUCTION

To date, little is known concerning the origin and regulatory mechanisms associated with the development of the coronary vessels at the surface of the myocardium. Combining data from several studies, it appears that the definitive coronary vessels may be composed of portions of several stage-specific attempts to vascularize the developing myocardial wall.[1] One of these components consists of a vascular plexus that forms within the interspace between the basal surface of the epicardium and the external surface of the myocardium. Using a marker specific for endothelial cells (QH1),[2] we have shown that the endothelial cells of the plexus appear to be derived from precursors located within the mesenchyme of the dorsal mesocardium.[3] Upon entering the myocardial/epicardial interface, these vascular precursors are surrounded by an extracellular matrix enriched in fibronectin and containing adheron-like complexes[3] similar to those observed within inductively active areas of the developing heart.[4] Consequently, we propose that coronary vessel vasculogenesis is derived from reciprocal tissue interactions between adjacent progenitor tissues: the epicardium, myocardium, and dorsal mesocardium. A culture model was developed to provide a bioassay for examining the mechanisms involved in the proposed vasculogenic tissue interactions.

METHODS

Intact hearts, partially invested with epicardium, were removed from stage 18 quail embryos and explanted onto lattices of hydrated collagen.[5] The cultures were observed daily using Hoffman modulated contrast or phase optics. The explants were

[a]This work was supported by the Wisconsin Heart Association, 85-GA-32.

removed at day 4 and cultures allowed to proceed for a total of 6-14 days. At the end of the culture period, some of the cultures were fixed (3% glutaraldehyde), embedded in plastic, and sectioned to examine for the presence of vascular structures. Selected cultures were fixed (2% paraformaldehyde), immunostained as whole mounts using QH1, and examined with epifluorescent optics.

RESULTS AND DISCUSSION

During the first day in culture, an outgrowth of epithelial cells extended from the cut ends of the explant onto the surface of the collagen lattice (FIG. 1). Within four days, the outgrowth completely surrounded the explanted heart. The epithelial cells generated a population of mesenchymal cells that migrated into the collagen lattice as dispersed cells or as radiating tracts of cells that were arranged end-to-end (FIG. 2). This latter pattern of migration was distinctly different from the exclusively dispersed migration observed for cardiac mesenchymal cells derived from the AV endothelium.[5] Proliferation of both epithelium and mesenchyme did not appear to be affected by explant removal at day 4. By the end of the first week of culture, some of the mesenchymal cells began to interconnect forming cellular networks (FIG. 3). In contrast to the results just described, only scant surface outgrowth and limited mesenchyme formation was observed even after several days in culture when hearts from stage 15 embryos (prior to epicardial formation) were explanted onto collagen gels.

A subpopulation of the mesenchymal cells located within the collagen lattice reacted positively with QH1. Positive staining was observed in the dispersed cells as well as those in end-to-end alignment (FIG 4). During the second week of culture, some of the QH1-positive endothelial cells lined vascular-like structures located within the gel. Some of these became interconnected into primitive vascular networks (FIG. 5). Examination of sections of cultures revealed that the vessel-like structures contained a continuous endothelial lining surrounded externally by rounded or fusiform shaped cells resembling pericytes (FIG. 6). These observations strongly suggest that the vascular-like structures formed by the anastomosing endothelial cells are true capillaries. Explants of dorsal mesocardium generated an enriched outgrowth of mesenchyme cells, many of which were also connected in an end-to-end arrangement. Moreover, vascular-like structures were present within the collagen lattice toward the end of week one in culture. The culture studies using explants of dorsal mesocardium reinforce the idea[3] that this embryonic tissue is the immediate progenitor tissue for the coronary vessel precursors.

To our knowledge, this is the first time that primary vasculogenesis, certainly associated with the coronary vessels, has been accomplished *in vitro*. If parallel studies show that it faithfully duplicates vessel formation *in vivo*, the culture model will provide a useful bioassay for studying the cellular and molecular mechanisms mediating tissue interactions during vasculogenesis.

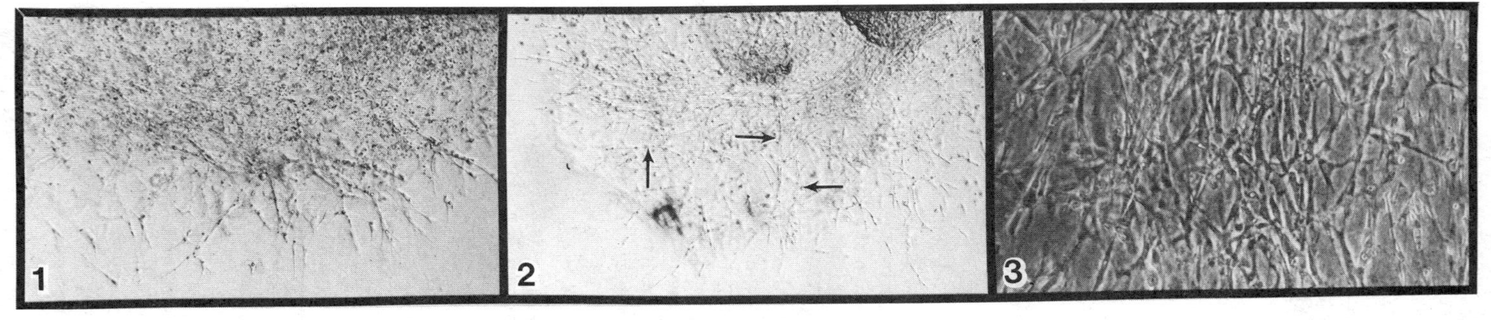

FIGURE 1. A view of the epithelial outgrowth on the surface of the collagen lattice. Mesenchyme cells extend from the periphery of the epithelium. $\times$ 75; reduced here by 30%.

FIGURE 2. Mesenchyme cells within the collagen lattice below the epithelium observed by optical sectioning with Hoffman optics. Many of the cells are dispersed, whereas others are abutted in a unique end-to-end arrangement (arrows). $\times$ 75; reduced here by 30%.

FIGURE 3. A view of the mesenchyme from a 6 day culture. Many of the cells have joined to form a cellular network. $\times$ 150; reduced here by 30%.

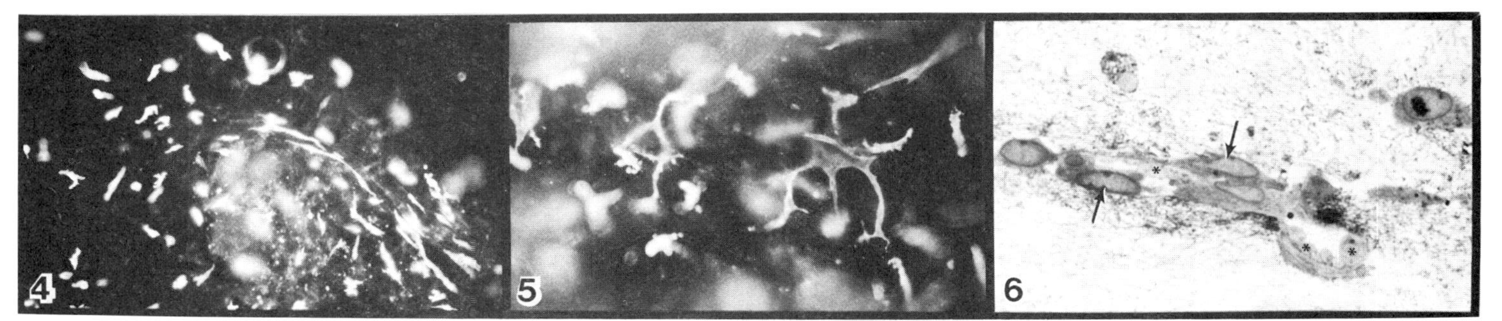

FIGURE 4. A 6 day culture stained as a whole mount with QH1. Although only a subpopulation of the mesenchyme stains positively with the antibody, it contains both dispersed and aligned cells. $\times$ 75; reduced here by 30%.

FIGURE 5. A higher power view of a culture stained with QH1. Some of the cells appear to be interconnected into a primitive vascular network. $\times$ 150; reduced here by 30%.

FIGURE 6. A plastic embedded section of a 14 day culture showing a vascular-like structure in cross section. The putative capillary is lined with a continuous endothelium (asterisks) that is surrounded externally by flattened cells (arrows). $\times$ 2000; reduced here by 30%.

REFERENCES

1. TOKUYASU, K. T. 1985. Development of myocardial circulation. *In* Cardiac Morphogenesis. V. Ferrans, G. Rosenquist & C. Weinstein, Eds.: 226-237. Elsevier. New York.
2. PARDANAUD, L., C. ALTMAN, P. KITOS, F. DIETERLEN-LIEVRE & C. A. BUCK. 1987. Vasculogenesis in the early quail blastodisc as studied with a monoclonal antibody recognizing endothelial cells. Development (Camb.) **100:** 339-349.
3. OLSON, M. D., D. L. BOLENDER & R. R. MARKWALD. 1989. Origin of coronary vessel presursors. Anat. Rec. **223:** 85-86.
4. MJAATVEDT, C. H., R. C. LEPERA & R. R. MARKWALD. 1987. Myocardial specificity for initiating endothelial-mesenchymal cell transition in embryonic chick heart correlates with a particulate distribution of fibronectin. Dev. Biol. **119:** 59-67.
5. BERNANKE, D. H. & R. R. MARKWALD. 1982. Migratory behavior of cardiac cushion tissue cells in a collagen lattice culture system. Dev. Biol. **91:** 235-245.

Myofibrillogenesis and Myosin ATPase Activity of the Embryonic Chick Heart[a]

JENNIFER L. BRECKLER

Department of Biology
San Francisco State University
San Francisco, California 94132

During early myocardial development, the assembly and cellular organization of the myofibril contractile elements take place. Cardiac ventricular muscle from embryonic chicken was examined in day 4-20 embryos, in order to determine the ultrastructural patterns of myofibril assembly. Cardiac tissue was prepared for transmission electron microscopy (TEM) according to Johnson,[1] by dissection on ice. Relaxation was produced in the presence of tetrodotoxin (10^{-6}M TTX), pH 7.4, in PBS buffer. Tissue was fixed in 4% formalin/2% glutaraldehyde, postfixed in osmium, and then embedded in LR White. Sarcomere assembly at days 4-6 occurred primarily along the longitudinal axis of developing cardiac myocytes, close to the sarcolemma. By day 6, lateral alignment of myofibrils began to occur, in conjunction with the appearance of intermediate filaments associated with the Z-disc. Subsequent changes consisted of mitochondrial reorganization relative to the myofibrils, while the number of myofibrils per cell increased.

In order to determine the biochemical character of the contractile proteins during this period of myofibril organization, we examined the enzymatic activity of myosin, the major contractile protein of the myofibrils. Myosin from whole hearts was purified[2] at days 7, 10, 13, 16, and 19 of embryonic development. The levels of calcium-activated embryonic myosin ATPase activity obtained (see FIG. 1) were significantly different from the adult ventricular myosin ATPase value (0.24 $\pm$ 0.03 micromols Pi/mg/min) only at day 13 (0.16 $\pm$ .02 micromols Pi/mg/min). Myosin ATPase activity reached a maximum value at day 10 (0.30 $\pm$ .02 micromols Pi/mg/min). These minor fluctuations in myosin ATPase activity correspond approximately to the timing of the establishment of cholinergic innervation.[3] The light chain pattern of myosin was then determined using SDS-PAGE and was virtually identical to the adult pattern of 2 major light chains (LCS_1 and LCS_2) throughout development (days 10, 13, 16, and 19). This result suggests that the differences that we observe in the myosin ATPase activity during development may be due to variations in the heavy chain portion of the myosin molecule.

We used an immunological approach in order to further characterize myosin properties during cardiac development. Antibodies to myosin were prepared by several injections of either SDS-PAGE-purified embryonic myosin heavy chain (MHC) or

[a]This work was supported in part by the American Heart Association, California affiliate.

myosin light chain (LCS_1) into rabbits. Frozen tissue sections of developing chicken hearts were then examined for the presence of MHC and LCS_1 using indirect immunofluorescence (fluorescein-labeled goat anti-rabbit IgG). The LCS_1 antibody reacted strongly with myofibrillar A-bands in chick ventricular cells throughout development. This result is consistent with the myosin light chain pattern findings, which showed no differences in the light chains throughout development. On the other hand, anti-MHC showed the strongest fluorescence in day 6 embryonic hearts, which markedly diminished throughout development (see FIG. 2). Only background levels of binding were detectable by the time of hatching at day 21. A specificity control experiment was done using anti-MHC antibodies that were preabsorbed with purified heavy chain and showed no binding to myocardial cells. Thus, the anti-MHC result suggests that a unique embryonic myosin heavy chain is produced during early myocardial development, at a time when we observe the alignment of the myofibrils in the myocyte; its synthesis is gradually reduced in amount as embryonic development proceeds. Similar findings of unique embryonic myosin isozymes have been reported for developing skeletal muscle in mammals.[4]

CONCLUSION

Embryonic chicken myocardial cells, a few days prior to hatching, showed myofibril organizational patterns that resembled adult myocardial cells. Purified cardiac myosin ATPase activity in day 13 embryos was different than adult ventricle. Embryonic myosin heavy chain antibody binding was high in day 6 embryos.

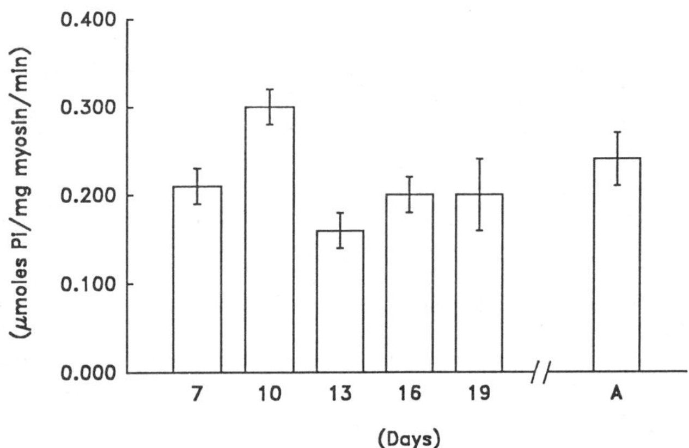

FIGURE 1. Myosin ATPase activity (mean ± SD) of chick embryonic myocardium compared to adult ventricle. Measurement of calcium-activated ATPase activity was repeatedly performed at 50 mM KC1, 25° C, for day 7 (n=8), day 10 (n=10), day 13 (n=13), day 16 (n=7), day 19 (n=6) embryos, and adult ventricle (n=9).

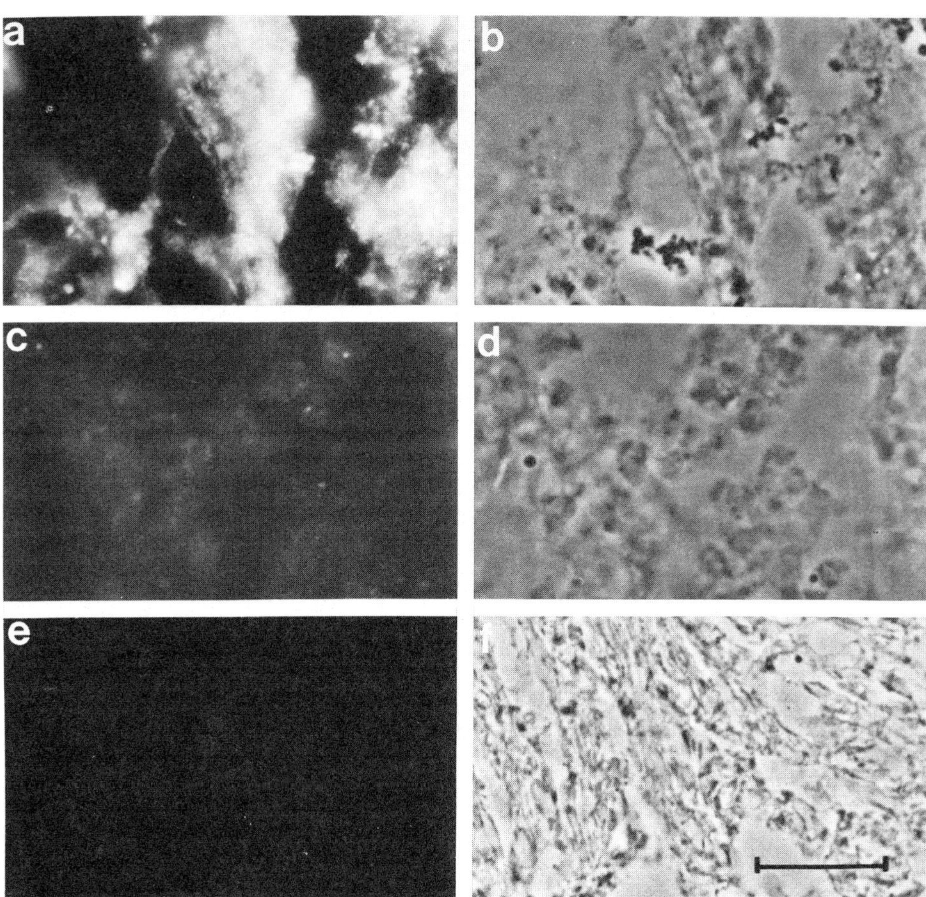

FIGURE 2. Antimyosin heavy chain binding on frozen sections of chick embryonic ventricular tissue, visualized with indirect immunofluorescence. Phase contrast (b,d,f) and fluorescent (a,c,e) micrographs are shown for day 6 (a,b), day 8 (c,d), and day 12 (e,f) embryos. Bar represents 5 microns. Immunoautoradiography showed high specificity of antibody used (result not shown).

ACKNOWLEDGMENTS

The author wishes to acknowledge the laboratory assistance of Mary Eaton, Elizabeth Narron, Geraldine Ryan, and Robert Winters.

REFERENCES

1. JOHNSON, J. 1983. Current trends in morphological techniques. R. Adelman & G. Roth Eds.:216-245. CRC Press. Boca Raton, FL.
2. MOMMAERTS, W. F. H. M., A. J. BULLER & K. SERAYDARIAN. 1969. The modification of some biochemical properties of muscle by cross-innervation. Proc. Natl. Acad. Sci. USA **64:** 128-133.
3. RICKENBACHER, J. & E. MULLER. 1979. The development of cholinergic ganglia in the chick embryo heart. Anat. Embryol. **155:** 253-258.
4. WHALEN, R. B., S. M. SELL, G. S. BUTLER-BROWNE, K. SCHWARTZ, P. BOUVERET & I. PINSET-HARSTROM. 1981. Three myosin heavy-chain isozymes appear sequentially in rat muscle development. Nature (London) **292:** 805-809.

Stretch-Activated Ion Channels in Neonatal Ventricular Myocytes

V. K. CHEN [a]

Department of Biophysics
State University of New York at Buffalo
Buffalo, New York 14260

Patch clamp recordings from ventricular myocytes of neonatal rats showed ionic channels that open in response to membrane stretch due to applied negative pressures of 1-6 cm Hg in the patch electrode. The electrical response to stretch, consisting of markedly increased channel opening frequency, was maintained with some bursting during stretch applications as long as, or longer than, 40 seconds. The channels have a conductance averaging 120 pS in isotonic KCl, have a mean reversal potential of 31 mV depolarized from resting membrane potential, and do not require external calcium for activation (because recordings are done in the absence of external calcium). The channels behave ohmically to applied voltage. The channels appear to be relatively nonselective for cations based upon measured reversal potential. Patches were excised from viable unattached myocytes that were round to oval (approximately 20 microns in diameter) in shape. The excised patch had noticeable bursting, and bunching of the channeling openings could be recorded in comparison to the cell attached patch recordings (FIG. 1). The altered bursting interval could be attributed to the damage

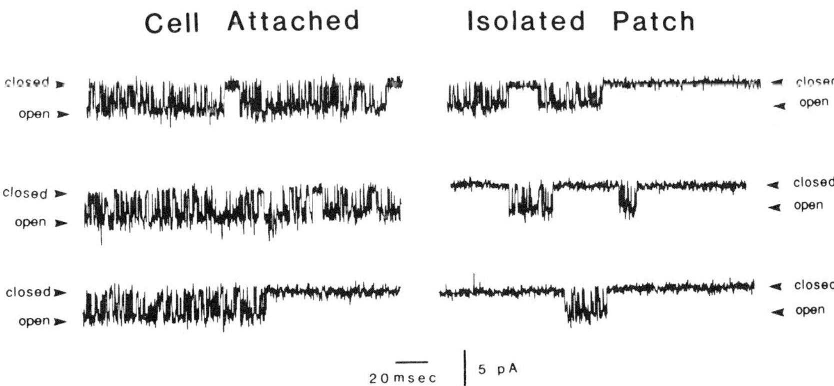

FIGURE 1. Comparison of current records of cell attached and excised patch and the presence of long durations of channel closing in the excised patch records.

[a] Address for correspondence: V. K. Chen, Box 21, Amherst, NY 14226.

caused by excision, this bunching expected from the cell-attached patch data[1] in these cells, as well as the excised patch data of other cells.[2-4] This alteration may suggest how cytoskeletal elements play a role in force transmission to channel. Notice that the channel conductance and the shortest opening times were apparently unchanged. This control system may have a role in the development of specific regions of the heart. The stretch-activated ion channels have been described in frog skeletal muscle,[5] chick myoblasts,[4] and snail heart cells.[2,3] Although there is little evidence linking stretch sensitivity to any macroscopic currents in the heart, stretching a chick embryonic ventricle induces a pacemaker current,[6] which increases ventricular contractility.[7] Because they are gated by physiological levels of tension, stretch-activated ionic channels may represent a cellular control system wherein beat-to-beat tension as well as osmotic balance modulate a portion of membrane conductance.

REFERENCES

1. CRAELIUS, W., V. CHEN & N. EL-SHERIF. 1988. Biosci. Rep. **8:** 407-414.
2. BREZDEN, B. L., D. R. GARDNER & C. F. MORRIS. 1985. J. Exp. Biol. **123:** 175-189.
3. SIGURDSON, W. J., C. F. MORRIS, B. L. BREZDEN & D. R. GARDNER. 1986. J. Exp. Biol. **127:** 191-209.
4. GUHARAY, F. & F. SACHS. 1984. J. Physiol. (London) **352:** 685-701.
5. BREHM, P., R. KUHLBERG & F. MOODY-CORBETT. 1984. J. Physiol. (London) **350:** 631-648.
6. RAJALA, G. M., M. J. PINTER & S. KAPLAN. 1977. Dev. Biol. **61:** 330-337.
7. McGAUGHEY, T., Y. KUARCHI, A. NOMA & H. IRISAWA. 1984. Pfluegers Arch. **402:** 248-257.

Intrinsic Heart Rate Maximizes Dorsal Aortic Blood Flow in the Stage 24 Chick Embryo

BETTINA CUNEO, SHARON HUGHES, AND
D. WOODROW BENSON JR.

Children's Memorial Hospital
Northwestern University
Chicago, Illinois 60614

Although the determinants of heart rate (HR) during cardiovascular development have not been completely defined, the effects of HR on flow (Q) and stroke volume (SV) have been demonstrated.[1,2] In the chick embryo, HR increases from 90/min at initiation of contraction (Hamburger-Hamilton stage 10) to 210/min at piping. There appears to be a precise HR for specific stages of development. We hypothesized that at specific developmental stages maximal Q and SV would occur at intrinsic HR.

METHODS

Fertile white Leghorn chicken eggs were incubated to Hamburger-Hamilton stage 24; embryos were exposed by opening the shell and its membranes. Temperature was maintained at 37-38° C with a heated sand bath and radiant warmer. The intrinsic HR (I) was determined. Then the sinus venosus was paced (2 ms duration, < 4 mA) at intrinsic HR (P:I), at HR increased to 125% (P:125%I) and 150% (P:150%I) of intrinsic, and at HR decreased by paired pacing to 75% (P:75%I) and 50% (P:50%I) of intrinsic. A recovery period was permitted between each paced change. Aortic flow velocity (measured with a 20 mHz pulsed Doppler velocity meter) and aortic cross-sectional area were measured in each embryo; then Q (aortic cross-sectional area times velocity) and SV (Q/HR) were calculated at each HR. A complete pacing study was performed in less than 8 minutes; only embryos whose HR recovered to intrinsic rates after pacing were included. Data was digitally sampled at 2 ms intervals, stored on a Bernoulli disc, and analyzed with a software package from RC Physiorecorder. Data were evaluated by one way ANOVA and Scheffe.

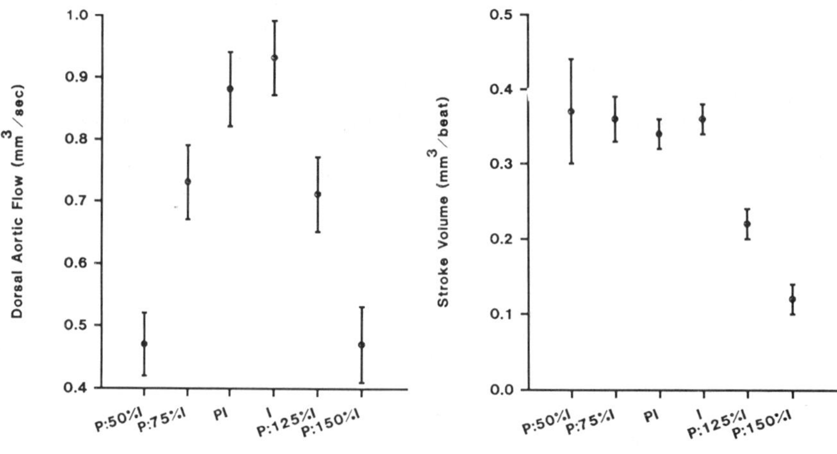

FIGURE 1. Dorsal aortic flow and stroke volume (mean ± SEM) versus heart rate (% of intrinsic). Flow and stroke volume were measured at intrinsic heart rate (I), during sinus venosus pacing at intrinsic heart rate (P:I), and at paced rates faster (P:125%I, P:150%I) and slower (by paired pacing) (P:75%I, P:50%I) than intrinsic rate.

RESULTS

Results of this study showed that pacing at the intrinsic rate did not significantly alter Q or SV from intrinsic values. Q was maximal at intrinsic HR and decreased proportionally to HR at both paced increase and paced decrease HR ($p < .001$). SV decreased in a linear fashion at increased HR ($p < .001$) but was unchanged from intrinsic values at slower HR ($p =$ NS) (see FIG. 1). SV and Q (mean and SEM) at increased and decreased HR are summarized in TABLE 1.

DISCUSSION

From this study we concluded that in the stage 24 chick embryo, pacing-induced HR increase and decrease exert a profound effect on Q, and maximal Q occurs at the intrinsic HR. As previously demonstrated,[2,3] SV decreased with a paced increase in HR. When HR is decreased to 50% and 75% of intrinsic HR by paired sinus venosus pacing, however, SV is unchanged from intrinsic values. The failure of SV to increase at slow HR may result from decreased ventricular compliance or because paired pacing restricts end diastolic volume by interfering with atrioventricular synchrony.

TABLE 1. Mean Stroke Volume and Flow at Different Heart Rates

	I (n = 23)	P:50%I (n = 10)	P:75%I (n = 16)	P:I (n = 22)	P:125%I (n = 23)	P:150%I (n = 10)
SV	.36 ± .02	.37 ± .07	.36 ± .03	.34 ± .02	.22 ± .02	.12 + .02
Flow	.93 ± .06	.47 ± .05	.73 ± .06	.88 ± .06	.71 ± .06	.47 + .06

REFERENCES

1. NAKAZAWA, M., S. MIYAGAWA, A. TAKAO, E. B. CLARK & N. HU. 1986. Hemodynamic effects of environmental hyperthermia in stage 18, 21, and 24 chick embryos. Pediatr. Res. **20:** 1213-1215.
2. DUNNIGAN, A., N. HU, D. W. BENSON JR. & E. B. CLARK. 1987. Effect of heart rate increase on dorsal aortic flow in the stage 24 chick embryo. Pediatr. Res. **22:** 442-444.
3. BENSON, D. W., JR., S. HUGHES, N. HU & E. B. CLARK. 1989. Effect of heart rate increase on dorsal aortic flow before and after volume loading in the stage 24 chick embryo. Pediatr. Res. **26:** 438-441.

Subpopulations of Cardiomyocytes in the Embryonic Chicken Heart

F. DE JONG, T. OPTHOF,[a] A. A. M. WILDE,[a]
M. J. JANSE,[a] W. H. LAMERS, AND
A. F. M. MOORMAN

Department of Anatomy and Embryology
[a]*Department of Clinical and Experimental Cardiology*
AMC, Meibergdreef 15
University of Amsterdam
1105AZ, Amsterdam, the Netherlands

Embryonic chicken hearts function without a morphologically recognizable conduction system, although they show an adult-like ECG.[1] Combined immunohistochemical and electrophysiological studies revealed that during the septational period, four subpopulations of cardiomyocytes can be detected that appear to be responsible for a coordinated contraction pattern.

Serial sections of whole chicken embryos between 3 and 7 days of development were alternately incubated with 3 monoclonal antibodies (Mab). Two Mabs were specific for the adult atrium myosin heavy chain (MHC) fraction (reactive with either A1- or with A2-isomyosins), and the third Mab was specific for the adult ventricle MHC fraction (reactive with V-isomyosins)[2] (FIG. 1). Isolated chicken hearts were explored, at comparable stages, with extracellular electrodes consisting of two terminals glued together. Conduction velocities in the myocardium were calculated by dividing the distance between the terminals (140 μm) by the time delay measured between the activation moments underneath the terminals. Simultaneous recordings of intracellular and extracellular signals proved the validity of the signal interpretation in the extracellular recordings (FIG. 2).

Subpopulation I (expressing V-isomyosin) is found as the compact myocardial layer of the ventricular free walls and in the core of the emerging ventricular septum. Subpopulation II (expressing A1- and A2-isomyosins) comprises the atrial free walls, the atrial septum (except its rim), and the sinus node area. Subpopulations I and II (except the sinus node area) form the working myocardium of the ventricles and the atria, respectively. They show fast rising action potentials (AP) (FIG. 2). Subpopulation III (expressing V- and A1-isomyosins) emerges in the ventricular trabeculae. It is indicated that this subpopulation is activated slightly before subpopulation I. Subpopulation IV (expressing V-, A1- and A2-isomyosins) forms the source from which developmentally regulated subpopulation I, large parts of subpopulation II, and subpopulation III emerge when the expression of (one or both) atrial or ventricular isomyosins is lost. Strategically positioned areas of subpopulation IV, however, remain in (1) the sinus venosus and contiguous parts of the atria, including the rim of the atrial septum; (2) the atrioventricular junctional area; and (3) the myocardium of the outflow tract (OFT) (FIG. 1). Subpopulation IV conducts the activation impulse

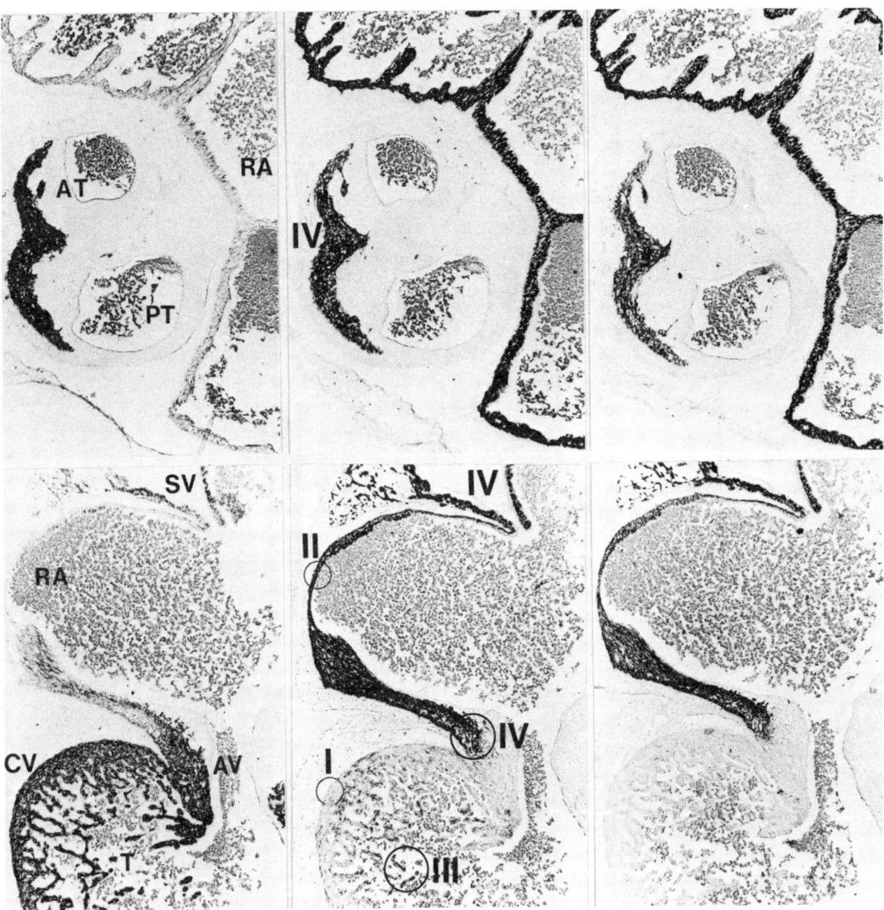

FIGURE 1. Isomyosin distribution in an embryonic chicken heart at 6 days of development. Two series of three consecutive transverse tissue sections through the OFT region (top row) and through the AV region (bottom row) were alternately incubated with monoclonal antibodies reactive with V- (left column), A1- (central column), and A2- (right column) isomyosins. I-IV = subpopulations I-IV; SV = sinus venosus; RA = right atrium; AV = atrioventricular junctional area; T = ventricular trabeculae; CV = compact ventricular myocardium; AT = aortic trunk; PT = pulmonary trunk.

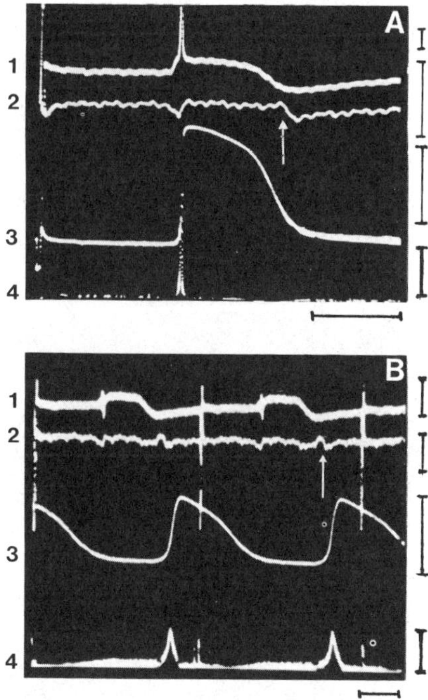

FIGURE 2. Panels A and B show unipolar electrograms of a 4-day-old embryonic chicken heart recorded on the ventricle (traces 1) and on the OFT (traces 2), whereas traces 3 show simultaneously recorded action potentials in the ventricle and in the OFT (close to the extracellular electrode), respectively. Traces 4 are the first-time derivatives of the action potentials. In panel A vertical bars indicate 0.1 mV (traces 1 and 2), 50 mV (trace 3), and 25 V/s (trace 4). In panel B vertical bars indicate 0.5 mV (traces 1 and 2), 50 mV (trace 3), and 5 V/s (trace 4). Horizontal bars indicate 50 ms. Notice that the OFT activation (indicated by arrows in traces 2) is not a remote ventricular repolarization signal but that it is caused by typical, slowly rising, action potentials with an amplitude of about 50 mV and a maximum upstrike velocity of about 5 V/s.

very slowly (< 1.5 cm/s) and shows slowly rising long-lasting APs with repolarization phases that in the OFT continue during the next heart cycle (FIG. 2). These results indicate that subpopulation III evolves into the fast conducting elements of the conduction system and that subpopulation IV remains in the slow conducting elements of the conduction system.

REFERENCES

1. VAN MIEROP, L. H. S. 1967. Am. J. Physiol. **212:** H407–415.
2. DE JONG, F., I. J. M. DE GROOT, W. J. C. GEERTS, A. WESSELS, A. W. PESCHAR, W. H. LAMERS & A. F. M. MOORMAN. 1988. Sarcomeric and nonsarcomeric muscles: Basic and applied research prospects for the 90's. U. Carraro, Ed.: 299–304. Unipress Padova.

The Developmental Relation between Pulmonary Vascularization and the Pulmonary Arch Artery

M. C. DE RUITER, A. C. GITTENBERGER-DE GROOT,
R. E. POELMANN, AND S. RAMMOS [a]

Department of Anatomy and Embryology
University of Leiden
2300 RC Leiden, the Netherlands

[a]*Department of Pediatric Cardiology*
Düsseldorf, Federal Republic of Germany

Except for the muscular morphology of the ductus arteriosus, which arises from the pulmonary arch artery, the other derivatives of the branchial arch system are elastic in nature. So the ductus arteriosus deserves a special place in the branchial arch system. Even the most complete studies of the development of the human aortic arch system disregard the unique histology of the ductus. Study of congenital heart malformations like pulmonary atresia revealed that certain aortopulmonary collaterals have a marked similarity in histology with the ductus arteriosus. To enhance our understanding of these phenomena we studied the development of the aortic arch and the pulmonary arteries in rat embryos, cultured *in vitro* from 10-12 days p.c. These were injected with India ink to visualize developing vascular sprouts in serial sections.[1] The experiments show that, at the time of the development of the second to fourth arch artery, the primitive pulmonary plexus is connected to the dorsal aortae by an extensive though transient system of ventral segmental arteries (FIG. 1). The most cranial vessel of this system becomes part of the most caudal developing branchial arch artery, that is, the sixth or pulmonary arch artery. In time this immediately follows the formation of the complete fourth arch. A well-formed paired sixth arch, as is depicted in most textbooks, is never seen. The proximal part of the sixth arch is a plexus-like structure (FIG. 2), which very rapidly seems to be incorporated into the aortic sac region. This results in a very close but separate entrance of the right and left ductus arteriosus with the slender right and left pulmonary arteries, respectively. This is followed in time immediately by the disappearance of the right ductus, leaving the right pulmonary artery connected to the pulmonary trunk region of the aortic sac. It is postulated that, with maldevelopment of the pulmonary arch artery (which seems to relate to abnormalities in the pulmonary outflow tract), ventral segmental arteries connecting with the pulmonary plexus many persist as aortopulmonary collaterals. The pulmonary arch artery, and in particular the part that forms the ductus arteriosus, should be considered as the first ventral segmental artery, instead of the last branchial artery.

FIGURE 1. Schematic representation of the developing branchial arch system. The second (II) and third (III) arches are complete. The fourth arch is not complete yet. At the level of the pulmonary plexus, several ventral segmental arteries (arrows) are indicated.

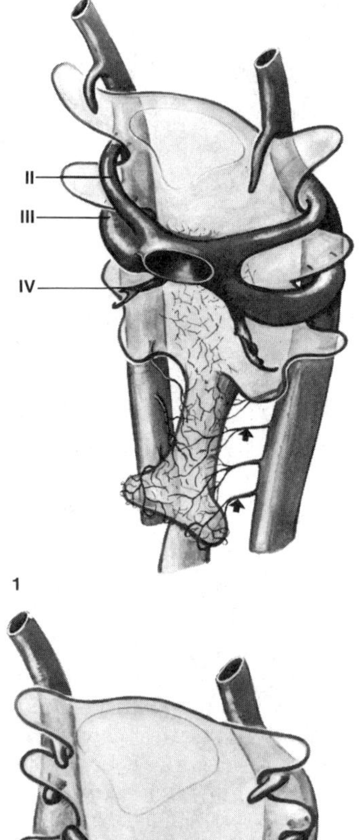

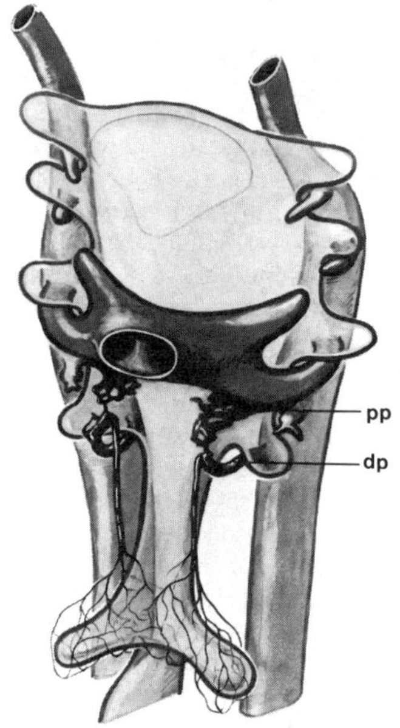

FIGURE 2. Schematic representation of the stage at which the sixth artery has just formed. The proximal part (pp) connecting to the aortic sac is still plexus-like; the dorsal part (dp) (the future ductus arteriosus on the left side) is formed by the most cranial vessel of the ventral segmental arteries. The other connections (see FIG. 1) have disappeared.

REFERENCE

1. DE RUITER, M. C., A. C. GITTENBERGER-DE GROOT, S. RAMMOS & R. E. POELMANN. 1989. The special status of the pulmonary arch artery in the branchial arch system of the rat. Anat. Embryol. **179:** 319–325.

The Early Development of the Tunica Media in the Expanding Vascular System

M. C. DE RUITER, A. C. GITTENBERGER-DE GROOT,
R. E. POELMANN, AND L. VAN IPEREN

Department of Anatomy and Embryology
University of Leiden
2300 RC Leiden, the Netherlands

Histogenesis of the vascular system starts with the formation of an endothelial tube within a seemingly undifferentiated mesenchymal surrounding. The outer layer of the larger vessels, the media, differentiates later on in development. Because the vascular system is continuously growing and remodeling, this is a factor to be dealt with in studying vascular histogenesis. In the rat embryo the vessel wall consists solely of endothelial cells. The first indications of the tunica media formation are found light-microscopically as mesenchymal condensations encircling both dorsal aortae at 12.5 days p.c. As markers for early media differentiation α-actin[1] and collagen type IV have been used. Immunohistochemistry on 20 rat embryos, ranging from 11-15 days p.c., reveals that the actin filaments are detectable in the dorsomedial and lateral quadrant of the dorsal aortic wall (FIG. 1). Immunoelectronmicroscopy provides the evidence that the endothelial cells do not contain actin. The first adjoining layer of mesenchymal cells, however, are positive from the 11 day stage onwards. This implies that 1.5 days before the mesenchymal condensations are detectable, a layer of actin-positive cells have differentiated. In 12-day-old embryos most of the mesenchymal cells surrounding the dorsal aortae are actin-positive. The exception is formed by those cells in the region where the aortae have vascular connections to peripheral organs such as the branchial arch system, the dorsal intersegmental arteries, and the aortopulmonary plexus. From 13 days onwards the layer of actin-containing cells keeps expanding, also encircling peripheral vessels such as the subclavian and vertebral vessels.

The development of the endothelial basal lamina, as demonstrated immunohistochemically with an antibody against collagen type IV, corresponds very closely with the actin patterns. The basal lamina is formed first in the dorsomedial part of the aortae, gradually spreading to the lateral and ventral sides. Thus, the media differentiation starts in that part of the dorsal aortae where no major vessels are connected. The actin-negative areas are involved in extensive remodeling, implying formation of new vessels, as well as disconnecting previously existing ones. We hypothesize that differentiation of the media and local remodeling of the vascular system are mutually exclusive, probably because the endothelium in these regions is not confined to its locations, but is active in the remodeling process.

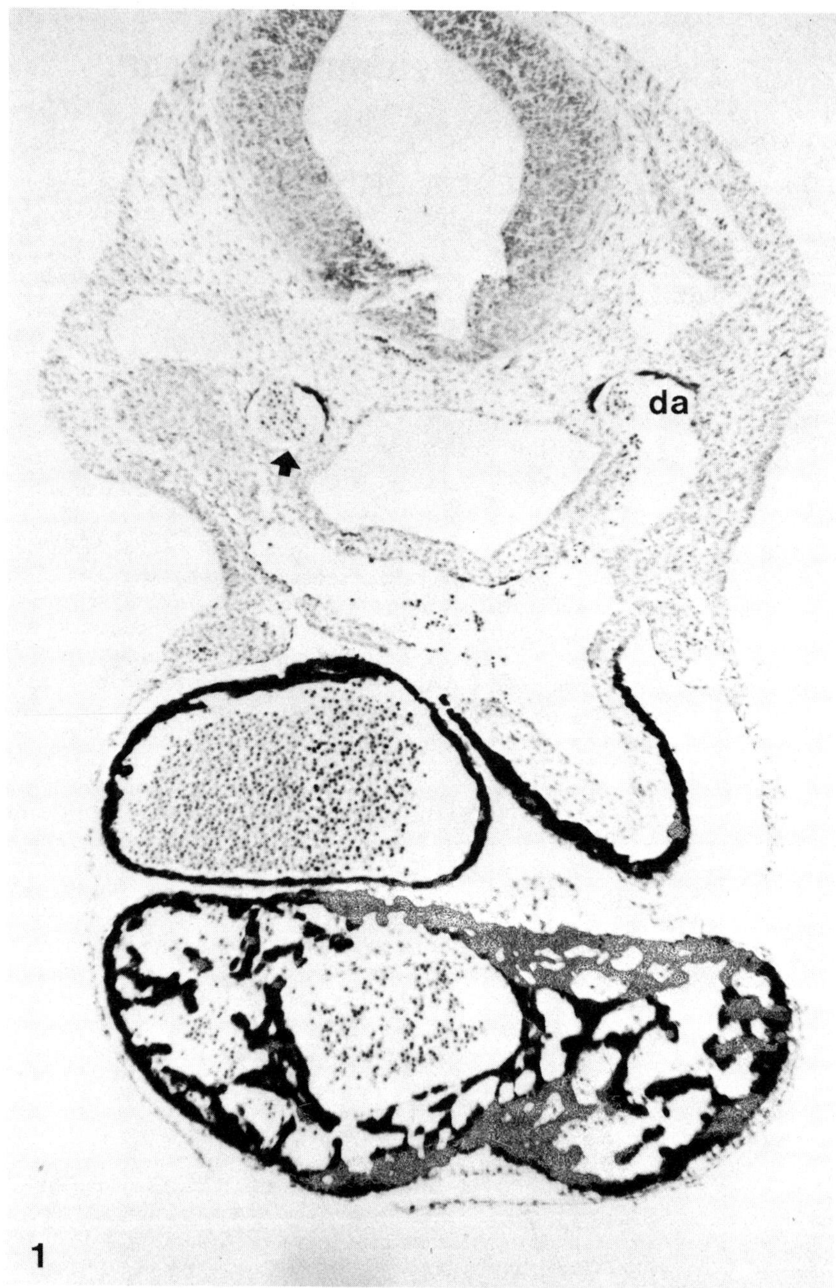

FIGURE 1. Transverse section of an 11.5 day rat embryo incubated with an anti-actin antibody, showing positive cells surrounding part of the dorsal aortae (da). Note the ventrally located, negative region between two branchial arch arteries (arrow). The myocardium is positive as well. On the right side the third arch artery connects to the dorsal aorta.

REFERENCE

1. TSUKADA, T., M. A. MCNUTT, R. ROSS & A. M. GOWN. 1987. HHF35, a muscle actin-specific monoclonal antibody. Am. J. Pathol. **127:** 389-402.

Murine Models of Cardiovascular Dysmorphogenesis

ERIC L. EFFMANN,[a,b] SANDRA A. WHITMAN,[a]
AND BRADLEY R. SMITH[a]

[a]Department of Radiology
and
[b]Department of Cell Biology
Duke University Medical Center
Durham, North Carolina 27710

The pathogenesis and ontogeny of most cardiovascular malformations is unknown. Although cardiac malformations may be induced by pharmacologic, teratologic, or mechanical insults, a single perturbation often results in a wide spectrum of malformations. Single or closely related lesions have been described in the few reports of naturally occurring (genetic) mammalian models of cardiovascular malformations. We have previously described[1,2] a method to efficiently study large numbers of mouse embryos for cardiovascular malformations. We describe potentially useful genetic murine models of pulmonary atresia with VSD and of persistent truncus arteriosus.

Embryos, prepared by the mating schemes described below, were studied by steriomicroradiography, histologic sectioning, and computer reconstruction methods following perfusion fixation and silver nitrate microangiography.[1,2]

Murine trisomy 13 was produced by a different breeding scheme than that originally used by Pexieder *et al.*[3] by mating Robertsonian translocation female mice, Rb(6.13)3Rna/Rb(5.13)70Lub, with all acrocentric (normal) NMRI males. Of 126 embryos analyzed thirty-seven embryos (29%) had trisomy 13. These ranged from stage[4] 16 (day 10) to stage 23 (day 16) and were compared with normal littermates and with normal NMRI embryos. Young trisomic embryos (stage 16-20) demonstrated narrowed ventricular outflow tracts, and all older embryos (stage 21-23) demonstrated pulmonary atresia with ventricular septal defect (FIGURES 1A and 2A). The pulmonary arteries received blood from the dorsal aorta by way of a persistent ductus arteriosus. Sequential stages of affected embryos demonstrated progressive attenuation of the ventricular outflow tract associated with enlarged conotruncal ridges.

Homozygous Splotch embryos were produced by mating heterozygous male and female Splotch mice (C57BL/6J-N Sp, Jackson Laboratory, Bar Harbor, Maine). The homozygous embryos were identified by the presence of caudal or caudal and cranial neural tube defects. Twenty-four (21%) of 112 embryos from 22 litters were homozygous for the neural crest mutant gene—Splotch. These embryos were staged and divided for analysis purposes into fifteen younger embryos (stages 19 and 20—days 11.5 and 12) and nine older embryos (stages 21 and 22—days 13 and 14). The truncus arteriosus was undivided in all but one affected embryo. This type I persistent truncus arteriosus (PTA) lesion appeared to be secondary to incomplete ingrowth of the aorticopulmonary septum to join the conotruncal ridges (FIG. 2B). There was pro-

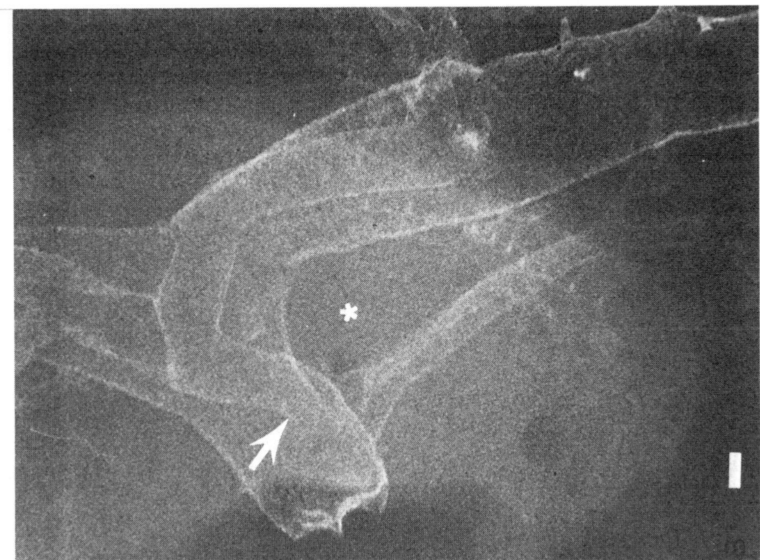

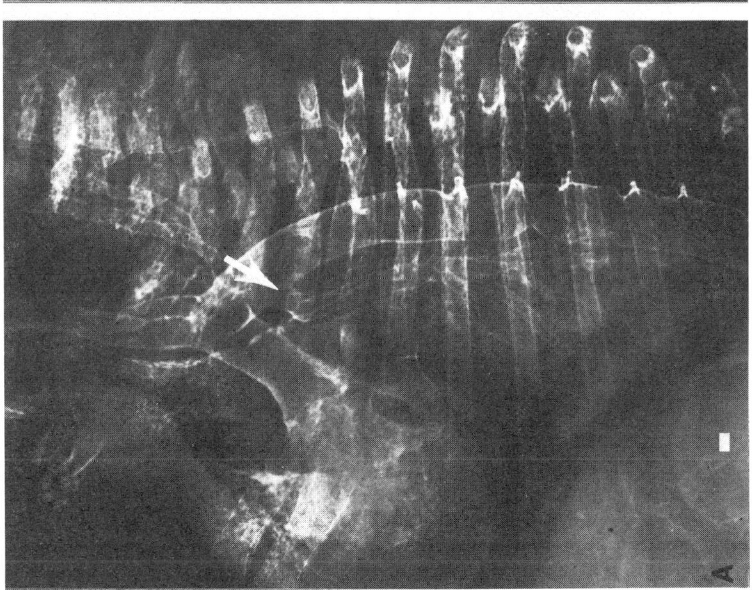

FIGURE 1. Lateral microradiographs of murine models of cardiovascular dysmorphogenesis. Bar = 100 μm. (A) Trisomy 13 (stage 22, day 14) demonstrates absence of right ventricular outflow and main pulmonary artery. Note the supply to the right and left pulmonary arteries by a small persistent ductal connection (white arrow). (B) Homozygous Splotch embryo (stage 21, day 13.5) demonstrates the origin of right and left pulmonary arteries from the truncus arteriosus. Note the absence of a ductus arteriosus in the expected location (*). Also, note the proximal origin of the right brachiocephalic vessel from a position close to the truncal valve (white arrow).

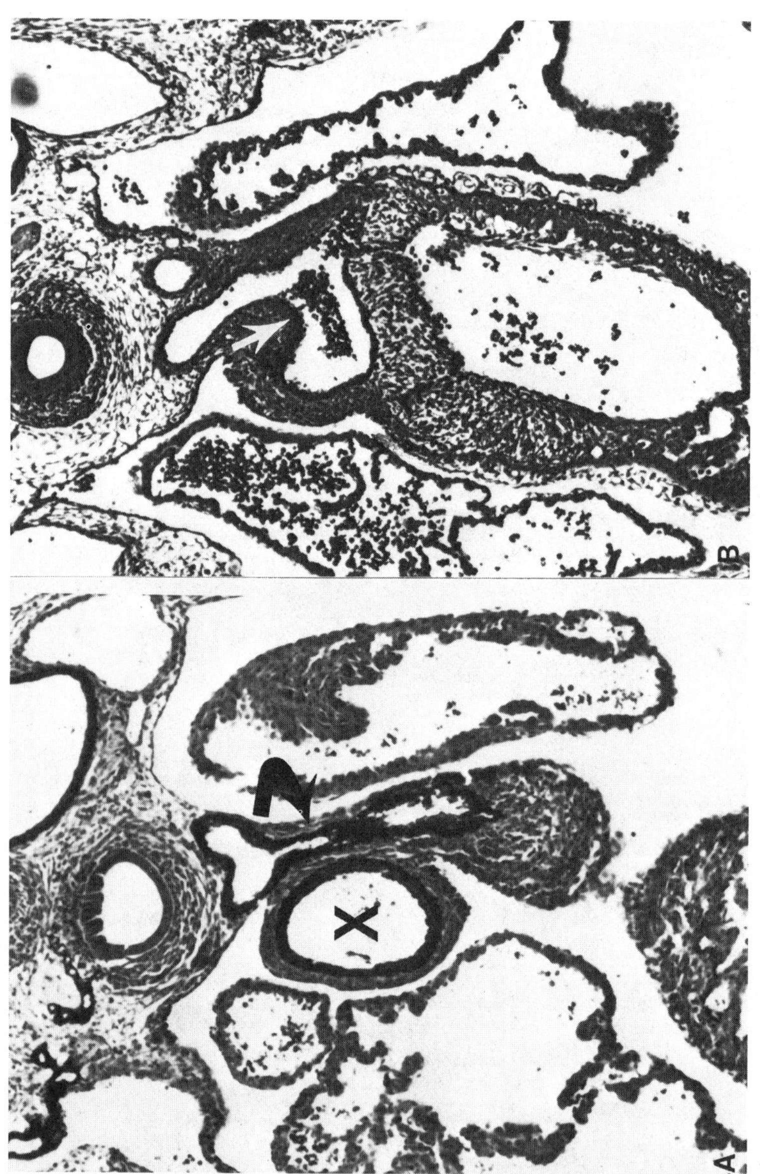

FIGURE 2. Transverse (axial) sections through the arterial outflow portions of the heart. (A) Trisomy 13 embryo (stage 22, day 14) demonstrates marked narrowing of the main pulmonary artery (curved black arrow) in comparison with the cross-section of the adjacent aorta (X). (B) Homozygous Splotch embryo (stage 21, day 13.5) demonstrates failure of ingrowth of the aorticopulmonary septum (white arrow) to divide the truncus arteriosus.

gressive attenuation and final disappearance of the dorsal sixth arch (ductus arteriosus) (FIG. 1B). The role of neural crest cell migration in the pathogenesis of PTA in homozygous Splotch embryos is unknown.

Two potentially useful murine models for studying the importance of genetic factors in cardiovascular dysmorphogenesis are described. Stereomicroradiography coupled with histological analysis is an efficient method of detecting other potentially useful models of cardiovascular disease.

REFERENCES

1. EFFMANN, E. L. 1982. Development of the right and left pulmonary arteries—A microangiographic study in the mouse. Invest. Radio. **17:** 529-538.
2. EFFMANN, E. L., S. WHITMAN & T. PEXIEDER. 1986. Stereomicroangiography in embryologic and teratologic investigation. Teratology **34:** 103-112.
3. PEXIEDER, T. *et al.* 1981. Congenital Heart Disease in Experimental (Fetal) Mouse Trisomies: Incidence. *In* Perspectives in Cardiovascular Research. T. Pexieder, Ed.: **5:** 389-399. Raven Press. New York.
4. THEILER, K. 1972. The House Mouse. Springer-Verlag. New York.

Familial Partial DiGeorge Syndrome

Unmasking of Hypoparathyroidism by EDTA Challenge

SAMUEL S. GIDDING, ANN L. MINCIOTTI, AND
CRAIG B. LANGMAN

Divisions of Cardiology and Nephrology
Department of Pediatrics
Children's Memorial Hospital
Northwestern University
Chicago, Illinois 60614

Neural crest cells participate in the embryonic development of aorticopulmonary and conotruncal septa, thymus, and parathyroid glands.[1] Inasmuch as the DiGeorge syndrome includes developmental anomalies of these tissues, a causal relation for abnormal neural crest development has been suggested.[2] This paper describes the unmasking of latent hypoparathyroidism by disodium EDTA infusion in two patients with conotruncal cardiac defects not previously suspected to have the DiGeorge syndrome.

SUBJECTS AND METHODS

Patient 1 was a 26-year-old woman with repaired tetralogy of Fallot. One of her four children had the complete DiGeorge syndrome and another had truncus arteriosus and normal parathyroid and thymic function. Patient 2 had repaired truncus arteriosus and was 5 years of age. Patient 3 had undergone repair of hemitruncus, had a twin with truncus arteriosus, and was 2 years of age. All subjects had normal resting ionized calcium (Ca^{2+}), parathormone (PTH), and lymphocyte function.

An intravenous infusion of EDTA (5% dextrose with 0.2% sodium chloride; 600 mL containing 3,000 mg of disodium EDTA and 2% lidocaine (0.3 mL/kg of body weight)) was administered at a rate of 5 mL/kg/h. Measurements were made at onset, 30 minutes, 1 h, 1½ h, 2 h, and 2½ h.[3] Blood-ionized Ca^{2+} and pH were measured with a Ca^{2+}-selective electrode. Serum total Ca^{2+}, phosphorus, and magnesium were measured according to standard methods. Serum PTH levels were measured by a sensitive midmolecule radioimmunoassay (INCSTAR, Stillwater, MN). Results from 11 normal adults were used as a comparison. The regression line and confidence limits to describe the relation between ionized Ca^{2+} and PTH were constructed using repeated measures analysis of variance. The patients' responses were then compared with that of the normal population.

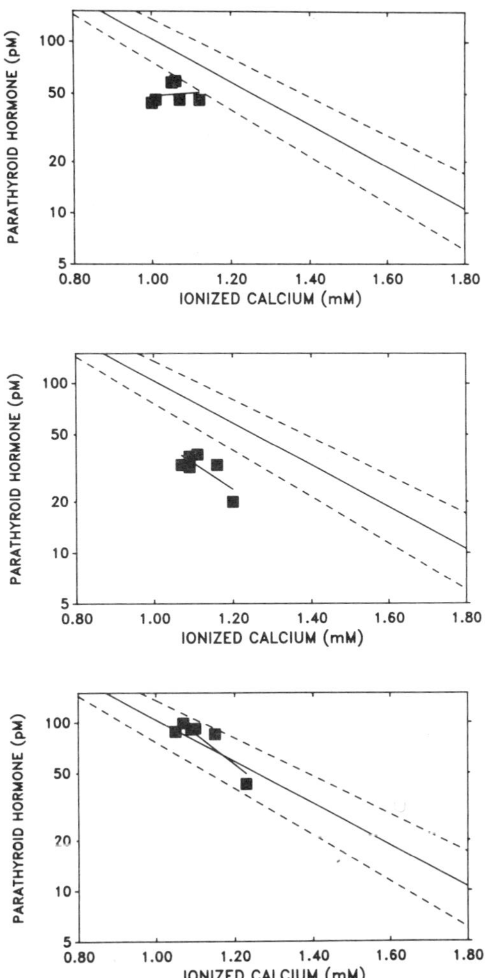

FIGURE 1. Level of mid-molecule parathyroid hormone in relation to blood-ionized calcium during EDTA infusion in the study patients (squares) and 11 normal subjects (regression line: thick line and thin lines, mean 2 SD, respectively). The vertical scale is logarithmic. The values in the patients represent mean determinations of duplicate ionized calcium and triplicate determinations of parathyroid hormone at each point; the regression line is the solid line between points. The slopes of the regression lines are significantly different from normal for patients 1 and 2 (top and middle panels) but not for patient 3 (bottom panel).

RESULTS

All three patients had normal resting ionized Ca^{2+} levels (1.12-1.25 mM) and PTH levels (23-43 pM). EDTA infusion caused progressive reduction in the blood-ionized Ca^{2+} levels and became significant two hours after infusion (minimum ionized Ca^{2+} levels, 1.01-1.05 mM). Two patients had abnormal PTH responses. Patient 1 had only a 22% increase from basal levels, which was less than the expected doubling (FIG. 1, top). Patient 2 had resting levels of PTH that were at the lowest limits of normal and increased PTH concentration by only 60% after achieving an ionized Ca^{2+} level of 1.07 mM (FIG. 1, middle). Patient 3 achieved the normal doubling of PTH in response to hypocalcemia (FIG. 1, bottom). Serum phosphorus concentrations remained normal. Serum magnesium concentrations remained low and unchanged in the two patients with abnormal PTH responses, but decreased significantly from normal in patient 3.

DISCUSSION

This study has shown that latent hypoparathyroidism, defined as an abnormal PTH response to hypocalcemia, may be present in selected patients with cardiac defects associated with DiGeorge syndrome. This observation strengthens the hypothesis that the etiology of these defects is related to an abnormality of neural crest development.[1,2,5] Further, we have shown the transmission of the DiGeorge syndrome from generation to generation by unmasking latent hypoparathyroidism in a mother with tetralogy of Fallot who gave birth to two affected children—one with the DiGeorge syndrome and one with truncus arteriosus. One patient with familial truncus arteriosus had a normal response. EDTA infusion in selected patients may be helpful in elucidating the inheritance of the DiGeorge syndrome and the development of certain conotruncal cardiac defects.

REFERENCES

1. KIRBY, M. L. & D. E. BOCKMAN. 1984. Neural crest and normal development: A new perspective. Anat. Rec. **209:** 1-6.
2. VAN MIEROP, L. H. & L. M. KUTSCHE. 1986. Cardiovascular anomalies in DiGeorge syndrome and importance of neural crest as a possible pathogenetic factor. Am. J. Cardiol. **58:** 133-137.
3. TSANG, R. C., I. W. CHEN, P. MCENERY et al. 1976. Parathyroid function tests with EDTA infusions in infancy and childhood. J. Pediatr. **88:** 250-256.
4. GIDDING, S. S., A. L. MINCIOTTI & C. B. LANGMAN. 1988. Unmasking of hypoparathyroidism in familial partial DiGeorge syndrome by challenge with disodiumedetate. N. Engl. J. Med. **319:** 1589-1591.
5. LAMMER, E. J. & J. M. OPITZ. 1986. The DiGeorge anomaly as a developmental field defect. Am. J. Med. Genet. Suppl. **2:** 113-127.

Hemodynamic Mechanisms in Cardiovascular Teratogenesis

ENID F. GILBERT-BARNESS,[a] STEVE KARGAS,[a]
GEORGE KARGAS,[a] AND HAROLD BRUYERE[b]

[a]Department of Pathology and Laboratory Medicine
University of Wisconsin
Madison, Wisconsin 53792
and
[b]Department of Pharmacy
University of Wyoming
Laramie, Wyoming 82071

Adverse hemodynamic changes during cardiogenesis and vascular development predispose to abnormal morphogenesis of the cardiovascular system. It has been demonstrated that the embryonic chick circulation is pharmacologically responsive to drugs that we have shown induce cardiovascular defects in the chick embryo. These include, in particular, β-adrenergic stimulants and methylxanthines.[1-3] Previous techniques are, however, invasive, and embryos have not survived the trauma produced by the methodology. Our approach to determination of pathophysiologic mechanisms of teratogenesis is unique in that embryos subjected to microcinephotoanalysis survive to an age when cardiac development is complete and hearts and vessels are large enough to determine structural defects by gross examination. In this study, embryos were noninvasively examined using microcinephotoanalysis (Hamburger-Hamilton stages 18-21). Cardiac function determinations may be conducted during a major period within the interval of early heart morphogenesis.[4-6]

Cardiovascular malformations can be related to alterations in hemodynamic function as shown by decrease in end-diastolic volume, end-systolic volume, stroke volume, heart rate, cardiac output, and a rapid and sustained increase in ejection fraction. Alterations in hemodynamic function have been correlated with abnormalities in cardiac embryogenesis (FIG. 1).

Clinically significant cardiovascular anomalies have been induced with exposure of chick embryos to cardioactive drugs. Malformations have included tetralogy of Fallot (FIG. 2A), truncus arteriosus (FIG. 2B), double outlet right ventricle, isolated ventricular septal defect, interruption of the aortic arch with subpulmonic ventricular septal defect and posterior deviation of the subpulmonic conus, and dextroposition of the aorta.

We have further shown that β-1 receptor activity plays an important role in the teratogenic process.[7] Pretreatment with β-receptor blocking agents significantly reduces the incidence of malformations.[8]

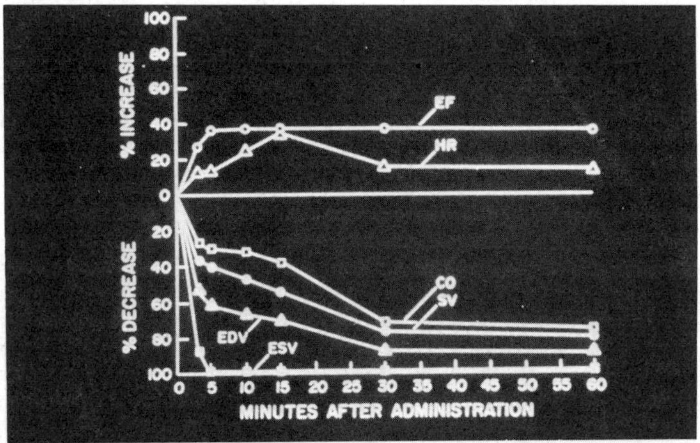

FIGURE 1. Relative percent changes in cardiac function preceding epinephrine-induced interrupted aortic arch. The effects of caffeine with time on (A) stroke volume, (B) ejection fraction, (C) cardiac output, and (D) cardiac rate in the stage 19 chick embryo. Each point represents the mean of 6 or 7 determinations.

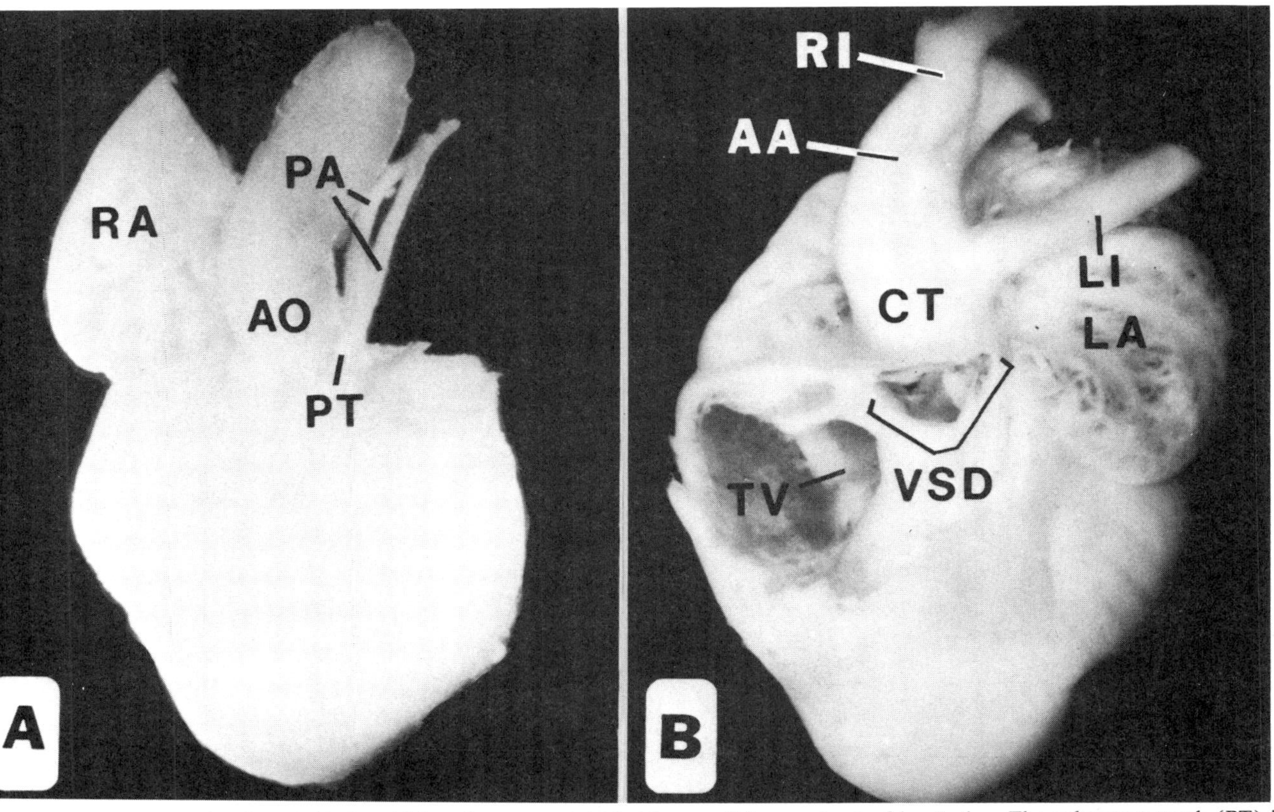

FIGURE 2. A. Tetralogy of Fallot. A 13 day chick embryo treated with 4.1 mg caffeine on day 3 of incubation. The pulmonary trunk (PT) is markedly stenotic with severely hypoplastic pulmonary arteries (PA). Examination of the heart showed a ventricular septal defect with an overriding aortic valve. RA, right atrium; AO, aortic root. **B.** Truncus arteriosus. Right ventricular view of 17 day chick embryo exposed to 4.1 mg caffeine on day 3 of incubation. Examination of this heart showed a common aorticopulmonary trunk (CT) with a large ventricular septal defect (VSD). RI, right innominate; LI, left innominate; AA, aortic arch; LA, left atrium; TV, tricuspid valve. (Bruyere *et al.*:[4] With permission from Alan R. Liss Inc.)

REFERENCES

1. HODACH, R. J., E. F. GILBERT & J. F. FALLON. 1974. Teratology **9:** 203-210.
2. GILBERT, E. F., H. J. BRUYERE, JR., S. ISHIKAWA, M. O. CHEUNG & R. J. HODACH. 1977. Teratology **16:** 47-52.
3. BRUYERE, H. J., JR., R. MATSUOKA, E. CARLSSON, M. O. CHEUNG, R. DEAN & E. F. GILBERT. 1983. Teratology **23:** 75-82.
4. Bruyere, H. J., Jr., T. Nishikawa, H. Uno, J. E. Gilbert & E. F. GILBERT. 1987. Experimentally induced cardiovascular malformations in the chick embryo. *In* Genetic Aspects of Developmental Pathology. BD: OAS. E. F. Gilbert & J. M. Opitz, Eds. Vol. **23:** 443-448. Alan R. Liss, Inc. New York.
5. GILBERT, E. F., H. J. BRUYERE, JR., S. ISHIKAWA & M. O. CHEUNG. 1980. The role of catecholamines and other cardiac stimulants in cardiovascular teratogenesis: recent observations and proposed mechanisms. *In* Perspectives in Cardiovascular Research. T. Pexieder, Ed. Vol. **5:** 473-484. Alan R. Liss, Inc. New York.
6. BRUYERE, H. J., B. J. MICHAUD, E. F. GILBERT & J. D. FOLTS. 1987. J. Appl. Toxicol. **7(3):** 197-203.
7. GILBERT, E. F., S. ISHIKAWA & H. J. BRUYERE, JR. 1979. Spectrum of cardiovascular malformations in embryonic chicks induced by β stimulating agents. *In* Proceedings of the Symposium on Etiology and Morphogenesis of Congenital Heart Disease. R. Van Praagh & A. Takao, Eds. 155-175. Futura Press. New York.
8. GILBERT, E. F., H. J. BRUYERE, JR., S. ISHIKAWA, M. O. CHEUNG & R. J. HODACH. 1977. Teratology **15:** 317-324.

Endocardial Surface Changes during Hamster Atrium Development

A TEM, SEM, and ANF Immunoelectron Microscopic Study[a]

JACQUES GILLOTEAUX AND DAVID LINZ

Anatomy Department
Northeastern Ohio Universities College of Medicine
Rootstown, Ohio 44272

The mammalian atria have not been well-characterized morphologically with respect to development and aging. Several transmission (TEM) and scanning electron microscopy (SEM) studies have focused on the embryology of septation. Only a handful of mammalian models, however, were studied with regard to the endocardium ultrastructure,[1-6] whereas a large amount of information was obtained from embryological studies of chick development.[7,8] The newly recognized endocrine function of the atria[9] and the availability of antiserum against atrial natriuretic factor (ANF) presents an opportunity to correlate ultrastructural morphology with endocrine function.

This report describes and complements other observations obtained in pre-, neo- and postnatal development of the Syrian hamster atria as they pertain to the functions of the endocardial endothelium.

Fifteen Syrian hamster embryos, thirteen-day gestation, and fifteen neonates (1 d old) from three pregnant mothers (F1B strain) from BioBreeders (Watertown, MA) were used. Following Na barbital anesthesia and euthanasia (5 mg/100 g body weight, i.p.), all the developing fetuses were quickly removed from their placental membranes and immersed in aerated lactated Ringer solution. Ten embryos were dissected, and entire hearts, showing contractility, were excised and fixed for 1 h in 2% buffered glutaraldehyde (0.15 M Na cacodylate, pH 7.3) solution. Five others were fixed for immunoelectron cytochemistry [IEM] in 4% paraformaldehyde and 1% glutaraldehyde buffered solution (0.1 M phosphate). Fifteen neonate hearts were subdivided similarly in two groups (TEM and IEM) and fixed after anesthesia was performed (50 µL i.p. Na barbital). Following a rinsing step in the same buffer, the right atria were isolated and postfixed in 1% aqueous OsO_4. Samples were dehydrated and either prepared for SEM (n = 5) or for TEM. The atria to be studied by IEM were not postfixed in osmium but embedded in epoxy resin after dehydration. Samples for TEM and IEM were contrasted by uranyl and lead salts before being examined. For immunoelectron microscopy, the De Mey *et al.*[10] procedure was used and, following

[a] This research was supported by the American Heart Association, Inc., Akron chapter and by the Ohio Board of Regents Research Challenge Fund to NEOU College of Medicine.

TABLE 1.

	Fetuses		Newborn	Adult
Age (days)	−5	−2	1	60
ANF granules diameter (nm +/− SEM)	138 (15)	149 (43)	173 (41)	187 (48)
		ns	$p < 0.05$	$p < 0.1$
Immunogold density (no. gold/μm^2)	119	224	328	430
	$p < .05$	$p < .005$	$p < 0.005$	
no. granules measured	n = 160	n = 109	n = 130	n = 132

incubation, ultrathin sections with anti-alpha ANF (gift of Dr. L. Jennes, Wright State University, Dayton) and immunolabeling revealed anti-rabbit IgG labeled with colloidal gold particles of 15 nm diameter (Janssen Pharmaceuticals, NJ). Specificity tests were described in a previous report.[11] Atrial granule size, immunolabeling density of gold particles per μm square surface of atrial granules, and significance of comparisons between average values obtained for each age group are reported (Student *t* test) in TABLE 1.

From 13 embryonic days (ed) of development until birth, we found that the atrial endothelium was composed of a simple squamous epithelium delimited from the subendocardial layer by its own primitive basal lamina. The endothelium displays bulging to rounded cells up to 6 μm thick (perikaryal region) or squamous-like morphology of less than 1 μm in thickness (FIGURES 1 and 2). It is not uncommon to observe endocardial cells (FIG. 4) or adjacent atrial myocytes (FIG. 2) undergoing mitotic activity. In these developmental stages the nuclei are always euchromatic, and the cytoplasms contain numerous free ribosomal-like particles, or aggregates, and RER cisterns (FIGURES 1 and 4). It is interesting to report that up to 13 ed, the endothelial lining is rudimentary and shows fenestrations and large gaps or discontinuities as illustrated by FIGURES 1 (TEM) and 3 (SEM). The basal laminae are not as clearly delineated as in the neonate. In addition, the endothelial surface is covered by scarce microvilli and blebs in the fetal stages (*e.g.* FIG. 3), whereas endocardial cells of neonates display many microvilli (FIG. 4)

The myoblasts differentiate until birth, and they are attached to each other by small, macular intercalated junctions ranging from 0.1 (13 ed) to at least 2 μm (neonate) in length. Lipid droplets are visible, as well as many mitochondrial profiles (some appear as empty spaces in the neonate (FIG. 4)). Myofilaments are scarce, but sarcomere formation of small bundles of myofilaments is detected. By contrast, myofibrils are more abundant in the neonate and fill a large part of the sarcoplasm.

Atrial granules are observed throughout the sarcoplasmic spaces of all the atrial myocytes examined. The atrial granules are scarce in the fetal stages, although they are quite abundant in the neonates. These atrial granules become visible before the

---

FIGURES 1-5. Ultrastructural aspects of hamster right atrial endocardium. FIGURES 1-3: Thirteen-day-old embryonic heart. In 1 and 3, large arrows point toward endocardial discontinuities. Small arrows point toward some atrial granules. Bars = 1 μm. FIGURE 2: ANF immunolabeling in atrial granules (15 nm diameter gold labels; small arrows) in a mitotic

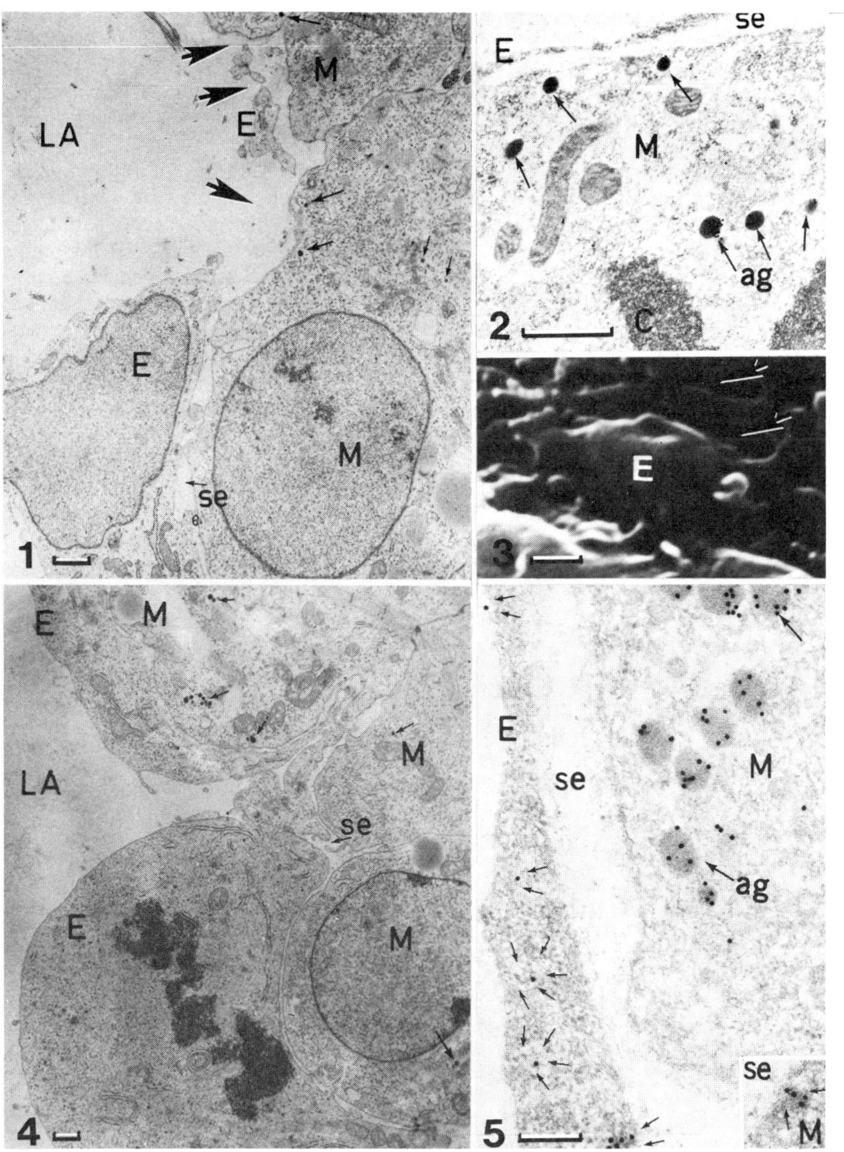

myoblast. Bar = 0.5 μm. FIGURE 3: SEM of endocardial surface. FIGURES 4-5: Neonate (1 d old) heart. In 4: Continuous endocardial lining with a mitotic endothelial cell. Atrial granules are arrowed. Bar = 1 μm. In 5: ANF immunolabeling in atrial granules (15 nm diameter gold labels) and in endocardial endothelial cell (arrowed). Labels are detected at the basal side, in vacuoles, and at the endothelial surface. Inset: close-up of atrial granule exocytosis from the myocyte of the main FIGURE 4 cut out from an adjacent site of FIGURE 4. Bar = 200 nm. ag: atrial granule; C: chromatin; E: endocardial endothelium; LA: lumen atrial chamber; M: atrial myocyte; se: subendocardial space.

myofibrils develop. They range from 50 to 330 nm in diameter (TABLE 1), and their ANF content is identified by the gold labeling (15 nm gold particles; FIGURES 2 and 5). In the neonate, ANF immunoreactivity is detected on the basal side, in vacuoles and at the apical surface of the endocardial cells (FIG. 5) after ANF-containing secretory product has been liberated in the endomysium and in the subendocardial spaces (insert of FIG. 5).

Because the endocardium is discontinuous until the 13th day of embryonic development, one can hypothesize that the early stages of Syrian hamster atrial myocardial development would be more susceptible to the effects of pathogenic compounds than the later stages of development.[13] Immunolabeled ANF-containing granules can be employed as a marker for undifferentiated atrial myocytes because they appear before the sarcomeres of the contractile machinery are expressed and organized.[12] While the atrial tissues are developing and differentiating, the myocytes produce and secrete proANF, which has to be activated into ANF. Although it is not clear where this activation occurs, it is significant to note that the endocardial endothelium is the only barrier between the endocrine myocytes and the blood.[12–14]

This report and others[12–14] suggest that the endocardium is not only involved in morphogenetic functions but that it also protects against noxious compounds and may also play a role in the processing of proANF into ANF and/or at least in controlling the rate of its secretion in the blood. Moreover, and because of the discontinuous endocardial lining observed until day 13 in the Syrian hamster, one could speculate that during early cardiac development, inactive proANF (1-126) is found in the blood along with ANF (98-126).

REFERENCES

1. CANDIOLLO, L. 1963. Z. Zellforsch. **61:** 486-492.
2. CHALLICE, C. E. & S. VIRÁGH 1973. *In* Ultrastructure of the mammalian heart. C. E. CHALLICE & S. VIRÁGH, Eds.: 91-126. Academic Press. New York.
3. HARASAKI, H., H. SUZUKI, H. HANANO & M. TORISU. 1975. Arch. Histol. Jpn. **38:** 71-84.
4. MANASEK, F. J. 1979. The cardiovascular system. *In* Handbook of Physiology. R. M. BERNE, N. SPERELAKIS & S. R. GEIGER, Eds. Vol. I: 29-42. American Physiological Society. Bethesda, MD. (sect. 2).
5. MELAX, H. & T. S. LEESON. 1967. Cardiovasc. Res. **1:** 349-355.
6. SONG, S. H. 1977. Acta Anat. (Basel) **99:** 67-78.
7. PEXIEDER, T. 1977. Bibl. Anat. **15:** 531-534.
8. PEXIEDER, T. 1981. Scanning Electron Microsc. **II:** 223-253.
9. DE BOLD, A. J. 1987. Can. J. Physiol. Pharmacol. **65:** 2007-2012.
10. DE MEY, J., M. MOEREMANS, M. DE WAELE, G. GEUENS & M. DE BRABANDER. 1981. Cell Biol. Int. Rep. **5:** 889-899.
11. SCOTT, J. N. & L. JENNES. 1987. Cell Tissue Res. **248:** 479-481.
12. GILLOTEAUX, J. & D. LINZ. 1989. Am. J. Anat. **184:** 323-335.
13. GILLOTEAUX, J. 1989. Anat. Embryol. **179:** 227-236.
14. GILLOTEAUX, J., R. MENU, L. JENNES & J.-J. VANDERHAEGHEN. 1988. J. Cell. Biochem. (Suppl.) **12A:** 103.

Development of the Coronary Arterial Orifices

A. C. GITTENBERGER-DE GROOT,[a]

A. J. J. C. BOGERS,[c] R. E. POELMANN,[a]

B. M. PÉAULT,[d] AND H. A. HUYSMANS[b]

[a]*Department of Anatomy and Embryology*
[b]*Department of Thoracic Surgery*
University of Leiden
2300 RC Leiden, the Netherlands

[c]*Department of Thoracic Surgery*
Thorax Center
Dijkzigt University Hospital
Rotterdam, the Netherlands

[d]*Institut d'Embryologie du CNRS et du College de France*
Nogent-sur-Marne, France

Coronary artery origin and course show a rather constant pattern, but frequently anomalies occur. In order to investigate the normal and abnormal coronary arterial patterns, a development of the orifices and proximal parts of the coronary arteries was performed. Using conventional histological techniques in human and rat embryos, the conclusion was drawn that neither the theory of direct influence of outlet septation,[1] nor the theory of multiple coronary arterial sprouting[2] adequately explain normal and abnormal coronary arterial development.[3] A technical limitation of the conventional techniques was found in the difficulty to detect endothelial cells in the earliest stages of vessel development. Using a monoclonal anti-endothelial staining in quail embryos, anti-MB_1,[4] however, endothelium in all stages could be investigated. Fifteen quail embryos of 5-10 days after fertilization were studied. In these we never observed more than two coronary orifices emerging at 7-9 days after fertilization. Coronary orifices (FIG. 1) were invariably present beyond those stages. The coronary orifices were always situated in the facing sinuses of the aorta.[5] A coronary orifice, when present, was always connected to the proximal coronary arterial vasculature in the peritruncal ring. Furthermore, in several specimen, coronary arteries were observed penetrating the aortic media from the peritruncal ring. In two specimens the coronary artery even contacted the still intact lining of the aorta. On the basis of these data the conclusion is drawn that there is evidence that the coronary arteries grow into and not, as is generally supposed, out of the aorta.

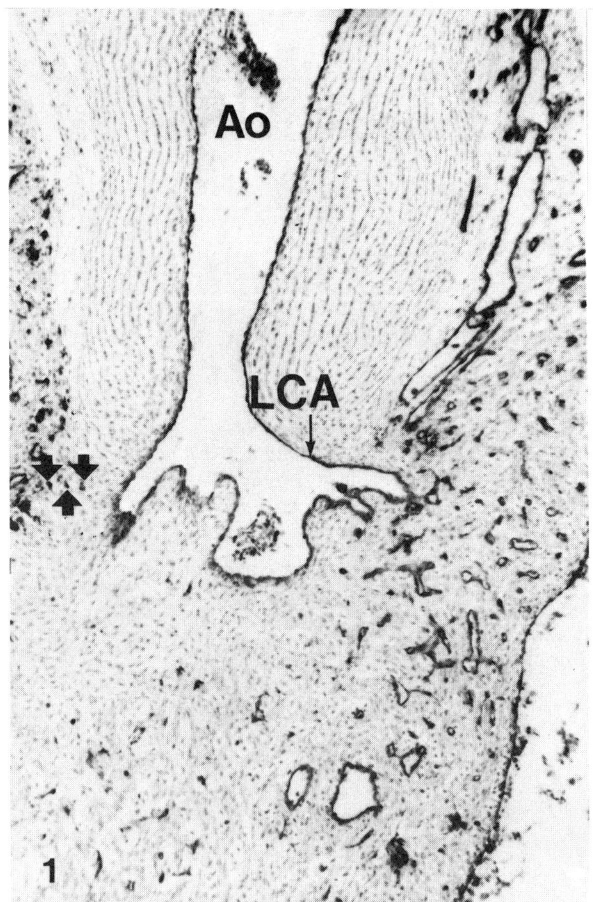

FIGURE 1. Section of the aortic orifice level of a quail heart 8 days after fertilization. The left coronary artery (LCA) connects the aorta (Ao) to the peritruncal ring coronary vasculature. Three little dots (arrows) indicate the site of the developing right coronary artery. Staining: anti-MB$_1$ antibody; × 35.

REFERENCES

1. ABRIKOSOFF, A. 1911. Aneurysma des linken Herzventrikels mit abnormer Abgangstelle der linken Koronararterie von der Pulmonalis bei einem fünfmonatlichen Kinde. Virch. Arch. Pathol. Anat. **203:** 413–420.
2. HACKENSELLNER, H. A. 1956. Akzessorische Kranzgefassanlagen der Arteria Pulmonalis unter 63 menschlichen Embryonen-Serien mit einer groszten Länge von 12 bis 36 mm. Z. Mikrosk. Anat. Forsch. **62:** 153–164.
3. BOGERS, A. J. J. C. & A. C. GITTENBERGER-DE GROOT. 1988. The inadequacy of existing theories on development of the proximal coronary arteries and their connections with the arterial trunks. Int. J. Cardiol. **20:** 117–122.

4. PÉAULT, B. M., J. P. THIERY & N. M. LE DOUARIN. 1983. Surface marker for hemopoietic and endothelial cell lineages in quail that is defined by a monoclonal antibody. Proc. Natl. Acad. Sci. USA **80:** 2976-2980.
5. GITTENBERGER-DE GROOT, A. C., U. SAUER, A. OPPENHEIMER DEKKER & J. M. QUAE-GEBEUR. 1986. Coronary arterial anatomy in transposition of the great arteries: a morphologic study. Pediatr. Cardiol. **4:** 15-24.

Fetal Manifestations of Cardiovascular Hypertrophy in Spontaneously Hypertensive Rats[a]

SARAH D. GRAY

Department of Human Physiology
School of Medicine
University of California
Davis, California 95616

INTRODUCTION

Spontaneous (genetic) hypertension in the rat (SHR) has been characterized with respect to structural and functional changes in the heart and blood vessels in the adult stage. In comparison to normotensive control Wistar-Kyoto (WKY) rats, SHR have greatly thickened ventricular and arterial walls. Blood pressure has been thought to rise only after about 6-7 weeks of age, and the hypertrophy has been considered to occur as an adaptive response to the rising pressure, but cardiac hypertrophy can be detected in the neonate.[1] Although it is still unclear whether the increased wall thickness is due to adaptation or is a primary defect of genetic hypertension, it is apparent that it occurs early in development. Also, humoral factors associated with the hypertensive state have been described, which are thought to affect tranpsort processes in the vessel walls and facilitate functional vasoconstriction by increasing available calcium in smooth muscle cells; the increased vasoconstriction raises vascular resistance and thereby increases the blood pressure.

The present study characterizes the course of development of ventricular and arterial wall mass in fetal and neonatal SHR and uses embryo cross-transfer to expose animals of both strains to the opposite *in utero* environment. The animals are developed to term in order to determine the importance of circulating hypertensive factors in wall development.

METHODS

SHR and WKY pregnant dams were anesthetized with Na-pentobarbital (3.5 mg/ body weight), and fetuses were removed for analysis of ventricular and aortic weights, and aortic and carotid artery wall and lumen dimensions; neonates were also studied.

[a] This work was supported by NIH Grant HL 29880.

TABLE 1.

Ventricular Development		
17 Days Gestation	WKY (n=115)	SHR (n=147)
VW, mg	2.50 ± 0.03	2.28 ± 0.02
VW/BW, mg/g	5.17 ± 0.04	6.52 ± 0.05
One day old	WKY (37)	SHR (22)
VW, mg	23.46 ± 0.30	26.23 ± 0.37
VW/BW	4.02 ± 0.04	4.93 ± 0.04
Aortic and Carotid Artery Development		
Normal, one day old	WKY (7)	SHR (7)
Aortic MA/LA	0.174 ± 0.010	0.237 ± 0.035
Carotid MA/LA	0.217 ± 0.022	0.317 ± 0.051
Cross-transferred, one day old	WKY (30)	SHR (28)
Aortic MA/LA	0.202 ± 0.009	0.307 ± 0.019
Carotid MA/LA	0.279 ± 0.013	0.412 ± 0.028

Embryo transfer between SHR and WKY[2] was carried out on days 4-5 of gestation: SHR embryos were transferred to pseudopregnant WKY dams and WKY embryos to pseudopregnant SHR dams; all were allowed to develop to term. Vessels were perfusion-fixed with Zamboni's fixative, postfixed with 1% osmium tetroxide, embedded in plastic, and sectioned at 1 μm thickness. Cross-sectional areas of vessels were determined on the Zeiss Image Analyzer: lumen area (LA) and medial area (MA). Wall/lumen ratios were expressed as MA/LA.

RESULTS

Analysis of normal fetal and neonatal ventricular development in SHR and WKY revealed higher ventricular weight/body weight ratios in SHR at 17 days gestation and the first postnatal day. Development of the large arteries was also characterized by an increased wall/lumen ratio in SHR at 1 day of age, both in normally developing animals and in those that were transferred to WKY dams. Linear regression analysis of the log of VW on log BW in late gestation (17-22 days) yielded a greater y intercept for SHR (0.752 vs. 0.675), predicting that at any body weight, ventricular weight will be higher in SHR. The differences in dimensions in the large conduit vessels are largely in wall thickness, rather than lumen size. There are slightly more elastic laminae present in SHR (9.51 ± 0.19 vs. 7.79 ± 0.18), so the increased wall thickness is probably due to increases in both cellular and connective tissue elements.[3]

DISCUSSION

The data indicate that ventricular mass is increased in SHR over that of WKY by 17 days *in utero.* Aortic/carotid artery wall mass is also increased relative to lumen size during both the fetal and neonatal stages, as indicated by the greater medial area/lumen area ratios in SHR. Although it is not clear what the blood pressure is *in utero,* it is possible that these effects may be primary defects rather than adaptive. The data suggest that circulating hypertensinogenic factors in hypertensive animals do not modify the early developmental pattern of the vascular wall in WKY, and the lack of such factors does not prevent the genotypic pattern in SHR.

REFERENCES

1. GRAY, S D. 1984. Clin. Exp. Hyperten. **A6:** 755-781.
2. GRAY, S. D. & C. C. LAWRENCE. 1984. Clin. Exp. Hyperten. **B2:** 351-369.
3. IREDALE, R. B., C. A. ECCLESTON-JOYNER, R. B. RUCKER & S. D. GRAY. 1989. Clin. Exp. Hyperten. **A11:** 173-187.

Noninvasive Ultrasonic Assessment of Chick Embryo Cardiac Function

JAMES C. HUHTA, AGOSTINHO BORGES,
GRACE Y. YOON, KENNETH A. MURDISON, AND
DENNIS C. WOOD

The Division of Cardiology
Department of Pediatrics
The University of Pennsylvania School of Medicine and
The Children's Hospital of Philadelphia
Philadelphia, Pennsylvania 19104

Functional assessment of the heart during early morphogenesis has been hampered by the fact that all existing experimental preparations require an invasive approach. Current pulsed Doppler technology for chick embryo evaluation requires physical penetration of the embryonic membranes to place the probe directly on the embryo and uses zero-crossing technology, not state-of-the-art discrete Fourier transform spectral analysis of blood velocity.[1-3] Therefore, quantitative assessment of intracardiac blood velocities has not been done. A noninvasive methodology would allow longitudinal studies of functional changes of normal embyronic physiology during a period of time that the heart is undergoing dramatic morphologic change. For example, functional assessment of the atrioventricular and semilunar cushions by Doppler technology would allow testing of the hypothesis that valvar regurgitation and congestive heart failure is a pathway by which disordered morphology may lead to embryo wastage.

High frequency imaging/Doppler equipment was adapted for this application and applied to the chick embryo model of normal morphogensis with the goal of describing the normal cardiovascular functional phenotype, that is, blood flow and myocardial/valvular function during normal development. Fertile White Leghorn chicken eggs were incubated blunt end up in a forced-draft constant humidity incubator to Hamburger-Hamilton stage 18-32 (3-6 days), and the noninvasive imaging and Doppler evaluation was performed daily by way of a very thin plastic window in the egg shell without removing the overlying membranes of the embryo (FIG. 1).

Maximal outflow and inflow tract velocity waveforms (n = 159) were obtained from 76 embryonic hearts by optimizing the embryo position using 7.5 MHz ultrasonic imaging direction. Doppler signals were analyzed by real-time chirp-z transformation.[4] Doppler signals of adequate amplitude for analysis were obtained in all embryos from the point of first detection of heart rate by imaging, and 26 were followed longitudinally for three or more days. Peak outflow velocity increased from 15 ± 7 to 50 ± 6 cm/s ($p < 0.001$), whereas average heart rate increased from 156 to 220 beats per minute. Cross-sectional and longitudinal analysis of peak outflow tract velocity showed similar patterns of change in blood velocity with increasing embryo age: a linear increase in velocity until mid gestation and a decrease thereafter (FIG. 2).

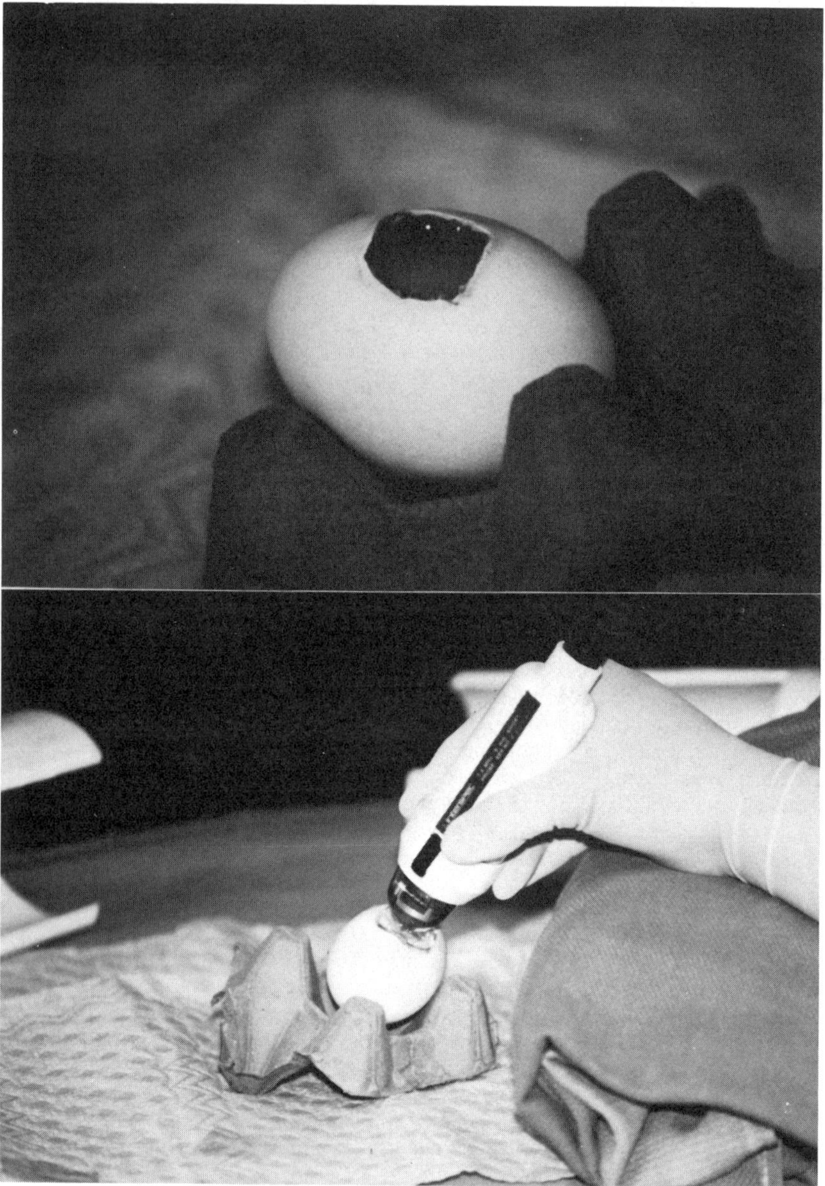

FIGURE 1. Technique of creating a window in the egg shell for Doppler evaluation of the chick embryo heart (upper panel). The window is sealed with a thin plastic, and the ultrasonic transducer is placed over it to obtain images and Doppler of the developing chick heart (lower panel).

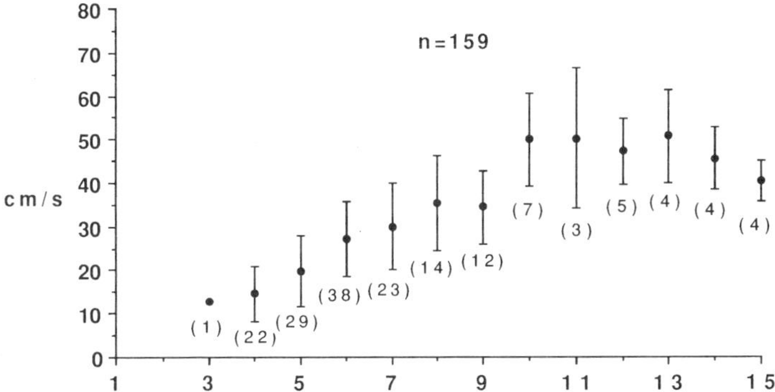

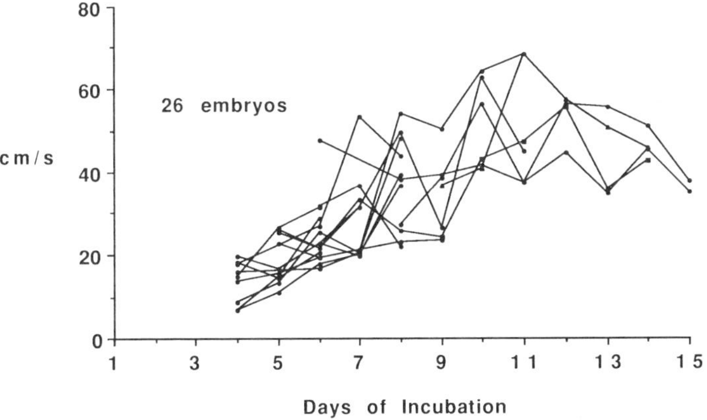

FIGURE 2. Peak ventricular outflow velocities noninvasively determined by image-directed pulsed Doppler. The cross-sectional data showed an increase of the outflow velocity during the first half of gestation (upper panel). The longitudinal outflow velocity data from serial evaluation of 26 embyros showed similar results (lower panel). cm/s = centimeters per second.

We conclude that state-of-the-art ultrasonic Doppler and imaging technology can be used to evaluate the hemodynamics of chick embryo cardiac development noninvasively. Peak outflow velocity increased with increasing age. No valvular regurgitation was detected. This longitudinal measurement technique will allow the evaluation of the functional effects of interventions designed to disturb normal cardiac embryogenesis.

ACKNOWLEDGMENT

We thank the Interspec Corporation for technical support for this study.

REFERENCES

1. DUNNIGAN, A., N. HU, D. W. BENSON & E. B. CLARK. 1987. Effect of heart rate increase on dorsal aortic flow in the stage 24 chick embryo. Pediatr. Res. **22:** 442-444.
2. HARTLEY, C. J. & J. S. COLE. 1974. An ultrasonic pulsed Doppler system for measuring blood flow in small vessels. J. Appl. Physiol. **37:** 626-629.
3. CLARK, E. B. & N. HU. 1982. Developmental hemodynamic changes in the chick embryo from stage 18 to 27. Circ. Res. **51:** 810-815.
4. OPPENHEIM, A. & R. SCHAFFER. 1975. Computation of the discrete Fourier Transform. *In* Digital Signal Processing. 321-326. Prentice Hall. Englewood Cliff, N. J.

All-Trans Retinoic Acid Induced Cardiovascular Malformations

KAZUO IRIE, M. ANDO, AND A. TAKAO

Department of Pediatric Cardiology
The Heart Institute of Japan
Tokyo Women's Medical College
Shinjuku-ku, Tokyo, 162 Japan

The purpose of this study was to determine the effect of *all-trans* retinoic acid (t-RA) on the developing cardiovascular system (CVS)[1-3] in mice. A single dose of 5-100 mg/kg tRA in 0.1 mL DMSO was given to ICR mice intraperitoneally on days 6, 7, 8, or 9 of gestation (plug day = day 0). Controls received 0.1 mL DMSO. Fetuses were removed on day 18 and examined for cardiovascular malformations (CVM) under a dissection microscope.

Controls had very few CVM. Treated mice produced CVM in 36% (day 6), 13% (day 7), 91% (day 8), or 67% (day 9) of the examined fetuses in ICR mice (TABLE 1). Moreover, t-RA induced stage-specific CVM: visceral heterotaxia (day 6); transposition of the great arteries (TGA) and double outlet right ventricle (DORV) (day 8); truncus arteriosus communis (TAC), tetralogy of Fallot (TOF), and interrupted aortic arch (IAA) (type B) with thymic abnormalities (TA) (day 9) (TABLE 2).

In conclusion, t-RA has a teratogenic effect on the developing CVS and produces the stage-related CVM in mice.

TABLE 1. Effects of tRA on the Developing CVS in ICR Mice

GD	Dose mg/kg	No. in litter	No. of implants	Mortality (percent)	No. examined F	CVM (percent)	TA (percent)
6	10	7	98	22(22)	76	17(22)[a]	0
	20	9	115	61(53)	53	19(36)[a]	0
7	5	7	92	19(21)	73	7(10)[a]	0
	10	5	61	37(61)	24	3(13)[a]	0
8	60	16	191	71(37)	123	87(71)[a]	2
	80	9	119	53(45)	70	64(91)[a]	3
9	80	8	103	13(13)	90	17(19)[a]	74
	100	10	130	41(32)	114	76(67)[a]	89

[a] $p < 0.05$, compared to controls with DMSO.

TABLE 2. Distribution of CVM Induced by tRA.

Percent GD	6		7		8		9	
Dose	10	20	5	10	60	80	80	10
Visceral heterotaxia	13	15	1					
TGA	5	9	1		35	64		2
DORV	1	9	1	4	15	19	3	3
TAC					2	4		12
TOF					1		3	4
IAA (B)					2		2	17
Vascular ring							4	4
VSD	3	2	4	0	7	4	6	15
miscellaneous	0	1	3	9	9	0	1	10

REFERENCES

1. SHENEFELT, R. E. 1972. Morphogenesis of malformations in hamsters caused by retinoic acid : Relation to dose and stage of treatment. Teratology 5: 103-118.
2. TAYLOR, I. M., M. J. WILEY & A. AGUR. 1980. Retinoic acid induced heart malformations in the hamster. Teratology 21: 193-197.
3. DAVIS, L. A. & T. W. SADLER. 1981. Effects of vitamin A on endocardial cushion development in the mouse heart. Teratology 24: 139-148.

Neural Crest Ablation Does Not Alter Ventricular Pressure or Estimated Cardiac Output Despite Altered Morphology[a]

WILLIAM F. JACKSON,[b,c] HAROLD E. GAULDIN,[d]
HITOSHI TOMITA,[d] AND LINDA LEATHERBURY[e]

[b]Department of Physiology and Endocrinology
[d]Department of Anatomy
[e]Department of Pediatric Cardiology
Medical College of Georgia
Augusta, Georgia 30912

INTRODUCTION

Cranial neural crest cells are required for normal heart development. Experimental ablation of these cells results in a number of morphological alterations of the heart and outflow tract such as persistent truncus arteriosus and double outlet right ventricle.[1,2] Recently, Stewart *et al.*[3] reported that neural crest ablation depresses systemic blood pressure in stage 18 chick embryos. Loss of premigratory neural crest cells is associated with altered development of the aortic arch arteries at this stage of development. In particular loss of neural crest cells that will migrate through aortic arches 3 and 4 results in hypoplasia or lack of development of arch arteries in that region.[2,4] This loss of vessels could increase the resistance to blood flow offered by the arch arteries and could increase the pressure drop across these vessels. This might explain the low systemic pressure recorded in neural crest-ablated embryos.[3] Alternatively, loss of premigratory neural crest cells could result in depressed cardiac function, and this might explain the results of Stewart *et al.*[3] The purpose of the present study was to test these hypotheses by measurement of ventricular and dorsal aortic pressures and cardiac output in control and neural crest-ablated embryos.

[a]This work was supported by a National Heart, Lung, and Blood Institute Grant, HL 36059.

[c]Present address: Department of Biological Sciences, 5020 McCracken Hall, Western Michigan University, Kalamazoo, MI 49008.

METHODS

Fertilized Arbor Acre chicken eggs were incubated and prepared for microsurgery as reported previously.[1,2] Surgical ablation of premigratory neural crest cells from the mid-otic placode to the caudal portion of somite two was performed at Hamburger-Hamilton[5] stage 9-11 as described previously.[1,2] These operated embryos (experimental) along with unoperated controls were then allowed to develop to Hamburger-Hamilton stage 18. We then used high speed microcinephotography (100 frames/s) to estimate cardiac volumes and the servo-null technique to measure intraventricular and dorsal aortic pressures.

RESULTS

Experimental animals displayed no significant change in heart rate, peak ventricular pressure, or end diastolic pressure compared to controls (FIG. 1). Dorsal aortic pressures measured in some animals were also not significantly different. In control animals systolic and diastolic dorsal aortic pressures were 0.91 ± 0.04 mm Hg and 0.51 ± 0.04 mm Hg (n = 22), respectively. Dorsal aortic pressures in experimental embryos were 0.92 ± 0.05 mm Hg and 0.44 ± 0.03 mm Hg (n = 15) for systolic and diastolic pressures, respectively.

There was significant dilatation of the primitive ventricles in the experimental group: traced ventricular areas at end diastole and end systole were significantly greater in the experimental group (FIG. 2). The change in ventricular cross-sectional area, however, during the cardiac cycle (*i.e.,* end diastolic area–end systolic area), an estimate of stroke volume, was unchanged (FIG. 2). In agreement with the area data presented in FIGURE 2, calculated cardiac outputs were similar in control (28.1 ± 3.1 μL/min, N = 14) and experimental (32 ± 3.4 μL/min, N = 12) groups.

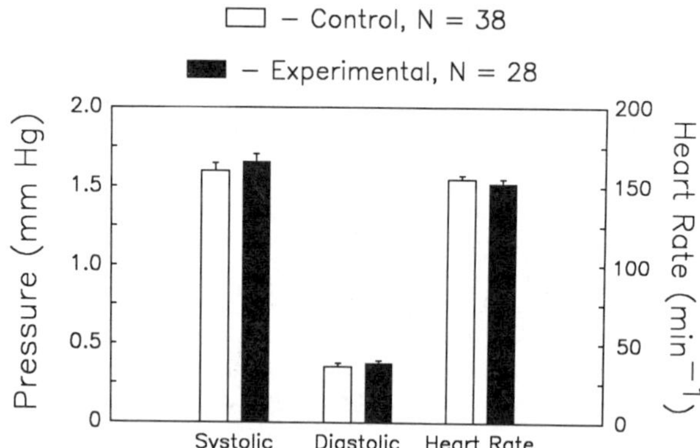

FIGURE 1. Lack of effect of neural crest ablation on ventricular pressures and heart rates. Data are means ± SE with the number of embryos given. Pressures were measured using the servo-null method at stage 18 after neural crest ablation at stage 9-11 (experimental) or in control embryos at the same stage. See text for more information.

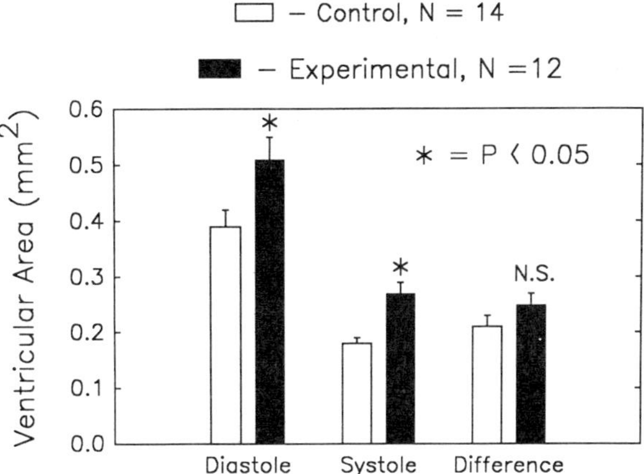

FIGURE 2. Effect of neural crest ablation on ventricular cross-sectional area. Data are mean areas ± SE with the number of embryos shown. End systolic and end diastolic ventricular areas were determined by frame by frame analysis of cinephotographic images using a digitizing tablet. * = significant difference by analysis of variance and subsequent comparison of mean values; $p < 0.05$.

DISCUSSION

Thus, although dilated, the primitive ventricle in experimental animals produced normal pressures and cardiac output. Equal pressures and flows suggest that the blood flow resistance offered by the aortic arch arteries was similar in the two groups, in spite of known depression or lack of blood flow in arch artery 4 in the experimental group (Leatherbury and Gauldin, unpublished observations). These data suggest that the embryonic cardiovascular system has considerable ability to compensate for and adapt to altered structure to maintain function within the normal range.

In the present study we found no significant effect of cardiac neural crest ablation on dorsal aortic pressure. This is in contrast to the observations of Stewart *et al.*[3] who found significant depression of vitelline artery pressure in neural crest-ablated embryos. Unless ablation of cardiac neural crest alters vitelline artery pressure independent of dorsal aortic pressure, these data are difficult to reconcile. It should be noted, however, that the neural crest lesion used by Stewart *et al.*[3] was more extensive than that used in the present study. Also heart rates in the earlier study were very low (80-90 bpm) compared to 150-160 bpm in the present study.

The cause of the ventricular dilation is also not clear. Calculated wall stress was elevated in the experimental group[6] despite normal pressures and estimated outflow resistance. This could mean that the compliance of the primitive ventricle is somehow altered by neural crest ablation such that at similar pressures, the ventricles in experimental embryos are distended more than the control ventricles.

REFERENCES

1. KIRBY, M. L., T. F. GALE & D. E. STEWART. 1983. Neural crest cells contribute to normal aorticopulmonary septation. Science **220:** 1059-1061.

2. NISHIBATAKE, M., M. L. KIRBY & L. H. S. VAN MIEROP. 1987. Pathogenesis of persistent truncus arteriosus and dextroposed aorta in the chick embryo after neural crest ablation. Circulation 75(1): 255-264.
3. STEWART, D. E., M. L. KIRBY & K. K. SULIK. 1986. Hemodynamic changes in chick embryos precede heart defects after cardiac neural crest ablation. Circ. Res. 59(5): 545-550.
4. BOCKMAN, D. E., M. E. REDMOND, K. WALDO, H. DAVIS & M. L. KIRBY. 1987. Effect of neural crest ablation on the development of the heart and arch arteries in the chick. Am. J. Anat. 180: 332-341.
5. HAMBURGER, V & H. L. HAMILTON. 1951. A series of normal stages in the development of the chick embryo. J. Morphol. 88: 49-92.
6. LEATHERBURY, L., D. S. BRADEN, H. TOMITA, H. E. GAULDIN & W. F. JACKSON. 1990. Hemodynamic changes-wall stresses and pressure gradients in neural crest-ablated chick embryos. N. Y. Acad. Sci. This volume.

Troponin T Isoform Switching during Heart Development

J.-P. JIN, J. L.-C. LIN, AND J. J.-C. LIN

Department of Biology
University of Iowa
Iowa City, Iowa 52242

Myocardial development proceeds by a sequential and/or overlapping expression of many myofibrillar protein isoforms.[1,2] The regulation of isoform switching and the functional differences of isoforms are not completely understood. With specific antibodies, we[3] and others[4] have detected an isoform switching of troponin T (TnT) during rat heart development. Using DNA cloning, Cooper and Ordahl[5] have shown that a single cardiac TnT gene in chicken can generate two mRNAs by way of developmentally regulated alternative splicing. Although the proteins are not demonstrated yet, these two mRNAs are expectedly translated into two isoforms of chicken cardiac TnT. In this study, we have compared expression patterns of TnT isoforms in both rat and chicken hearts during development. Through the isolation and characterization of cDNA clones, we have found that the two isoforms of rat cardiac TnT are also derived from a single gene.

Rat cardiac TnT isoform switching appears to begin between 3 days and 5 days after birth (lane 4 and 5 in FIG. 1B) and reaches completion in the rats at about two weeks of age (lane 7 in FIG. 1B). On the contrary, a significant amount of the adult isoform of TnT is already observed in chicken hearts of 10-day-old embryos (lane 2 in FIG. 1D). In fact, the TnT isoform switching in chicken hearts starts as early as the 5-day-old embryo and completes switching within the first week posthatch (data not shown). These results may suggest that chicken embryonic heart is developmentally more advanced in its differentiation than rat fetal heart. In addition, this difference in time course of switching may reflect a difference in the environments that surround rat fetus or chicken embryo. In rat, a fluctuation in maternal health will have some effects on the performance of fetal hearts, whereas there is no such effect in chicken embryo. Thus, if the embryonic isoform of cardiac TnT can confer different Ca^{2+} sensitivity for thin filaments or provide more resistance to various inotropic stimuli and acidosis, a delay onset of isoform switching until postpartum in rat would be advantageous for the survival of fetus during perinatal period. In this context, Solaro *et al.* have demonstrated that the isoform switching of TnT and possibly troponin I in the myofilaments may be related to the observed functional difference between fetal and adult hearts of dogs[6] and rats.[7]

To determine the structural difference between the embryonic and adult isoforms of rat cardiac TnT, several cDNA clones have been obtained from an expression library constructed from young rat heart poly(A)$^+$ RNAs. DNA sequencing reveals that there are two classes of TnT cDNA clones existing in the library with difference in the presence or absence of a 30 base pair fragment in the coding sequence. This region would translate into a highly acidic decapeptide at residues 18-27 of the

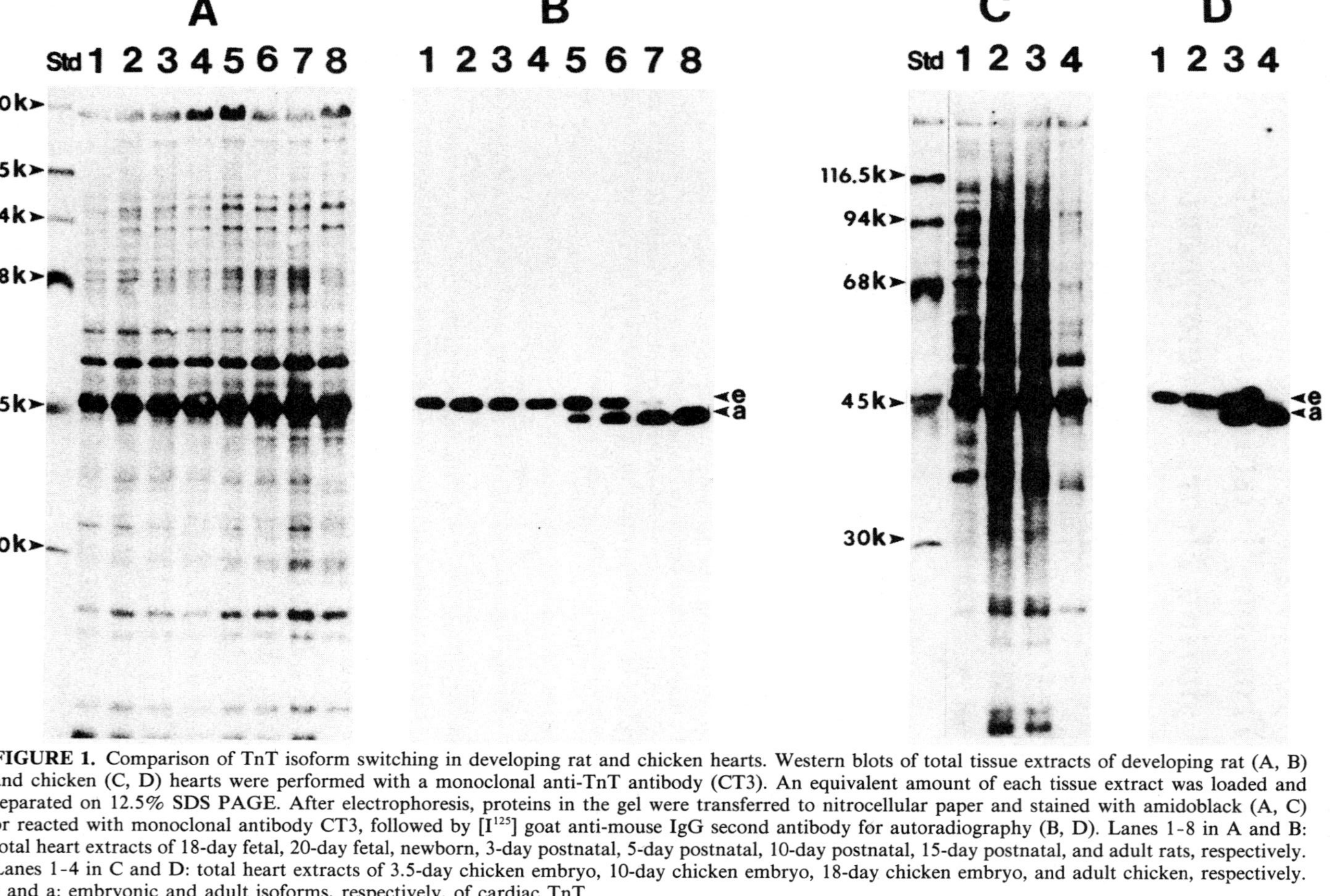

FIGURE 1. Comparison of TnT isoform switching in developing rat and chicken hearts. Western blots of total tissue extracts of developing rat (A, B) and chicken (C, D) hearts were performed with a monoclonal anti-TnT antibody (CT3). An equivalent amount of each tissue extract was loaded and separated on 12.5% SDS PAGE. After electrophoresis, proteins in the gel were transferred to nitrocellular paper and stained with amidoblack (A, C) or reacted with monoclonal antibody CT3, followed by [I^{125}] goat anti-mouse IgG second antibody for autoradiography (B, D). Lanes 1-8 in A and B: total heart extracts of 18-day fetal, 20-day fetal, newborn, 3-day postnatal, 5-day postnatal, 10-day postnatal, 15-day postnatal, and adult rats, respectively. Lanes 1-4 in C and D: total heart extracts of 3.5-day chicken embryo, 10-day chicken embryo, 18-day chicken embryo, and adult chicken, respectively. e and a: embryonic and adult isoforms, respectively, of cardiac TnT.

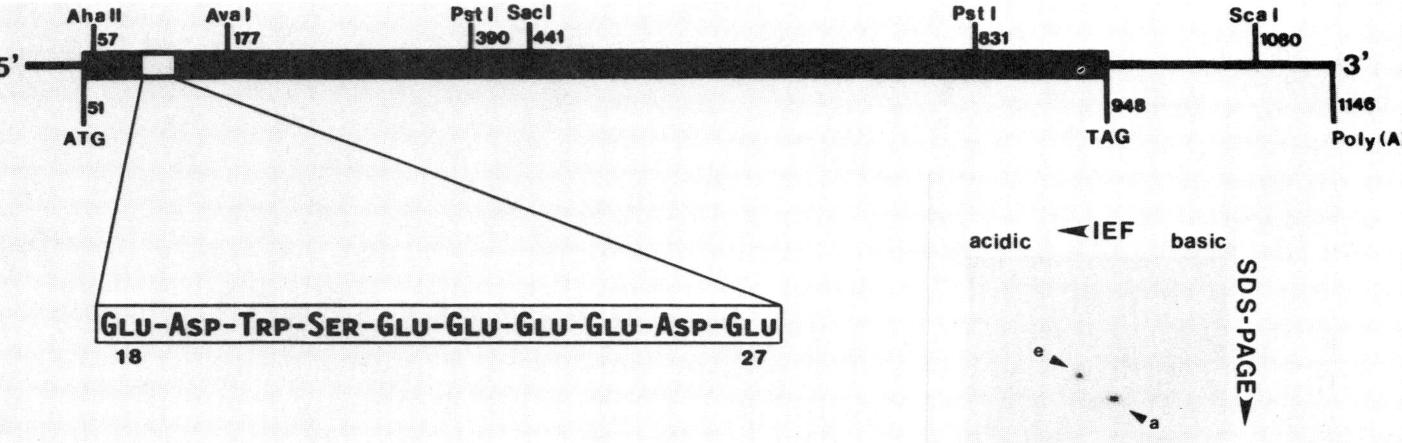

FIGURE 2. Sequence difference between the embryonic and adult isoforms of rat cardiac TnT. A composite restriction enzyme map of the cDNA, representing rat cardiac TnT mRNA, was derived from sequencing data of three independent cDNA clones and from S1 nuclease protection analysis of mRNAs. The numbers at each restriction site, ATG, TAG, and poly (A) site indicate the residue numbers in the nucleotide sequence. The wide bar region represents the coding region. The open box within the coding region is the sequence found only in the embryonic isoform cDNA and corresponds to residue 18 to 27 in the embryonic TnT protein, which contains a highly acidic decapeptide. The two-dimensional gel protein profile at the lower right shows the differences in both molecular mass and isoelectric point between the embryonic and adult isoforms of rat cardiac TnT. IEF, isoelectric focusing; SDS PAGE, SDS polyacrylamide gel electrophoresis; e, embryonic isoform; a, adult isoform. The sample for the 2D gel was the immunoprecipitate of *in vitro* translation products of poly(A)$^+$ RNA from young rat hearts by anti-TnT antibody.

embryonic isoform of rat cardiac TnT (FIG. 2). S1 nuclease mRNA mapping has further confirmed this conclusion.[8] The properties of the predicted TnT proteins are consistent with our 2D gel data that the embryonic rat cardiac TnT isoform is larger and more acidic than the adult isoform (FIG. 2). These results suggest that developmentally regulated alternative RNA splicing generates two isoforms of rat cardiac TnT from the same gene product.

REFERENCES

1. CAPLAN, A. I., M. Y. FISZMAN & H. M. EPPENBERGER. 1983. Science **221:** 921-927.
2. SWYNGHEDAUW, B. 1986. Physiol. Rev. **66:** 710-771.
3. JIN, J.-P. & J. J.-C. LIN. 1988. J. Biol. Chem. **263:** 7309-7315.
4. SAGGIN, L., S. AUSON, L. GORZA, S. SARTORE & S. SCHIAFFINO. 1988. J. Biol. Chem. **263:** 18488-18492.
5. COOPER, T. & C. ORDAHL. 1985. J. Biol. Chem. **260:** 11140-11148.
6. SOLARO, R. J., P. KUMAR, E. M. BLANCHARD & A. F. MARTIN. 1986. Circ. Res. **58:** 721-729.
7. SOLARO, R. J., J. A. LEE, J. C. KENTISH & D. G. ALLEN. 1988. Circ. Res. **63:** 779-787.
8. JIN, J.-P. & J. J.-C. LIN. 1989. J. Biol. Chem **264:** 14471-14477.

Optical Indications of Spontaneous Electrical Activity and Functional Organization of Pacemaking Area in the Early Embryonic Chick Heart

KOHTARO KAMINO, HITOSHI KOMURO,
TETSURO SAKAI, AND AKIHIKO HIROTA

Department of Physiology
Tokyo Medical and Dental University
School of Medicine
Bunkyo-ku, Tokyo 113, Japan

In the early phases of cardiogenesis of the chick embryo, paired cardiac primordia are brought together at the midline and begin to fuse with each other at the 7-somite stage of development. This process results in the formation of the primitive tubular heart, which begins beating spontaneously at the middle period of the 9-somite stage in the embryo. In these early stages, however, because the myocardial cells are extremely small and fragile, it is technically difficult or impossible to impale them with microelectrodes. This problem has seriously hampered conventional electrophysiological studies on the very early embryonic heart.

Using a 10 × 10- or 12 × 12-element photodiode array and a voltage-sensitive merocyanine-rhodanine dye, we have monitored spontaneous electrical activity (FIG. 1), and, with a combination of multiple-site optical recording and graphic methods, we have assessed quantitatively the pacemaking area in the early embryonic precontractile chick heart (FIG. 2). Thus we were able to monitor spontaneous action potentials optically, for the first time, in the prefused chick cardiac primordium at the 6-somite stage of development.[1] The action-potential-related optical signals detected from the cardiac primordium were extremely small in size and were concentrated in a small well-defined area. These results show that spontaneous electrical activity is generated first in the prefused cardiac primordium. As development proceeds to the 9-somite stage, both the size of the action potential-related optical signal and the extent of the electrically active area increase dramatically, and the pacemaker site can be identified. The pacemaking area is basically circular in shape with a size estimated to be about 1200-3000 μm^2.[2] In the 7- to early 8-somite embryonic hearts, the location of the pacemaking area is not uniquely determined, and as development proceeds to the 9-somite stage, the pacemaking area becomes confined to the left preatrial tissue. These observations suggest that the pacemaking area is composed of about 60-150 cells in the early embryonic precontractile chick heart, and that a population of pacemaking cells, rather than a single cell, serves as its rhythm generator.

In addition, the regional gradient of pacemaker activity in the early embryonic precontractile chick heart was determined quantitatively.[3] The absorption changes

397

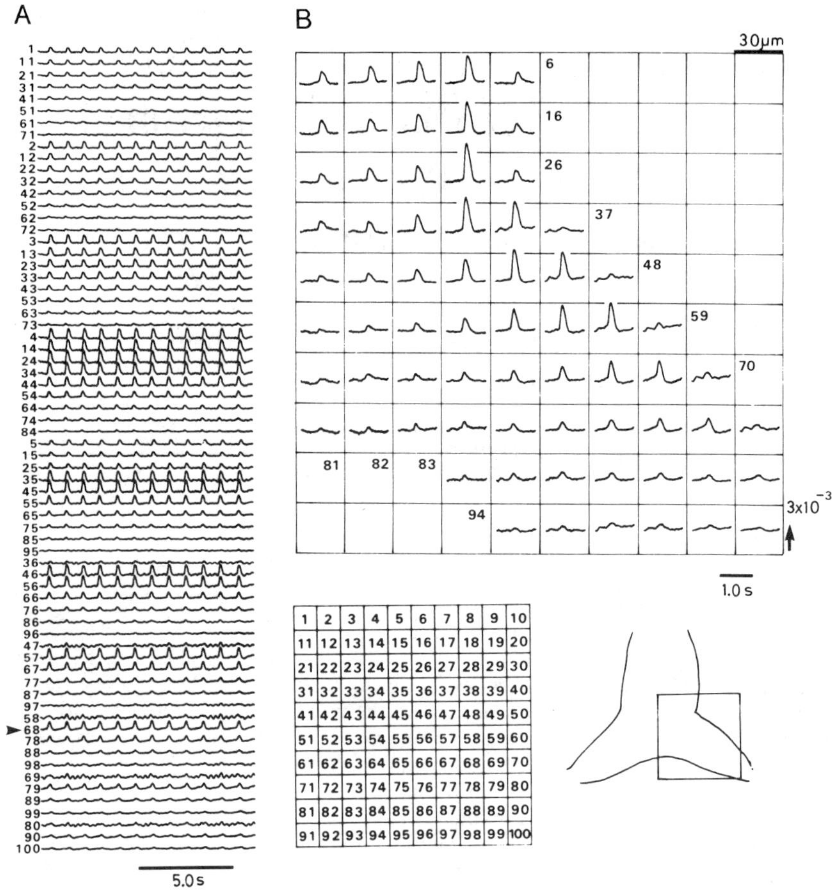

FIGURE 1. Two examples of simultaneous optical recordings of spontaneous action potentials from sixty-eight contiguous loci of a 9-somite embryonic precontractile chick heart.[3] The 10 × 10-element photodiode array was positioned over a 50x magnified image of the left preatrial tissue of the heart and a part of the left ventricle. The preparation was stained with a voltage-sensitive merocyanine-rhodanine dye (NK2761). The measurements were made with a 702 ± 13 nm interference filter at 36.8-37.1° C in a single sweep. The traces are displayed in parallel in A, and the signals are displayed according to the arrangement of the photodiode in B. The relative location of the photodiode array on the image of the heart is illustrated on the lower right. In A, numerals to the left of the optical traces indicate numbers of the elements of the photodiode array, corresponding to the illustration on the bottom. In B, the direction of the arrow to the right of the recording indicates a decrease in transmission (increase in absorption), and the length of the arrow represents the stated value of the change in intensity divided by the DC background intensity (=fractional change). In recording A, small delays in firing time were observed in traces of the nearly synchronized optical signals. These delays correspond to the conduction time, and the earliest action signal appeared in the trace indicated by the arrowhead. In recording B, it was evident that the action potential signal was first detected at position 68 on the left preatrial tissue. This position was considered as the pacemaker site in this heart, and the excitation spread over the heart from this site.

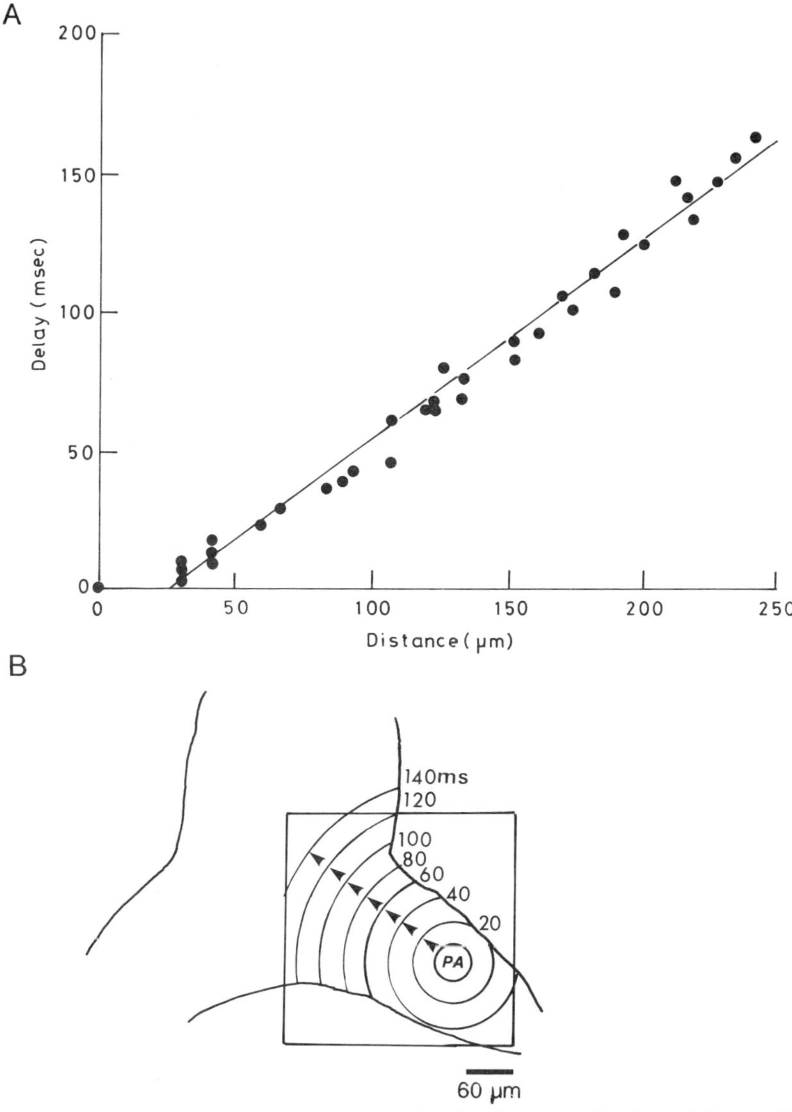

FIGURE 2. The delay in the foot of the optical action signal as a function of distance from the center of the pacemaker area (A). Data were obtained from the recording shown in FIGURE 1.[3] The center of position 68 is regarded as the zero-point reference for the delay and the distance. The delay and distance were related by a single straight line. Thus, using this graph, we assessed the shape and size of the pacemaking area. An extrapolated value of this line on the distance axis (X-axis) was about 26 μm. From this graphic representation, we concluded that the shape of the pacemaking area was circular with a radius of about 26 μm, and that the excitation that appeared in this circular pacemaking area (PA) was spread radially, at a uniform rate, over the heart. From the reciprocal of the slope of this line, the conduction velocity was calculated to be about 1.4 mm/s. In B the location, shape, and relative size of the pacemaking area and the conduction pattern are illustrated; one contour interval represents the conduction distance per 20 ms, and the pacemaking area was estimated to be about 2122 μm^2.

related to the slow diastolic depolarization were detected, and they were concentrated in and near the pacemaker. The region, in which these absorption changes related to slow diastolic depolarization were detected, increased in size as development proceeded. The slope of the absorption change related to diastolic depolarization was measured as an indicator of the pacemaker activity. The slope was largest in the pacemaking area and gradually decreased towards the periphery. The maximum slope of the optical change, related to the slow diastolic depolarization, also increased as development proceeded and was related to early development of the heart rate. Thus, these results suggest that formation of a regional gradient of pacemaker activity gives rise to the functional architecture of the pacemaking area during the early phases of cardiogenesis.

REFERENCES

1. HIROTA, A., K. KAMINO, H. KOMURO & T. SAKAI. 1987. Mapping of early development of electrical activity in the embryonic chick heart using multiple-site optical recording. J. Physiol. (London) **383:** 711–728.
2. KAMINO, K., H. KOMURO, T. SAKAI & A. HIROTA. 1988. Functional pacemaking area in the early embryonic chick heart assessed by simultaneous multiple-site optical recording of spontaneous action potentials. J. Gen. Physiol. **91:** 573–591.
3. KAMINO, K., H. KOMURO & T. SAKAI. 1988. Regional gradient of pacemaker activity in the early embryonic chick heart monitored by multisite optical recording. J. Physiol. (London) **402:** 301–314.

Characterization of Ca-Deficient Hypertension in Chick Embryos

Adrenergic Regulation of Cardiovascular Function and Cellular Ca Handling[a]

MASAFUMI KOIDE AND ROCKY S. TUAN

Department of Biology
University of Pennsylvania
and
Departments of Orthopaedic Surgery
and Biochemistry and Molecular Biology
Thomas Jefferson University
Philadelphia, Pennsylvania 19107

The developing chick embryo derives the majority of its required Ca from the eggshell.[1] Chick embryos rendered Ca-deficient by long-term culture outside the eggshell develop hypertension and tachycardia, conditions that are ameliorated with Ca repletion.[2] To characterize the hypertension of cultured shell-less (SL) chick embryos, we have compared their cardiovascular response to adrenergic drugs with normal (NL) embryos at day 14 of incubation. Blood pressure and pulse rate of the embryos were measured[2] before and after administration of noradrenaline (NA), phentolamine (PA), isoproterenol (IP), and propranolol (PP) directly applied onto the chorioallantoic membrane. In addition, the cellular basis of adrenergic regulation was examined using erythrocytes (RBC) from these embryos by analyzing adrenergic drug effects on ^{45}Ca uptake[3] by RBC treated with *p*-chloromercuriphenyl sulfonate (PCM), inasmuch avian RBC have a catecholamine-sensitive adenylate cyclase.[4]

Baseline blood pressures (systolic/diastolic) and pulse rate were uniformly higher in SL (23.2 ± 0.6/13.4 ± 0.4 mm Hg and 195 ± 2/min) than in NL (20.3 ± 0.4/11.9 ± 0.3 and 170 ± 4) embryos. In both embryos, blood pressure was elevated by NA and PP, but lowered by IP and PA; pulse rates were decreased by PP and PA, and increased by NA and IP. Pharmacological sensitivity to NA and PA, based on their effective dosages and magnitude of response in blood pressure and pulse rate, was higher in SL embryos (FIG. 1). On the other hand, the embryos did not differ significantly in their sensitivity to IP and PP. The plasma concentration of catecholamines was considerably higher in SL embryos (TABLE 1). Although serum Ca was lower in SL embryos, myocardial Ca content was not significantly different, and plasma volume was not expanded in SL embryos (TABLE 1). These data suggest that the

[a] This work was supported in part by Grants from the NIH (HD15306 and HD21355), March of Dimes (1-1146), and USDA (88-37200-3746). M.Koide is an International Rotary Scholar.

hypertension of SL embryos is primarily due to Ca deficiency, but not to Na retention, and that the cardiovascular function of SL embryos is under more sensitive and potentiated α-adrenergic regulation, perhaps a result of different cellular Ca handling.

At a cellular level, in the absence of adrenergic modifiers, ^{45}Ca uptake by PCM-treated RBC was similar in the two embryos with respect to rate and total accumulation (rate: SL, 8.9 $\pm$ 0.9, NL, 10.8 $\pm$ 2.0 pmol/min/μL cell vol.; total accumulation: SL, 2.4 $\pm$ 0.3, NL, 2.5 $\pm$ 0.5 nmol/μL cell vol.) Both parameters were increased by PA (SL, 50.0 $\pm$ 2.9 and 5.7 $\pm$ 0.2; NL, 94.6 $\pm$ 8.2 and 6.8 $\pm$ 0.2, respectively) and PP (SL, 78.2 $\pm$ 7.5 and 3.6 $\pm$ 0.1; NL, 123.6 $\pm$ 5.7 and 5.3 $\pm$ 0.3, respectively), the effects being greater in NL embryos. On the contrary, NA and IP treatment did not increase RBC Ca uptake. Because PCM acts extracellularly and affects primarily Ca influx, but not the plasma membrane Ca-ATPase, these results suggest that the observed effects of adrenergic blockers are due to their actions on Ca-ATPase-mediated Ca extrusion. Therefore, the relatively lower net Ca uptake by blocker-treated RBC of SL embryos may reflect a higher Ca pumping activity. Taken together with the data from *in vivo* experiments, this feature of cellular Ca handling in SL embryos may be functionally related to their intrinsically higher α-adrenergic sensitivity. For example, upon PA treatment, the SL embryo would exhibit more sensitive vascular dilatation as mediated by lower cellular Ca.

In conclusion, these properties of the SL chick embryo indicate that it is a novel and useful experimental system to study the relationship between Ca homeostasis, development of hypertension, and adrenergic regulation of cardiovascular/cellular functions.

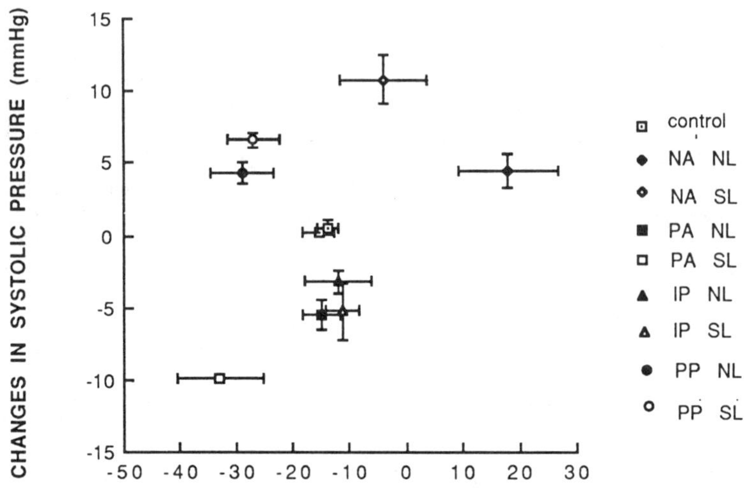

FIGURE 1. Schematic summary of the effects of adrenergic drugs on systolic pressure and pulse rate of NL and SL chick embryos. Values represent changes (mean $\pm$ SE) in systolic blood pressure and pulse rate at 6 min after the administration of each adrenergic drug. Dosages indicated here are 10 μg for NA, 1000 μg for PA, 300 μg for IP, and 30 μg for PP. The highest dosage of IP used was chosen, because typical β-1 action was barely observable at the lower dosages.

TABLE 1. Analysis of Electrolytes, Catecholamines, and Plasma Volume in NL and SL Chick Embryos[a]

Embryos	Serum calcium (mg/dL)	Myocardial calcium (μg/100 mg)	Serum sodium (mEq/L)	Plasma volume (mL)	Plasma catecholamines		
					Dopamine (ng/mL)	Noradrenaline (ng/mL)	Adrenaline (ng/mL)
NL	9.2 ± 0.2	4.1 ± 0.2	118.0 ± 0.5	1.17 ± 0.06	5.94	0.62	0.42
SL	5.6 ± 0.2[b]	4.6 ± 0.2	126.0 ± 0.6[b]	0.85 ± 0.05[b]	11.04	17.36	1.44

[a] Values are mean ± SE. Serum and heart data were derived from 40 NL and 54 SL embryos. Plasma volumes were from 7 NL and 6 SL embryos. Plasma samples from more than 10 embryos were combined for the measurement of catecholamines.

[b] Statistical significance (SL vs NL; $p < 0.01$) was evaluated by the Student t test.

REFERENCES

1. TUAN, R. J. 1987. Exp. Zool. Suppl. **1:** 1-13.
2. TUAN, R. & H. NGUYEN. 1987. J. Exp. Med. **165:** 1418-1423.
3. TUAN, R., M. CARSON, J. JOZEFIAK, K. KNOWLES & B. SHOTWELL. 1986. J. Cell Sci. **82:** 73-84.
4. KREGENOW, F. 1977. *In* Membrane Transport in Red Cells. J. Ellory & V. Lew, Eds.: 383-426. Academic Press. New York.

Fine Structural Features of Coronary Vasculogenesis in Collagen Lattices

J. KEVIN LANGFORD, DON A. HAY,[a] AND
DAVID L. BOLENDER [b]

Department of Biology
Stephen F. Austin State University
Nacogdoches, Texas 75962
and
[b]*Department of Anatomy and Cellular Biology*
Medical College of Wisconsin
Milwaukee, Wisconsin

INTRODUCTION

The morphogenetic events leading to the formation of coronary circulation have been previously described,[1] but the developmental mechanisms involved are still poorly understood. We have proposed that coronary vasculogenesis results from interactions between primary precursor tissues that include the myocardium, dorsal mesocardium, and the epicardium.[2] In order to analyze the mechanisms involved in these putative tissue interactions, a tissue culture model was established (cf Bolender *et al.,* this volume). We report here further characterization of the culture model at the ultrastructural level.

METHODS

Whole chick hearts between stages 15-22 HH were explanted onto collagen gels, grown for four days, at which time the explant was removed. Additional cultures were established by explanting the villus-like processes from the dorsal mesocardium (DM; FIG. 1) that have been shown to contain vascular precursors.[2] After seven days in culture, collagen gels were thoroughly rinsed with buffer and fixed in 2% glutaraldehyde. Following postfixation in osmium, tissues were embedded in Spurr-Lecithin, sectioned, and examined.

---

[a] Corresponding author.

RESULTS AND DISCUSSION

Examination of the cultures originating from stage 17-22 embryos revealed a multilayered outgrowth on the surface of the collagen lattice and mesenchymal cells dispersed within the gel. After a week in culture, vascular-like structures were observed either extending from the surface deep into the gel (FIG. 2) or coursing beneath yet parallel to the surface before penetrating the gel. These vessel-like structures had what appeared to be a continuous lining of endothelial cells surrounded externally by flattened cells resembling pericytes. When atria, ventricles, or DM of stage 15 embryos were cultured separately for seven days, DM explants produced extensive vascular plexuses. No vessels developed from stage 15 atrial or ventricular cultures.

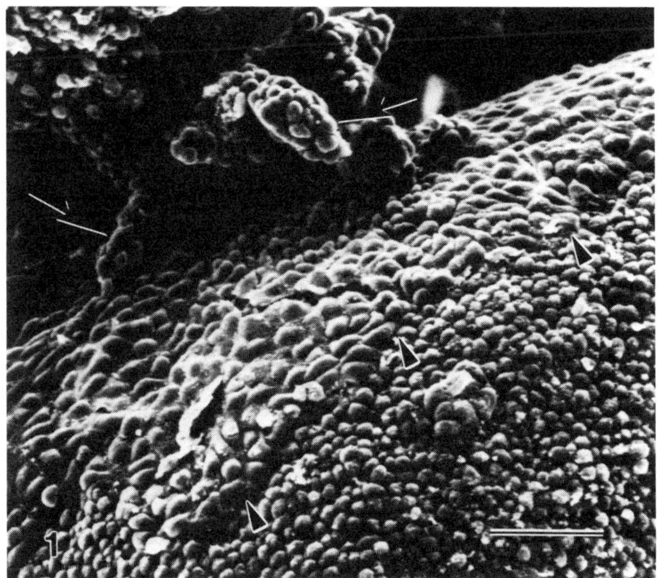

FIGURE 1. The dorsal surface of a three-day (HH stage 18) embryonic chick heart exhibits a cluster of villus-like projections (arrows) that constitute the dorsal mesocardium at the atrio-ventricular junction. A layer of epicardium extends from the villi over the myocardial surface. Arrowheads denote leading edge of epicardium. Bar = 40 μm.

Cellular debris filled the lumina of smaller vessels, whereas in larger vessels debris was absent. The consistent appearance of such debris in the smallest vessels suggests that programmed autolysis may be responsible for vascular patency. Phagolysosomes were found within endothelial cells and undifferentiated pericytes. Cells resembling thrombocytes (FIG. 5) that were restricted to the lumina also contained phagolyso-somes. This suggests that the process of debris removal is accomplished by phagocytosis. Vessels were lined with highly attenuated cells possessing multivesicular bodies and fenestrae (FIG. 4) and were connected by adhering junctions (FIG. 3). Pinocytotic vesicles were absent.

Explants of the dorsal mesocardium contained endodermal derivatives as well as differentiated myocardial cells. Some of the vascular-like structures in these cultures contained polymorphonuclear leukocytes (FIG. 6) and thrombocytes. In the embryo, portions of some vessels retain hemopoietic potential, a fact that could explain the presence of these cells within the cultures. Moreover, the interaction of mesoderm and endoderm is considered to be necessary for the initiation of vasculogenesis and hemopoiesis.[3]

In summary, the vessels that developed within our culture system appear similar to those associated with the heart *in vivo*. These observations suggest that explanting coronary vessel precursor tissues onto collagen gels might provide a useful model with which to identify the mechanisms responsible for coronary vasculogenesis.

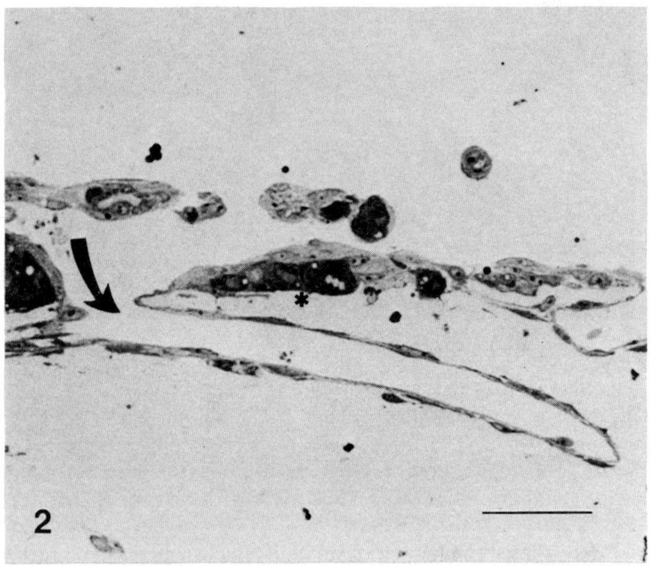

FIGURE 2. A light micrograph of a seven-day DM explant illustrating the origin (curved arrow) and course of a vessel that extends deep within the lattice. Large dark cells (*) surrounding the vessel opening resemble differentiating endodermal cells (hepatocytes ?). Bar = 10.7 μm.

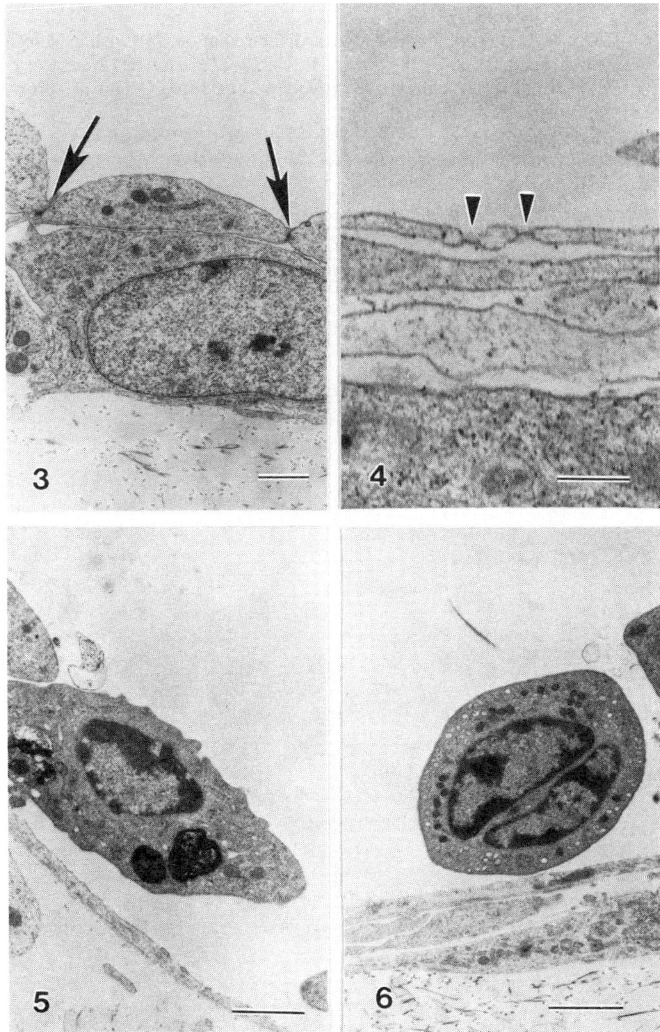

FIGURE 3-6. Characteristic features of all vessels derived from explants. Adjacent endothelial cells (FIG. 3) are attached by adhering junctions (arrows). Bar = 1.0μm. Attenuated endothelial cells (FIG. 4) exhibit fenestrae (arrowheads). Bar = 0.25μm. Elliptical cells (FIG. 5) resembling avian thrombocytes and containing secondary lysosomes populate the vessels. Bar = 1.0μm. Bilobed cells (FIG. 6) are similar to polymorphonuclear leukocytes and inhabit vessel lumina. Bar = 1.9 μm.

REFERENCES

1. TOKUYASU, K. T. 1985. Development of myocardial circulation. *In* Cardiac Morphogenesis. V. Ferrans, G. Rosenquist & C. Weinstein, Eds. 226-237. Elsevier. New York.
2. OLSON, M. D., D. L. BOLENDER & R. R. MARKWALD. 1989. Origin of coronary vessel precursor. Anat. Rec. **223:** 85-86.
3. PARDANAUD, L., F. YASSINE & F. DIETERLEN-LIEVRE. 1989. Relationship between vasculogenesis, angiogenesis and haemopoiesis during avian ontogeny. Development **105:** 473-485.

Induction of Myofibrillogenesis in Cardiac Mutant Axolotls by RNA from Normal Embryonic Endoderm[a]

LARRY F. LEMANSKI, LYNN A. DAVIS,[b]
PEI SHEN SHEN, SHERRIE M. LA FRANCE, AND
MARGARET E. FRANSEN

*Department of Anatomy and Cell Biology
State University of New York
Health Science Center
Syracuse, New York 13210*

[b]*Department of Anatomy and Cell Biology
University of Virginia School of Medicine
Charlottesville, Virginia 22908*

Recessive mutant gene *c*, for "cardiac nonfunction" in the axolotl results in an absence of heart function.[1] Skeletal muscle does not appear to be defective. Morphological studies comparing normal and mutant heart development from stage 34 (heart beat stage) through 41 (when mutant embryos die) have been reported.[2] Electron microscopy reveals that normal ventricular heart myocytes contain organized sarcomeric myofibrils at stage 34-35. By stage 41, the normal ventricular myocardium shows trabeculae formation and contains well-differentiated muscle cells. The mutant myocardium does not trabeculate and remains a single cell layer in thickness. Mutant heart ventricular cells contain a few scattered thin (6 nm) and thick (15 nm) filaments and occasional Z bodies. Some mutant cells show a partial organization of myofilaments; however, distinct sarcomeric myofibrils are not observed. Mutant cells, instead, show amorphous proteinaceous collections in their peripheral cytoplasm where myofibrils initially organize in normal cells.

Humphrey[1] performed heart transplant experiments and showed that mutant hearts transplanted into the heart regions of normal embryos began to beat. In reciprocal transplants, normal into mutant, the normal organs failed to beat. These experiments suggested that gene *c* might exert its effect by way of abnormal induction or inhibitory processes in the heart region of mutant embryos. It is well-established that anterior endoderm in amphibians is an important heart inductor tissue.[3–5] Inasmuch as Humphrey's[1] transplantation experiments were suggestive of abnormal inductive processes in cardiac mutant embryos, we performed experiments to determine whether the cardiac defect could be corrected by culturing mutant (c/c) hearts with normal (+/+) anterior endoderm or by medium conditioned by the preculture of normal

[a]Supported by NIH Grants HL-32184 and HL-37702 and a Grant-in-Aid from the American Heart Association to L.F.L.

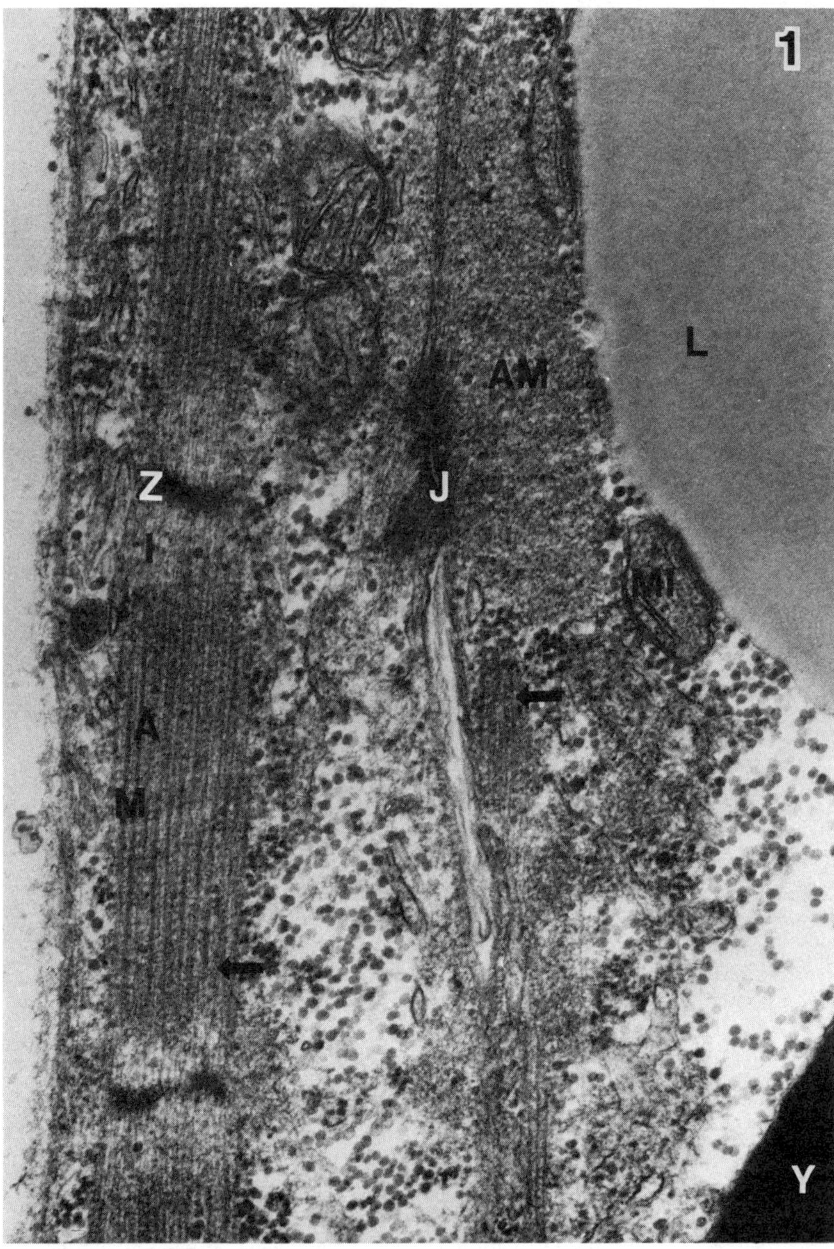

FIGURE 1. Transmission electron micrograph of a mutant axolotl heart explanted at stage 35 and cultured for several days in Holtfreter's salt solution in the presence of anterior endoderm explanted from a normal stage 28 embryo. The amount of amorphous proteinaceous accumulations (AM) so characteristic of the mutant myocardium is reduced as a result of this treatment. Instead, myofibrils appear (arrows) with a normal array of sarcomeric components (I-band, Z-line, A-band, M-line). Mitochondria (MI), cell junction (J), yolk platelet (Y), and lipid droplet (L).

endoderm. Mutant (c/c) hearts cultured with normal ($+/+$) endoderm or endoderm-conditioned media contracted throughout their lengths by 24 hours in culture. After 48 hours in culture, the ventricular portions of the "rescued" mutant hearts were examined by electron microscopy and were found to contain well-organized sarcomeric myofibrils of normal morphology (FIG. 1). By contrast, no organized sarcomeres could be found in the mutant hearts cultured with a variety of nonanterior endoderm tissue. These experiments suggest that a diffusible substance from normal ($+/+$) anterior endoderm corrects the heart defect in cardiac lethal embryos and in essence transforms genotypic mutant hearts into phenotypic normals.

In an attempt to define the diffusible factor in the conditioned medium, enzyme inactivation studies using insoluble enzymes were performed. Only RNAase (not trypsin or neuraminidase) eliminated the ability of the endoderm-conditioned medium to rescue mutant hearts.[6] When total RNA was extracted from stage 29 normal anterior endoderm and cultured with mutant hearts at stage 34-35, again the mutant hearts contracted vigorously and formed myofibrils of normal morphology.[6] Hearts cultured with liver or brain RNAs did not beat or form myofibrils. Thus, RNA from normal anterior endoderm appears to induce myofibrillogenesis in cardiac mutant hearts. Molecular studies are currently in progress to further understand the actions of gene c and its relationship to the heart induction phenomenon.

REFERENCES

1. HUMPHREY, R. R. 1972. Dev. Biol. **27:** 365-375.
2. LEMANSKI, L. F. 1973. Dev. Biol. **33:** 312-333.
3. JACOBSON, A. G. & T. T. DUNCAN. 1968. J. Exp. Zool. **167:** 79-103.
4. FULLILOVE, S. L., 1970. J. Exp. Zool. **75:** 323-326.
5. JACOBSON, A. G. & A. K. SATER. 1988. Development **104:** 341-359.
6. DAVIS, L. A. & L. F. LEMANSKI. 1987. Development **99:** 145-154.

Abnormalities in Myofibril Organization and Cell Shape in Developing Cardiomyopathic Hamster Heart Cells in Culture[a]

JIAN LI, DOUGLAS R. ROBERTSON, AND
LARRY F. LEMANSKI[b]

Department of Anatomy and Cell Biology
State University of New York
Health Science Center at Syracuse
Syracuse, New York 13210

The cardiomyopathic (CM) hamster whose heredity is purportedly transmitted by an autosomal recessive gene,[1] is a reproducible, spontaneous model of cardiac hypertrophy, dilation, and congestive failure.[2] In previous studies, we report various abnormalities in myocardial cells, including myofibril disorientation, helical cell shape, and Z band irregularities.[3]

The specific aims of our studies address possible morphological differences between normal and cardiomyopathic myocytes during development in culture, and if there are alterations in cytoskeletal proteins. Primary cultures of cardiac myocytes from normal and cardiomyopathic newborn hamsters (strain UM-X7.1) were analyzed by indirect immunofluorescent microscopy after 3, 5, 7, and 9 days. After treatment with "microtubule stabilizing buffer," the cells were fixed in formaldehyde, then immunofluorescently single- or double-stained with various combinations of anti-tubulin, anti-α-actinin, or anti-actin.

Both normal and cardiomyopathic myocytes appeared round in shape after 3 days in culture. Tubulin staining is most intense immediately around the nucleus with fluorescent "rays" appearing to radiate out to the cell periphery, as well as circumferentially around the edges of most cells (FIG. 1). Double staining with tubulin and actin shows colocalization of these two proteins in some cells. There are no significant differences in cell shape or in tubulin, actin, and α-actinin distribution between normal and cardiomyopathic cells after 5 days in culture. As the size of the cells increase, more cytoplasmic projections are observed in normal hamster cardiac myocytes (FIG. 2A, C, E). By contrast, most of the cardiomyopathic myocytes show few cytoplasmic projections even as late as 9 days in culture (FIG. 2B, D, F) (Chi-square test; n=4; $x^2=20.76$; $p<0.01$). Thus, the number of projections per cell are much fewer in cardiomyopathic myocytes than in normal, especially after 7 and 9 days in culture,

[a]This work was supported by NIH Grants HL-32184 and HL-37702 and a Grant-in-Aid from the American Heart Association to L. F. Lemanski.

[b]To whom correspondence should be addressed.

(p <0.01). One obvious change during development of cardiomyopathic cells was an increase in cell surface area (p <0.05 after 7 days; p <0.01 after 9 days); however, the perimeter dimension of CM cells was less than in normal myocardial cells (FIG. 2G) . This peripheral cell dimension was significantly different at all stages of culture (p <0.01).

These results suggest that cardiomyopathic myocytes have abnormal shapes in culture and fail to form cytoplasmic projections as seen in normal cells. The cardiomyopathic cells also show hypertrophy *in vitro,* as seen with an increase in cell

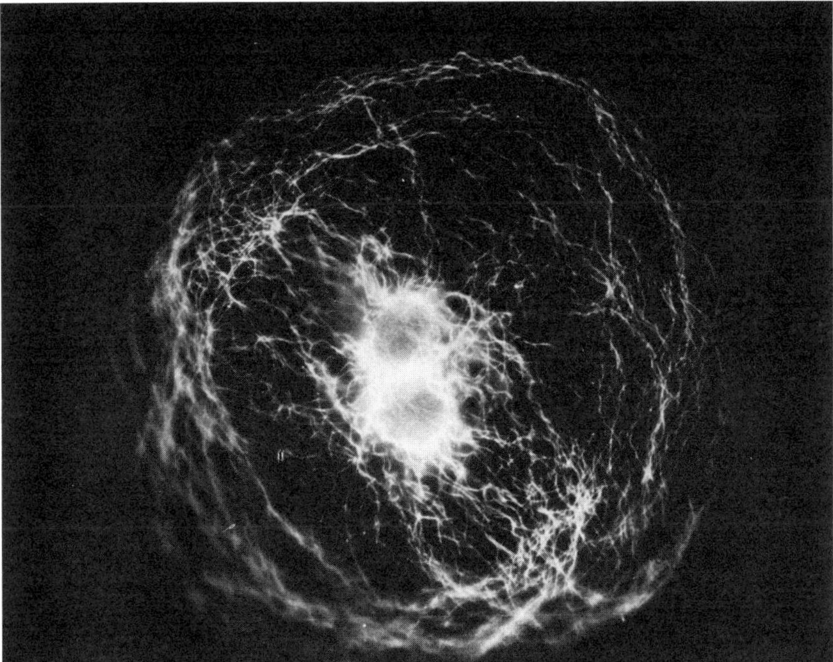

FIGURE 1. Immunofluorescent staining of cardiac myocytes from normal hamster after 3 days in culture using monoclonal anti-α-tubulin antibodies. The cells were isolated with 0.08% trypsin and 0.01% collagenase from 3-day-old newborn hamsters. After incubation in 15% fetal calf serum medium, the cells were treated with microtubule stabilizing buffer (0.1M PIPES, 0.5 mM MgCl, 0.1 mM EDTA at pH 6.9, 37° C, 5 min.), then permeabilized with 0.5% Triton X-100, and fixed with 2% formaldehyde. Microtubules in cardiac myocytes appear to be distributed around nucleus and circumferentially at the edges of the cells. There were no obvious differences in the distribution pattern of tubulin in normal and cardiomyopathic hamster heart cells at this stage of development.

surface area, but was not concomitant with an increase in the peripheral surface dimension. These observations are consistent with studies of isolated ventricle myocytes from adult hamster[4] and suggest that the lack of peripheral cell specialization may be an expression of abnormal internal cytoskeletal organization[2] and calcium accumulation in CM cells[5] or other published biochemical and physiological lesions in CM cells. Whether this unusual behavior is related to an abnormality of membranes, to the cytoskeletal system in cardiomyopathic heart cells, or to some other factor requires further study.

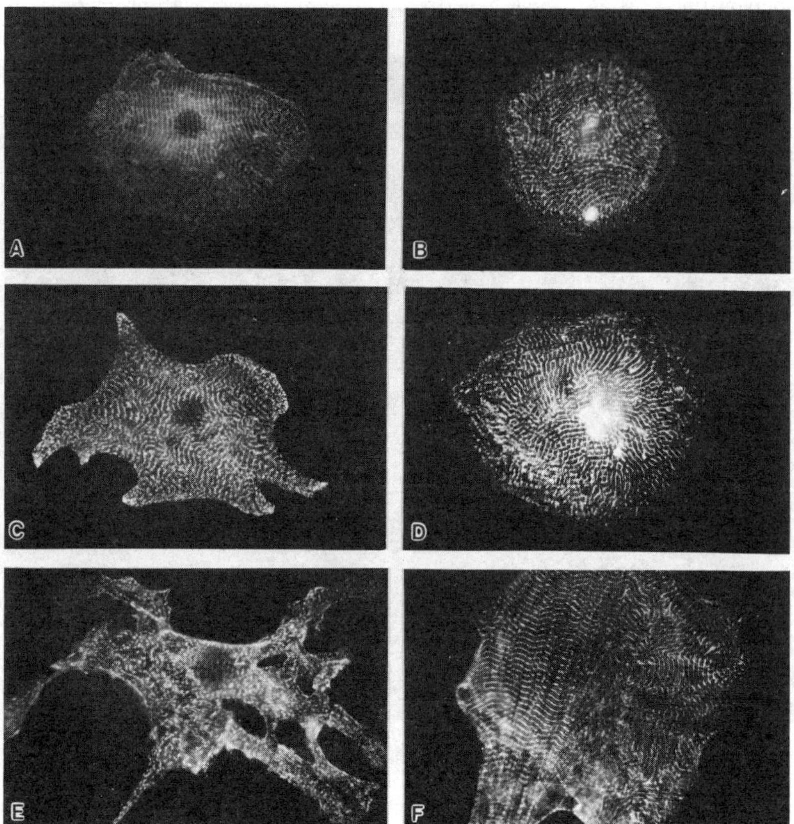

FIGURE 2A-F. Anti-α-actinin antibody stained hamster heart cells in culture. The left panels show an increase in the number and size of cytoplasmic projections in normal cells from 3 days to 9 days. By contrast, myocytes from cardiomyopathic hamster hearts (right panels) show fewer projections. In addition, the cardiomyopathic cells show myofibril disarray.

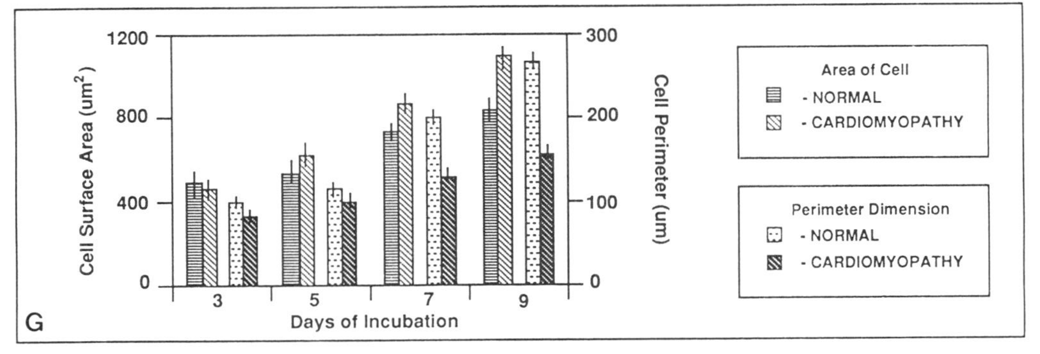

FIGURE 2G. Comparison of cell surface areas and perimeter dimensions of cardiac myocytes from normal and cardiomyopathic hamster hearts in culture. In general, cardiomyopathic heart cells showed an increased surface area but decreased perimeter dimensions during the later time periods in culture, while at the early stages, normal and cardiomyopathic cells were similar. These results were analyzed using a Student *t* test. There were no significant differences in surface area at 3 and 5 days ($p > 0.05$), but after 7 days in culture differences between normal and CM cells were significant ($p < 0.05$ at 7 days; $p < 0.01$ at 9 days). The perimeter dimensions of the cells were significantly different at all four stages of culture; ($p < 0.01$). (N=70 cells/column; mean ± 95% confidence interval).

REFERENCES

1. HOMBURGER, F. & J. BAKER. 1962. Arch. Intern. Med. **110:** 660-662.
2. PERLOFF, J. K. 1971. Mod. Concepts Cardiovasc. Dis. **40:** 23-26.
3. LEMANSKI, L. F. & Z. H. TU. 1983. Dev. Biol. **97:** 339-348.
4. SORENSON, A. L. & D. TEPPER. 1985. Cardiovas. Res. **19:** 793-799.
5. MA, T. S. & L. E. BAILEY. 1979. Cardiovas. Res. **13:** 487-498.

Fibronectin and Integrin Distribution on Migrating Precardiac Mesoderm Cells

KERSTI K. LINASK[a] AND JAMES W. LASH

*Jefferson Medical College and
University of Pennsylvania
Philadelphia, Pennsylvania 19104*

Directed movement of cells within the bilateral heart-forming regions (HFR) in stage 6 chick embryos signals the start of heart organogenesis. Biochemically the start of this movement is correlated with fibronectin (FN) synthesis in the lateral HFR. Fibronectin synthesis is accentuated, with increasing concentrations appearing in cephalad regions by stage 7.[1] The apparent cephalad to caudad difference in FN concentration along the length of the embryo suggested anterior-mesiad guidance of cell movement by way of a haptotactic mechanism. The significance of FN to cell movement was substantiated by experiments using FN antibodies to perturb cell-FN interactions[2,3] and by physically disrupting the FN concentration-dependent directionality by rotating the HFR 180 degrees.[3]

Subsequent studies have shown that both precardiac mesoderm and endoderm cells are able to synthesize FN and to secrete it in their environment as a dense meshwork of fibrils. In FIGURE 1A mesoderm cells from the HFR incubated in culture for 22 h are seen closely associated with fibrils immunostained with FN antibodies. This is similar to what is seen with endocardial cushion tissue cells and primordial germ cell migration, where the migrating cells synthesize the substratum upon which they migrate.[4] Conversely, neural crest cells do not synthesize FN, although they appear to recognize the molecule in their pathways during periods of migration.[5]

Seeking to confirm FN-based cell-matrix interactions, we have shown that migrating precardiac cells do possess an FN receptor that reacts with the cell-substratum attachment (CSAT) antibody that recognizes integrin, the 140,000 M_r FN receptor.[6] FIGURE 1B depicts a fluorescence microscopic image of a precardiac mesoderm cell spread out on a coverslip during incubation in culture. These permeabilized cells were immunostained with anti-integrin antibody to detect integrin. Treatment of early embryos with a pentapeptide containing RGD (0.4 mM), the peptide sequence in the FN cell-binding domain recognized by integrin, showed cardiabifida in relation to control embryos treated with pentapeptides having altered amino acid sequences whereby normal hearts developed.

Concomitant with FN synthesis, the precardiac cells are already becoming committed to specific differentiative pathways. In FIGURES 2A and 2B an explant of stage 5-6 embryonic quail precardiac mesoderm shows a cell population immunostaining

[a] Present address: Division of Cardiology, Department of Pediatrics, The Children's Hospital of Philadelphia and University of Pennsylvania School of Medicine, Philadelphia, PA 19104.

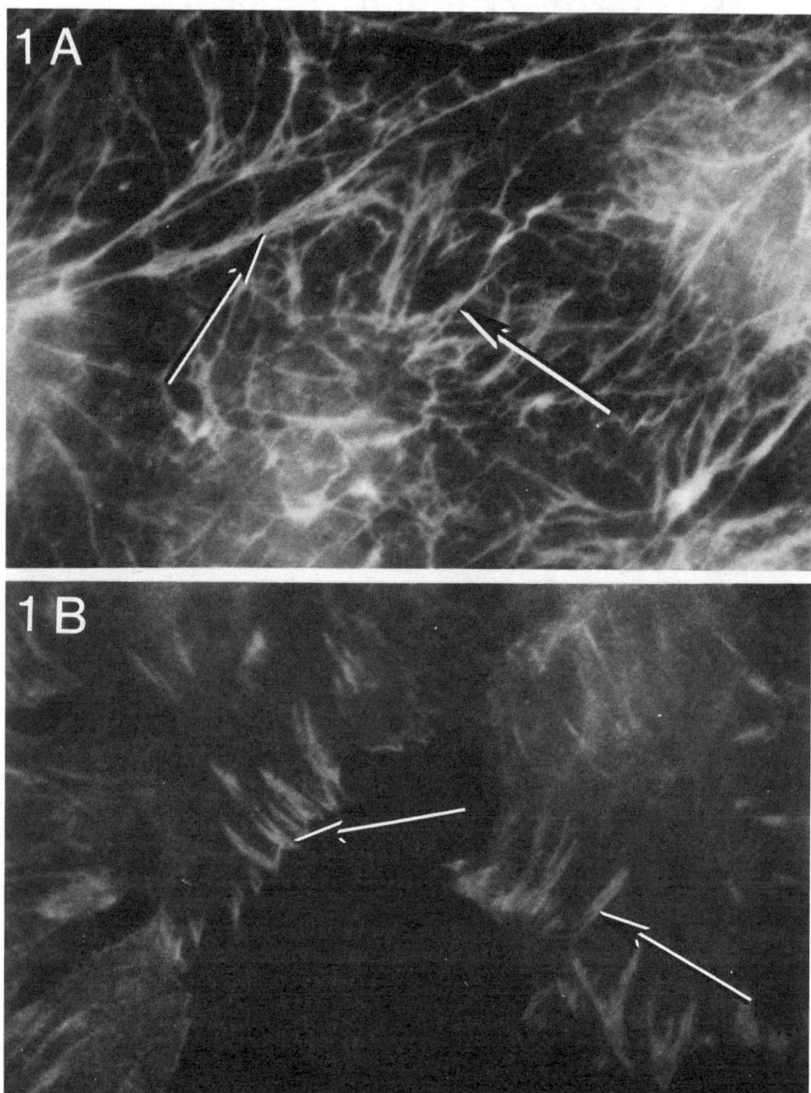

FIGURE 1. A: Precardiac mesoderm cells incubated in culture for 22 h are closely associated with a meshwork of fibrils immunostained with an FN antibody. **B:** Fluorescence microscopic image of a chick precardiac mesoderm cell that has migrated from an explant on a glass coverslip. After cell permeabilization, anti-integrin localizes to areas of close association with the substratum on the periphery of the cell (see arrows).

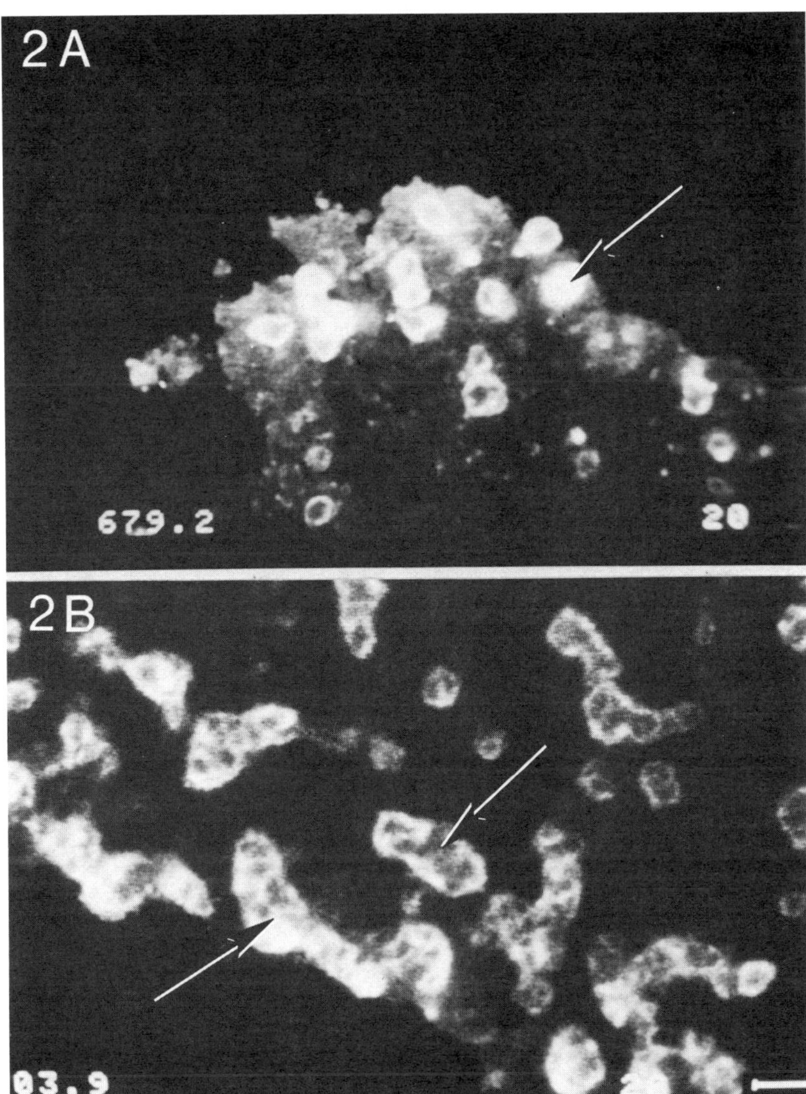

FIGURE 2. Confocal fluorescence microscopic image of a quail precardiac mesoderm explant immunostained with QH-1 monoclonal antibody that recognizes an endothelial cell antigenic determinant. Endothelial cells (arrows) are already differentiating during the earliest cell migration stages. **A:** Cells staining with QH-1 after 2 h incubation. **B:** Endothelial cells are beginning to associate with one another in clusters after 22 h of incubation.

with QH-1 monoclonal antibody indicating the presence of an antigenic marker for endothelial cells. These results suggest that precardiac cells are beginning to differentiate into a heterogeneous population of cells during the earliest cell migration stages of heart development.

Further studies are being planned to identify possible regulatory molecules, for example, growth factors, that may be responsible for initiating organogenic processes that include synthesis of both FN and its receptors, as well as gene activation leading to cell differentiation in the heart-forming regions of the early avian embryo.

REFERENCES

1. LINASK, K. K. & J. W. LASH. 1986. Dev. Biol. **114:** 89-101.
2. LINASK, K. K. & J. W. LASH. 1988. Dev. Biol. **129:** 315-323.
3. LINASK, K. K. & J. W. LASH. 1988. Dev. Biol. **129:** 324-329.
4. FFRENCH-CONSTANT, C. & R. O. HYNES. 1988. Development **104:** 369-382.
5. NEWGREEN, D. & J. P. THIERY. 1980. Cell Tissue Res. **211:** 269-291.
6. BUCK, C. A. & A. F. HORWITZ. 1987. Annu. Rev. Cell Biol. **3:** 179-205.

A Culture Model for Cardiac Morphogenesis[a]

JOHN W. LOUGH, DAVID L. BOLENDER, AND
ROGER R. MARKWALD

Department of Anatomy and Cellular Biology
Medical College of Wisconsin
Milwaukee, Wisconsin 53226

INTRODUCTION

Studies in amphibian and avian embryos have indicated that an inductive interaction between precardiac mesoderm and endoderm is required to establish a fully differentiated, functional heart.[1] The nature of the inductive stimulus is unknown. Although cell-cell interactions may be involved, it is likely that macromolecular factors secreted by the interacting tissues signal inductive changes in this and other developing systems.[2] To identify endodermal secretions that modulate cardiogenesis, an *in vitro* bioassay system is needed that ideally recapitulates the inductive processes necessary for three-dimensional heart morphogenesis. We report here that splanchnic mesoderm explanted onto hydrated collagen gel cultures with anterior endoderm from early embryos may provide such a model system.

METHODS

Precardiac (stage 6-8) mesoderm explanted without enzymes was placed on a 2 mm gel of hydrated collagen (1.5 mg/mL) with and without an overlay of collagen-coated 180 μm^2 mesh nylon (Nitex) containing a sheet of stage 6-8 anterior endoderm. The medium (M-199/ITS; Collaborative Research) was changed daily. Cultures were fixed in 3% glutaraldehyde/1% tannic acid and embedded in Spurr resin, from which thick (1 μm) and thin sections for light and electron microscopy were prepared.

[a]This work was supported by NIH Grant HL 39829.

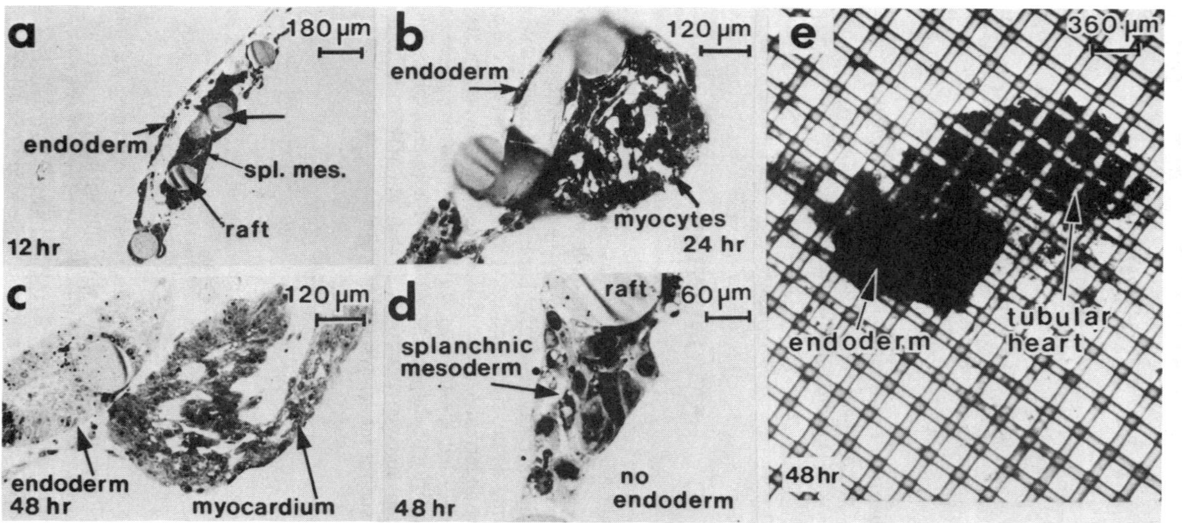

FIGURE 1. Light microscopy of mesoderm/endoderm cocultures. Stage 6-8 splanchnic mesoderm and endoderm were cultured on hydrated collagen gels for the indicated times, followed by fixation and sectioning (panels a-d). To facilitate removal, the endodermal cell-sheet was placed atop a nylon support screen (raft; FIG. 1a). Nonsectioned cells on a nylon raft are shown in panel e.

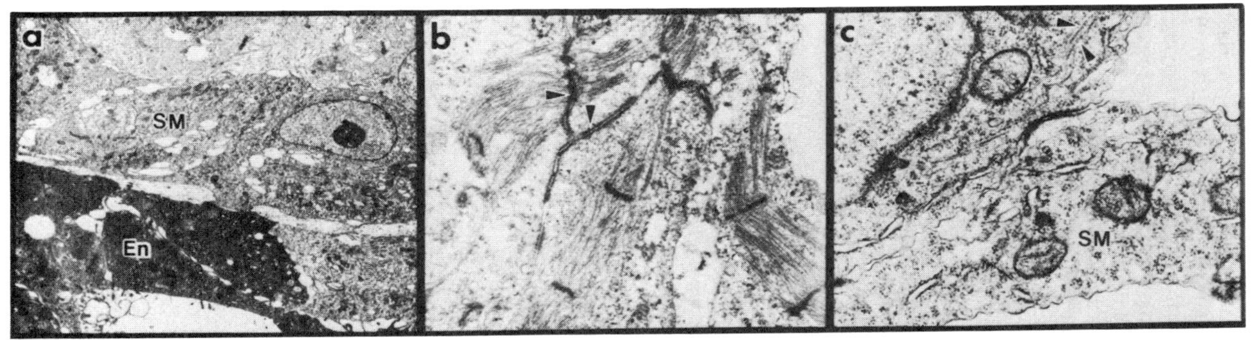

FIGURE 2. Electron microscopy of mesoderm/endoderm cocultures. Cultures were prepared as described above, followed by fixation and processing for electron microscopy. Panel a shows 12 h cocultured cells (SM, splanchnic mesoderm; En, endoderm). Panel b shows nascent sarcomeres and junctional complexes (arrowheads) in mesodermal cells of a 48 h coculture. Panel c shows 48 h mesodermal cells that had not been cultured with endoderm (SM, splanchnic mesoderm; arrowheads, putative myofilaments). Magnifications: a, ×6,000; b, ×25,000; c, ×12,000.

RESULTS AND DISCUSSION

In sectioned cultures, precardiac mesoderm cells overlaid with endoderm were arranged in several loosely knit layers by 12 h (FIG. 1a). By 24 h (FIG. 1b), the mesoderm cells had proliferated, migrating into the underlying gel (not visible in these micrographs) to form a pulsating vesicle-like structure resembling a primitive heart; the wall contained cellular cords reminiscent of myocardial trabeculae. By 48 h (FIG. 1c), endoderm and mesoderm had expanded. By contrast, mesoderm cells explanted without endoderm exhibited little evidence of cardiogenesis by 48 h (FIG. 1d), although contractions were noted. On the other hand, removal of the endodermal sheet after migration of mesoderm into the gel (24 h) had no effect on subsequent morphogenesis (not shown). A low power micrograph of a nonsectioned 48 h coculture is shown in FIGURE 1e.

FIGURE 2a is a transmission electron micrograph of a 12 h coculture. Higher magnification revealed that the extracellular space between the endoderm (En) and precardiac splanchnic mesoderm (SM) cells contained fibrogranular material that may attach to mesodermal processes, as well as the presence of myofilament bundles in the mesodermal cytoplasm. After 48 h (FIG. 2b), mesoderm cells contained nascent sarcomeres and junctional complexes resembling intercalated disks (arrowheads). FIGURE 2c shows mesoderm (SM) cells cultured without endoderm after 48 h; although these cells contained evidence of myofilaments (arrowheads) and were contractile, sarcomeres were not observed.

These results are consistent with other findings indicating an inductive role for endoderm during cardiac morphogenesis.[1] Although our results suggest, however, that endodermal secretions during the early stages of cardiogenesis are required for subsequent completion of the morphogenetic program, endoderm is not needed for mesoderm cells to become contractile. We are currently evaluating the effects of endoderm from noncardiac areas and characterizing the proteins synthesized by stage 6-8 endoderm, some of which migrate in SDS gels with M_rs similar to known growth factors.[3]

REFERENCES

1. JACOBSON, A. G. & A. K. SATER. 1988. Features of embryonic induction. Development **104:** 341-359.
2. EDELMAN, G. M. 1988. Topobiology. An introduction to molecular embryology. Basic Books. New York.
3. KOKAN-MOORE, N., D. L. BOLENDER & J. LOUGH. Unpublished observations..

Motility Patterns of Cultured Endothelial Cells Exposed to Physiological Levels of Fluid Shear Stress[a]

MICHITAKA MASUDA AND KEIGI FUJIWARA

Department of Structural Analysis
National Cardiovascular Center Research Institute
Suita, Osaka 565 Japan

Fluid shear stress affects the shape, alignment, and cytoskeletal organization of vascular endothelial cells (EC) *in situ* and *in vitro*.[1-3] We used cultured EC exposed to various levels of fluid shear stress as a model system for investigating how cells respond to mechanical forces. Using an optical flow chamber system,[4] we analyzed the motility pattern of EC and vascular smooth muscle cells (SMC) exposed to physiological levels of fluid shear stress.

When confluent bovine or canine arterial EC grown on type-I collagen-coated glass surface were exposed to 6-11 dynes/cm^2 (high shear) for over 36 h, the long axes of the EC and their stress fibers became aligned parallel to the direction of flow. Migration of EC biased preferentially in the downstream direction was apparent immediately after exposure to these levels of shear stress. With 4 dynes/cm^2 or less, they did not align or move in the direction of flow.

EC in sparse culture did not show these morphological changes even after exposure to the high shear level for 100 hours. After transition from a low shear to a high shear condition, however, sparsely cultured EC extended lamellipodia predominantly on the downstream side and began to migrate preferentially downstream. SMC in sparse or subconfluent cultures did not align or migrate in the direction of flow with shear stress levels of up to 10 dynes/cm^2. These results show that the motility pattern of a single EC, but not an SMC, can rapidly be affected by fluid shear stress and that the parallel orientation of the major axis of EC induced by high shear may require cell-cell interaction.

An analysis of the cell trails of sparsely cultured EC is summarized in TABLE 1 and suggests a possible mechanism for the biased cell locomotion observed under the high shear conditions. Consistent with a random walk model, EC exposed to low shear stress moved in all directions with the same velocity, and the magnitude of the turns was independent of the direction of cell movement. Although EC locomotion was slightly accelerated under high shear stress in the direction of flow, this level of acceleration could not account for the biased migration of EC under high shear.

[a] This work was supported by Grants for Cardiovascular Disease from the Ministry of Health and Welfare (Japan) and by the Ichiro Kanehara Foundation.

TABLE 1. Response of EC in Sparse Culture to Low (0.4 dynes/cm^2) and High (8 dynes/cm^2) Shear

		Direction of EC migration relative to the direction of flow			
	Shear level	Downstream	Perpendicular	Upstream	Average
Distribution	low	37	38	25	—
(percent)	high	80	14	6	—
Velocity (μm/h)	low	49	46	48	48
	high	55	51	49	54
Total turning angle	low	77	82	83	81
(°/20 min)	high	54	95	103	63

Rather, it was mostly due to a change in the turning property of EC. The total turning angle for EC migrating perpendicularly to or against the direction of flow was roughly doubled when compared to those moving downstream. Consequently, EC migrating in the perpendicular or the upstream directions tended to change their direction until they turned downstream. EC moving in the direction of flow tended to keep their original course.

Our results suggest that EC sense both the level and the direction of fluid shear stress. When the shear stress level is sufficiently high, EC respond to this physical force. The type of response appears to depend upon cell density of the EC culture.

REFERENCES

1. WHITE, G. E., M. A. GIMBRONE, JR. & K. FUJIWARA. 1983. J. Cell Biol. **97:** 416.
2. WHITE, G. E. & K. FUJIWARA. 1986. J. Cell Biol. **103:** 63.
3. WHITE, G. E., K. FUJIWARA, E. SHEFTON, C. F. DEWEY, JR. & M. A. GIMBRONE, JR. 1982. Fed. Proc. **41:** 321.
4. MASUDA, M. & K. FUJIWARA. 1988. Cell Struct. Function **13:** 638.

Migration of Cardiac Neural Crest Cells

A Temporal and Spatial Study in Early Quail-Chick Chimeras

SACHIKO T. MIYAGAWA,[a,b] KAREN WALDO,[b]
HITOSHI TOMITA,[b] AND MARGARET L. KIRBY [b]

[a]*Department of Pediatric Cardiology*
Heart Institute of Japan
Tokyo Women's Medical College
Tokyo, Japan

[b]*Department of Anatomy*
Medical College of Georgia
Augusta, Georgia 30912-2000

It has been shown that the cardiac neural crest from the level of the midotic placode to the rostral limit of somite 4 contributes to the septation of the outflow tract of the heart in chick embryos.[1] The cardiac neural crest can be divided into three regions: arch 3 (adjacent to the midotic placode to the rostral limit of somite 1), arch 4 (adjacent to somites 1 and 2), and arch 6 (adjacent to somite 3). The crest cells derived from the arch 4 region contribute four times as many cells to the outflow septation as the arch 3 or 6 regions.[2,3] The precise migration route of the neural crest is not clear, however. This study investigated the migration of the cardiac neural crest in quail-chick chimeras from stages 18 to 25.

Fertilized Arbor Acre chicken eggs (Seaboard Hatchery, Athens, GA) and Japanese quail eggs (HDG, Medical College of Georgia, Augusta, GA) at stages 8 to 11[4] were used to construct quail-chick chimeras. The embryos were prepared for microsurgery as has been described previously.[5] Eighty-nine chimeras were made by transplanting premigratory neural crest from these three regions bilaterally or unilaterally. In bilateral arch 3 or 4, chimeras at stage 24, the quail neural crest cells mainly surrounded the third (FIGURES 1, 2) or fourth pharyngeal arch arteries bilaterally. In bilateral arch 6 chimeras, the quail cells were located around the sixth pharyngeal arch arteries and the pulmonary arteries. After unilateral transplants, quail cells were located mainly in the ipsilateral side of the pharyngeal arch. The data further illustrates the precise time of migration of cardiac neural crest cells through the pharyngeal apparatus.

[a]Address correspondence to Sachiko T. Miyagawa, c/o Dr. Margaret L. Kirby, Department of Anatomy, Medical College of Georgia, Augusta, GA 30912-2000.

427

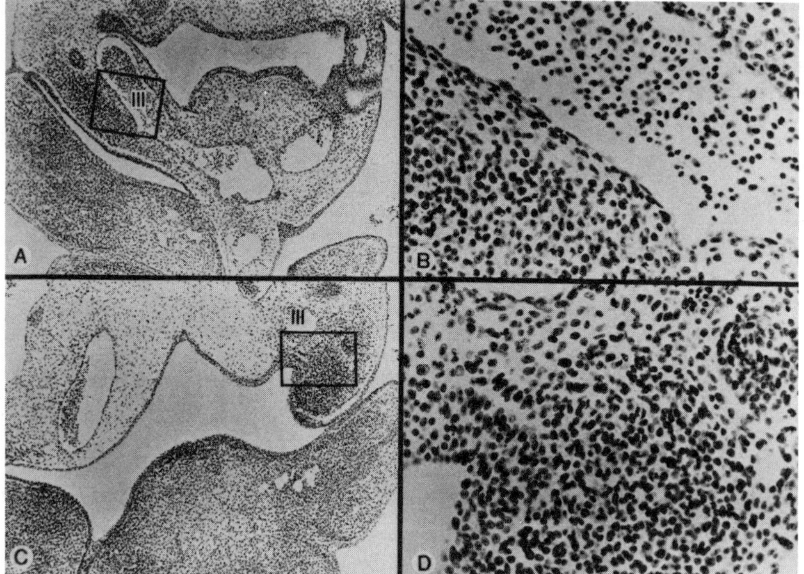

FIGURE 1. Transverse sections of a bilateral arch 3 chimera (stage 24). The quail cells surround the third pharyngeal arch arteries. A and B: the right third pharyngeal arch artery. C and D: the left third pharyngeal arch artery.

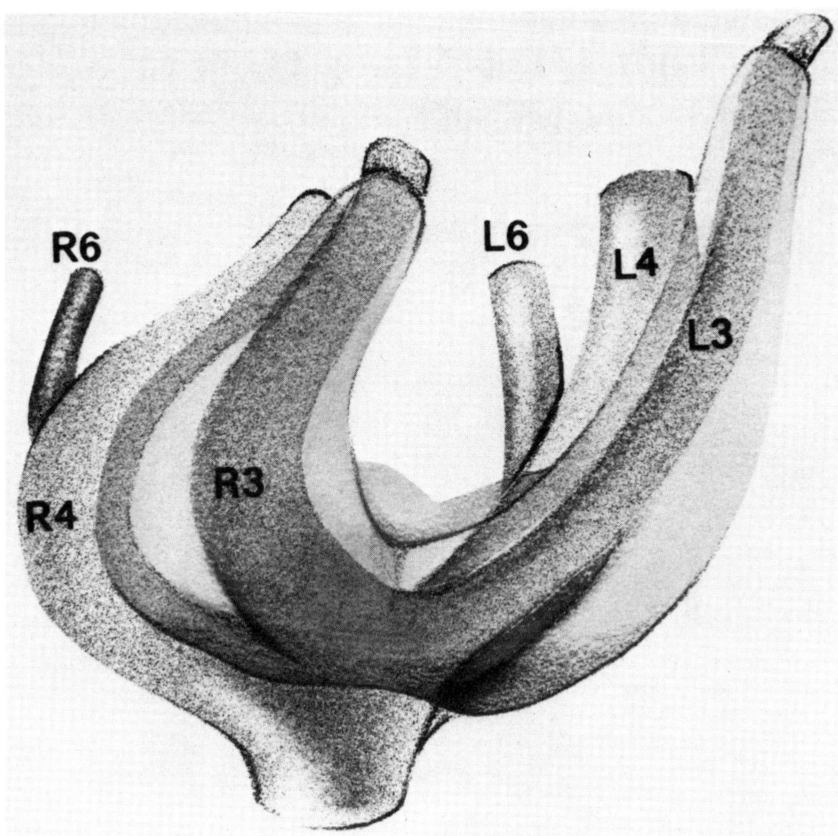

FIGURE 2. A schematic representation of the same chimera as FIG. 1. Frontal view. The quail cells form tubes that ensheathe the third pharyngeal arch arteries.

REFERENCES

1. KIRBY, M. L. 1987. Cardiac morphogenesis-recent research advances. Pediatr. Res. **21**(3): 219-224.
2. KIRBY, M. L., K. L. TURNAGE & B. M. HAYS. 1985. Characterization of conotruncal malformation following ablation of "cardiac" neural crest. Anat. Rec. **213**: 87-93.
3. PHILLIPS, M. T., M. L. KIRBY & G. FORBES. 1987. Analysis of cranial neural crest distribution in the developing heart using quail-chick chimeras. Circ. Res. **60**: 27-30.
4. HAMBURGER, V. & H. L. HAMILTON. 1951. A series of normal stages of the chick embryo. J. Morphol. **88**: 49-92.
5. KIRBY, M. L., T. F. GALE & D. E. STEWART. 1983. Neural crest cells contribute to normal aorticopulmonary septation. Science **220**: 1059-1061.

Long QT and Long QT with Deafness Syndrome

Beginning a Neural Analysis in an Embryonic Chick Model

M. J. MULROY, H. B. HOTELLING, AND
T. A. HARRISON

*Department of Anatomy
Medical College of Georgia
Augusta, Georgia 30912-2000*

Recent studies show that unilateral lesions of the nodose placode at 30-36 hours of incubation can produce prolonged QT intervals in the electrocardiograms (ECGs) recorded from 17 day embryonic chicks.[1] This lesion destroys the placodal precursors of the nodose ganglion neurons, some of whom provide the vagal sensory innervation of the heart. In this report, we have extended the initial observations to a total of 71 chick embryos, 48 with lesions and 23 sham-operated controls. Lesions of the right nodose placode were made by hot needle ablation in 30-36 hour embryos. For sham operated controls, the vitelline membrane was broken but no ablation was performed. On embryonic day 17, ECGs were recorded by inserting four silver wires through very small holes made in the shell, and QT and RR intervals were measured. FIGURE 1 shows the resulting distribution of corrected QT intervals[2] for sham and lesioned chicks. The lesioned embryos showed longer QTs than the shams, although not all lesions resulted in a long QT.

A few embryonic chicks were found to fit the Jervell and Lange-Nielsen pattern of long QT with deafness syndrome. After ECG evaluation, responses to clicks and pure tones at 80-130 dB were recorded in Nembutal-anesthetized chicks by way of a recording electrode near the round window membrane. In four animals, no cochlear response was present, even with the loudest stimuli. We presume that in these animals the lesion extended to the otic placode, which is adjacent to the nodose placode early in development, and we suggest that a similar mechanism may relate human deafness and long QT disorders.

We have begun to exploit these animal models of human Romano-Ward (long QT) and Jervell and Lange-Nielsen (long QT with deafness) syndromes to investigate the neurological basis for the observed cardiac and auditory disfunctions. Our initial studies focus on the nodose ganglion itself. The ganglion was dissected, embedded in historesin, sectioned, mounted, and stained with toluidine blue. Morphometric measurements were then carried out. Preliminary results of these studies are summarized in TABLE 1. In a few lesioned animals, the nodose ganglion either could not be

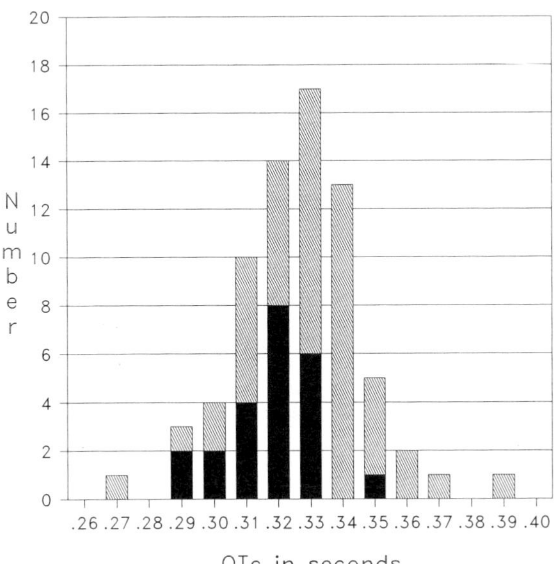

FIGURE 1. Frequency distribution of QTc. Histogram comparing the distribution of QTc intervals in 17 day chick embryos from which tissue had been removed in the region of the right nodose placode at 30-36 h of incubation (stage 10). These data indicate that the lesion can produce embryos with long QT intervals (defined as > 0.330 s, which was one standard deviation above the mean for an independent control group of normal chick embryos[1]); however, not all attempted lesions produced abnormally long QT intervals. The means of the two groups are significantly different at the .05 level using a two-tailed *t* test. ■, sham operated; ▨, right nodose removed. Sham operated: n = 23; SD = ±0.0131; mean = 0.316, 4% with long QT. Right nodose removed: n = 48; SD ±0.0205, mean = 0.325; 46% with long QT.

identified at all, or was present but contained either no cells, or a few cells in isolated patches. In most lesioned embryos, the ganglion did develop, appeared normal in size, but was reduced in volume. Cell size distributions show that there was a shift toward small cells in experimental ganglia.

We are currently extending these morphometric studies to include more cases and to include the sympathetic and parasympathetic ganglia supplying the heart. Previous studies indicate that disruption of one component of cardiac innervation during development results in compensatory changes in other components.[3] Thus, we must evaluate changes in all components to understand the causes of the long QT in this model. Studies of morphological changes in the cochlea, which occur with lesion-induced deafness, have also begun.

TABLE 1. Summary to Date of Observations on the Effects of Right Nodose Placode Lesions on QT Interval, Hearing, and the Integrity of the Right Nodose Ganglion[a]

| | | Nodose Ganglion Histology | |
Surgery	Result	Gross Evaluation	Volume
Sham	Normal QT	present, normal size (n = 5)	$656 \times 10^6 \ \mu m^3$ (n = 1)
Lesion	Long QT	absent (n = 2)	0
		present, small (n = 2)	$> >$ [b]
		present, normal size (n = 12)	$214 \times 10^6 \ \mu m^3$ (n = 1)
	Long QT and Deafness	present, normal size (n = 4)	$356 \times 10^6 \ \mu m^3$ (n = 1)

[a] Compared to sham-operated controls, experimental ganglia were reduced in size to varying degrees. Some were totally absent. Others appeared normal to gross evaluation, but were found to contain either no cells or very few, or to be greatly reduced in the volume of tissue containing ganglion cells. Cell size distributions in ganglia with cells showed a shift to small cells in the experimental ganglia. The mean areas of ganglion cells in μm^2 ± standard deviations were as follows: sham-operated controls, 557 ± 192.7; long QT with normal appearing ganglion, 306 ± 100.9; and long QT with deafness, 316 ± 137.0.

Tissue sections containing ganglion cells were drawn from the microscope slide with the aid of a drawing tube attachment. The drawings were digitized and areas calculated and summed using SigmaScan software. Volumes were calculated by multiplying total areas by section thickness (4 μm). Cell size distributions were produced by digitizing the areas of cell profiles containing nucleoli in sections constituting 10% of the total volume of each ganglion, sampled at equal intervals through the ganglion.

[b] Ganglion volume was not measured. Ganglion cells were either scattered along the nerve, not in the swelling identified as the ganglion, or only a few cells were found in the entire ganglion.

REFERENCES

1. CHRISTIANSEN, J. L. *et al.* 1989. Pediatr. Res. **26:** 11-15.
2. BAZETT, H. C. 1920. Heart **7:** 353-370.
3. KIRBY, M. L. *et al.* 1987. Cell Tissue Res. **247:** 489-496.

Effect of Bisdiamine Given to Pregnant Rats on Hemodynamics of Their Embryos

MAKOTO NAKAZAWA, SACHIKO M. TOMITA,
MAKOTO NISHIBATAKE, ATSUYOSHI TAKAO,
AND SEIJI MIURA

Department of Pediatric Cardiology
The Heart Institute of Japan
Tokyo Women's Medical College
8-1 Kawada-cho, Shinjuku-ku
Tokyo, Japan

INTRODUCTION

Developmental abnormalities of neural crest cells (NCC) produce congenital heart defects as well as an abnormal autonomic nervous system in chick embryos.[1,2] Ablation or excision of NCC in the chick embryo is also associated with hemodynamic changes[3] or altered response to cholinergic stimulation.[4] Bisdiamine may affect the NCC system in the rat, producing conotruncal anomalies. Thus, we hypothesized that hemodynamic alteration may be produced in embryos of bisdiamine-treated mother rats. The specific aim of the present study was to clarify the effect of bisdiamine given to mother rats on baseline hemodynamics in their embryos and on hemodynamic responses to acetylcholinc.

SUBJECTS AND METHODS

Bisdiamine at the dose of 200 mg or a solvent was given to pregnant Wistar rats at gestational day 10. Each embryo with the placenta was excised at gestational day 12 and immersed in Hanks' solution at 37° C. The yolk sac was windowed; then the umbilical artery was punctured with a micro-glass-pipette, and blood pressure was measured by a servo-null micro-pressure system. Blood flow velocity was measured at the truncus of the heart with a 20 MHz pulsed Doppler velocity meter. The change of the flow would represent the change of cardiac output in an assumption that the diameter of the truncus did not significantly change during interventions.[5] Acetylcholine, 0.5 μg diluted in 100 nL of distilled water, was infused into the placenta with a microinjector.

RESULTS

Baseline hemodynamics were similar in the bisdiamine-treated and control embryos in which solvent was given (FIG. 1). Acetylcholine slowed heart rate in both groups, and the decrement was significantly less in the bisdiamine-treated group than in the control (FIG. 2). Mean artery blood pressure and mean flow velocity, a measure of cardiac output, did not change on the drug, but stroke volume index (mean flow velocity/heart rate) increased. The increase of stroke volume index was less in the treated embryos than in the controls.

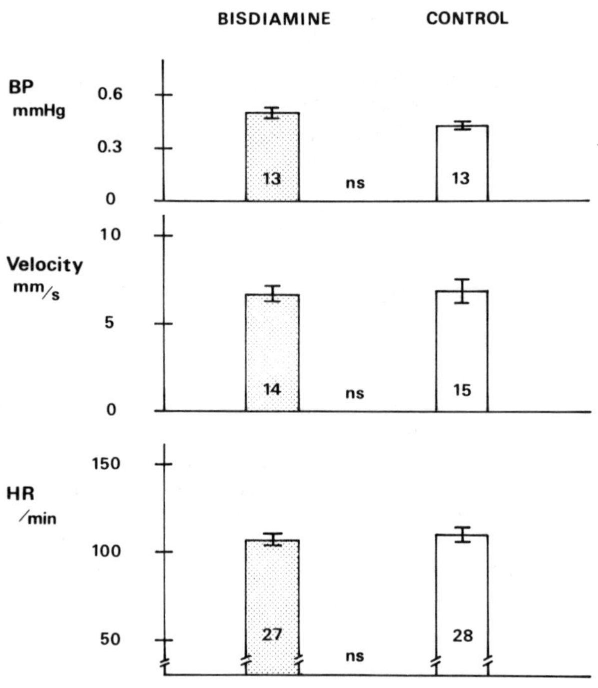

FIGURE 1. Blood pressure, blood flow velocity at the truncus, and heart rate were not different between the bisdiamine-treated and control embryos.

COMMENTS AND CONCLUSIONS

Bisdiamine given to pregnant mother rats did not affect baseline hemodynamics in their embryos, whereas the responses of heart rate and stroke volume to acetylcholine were altered. The response of heart rate was qualitatively similar to that seen in NCC-excised chick embryos.[4] These observations suggest a subtle alteration of pacemaker cell function and myocardial mechanical function in these embryos and that bisdiamine may possibly affect NCC, thus resulting in both abnormal cell function and abnormal morphogenesis.

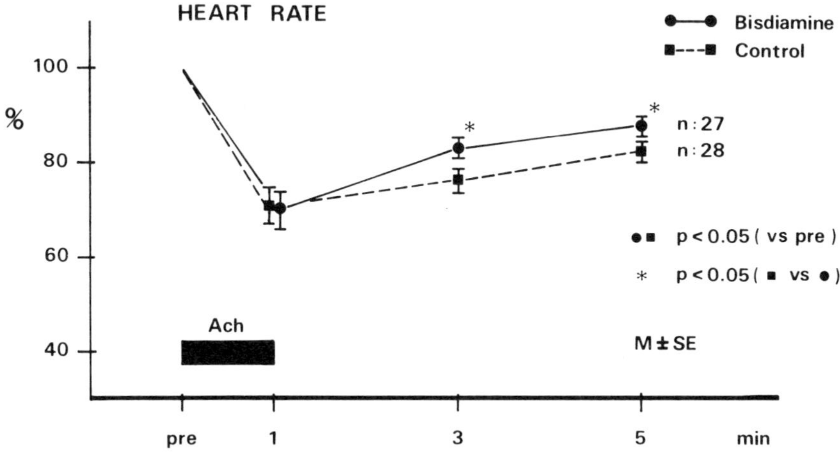

FIGURE 2. Heart rate was reduced by acetylcholine (Ach) injection. The reduction was less in the bisdiamine-treated embryos than in the controls.

REFERENCES

1. KIRBY, M. L. 1987. Pediatr. Res. **21:** 219-224.
2. KIRBY, M. L., R. S. ARONSTAM & J. J. BUCCAFUSCO. 1985. Circ. Res. **56:** 392-401.
3. STEWART, D. E., M. L. KIRBY & K. K. SULIK. 1986. Circ. Res. **59:** 545-550.
4. NAKAZAWA, M., S. MIYAGAWA, M. NISHIBATAKE, K. IKEDA & A. TAKAO. 1988. Heart Vessels **4:** 136-140.
5. NAKAZAWA, M., S. MIYAGAWA, T. OHNO, S. MIURA & A. TAKAO 1988. Pediatr. Res. **23:** 200-205.

Changes in Acetylcholinesterase Molecular Form Expression during Rat Heart Development

CYNTHIA NYQUIST-BATTIE AND
KARL T. SALTZMAN

Structural and Systems Biology
School of Basic Life Sciences
University of Missouri-Kansas City
Kansas City, Missouri 64108

Acetylcholinesterase (AChE) is a glycoprotein with multiple molecular forms that can be divided into two classes.[1] Asymmetric forms (A) contain catalytic subunits covalently bound to a collagen-helical peptide. The second class is termed globular(G) and consists of molecules that lack collagen tails. Globular forms exist as monomers (G_1), dimers (G_2), and tetramers (G_4) of the catalytic subunits. A and G forms of AChE are present in all chambers of rat heart, although most areas of the atria exhibit higher AChE-specific activities than the ventricles.[2,3] AChE is present in fetal rat heart before the onset of functional innervation.[4] To determine if the expression of AChE changes during the establishment of cholinergic innervation, a study of AChE molecular forms in developing rat heart was conducted.

TABLE 1. Contribution of the Individual AChE Molecular Forms to AChE Activity in Developing Whole Heart[a]

	$G_1 + G_2$	G_4	A_8	A_{12}
E1	43.0 ± 0.35	23.0 ± 0.24	9.60 ± 1.00	24.0 ± 0.10
E19	28.3 ± 1.25	29.3 ± 1.11	12.4 ± 1.91	30.9 ± 1.14
P2	45.3 ± 1.20	38.8 ± 1.10		15.9 ± 1.10
P7	42.9 ± 2.00	42.5 ± 1.48		14.3 ± 2.19
P14	36.9 ± 3.14	44.9 ± 1.13		14.9 ± 0.36
P21	37.1 ± 0.91	48.3 ± 0.92		14.4 ± 0.14
Adult	41.4 ± 1.98	47.8 ± 1.35		9.83 ± 1.13

[a] Values are means $\pm$ SEM (n = 3-6) and represent percentages of total gradient activity for each molecular form. AChE, extracted from rat heart, was separated into molecular forms by velocity sedimentation on linear sucrose gradients. Sedimentation coefficients (S) were determined relative to those of BSA (4.4S) and catalase (11.3S). G_1 AChE sedimented at 4.1S, G_2 at 6S, G_4 at 10.2S, A_8 at 12S, and A_{12} at 16S. In hearts from fetal animals, A_8 AChE formed a separate peak, but after birth A_8 AChE formed an insignificant shoulder on the G_4 peak. In our gradient system, G_4 and G_2 AChE were not resolved sufficiently to treat individually. E1 and E19 refer to embryonic days 1 and 19, whereas P2-P21 refer to postnatal days 2-21.

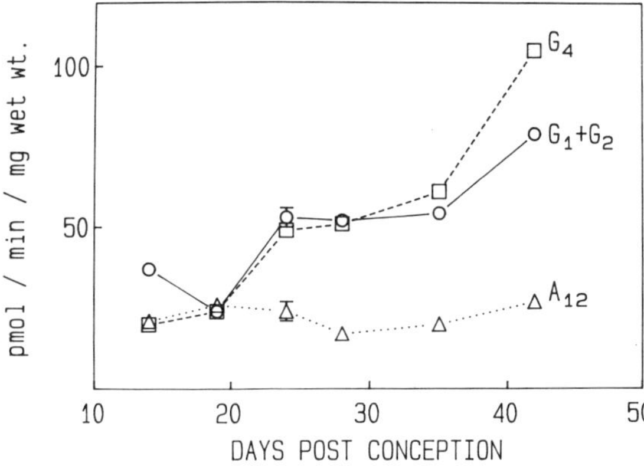

FIGURE 1. Activities per unit wet weight of the predominant AChE molecular forms in whole hearts removed from perinatal rats. Birth occurred between days 21 and 22, postconception.

AChE was solubilized from whole hearts of pre- and postnatal rats, using a method described previously.[2,3] Assays for AChE activity and the separation of AChE forms on linear 5-20% sucrose gradients were performed as outlined in our earlier work.[2,3]

The total activity per mg wet weight of cardiac AChE increased approximately threefold between postconception days 14-42, with values ranging from 86 ± 2 to 215 ± 4 pmol/min/mg wet weight. Analysis of the percent activities of AChE molecular forms during this period revealed a striking change in the ratio of A to G forms between the prenatal and postnatal periods (TABLE 1). After birth, asymmetric forms showed a significant decline in their percent activities. By contrast, the contributions of G_4 and $G_1 + G_2$ AChE increased during the perinatal period. Activities per mg wet weight for AChE forms are shown in FIGURE 1. These data illustrate that the activity of A_{12} AChE did not change significantly with age, but that the activities of the G forms did increase.

The major finding of this work is that during perinatal heart development, the levels of the globular forms of AChE increase, whereas that of A_{12} AChE remains relatively constant. The fact that the increased activities of globular AChE molecular forms coincides with the development of choline acetyltransferase[5] would suggest that the change in the composition of the pool of cardiac AChE is related to the development of the cholinergic nerves of the heart. Because globular AChE is associated with cholinergic nerves of the heart,[6] the increased globular AChE activity could be the result of the commencement of AChE expression by these nerves.

REFERENCES

1. MASSOULIE, J. & S. BON. 1982. Annu. Rev. Neurosci. **5:** 57-106.
2. NYQUIST-BATTIE, C., C. HODGES-SAVOLA & H. FERNANDEZ. 1987. J. Mol. Cell. Cardiol. **19:** 935-943.
3. NYQUIST-BATTIE, C. & K. TRANS-SALTZMANN. 1989. Circ. Res. **65:** 55-62.
4. LAMERS, W., A. KORTSCHOT, J. LOS & A. MOORMAN. 1987. Anat. Rec. **217:** 361-370.
5. MARVIN, JR., W., K. KERMSMEYER, R. McDONALD & R. ROSKOSKI, JR. 1980. Circ. Res. **46:** 690-695.
6. NYQUIST-BATTIE, C., R. T. DOWELL & H. FERNANDEZ. 1986. J. Cell Biol. **103:** 376a.

Hyaluronic Acid and Its Binding Protein, Hyaluronectin, as Morphogenetic Components during Formation of the Cardiac Jelly in Rat and Chicken Embryos

ROB E. POELMANN,[a]

ADRIANA C. GITTENBERGER-DE GROOT,[a]

MONICA M. T. MENTINK,[a]

J. CONNY VAN MUNSTEREN,[a]

BERTRAND DELPECH,[b] AND SZABOLCS VIRÁGH [c]

[a]*Department of Anatomy*
The University of Leiden
2300 RC, Leiden, the Netherlands

[b]*Centre Henri Becquerel*
Rouen, France

[c]*Department of Pathology*
Postgraduate Medical School
Budapest, Hungary

Early development of the heart depends not only on the formation of the endocardial tube, but also on the distribution and function of the extracellular matrix. During morphogenesis of the heart tube, scanning electron microscopy shows that extracellular fibers develop, located between the endocardium and the myocardium. This three-dimensional fibrous network is very prominent during cardiac looping. In the transmission electron microscope the fibers stain heavily after ruthenium red application. Immunohistochemistry on presomite to 30-somite embryos reveals the appearance of the various extracellular matrix components such as fibronectin, laminin, collagen type IV, and chondroitin sulphate.

Particular attention is paid to the role of hyaluronic acid (HA) and its binding protein, hyaluronectin (HN). In the cardiogenic plate an accumulation of HA and HN accompanies the formation of the endocardial tube. During further development, the locally enhanced presence of HA and HN precede formation of the cardiac jelly. HA (FIG. 1) has a widespread distribution in the embryo and the heart. HN, however, is preferentially located in, for example, the cephalic mesenchyme and in the cardiac jelly. It lines the myocardium and the endocardium as well as the fine fibrous strands, also visible in scanning and transmission electron microscopy (FIG. 2), that connect

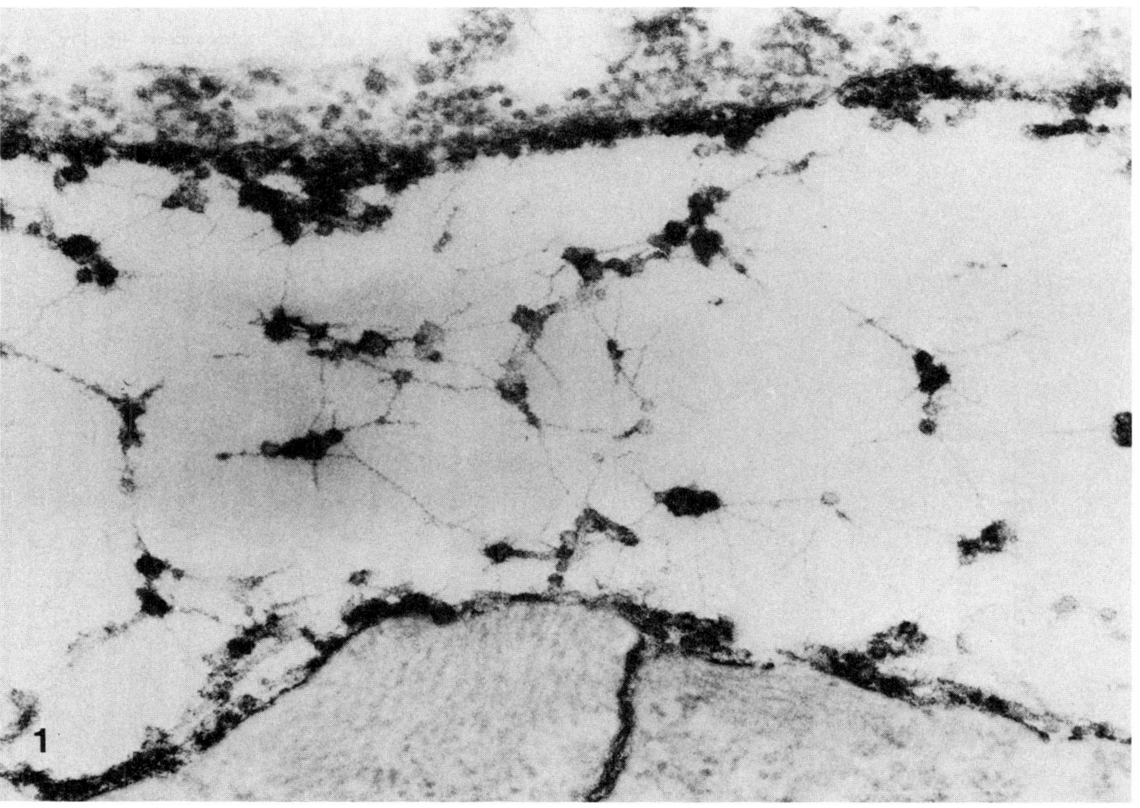

FIGURE 1. Ruthenium red-glutaraldehyde fixation results in the visualization of extracellular matrix fibers. The spaces in between are filled with hyaluronic acid.

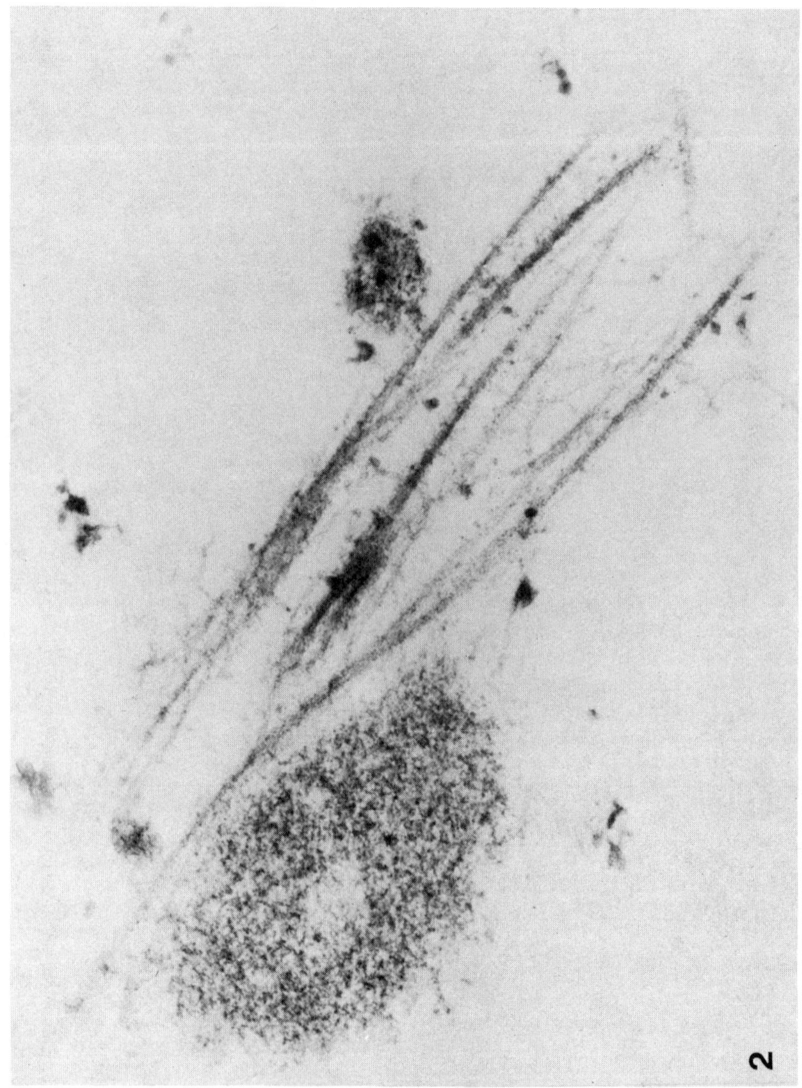

FIGURE 2. High-power electron micrograph revealing different components in the matrix, visualized as 20 nm fibers and globules.

both cellular layers. HA, with its water-binding capacity, is postulated to play an important role in cardiac looping. This is possible because of the asymmetric distribution of the cardiac jelly, as is shown after three-dimensional reconstruction of its distribution. Our results point also towards a component with a more restricted distribution, HN, serving as binding protein for the hygroscopic HA. In this process HN may function as a backbone for the otherwise gelatinous cardiac jelly.

Tissue Interaction and Signal Transduction in the Atrioventricular Canal of the Embryonic Heart[a]

R. B. RUNYAN, J. D. POTTS, D. L. WEEKS,[b]
R. V. SHARMA, C. L. LOEBER,[c] J. J. CHIANG, AND
R. C. BHALLA

Departments of Anatomy
[b]*Biochemistry and* [c]*Pediatrics*
University of Iowa
Iowa City, Iowa 52242

Mesenchyme formation in the atrioventricular (AV) canal of the heart was previously demonstrated to be the result of tissue interaction between the myocardium and the endothelium. Using an *in vitro* three-dimensional assay, it was shown that epithelial-mesenchymal transformation of avian AV endothelia could be produced by AV canal myocardium, an extract of cardiac AV canal extracellular matrix (ECM), or by conditioned media from a cell culture of AV canal myocardial cells. Inasmuch as analysis of the AV canal ECM suggested that one component of the stimulus might be a low molecular weight protein, we tested the effect of transforming growth factor-β (TGFβ) on competent AV canal monolayers. It was found that TGFβ1 (1-7 ng/mL), in combination with ventricular myocardium, produced an endothelial transformation. Neither TGFβ1 nor ventricular myocardium, alone, produced this effect. Further, normal AV endothelial transformation was blocked by an antibody against TGFβ when incubated with AV canal explants ($\geq 10 \, \mu g/mL$). Two separate antibody preparations against mammalian TGFβ demonstrated the presence of an immunoreactive molecule in the heart. Using a human TGFβ1 cDNA probe and mRNA from stage 16-17 chick embryos, a message size of 4.6 kb was found. These data suggest that a native member of the TGFβ family is one cofactor in a multifactorial ECM stimulus produced by the myocardium. In an additional approach, we have begun to explore the mechanism of signal transduction of the transforming stimulus. Epithelial-mesenchymal cell transformation in AV canal cultures was blocked by the phosphotyrosine inhibitor, genistein, and by the protein kinase C inhibitors H-7 and staurosporine. Activators of protein kinase C, PMA, and mezerein, produced a change in cell phenotype without stimulating invasion of the collagen gel. This change in phenotype appeared to be a partial transformation of the AV canal endothelium. Two bacterial endotoxins that perturb G proteins, cholera toxin and pertussis toxin, were also tested in the collagen gel transformation assay. Pertussis toxin, but not cholera

[a]This work was supported by NIH Grants HL 38645 to R. B. Runyan, GM 40308 to D. L. Weeks, and HL 35682 to R. C. Bhalla.

toxin, prevented epithelial-mesenchymal cell transformation by AV canal endothelia. Based upon these inhibitor studies, we proposed that signal transduction of the ECM stimulus is mediated by second messenger pathways that include free calcium. Examination of Ca^{2+} within endothelial cells with the fluorescent dye, fura 2, revealed that competent AV canal endothelial cells undergo a specific elevation of cytosolic calcium in response to a transformation stimulus from myocardially conditioned media. Incompetent AV canal monolayers and ventricular endothelia had little response to the transforming stimulus. These studies have demonstrated mechanisms that are involved in a critical element of cardiac valve and septal formation. Further analysis of these mechanisms may shed light on the malformations of valves and septa commonly found in the defective heart.

Distribution of Vitronectin and Its Receptor in Embryonic Human Heart[a]

H. SUMIDA, H. NAKAMURA,[b] AND Y. SATOW

Department of Geneticopathology
Research Institute for Nuclear Medicine and Biology
Hiroshima University
1-2-3 Kasumi, Hiroshima, 734 Japan

[b]*Department of Biology*
Kyoto Prefectural University of Medicine
Kyoto, Japan

During development of the heart, endocardial cells migrate into the conotruncal and atrioventricular (AV) cushions and become cushion mesenchymal cells.[1] As abnormal development of the cushions is one of the causes of cardiac malformations,[2] elucidation of mechanisms of endocardial cell migration is important. In the past decade, extracellular matrix in the cushions has been thought to be involved in migration of the endocardial cells. Our previous study, however, showed that fibronectin might not be involved in endocardial cell migration.[3]

Vitronectin (VN) is a glycoprotein containing the Arg-Gly-Asp sequence and is suggested to be involved in cell migration. In the present study, in order to elucidate whether VN mediates migration of the endocardial cells, we examined distribution of VN and its receptor (VN-R) in developing human hearts by immunohistochemistry.

Human embryos (Carnegie stages 14-20) that had been kept in the Department of Geneticopathology for 1-6 months in 10% formalin in 0.1 M phosphate buffer were used. These embryos were therapeutically aborted in Japan and were morphologically normal. The embryos were dehydrated and embedded in paraffin. Immunohistochemical procedure was performed routinely.[3] An anti-VN or an anti-VN-R antibody (Chemicon International Inc., CA) was used as a primary antibody. Specificity of the antibodies was checked by immunoblotting using the proteins from a human placenta.

In the embryos at all stages examined, immunoreactivity to the anti-VN antibody was recognized in the conotruncal and AV cushions. At stage 18 the aorticopulmonary (AP) septum was observed as a cellular condensation. At stage 20, the developing tunica media of the great arteries was clearly recognizable. At these stages, cushion mesenchymal cells were stained with the anti-VN-R antibody. The AP septum and tunica media of the great arteries were less stained with the anti-VN and anti-VN-R antibodies, whereas the tissue of the valves of the great arteries was stained. Intensity of staining at stage 14 and 18 was scored in TABLE 1.

[a] This work was supported in part by Inoue Foundation for Science (No. 01007 to H. Sumida).

444

These results suggest that VN is involved in migration of endocardial cells. Furthermore, contribution of VN and fibronectin (FN) to cardiogenesis may be different *in vivo,* because VN-poor tissues are FN-rich in the embryonic chick heart.[3] Thus, the distinctive distribution of VN and FN may be important in cardiac morphogenesis.

TABLE 1. Intensity of Staining at Stage 14 and 18

	AV cushion		Conotruncal cushion		AP septum		Myocardium	
	Stage 14	Stage 18	Stage 14	Stage 18	Stage 14	Stage 18	Stage 14	Stage 18
VN	+ +[b]	+ +	+ +	+ +	[a]	±	+ + +	+ + +
VN-R	+ +	+ +	+ +	+ +	[a]	±	+ + +	+ + +

[a] The AP septum is not formed at stage 14.

[b] Staining intensities were estimated subjectively on a scale, with ± being very slightly reactive and + + + intensely reactive.

REFERENCES

1. FUNDERBURG, F. M. & R. R. MARKWALD. 1986. Conditioning of native substrates by chondroitin sulfate proteoglycans during cardiac mesenchymal cell migration. J. Cell Biol. **103:** 2475-2487.
2. OKAMOTO, N. 1988. Cardiac morphogenesis and teratogenesis. Congenital Anom. **28** (Suppl.): S103-S117.
3. SUMIDA, H., H. NAKAMURA & Y. SATOW. 1989. The localization of fibronectin and 140 Kd fibronectin receptor in the truncus arteriosus of the chick embryonic heart. Arch. Histol. Cytol. **52:** 31-36.

Cell Differentiation Birthdates in the Embryonic Rat Heart[a]

R. P. THOMPSON, J. R. LINDROTH, A. J. ALLES,
AND A. R. FAZEL

Department of Anatomy and Cell Biology
Medical University of South Carolina
Charleston, South Carolina 29425

Regional differences in myocyte proliferation constitute but one of perhaps several factors that shape the vertebrate heart during embryonic and fetal morphogenesis. Interest in such cytokinetics has led to DNA-labeling studies of two distinct types. First, continuous labeling over several normal cell cycles has allowed the definition of subpopulations of myocytes in the embryonic chick heart that appear to have withdrawn from DNA-synthetic activity.[1,2] Second, in the experiments reported here, we have pulse-labeled DNA in embryonic rats and allowed development to proceed through birth, in an effort to detect persistence of such label due to slowed proliferation in restricted regions of the heart.

Each of fifteen timed-pregnant Long-Evans rats received a single intraperitoneal injection of bromodeoxyuridine (16 mg BrdU/100 gm, Sigma Chemicals) at daily or 6-hour intervals between 11 and 15 days of gestation, timed from 8 a.m. on the morning of sperm-positive vaginal smears. One day after normal delivery (day 21), hearts from 3-5 pups from each litter were processed[2] for immunohistochemical detection of labeled cells in serial sections 200 μm apart.

Of 31 hearts sectioned in the cardiac frontal plane, nine were processed for three-dimensional computer reconstruction[2-4] as shown in FIGURE 1. For quantitative comparisons, labeled nuclei in 8-10 sections from 12 hearts were tallied into nine anatomical categories. Although the greatest number of labeled cells were seen on day 13, the total number of labeled myocytes varied widely from heart to heart (300-1800), with no clear dependency upon age at labeling. In an effort to compensate for possible variations in initial labeling or uneven immunostaining, the tallies for each tissue were recalculated as percentages of all labeled cells seen in that heart. Means ($\pm$ SEM) of such normalized data for the principal chambers are presented in TABLE 1. Atrial labeling, low at the outset, appeared widespread in both atria by day 13, shifting markedly toward the left side by day 15. Such labeling was typically restricted to foci or networks of myocytes within the central trabeculae of the pectinate muscles, occasionally extending to the free walls. The percentage of cells in the right atrium (RA%) was low at 11 and 15 days but higher at day 13 ($p < 0.05$, Student t test); LA% increased dramatically by 15 days from low values at 11 days ($p \ll 0.01$). In the ventricles, label was largely confined to trabecular and subendocardial myocytes

[a] These studies were supported by an Established Investigator Award from the American Heart Association and NHLBI Grants 28936 and 37704.

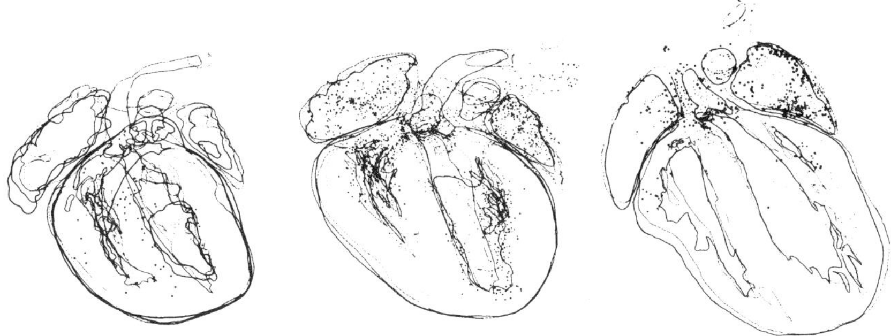

FIGURE 1. Computer reconstruction of the distribution of BrdU-positive-labeled cells in representative hearts labeled at 11, 13, and 15 days of gestation. Note emergence of atrial labeling at 13 days and its shift to the left side at 15 days. Note also labeled populations beneath the luminal surfaces of both ventricles and within the crux cordis. Bar = 500 μm.

along the septum and within the developing papillary muscles. Parietal myocardium and the central regions of the interventricular septum were typically devoid of staining. RV labeling percentages declined significantly between 11 and 15 days ($p << 0.01$); LV% appeared more variable, with a marginal decrease between 13 and 15 days ($0.1 > p > 0.05$). The remaining labeled myocytes were found in transitional zones surrounding the AV and semilunar valves and near the developing central fibrous body; though label was often clearly associated with central conducting and nodal tissue, the low number of sections available from these smaller anatomical regions precluded definition of temporal shifts in such areas.

This study demonstrates the existence and distribution of slowly proliferating subpopulations of subendocardial and trabecular myocytes that may serve a mechanical role in the molding of the interior of the heart during organogenesis and early growth, an electrical role in coordinating early cardiac contraction, or both. The regional temporal shifts observed in the distribution of labeling toward the upstream left quadrant during the period studied suggest early commitment of such cell populations in the right atrium, perhaps the right ventricle as well, compared to the left side of the heart. Further work may delineate more precise timing of such events in the preseptation period studied to date or more distinct divergence of myocardial proliferative rates at even earlier periods of gestation. The ability of some subpopulations to label throughout the period studied and the disappearance of label observed in siblings of these pups allowed to develop to 30 days of age suggest that these cells either die or continue to divide, if only slowly, throughout the fetal and neonatal period. They do not emerge as sharply or remain as nondividing differentiated tissues,

TABLE 1. Gestational Day of Labeling

	11 (n = 3)	13 (n = 3)	15 (n = 3)
RA%	10.8 ± 1.2	20.3 ± 2.9	10.2 ± 1.1
RV%	31.2 ± 3.8	22.7 ± 2.3	10.9 ± 1.1
LA%	5.9 ± 0.4	17.0 ± 4.3	34.2 ± 3.6
LV%	24.0 ± 3.9	26.2 ± 2.7	14.8 ± 3.5

as do the central neuronal cell populations described in earlier birthdating studies.[5] Preliminary confirmation of these findings in the heart with tritiated thymidine label, followed by autoradiography, provides confidence that the patterns reported here are not due to the known toxic or teratogenic effects of BrdU; thymidine radiolabeling, though more expensive and time consuming, may remain a more refined technique for quantitative estimation of label dilution rates. Finally, further study may establish whether the wide variations in total cell labeling observed here should be attributed to unevenness in delivery or detection of label or to fluctuations in cell-cycle synchrony in the mammalian heart, similar to those reported in the early chick.[6]

ACKNOWLEDGMENTS

We want to thank Donna Clark and Charlene Kerr for their expert technical assistance.

REFERENCES

1. JETER, J. R. & I. L. CAMERON. 1971. J. Embryol. Exp. Morphol. **25:** 405-422.
2. THOMPSON, R. P., J. R. LINDROTH & Y. M. WONG. 1989. Developmental Cardiology: Morphogenesis and Function. E. B. Clark & A. Takao, Eds. Futura Press. Mount Kisco, NY.
3. Wong, Y. M., R. P. Thompson & T. P. FITZHARRIS. 1983. Comput. Biomed. Res. **16:** 580-586.
4. LINDROTH, J. R., C. STARR, R. P. THOMPSON & A. ABUTALEB. 1986. Proceedings of the XII Northeast Bioengineering Conference. S. C. Orphanodoukis, Ed. 87-90. IEEE.
5. ALTMANN, J. & G. D. DAS. 1966. J. Comp. Neurol. **126:** 337-389.
6. STALSBERG, H. 1969. Dev. Biol. **20:** 18-45.

Septal Deficiency in Atrioventricular Septal Defect

J. P. VAN GRONINGEN, M. E. HARTEL, AND
A. C. G. WENINK

Department of Anatomy
University of Leiden
2333 AL Leiden, the Netherlands

In a morphometric study in which measurements of wall thicknesses of normal hearts were compared with those of hearts with congenital defects, the hearts with atrioventricular septal defect (AVSD) appeared more thin-walled than expected. Closer analysis revealed that this was possibly due to the fact that all measurements were divided by the apex/aorta length to provide an index that was independent of age. This measurement appeared to be abnormally long in hearts with an AVSD.

The abnormally small inflow/outflow ratio in AVSD hearts has long been known,[1,2] and though Rastelli[3] in his qualitative studies already spoke about the longer outlet, in recent years the small ratio was considered to be caused by an inlet deficiency.[1] When we placed our measurements on Rowlatt's[4] graphs of age/outlet and age/inlet of normal hearts, the AVSD inflow fell within the normal range, whereas the outlet appeared to be longer. Rowlatt's hearts, however, were fixed in formalin, whereas our collection was kept in an alcohol/glycerin mixture.

To substantiate these findings further, we measured the inlet length (apex/crux) and the outlet length of a larger number of AVSD hearts (n=34) and compared these with the same measurements in identically fixed normal hearts (n=27) of the same age range. Statistical analysis of our data with the Student t test revealed no difference between the inlet lengths of normal hearts and those of AVSD hearts ($p > 0.5$) (FIG. 1). The outlet lengths of AVSD hearts, however, showed a clear statistically significant difference from the normal outlet lengths ($p < 0.02$) (FIG. 2). No difference was found between complete and partial AVSD in inlet or outlet lengths. We contend therefore that the small inlet/outlet ratio in AVSD hearts is due to an abnormally long outlet. This is of great importance when searching for the causes of this developmental defect, although of course the septal "scoop" is definitely a septal deficiency.

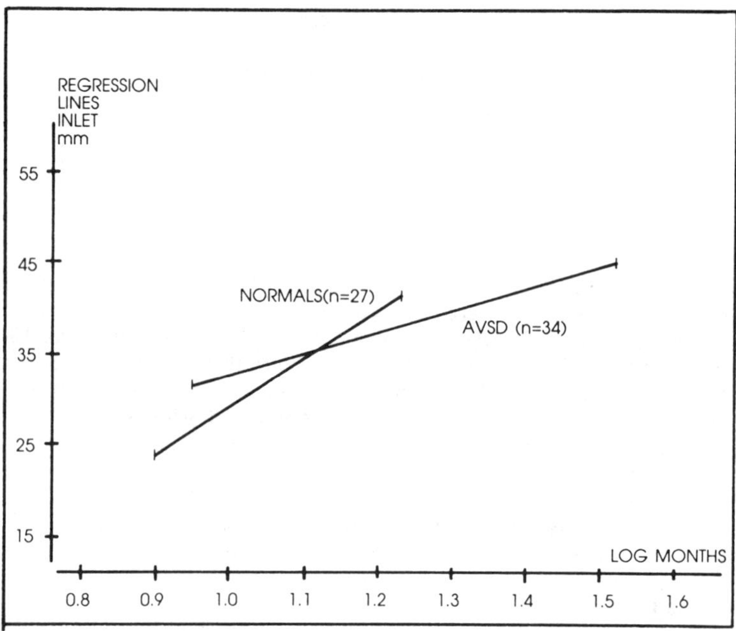

FIGURE 1. Regression lines of the *inlet* lengths of hearts with an AVSD as compared to the inlet lengths of normal hearts of children in the same age range. Statistical evaluation showed no significant difference between these two groups.

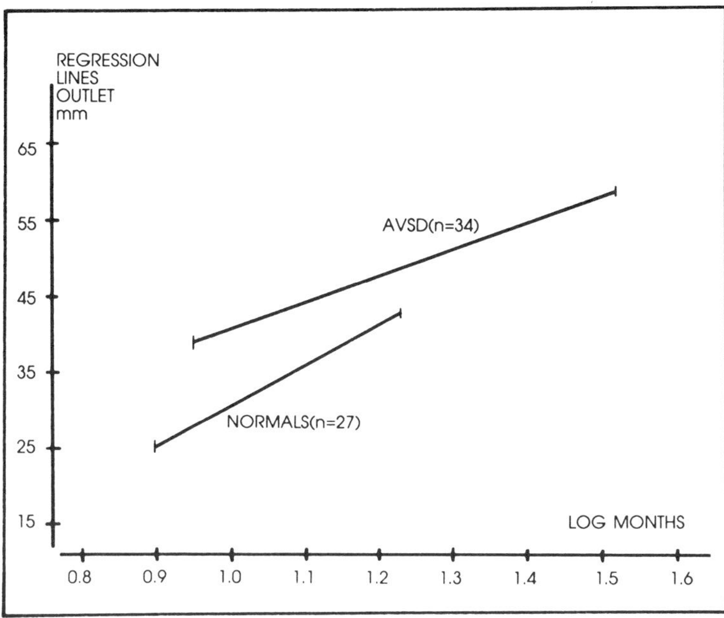

FIGURE 2. Regression lines of the *outlet* lengths of hearts with an AVSD as compared to the outlet lengths of normal hearts of children in the same age range. Statistical evaluation showed AVSD hearts to have significantly longer outlets.

REFERENCES

1. PICCOLI, G. P. *et al.* 1979. Morphology and classification of atrioventricular defects. Br. Heart J. **42:** 621-632.
2. PENKOSKE, P. A. *et al.* 1985. Further observations on the morphology of atrioventricular septal defects. J. Thorac. Cardiovasc. Surg. **90:** 611-622.
3. TITUS, J. L. & G. C. RASTELLI. 1976. *In* Atrioventricular Canal Defects. R. H. Feldt, Ed. W. B. Saunders Company. Philadelphia, PA.
4. ROWLATT, U. F. *et al.* 1963. The quantitative anatomy of the normal child's heart. Pediatr. Clin. North Am. **10:** 499-519.

Myocardial Hypertrophy in the Left Ventricle

J. P. VAN GRONINGEN AND A. C. G. WENINK

Department of Anatomy
University of Leiden
2333 AL Leiden, the Netherlands

A number of hypertrophic phenomena in the left ventricular outflow tract were studied in 47 normal hearts, 53 hearts with congenital anomalies, and 8 with hypertrophic cardiomyopathy. Based on the detailed anatomy of the subaortic outflow tract, we distinguished several subgroups within the group of normal hearts: hearts in which an anterolateral muscle bundle was wedged between aortic and mitral valves (ALM), hearts in which the anterior part of the septum showed a leftward curve so as to merge with the anterior free wall (AST), and hearts in which the normally smooth subaortic region was invested with prominent trabeculations (TRAB) (FIG. 1). A qualitative study revealed that all of the above phenomena appear not only in normal hearts, but also in hearts with various congenital defects, and in hearts with cardiomyopathy, without a clear pattern.

Therefore, we decided to study these hearts morphometrically. We measured wall thicknesses, indexed these by dividing all measurements by the outlet length, and found that anterior septal and wall thicknesses were significantly greater in the AST group than in the other normal hearts. Alternatively, AST hearts did not significantly differ from hearts with cardiomyopathy or from those with Eisenmenger defect or central muscular defect. The latter congenital malformations are characterized by the leftward septal curve and/or trabeculations mentioned above. For further information on this hypertrophic phenomenon we studied these hearts by routine histology and found a continuum of myocardial organization to disorganization, from normal hearts with an ALM, to normal hearts with an AST, to hearts with hypertrophic cardiomyopathy.

To get an insight in cell size at the sites measured during gross examination, we estimated the myocyte surface density (Sv) stereologically in 11 cases. Hereto we counted the number of transections of a specially designed grid with cell membranes in ten one micron thick epon-embedded sections of randomized cutting direction. The total (I) was submitted to the following stereologic formula:

$$Sv = 2 \times \frac{I}{L_p \times P} \times M$$

in which L_p is the length of a grid line, P the total number of grid lines, and M the magnification factor. Because these results were not corrected for heart size, they did show a relationship with age signifying physiological hypertrophy during postnatal heart growth.

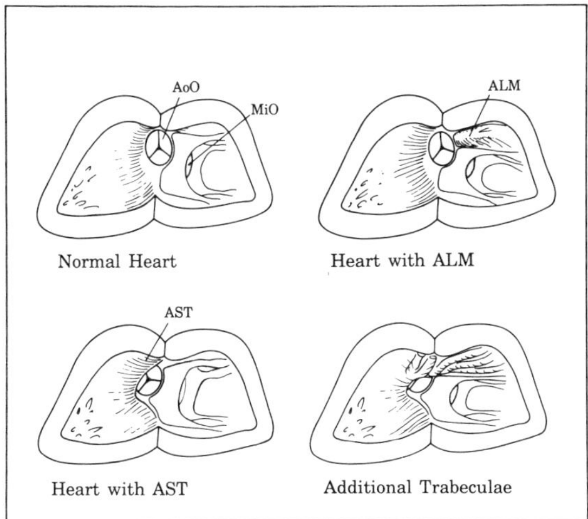

FIGURE 1. Anatomical variations of the outflow tract.

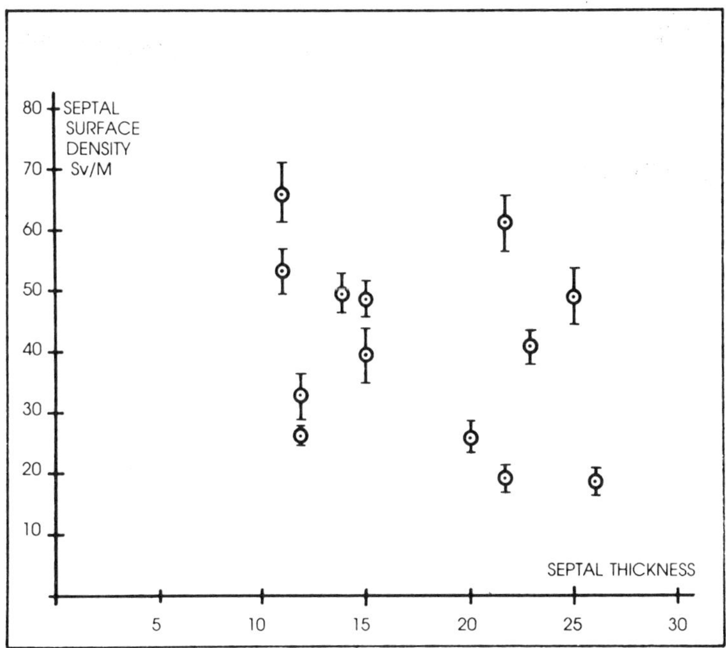

FIGURE 2. Myocyte surface density (as a parameter for cell size) of the anterior ventricular septum plotted against its macroscopic thickness. There is no correlation.

Surface density, however, and hence cell size, showed no relationship with septal thickness (FIG. 2). If these selected cases are representative for all our material, we conclude that macroscopic hypertrophy in childhood is not related to cell size, which means that gross hypertrophy in children could be any combination of cellular hyperplasia and hypertrophy. These results are of special importance in studying the nature of hypertrophy in congenital defects and hypertrophic cardiomyopathy in childhood and any possible relationship between these two.

Angiogenesis and Hematopoiesis in the Epicardium of the Vertebrate Embryo Heart

SZ. VIRÁGH,[a] F. KÁLMÁN,[a]
A. C. GITTENBERGER-DE GROOT,[b]
R. E. POELMANN,[b] AND A. F. M. MOORMAN [c]

[a]Department of Pathological Anatomy
Postgraduate Medical School
Budapest Pf 112 H-1389, Hungary

[b]Department of Anatomy and Embryology
University of Leiden
Leiden, the Netherlands

[c]Department of Anatomy and Embryology
University of Amsterdam
Amsterdam, the Netherlands

According to Manasek,[1] the term "myoepicardium," used to designate the primitive heart wall, is misleading, because the epicardium derives from a source other than the so-called myoepicardium. He suggested that Kurkiewicz's[2] original description, stating that in the bird heart the epicardium originates from the coelomic epithelium covering the sinus venosus and the septum transversum (ST), should be accepted. This concept has been supported in the mouse,[3–5] chick,[6] and Tupaia belangeri[7] embryos. The present communication summarizes the process of early angiogenesis and hematopoiesis as it relates to the origin and development of the epicardium in the quail, chick, mouse, and human embryo. Some aspects of this process in the human[8] and chick[9] embryo have already been published. The present results obtained with light microscope and electron microscope techniques, including the use of antiendothelial, antiembryonic, and adult hemoglobin markers, indicate that the proepicardial tissue coming from the septum transversum (ST) has a multipotential capacity. The micrographs substantiate that primitive blood cells enveloped by the mesothelial cells of the extracardiac epicardial blebs or vesicles (FIGURES 1 and 2) might be transferred to the surface of the heart tube. Extracellular matrix components like glycosaminoglycans and fibronectin, playing a role in the adhesion and migration of proepicardial cells, might also be transferred from the ST to the heart in this way. Some of the cells of the primary epicardium are able to detach from the outer layer and migrate in the originally acellular subepicardial space, which is the widest above the developing SA, AV, and IV grooves. The primary subepicardial layer in these grooves becomes populated first by mesenchymal cells able to transform into blood capillaries and blood cells. Before the opening of coronary artery orifices, hematopoietic and blood vessel-forming islands develop in the heart sulcuses. These islands form

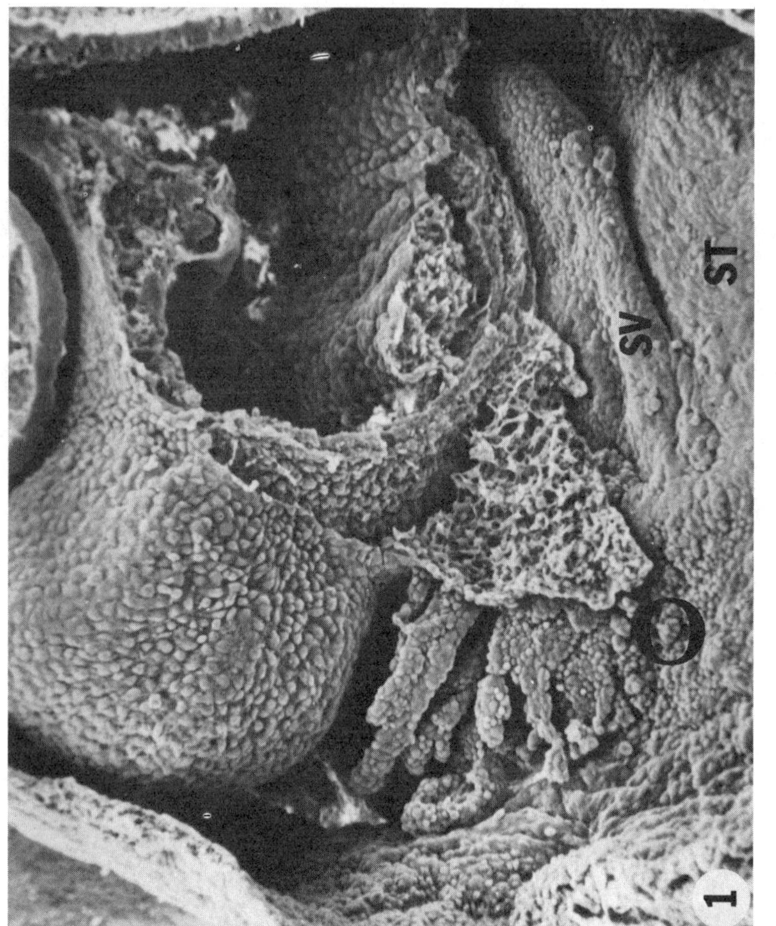

FIGURE 1. Dorsal aspect of a quail embryo (3 days 16 hours, HH stage 23) pericardial cavity. The ventricular loop of the heart was removed to expose several structures from the top to the bottom: a segment of the outflow tract, right atrium, atrioventricular canal, finger-like protrusions of the right subepicardial organ, sinus venosus (SV), septum transversum (ST), and an encircled epicardial bleb or vesicle. The transmission electron microscope (TEM) structure of a similar bleb is shown on FIG. 2; × 340.

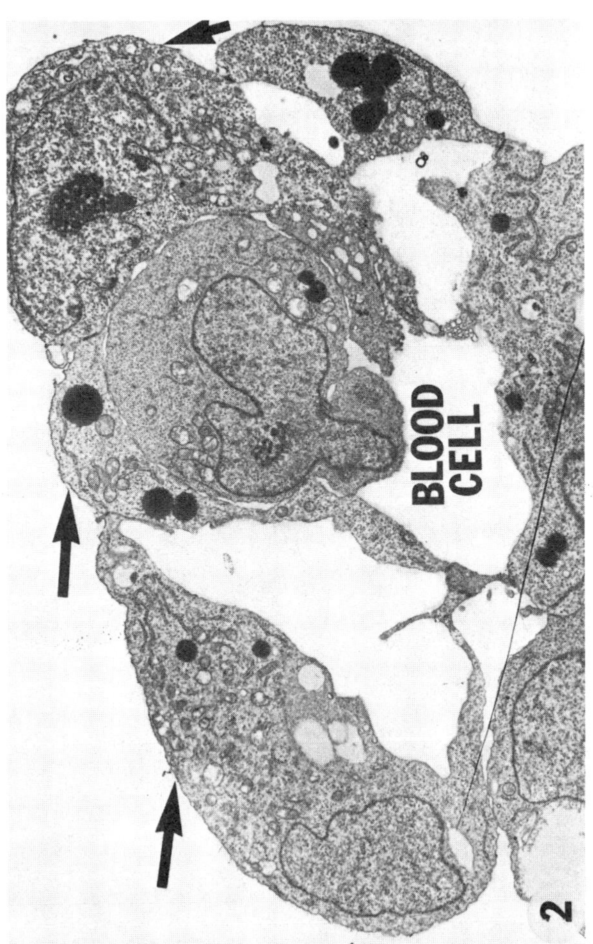

FIGURE 2. TEM micrograph of a proepicardial bleb or vesicle analogous to that shown on the surface of the septum transversum on FIG. 1. The superficial mesothelial cells (arrows) encircle a blood cell. 10.5 day mouse embryo; × 5000.

protuberances on the epicardial surface. In the quail heart the mesenchyme, having angio- and hematopoietic capacity, contributes to the formation of a paired subepicardial organ located bilaterally in the intersection of the SA and AV grooves (FIG. 1). In the early embryo heart capillaries are also formed by the evaginations of endocardial sinusoids in the subepicardial layer.[9] The primordia of the main branches of the coronary vessels are present before the opening of the coronary artery orifices.

REFERENCES

1. MANASEK, F. J. 1969. J. Embryol. Exp. Morphol. **22:** 333.
2. KURKIEWICZ, T. 1909. Bull. Acad. Sci. Cracovie **6:** 148.
3. VIRÁGH, SZ. & C. E. CHALLICE. 1973. J. Ultrastruct. Res. **42:** 1.
4. VIRÁGH, SZ. & C. E. CHALLICE. 1981. Anat. Rec. **201:** 157.
5. KOMIYAMA, M. *et al.* 1987. Anat. Embryol. **176:** 183.
6. HO, E. & Y. SHIMADA. 1978. Dev. Biol. **66:** 579.
7. KUHN, H-J. & G. LIEBHERR. 1988. Anat. Embryol. **177:** 225.
8. OBRUCNIK, M. *et al.* 1972. Folia Morphol. (Prague) **20:** 49.
9. RYCHTER, Z. & B. OSTADAL. 1971. Folia Morphol. (Prague) **19:** 113.

A New Perspective on the Development of the Coronary Arteries in the Chick Embryo

KAREN WALDO AND MARGARET L. KIRBY

Department of Anatomy
Medical College of Georgia
Augusta, Georgia 30912

Published accounts of coronary artery development describe the development of an endothelial evagination that "buds" the coronary artery from the site of the future coronary sinuses.[1,2] The purpose of this study was to confirm the appearance of the aortic "bud" in the chick embryo and to document the development of the coronary artery stems.

On embryonic day 6, 6.5, 7, 7.5, 9, and 10, Arbor Acre chicken embryos, incubated at 38° C and constant humidity, were injected with diluted India ink into the vitelline vein. After injection, each embryo was fixed *in situ* with Carnoy's fluid and removed from the egg. Each embryo's extraembryonic membranes were stripped away. The embryos were then placed in Carnoy's fluid for 24 hours and cleared in a 50:50 solution of benzyl benzoate:methyl salicylate. After clearing, the heart was removed from each embryo and the atria dissected away to allow full view of the outflow tract and the developing coronary arteries. Two ink-injected and cleared hearts were taken from each age group, embedded in paraffin, and serially sectioned for light microscopic examination.

On days 6, 6.5, and 7, a network of vessels circled the base of the heart and joined together to form a vascular ring around the bulbus. This advancing vascular network grew progressively each day superiorly toward the aortic and pulmonary valves, until on day 7 it had reached the level of the aortic cusps. An aortic endothelial evagination or bud was not observed. On day 7, a portion of the aortic endothelium of each cusp appeared denser and more granular in texture. Histologically, more ink particles appeared to have stuck to the endothelium in these areas.

On day 7.5, six out of nine hearts demonstrated one or both coronary artery stems. At higher magnification, and histologically in serial sections, these stems appeared to consist of one to three hair-thin channels that penetrated the aortic sinuses at the location of the roughened aortic endothelium. These channels originated from the bulbar vascular network. Two of the gross hearts demonstrated a "third" coronary artery penetrating the posterior noncoronary cusp. In serial section, one or more channels could be seen penetrating the roughened aortic endothelium just above the rim of the retreating myocardial cuff. Those hearts without coronary arteries failed to demonstrate aortic endothelial buds.

On day 9 many of the left coronary artery stems still consisted of two or three channels, one of which was always wider in diameter, longer and more dominant.

The right coronary artery stem was consistently short and broke into many branches. On day 10, the coronary artery stems had developed well-defined branches. Histologically, the left coronary artery still retained some regressing channels in addition to the one dominant channel.

It is significant that an aortic bud as described in the literature was never observed in this study and that the origin of the coronary artery appeared to be capillary branches from the bulbar vascular network. It is also significant that these capillary channels failed to penetrate the pulmonary artery or other sites on the aorta. This fact suggests that the development of the coronary artery represents a controlled invasion of the aorta by the capillaries of the bulbar vascular network. Moscatelli defines angiogenesis as a controlled invasion of a tissue by cells of another tissue.[3] Recent theory of angiogenesis states that new blood vessels can only originate from small venules or capillaries. If the theory of angiogenesis applies to the developing embryo, it should be impossible for the aorta to bud the coronary arteries. On the contrary, the coronary arteries must develop from a source of small venules or capillaries. We believe that source to be the bulbar vascular network.

REFERENCES

1. RYCHTER, Z. & B. OSTADAL. 1971. Mechanism of the development of coronary arteries in chick embryo. Folia Morphol. (Prague) No. 2 XIX: 113-124.
2. DBALY, J., B. OSTADAL & Z. RYCHTER. 1968. Development of the coronary artery in rat embryos. Acta Anat. 71: 209-222.
3. MOSCATELLI, D. & D. B. RIFKIN. 1988. Membrane and matrix localization of proteinases: a common theme in tumor cell invasion and angiogenesis. Biochim. Biophys. Acta 948: 67-85.

The Ontogenesis of Myosin Heavy Chain Isoforms in the Developing Human Heart[a]

A. WESSELS, J. L. M. VERMEULEN, SZ. VIRÁGH,[b]
AND A. F. M. MOORMAN

Department of Anatomy and Embryology
University of Amsterdam
Amsterdam, the Netherlands
and
[b]*Department of Pathology*
Postgraduate Medical School
Budapest, Hungary

The existence of two myosin heavy chain (MHC) isoforms in the human heart is well-established. In the adult situation, the heart-specific isoform, α-MHC, predominates in the atria, whereas β-MHC is the main isoform in the ventricles. Changes in the relative amounts of these isoforms take place during development and under certain pathological conditions. As it has been demonstrated that the MHC composition of a muscle and its contractile properties, for example, the maximum velocity of contraction, are closely correlated, it might be expected that insight in the MHC expression patterns will disclose the morphofunctional significance of the MHC expression patterns and the changes mentioned above. With this idea in mind, we have performed an immunohistochemical study on human embryonic, fetal, and neonatal hearts, using monoclonal antibodies against the α-MHC and β-MHC. In all stages examined, spatial heterogeneities in MHC distributions were observed. In the youngest embryo examined ($4\frac{1}{2}$ weeks of development, Carnegie stage 14), α-MHC is expressed in the atria, the ventricles, and the outflow tract (OFT) (FIG. 1a), whereas β-MHC is only expressed in the OFT and the ventricular myocardium (FIG. 1b), thereby marking the border between atrial and ventricular myocardium in the atrioventricular canal (AVC). In addition, β-MHC-expressing cells are observed in the sinoatrial (SA) junction. The strong coexpression of both MHC isoforms in the ventricles disappears after five weeks of development (FIG. 1c,d). After this stage no strong α-MHC expression in the ventricles is found anymore. As development proceeds the presence of β-MHC-expressing cells in the SA junctional area becomes more pronounced, thereby characteristically flanking the area of the developing SA node (SAN). In the SA-nodal cells themselves, however, only α-MHC can be detected (FIG. 2a,b). Characteristic MHC expression is also observed in the ventricular conduction system (VCS). At eight weeks of development a strong coexpression of both MHCs is observed in the area where the bundle of His is developing. As development proceeds, the area

[a]This work was supported by Grant 86-076h of the Dutch Heart Foundation.

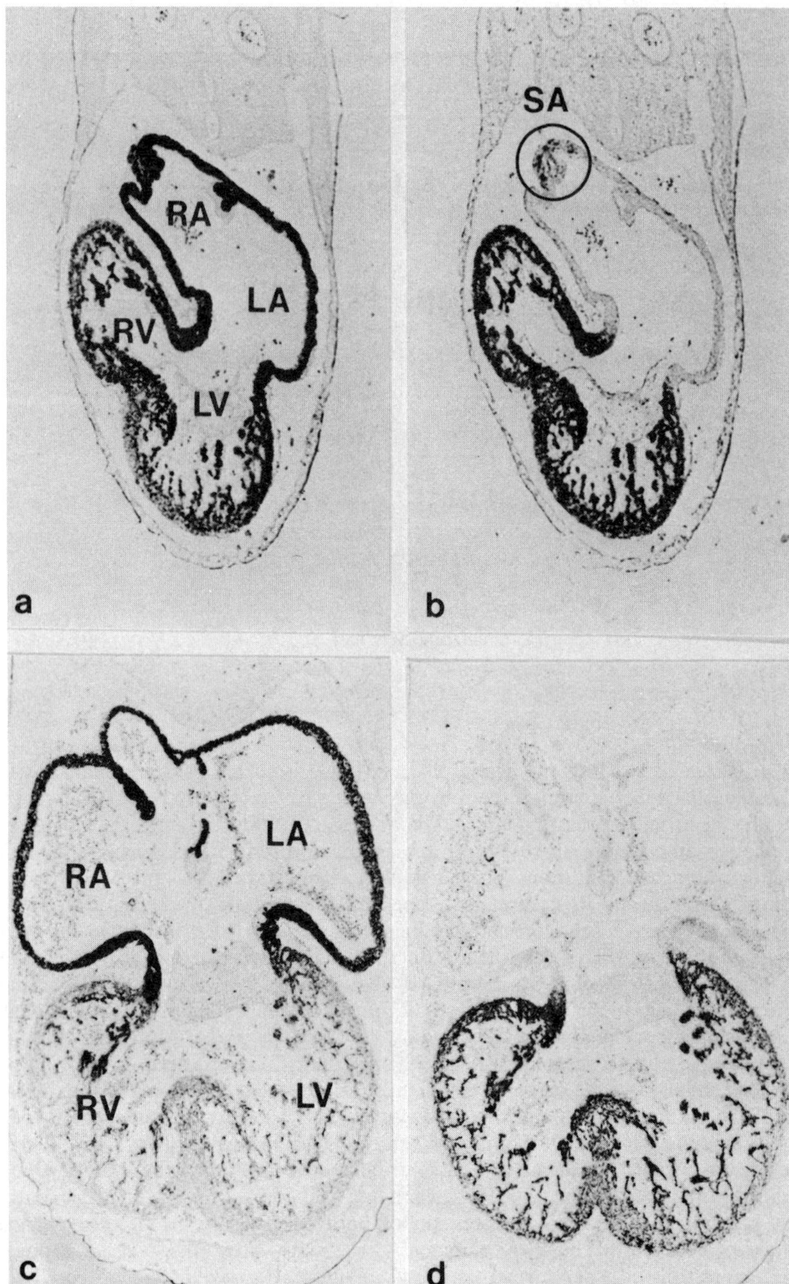

FIGURE 1. Immunohistochemical detection of myosin heavy chain (MHC) isoforms on serial sections of embryonic human hearts of 31-35 days (Carnegie stage 14) (a,b) and 35-38 days (Carnegie stage 15) (c,d) of development. At stage 14, α-MHC is expressed in the atria as well as in the ventricles (a), whereas in stage 15, α-MHC expression is restricted mainly to the atria (c). The expression of β-MHC is at both stages, however, confined to the ventricles (b,d). In addition, at both stages groups of β-MHC-expressing cells in the SA nodal area are observed (*e.g.* circled area in b). LA = left atrium, LV = left ventricle, RA = right atrium, RV = right ventricle, SA = sinoatrial junction.

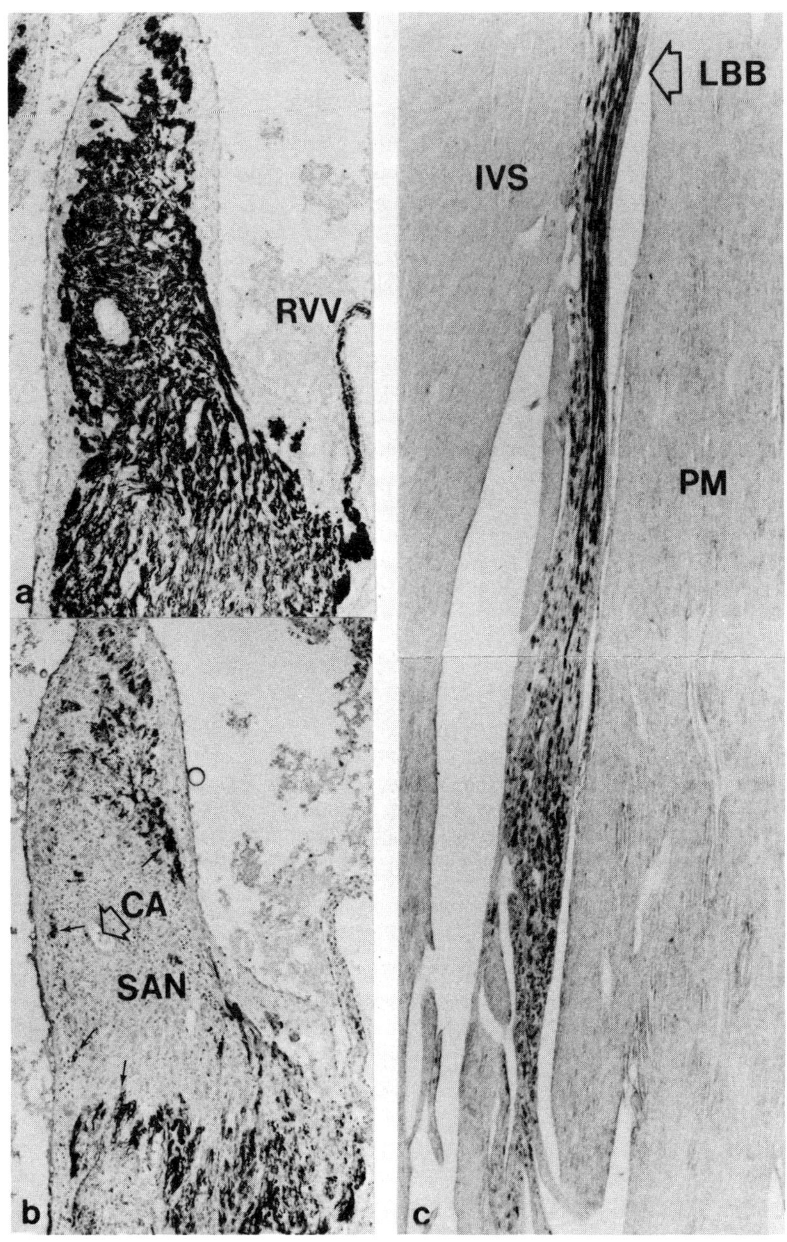

FIGURE 2. Myosin heavy chain (MHC) expression in the developing conduction system of the human heart. At 12 weeks of development the sinoatrial node (SAN) is characterized by the expression of α-MHC in the nodal and the surrounding cells (a) and the expression of β-MHC in cells flanking the SAN (b). Panel c shows a detail of a section of a neonatal heart (5 weeks old) incubated with anti-α-MHC. The left bundle branch and the Purkinje fibers show a strong reaction and are easy to discriminate from the ordinary working myocardium by the strong expression of this isoform. CA = central artery, IVS = interventricular septum, LBB = left bundle branch, PM = papillary muscle, RVV = right venous valve, SAN = sinoatrial node.

of coexpression grows, characteristically indicating the developing VCS. As a result, in the neonatal heart, the total VCS, including the bundle branches and the Purkinje fibers, is very easy to discriminate from the working myocardium by the strong expression of α-MHC (FIG. 2c) in addition to the expression of β-MHC.

DISCUSSION

The results presented in this paper illustrate that immunohistochemistry can be a very valuable tool for studying the development of the (human) heart. It offers us the possibility of detecting cells, or groups of cells, with characteristic features that are not so easy to discriminate from their surroundings with other methods. For example, the MHC isoform distributions indicate that the contractile properties of atrial and ventricular myocardium differ already very early in heart development (Carnegie stage 14), whereas the spatial distribution of the MHC isoforms combined with the distribution of other enzymes, such as the isoforms of creatine kinase, show that specialized myocardium is also found around the AV junctions and the developing semilunar valves.[1]

REFERENCE

1. WESSELS, A., J. L. M. VERMEULEN, SZ. VIRÁGH, F. KÁLMÁN, G. E. MORRIS, NGUEN THI MAN, W. H. LAMERS & A. F. M. MOORMAN. 1990. Spatial distribution of "tissue-specific" antigens in the developing human heart and skeletal muscle: (I) An immuno-histochemical analysis of creatine kinase isoenzyme expression patterns. Anat. Rec. In press.

Index of Contributors